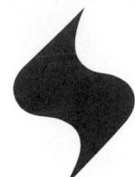

D1092409

Stedman's

INTERNAL MEDICINE

& GERIATRIC

WORDS

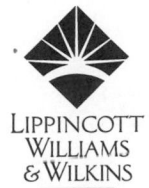

LIPPINCOTT
WILLIAMS
& WILKINS

Publisher: Rhonda M. Kumm, RN, MSN
Senior Manager: Julie K. Stegman
Senior Managing Editor: Nancy Wachter
Associate Project Manager: Heather A. Rybacki
Art Program: Jennifer Clements
Assistant Production Manager: Kevin Iarossi
Typesetter: Peirce Graphic Services, Inc.
Printer & Binder: Malloy Litho, Inc.

Printed in the United States of America

First Edition, 2002

Library of Congress Cataloging-in-Publication Data

Stedman's internal medicine & geriatric words / [editor, Kathy Rockel].
    p. cm.
  ISBN 0-7817-3832-6 (alk. paper)
    1. Internal medicine—Nomenclature.   2. Geriatrics—Nomenclature.   I. Title:
  Stedman's internal medicine and geriatric words.   II. Title: Internal medicine &
  geriatric words.   III. Rockel, Kathy.

RC41 .S834 2002
616'.001'4—dc21

2002066122
03
2 3 4 5 6 7 8 9 10

Stedman's

INTERNAL MEDICINE
& GERIATRIC
WORDS

Contents

Acknowledgments

An important part of our editorial process is the involvement of medical language specialists – as advisors, reviewers, and editors.

We extend special thanks to Kathy Rockel, CMT, and Nicole Peck, CMT, for editing the manuscript, helping to resolve many difficult content questions, and contributing and reviewing material for the appendix sections. We also extend special thanks to Helen Littrell, CMT, for performing the final prepublication review.

We are grateful to our Editorial Advisory Board members, including Harold Andrews; Pamela Bielanski; Sue Faris; Velva M. Flick, CMT; Jennie C. Frey, LPN; Kathy Hess, CMT; Julie Joviak; Sandy Kovacs, CMT; Anna Majoras, CMT; Susan Poirier; Diana Rezac, CMT; Cheryl Rittschof, MLS; Stephany Rue, CMT; and Suzanne Taubert, CMT. These medical transcriptionists and medical language specialists served as important contributors and advisors.

Other important contributors include Susan Bartolucci, CMT; Katharine Boggess, CMT; Linda A. Byrne, CMT; Jaimee A. Givens; and Heather Little, CMT, who focused on the appendix sections; Marty Cantu, CMT; Patty Gibson, MT; Robin Koza; Deborah S. Mahen, ALS, CPS, MLS; Tammy Meissner; Dana Sanford, MT; Gail D. Schoolcraft, CMT; and Annette Weiland, CMT.

Barb Ferretti played an integral role in the process by reviewing the content files for format, updating the database, and providing a final quality check.

As with all our *Stedman's* word references, this resource incorporates the suggestions and expertise of our many contacts in the medical transcriptionist community. Thanks to all of our advisory board participants, reviewers, and editors; AAMT meeting attendees; and others who have contacted us with requests and comments—keep talking, and we'll keep listening.

Editor's Preface

One of the characteristics of a good medical transcriptionist is a love of the medical language and medical terminology. We have an insatiable desire to increase our knowledge of the words used in medicine and to be able to use them appropriately in our work.

When I began medical transcription over 20 years ago, we were all so proud of the reference books on our desk. Each workstation was equipped with an English dictionary, a medical dictionary, a Physician's Drug Reference (PDR), and a book that was entitled "A Syllabus for the Surgeon's Secretary." We felt quite fortunate to have those few reference books with which to do our daily jobs. Then, one day, along came Stedman's, and we learned that, in addition to a medical dictionary, we could actually have books of words—and words for every specialty imaginable! I first had the opportunity to work with Stedman's several years ago on an edition of the OB/GYN book. I found it amazing that not only did this publisher have the foresight to do word books for medical transcriptionists, but they also had the novel idea to involve medical transcriptionists in the development of those books—imagine that!

If you look at any of the Stedman's word books, you will find this phrase: "Keep talking and we'll keep listening." And listen they have. Thus, the birth of a new book for the specialties of internal medicine and geriatrics. We asked, Stedman's listened, and it is now a reality. In this book, you will find thousands of words associated with these specialties. The appendices will provide you with several valuable resources, including sample reports, illustrations, and common tests within these specialties, as well as an "herbarium" listing a variety of natural remedies. I encourage you to familiarize yourself with this material so that you can benefit from the full value of the information.

I want to express my sincere thanks to the second editor of this book, Nicole Peck, CMT. She has been wonderful to work with on this project and has consistently demonstrated that insatiable quest for knowledge, as well as an ability to catch all of the details.

The staff at Stedman's has also been great. A special thanks to Heather Rybacki, Associate Project Manager, who managed our deadlines, kept us from straying off track, and exhibited great support for the entire project. It has been my honor to work with such a professional, intelligent team!

Enjoy this book, knowing that it is one more tool to be used in our profession and to quench that thirst for knowledge. And thank you, Stedman's, for always listening. We will continue to talk.

Kathy Rockel, CMT

Publisher's Preface

Stedman's Internal Medicine & Geriatric Words offers authoritative assurance of quality and exactness to the wordsmiths of the healthcare profession—medical transcriptionists, medical editors and copyeditors, health information management personnel, court reporters, and the many other users and producers of medical documentation.

In *Stedman's Internal Medicine & Geriatric Words,* users will find thousands of terms related to internal medicine/general practice, preventative care, and geriatric issues and conditions. Users will find terms for a variety of topics, including Alzheimer disease, nutrition, pain management, communicable diseases, diabetes, and rehabilitation medicine. Terms also include laboratory and diagnostic tests, therapeutic procedures, techniques, and medications, as well as equipment names and abbreviations with their expansions. The appendix sections provide anatomical illustrations with useful captions and labels, normal lab values, sample reports, and an "herbarium" listing a variety of natural remedies and their uses. For quick reference, we have also included lists of common abbreviations, common laboratory tests with descriptions, and expanded information on selected internal medicine and geriatric topics.

This compilation of more than 55,000 entries, fully cross-indexed for quick access, was built from a base vocabulary of approximately 36,000 medical words, phrases, abbreviations, and acronyms. The extensive A-Z list was developed from the database of *Stedman's Medical Dictionary, 27th Edition,* and supplemented by terminology found in current medical literature (please see list of References on page xvi).

We at Lippincott Williams & Wilkins strive to provide you with the most up-to-date and accurate word references available. Your use of this word book will prompt new editions, which we will publish as often as updates and revisions justify. We welcome your suggestions for improvements, changes, corrections, and additions—whatever will make this *Stedman's* product more useful to you. Please complete the postpaid card included in this book, and send your recommendations in care of "Stedman's" at Lippincott Williams & Wilkins.

Explanatory Notes

Medical transcription is an art as well as a science. Both approaches are needed to correctly interpret the dictation of a physician, whose language is a product of education, training, and experience. This variety in medical language means that there are several acceptable ways to express certain terms, including jargon. *Stedman's Internal Medicine and Geriatric Words* provides variant spellings and phrasings for many terms. These elements, in addition to complete cross-indexing, make *Stedman's Internal Medicine and Geriatric Words* a valuable resource for determining the validity of terms as they are encountered.

Alphabetical Organization
Alphabetization of main entries is letter by letter as spelled, ignoring punctuation, spaces, prefixed numbers, or other special characters. For example:

hydroxykynureninuria
5-hydroxyprogesterone
hydroxyproline

Terms beginning or ending with Greek letters show the Greek letter spelled out and listed alphabetically. For example:

alpha, α
    a. adrenergic agent
    a. antagonist
    a. 1 antitrypsin deficiency
    a. blocker
    a. chain disease
    interferon a.
    tumor necrosis factor-a. (TNF-alpha)

In subentry alphabetization, the abbreviated singular form or the spelled-out plural form of the noun main entry word is ignored.

Format and Style
All main entries are in **boldface** to expedite locating a sought-after term, to enhance distinction between main entries and subentries, and to relieve the textual density of the pages.

Irregular plurals and variant spellings are shown on the same line as the singular or preferred form of the word. For example:

scotoma, pl. scotomata
curette, curet

Hyphenation

As a rule of style, multiple eponyms (e.g., Addison-Biermer disease) are hyphenated. Also, hyphens have been added between a manufacturer's name and one or more eponyms (e.g., Vital-Metzenbaum dissecting scissors). Please note that in many cases, hyphenation is a question of style, not of accuracy, and thus is a matter of choice.

Possessives

Possessive forms have been dropped in this reference for the sake of consistency and conformance with the guidelines of the American Medical Association (AMA) and the American Association for Medical Transcription (AAMT). Please note, however, that in many cases, retaining the possessive, like hyphenating, is a question of style, not of accuracy, and thus is a matter of choice. To form the possessive of a word, simply add the apostrophe or apostrophe "s" to the end of the word.

Cross-indexing

The word list is in an index-like main entry-subentry format that contains two combined alphabetical listings:

(1) A *noun* main entry-subentry organization, which is typical of the A-Z section of medical dictionaries like *Stedman's:*

dermatosis
    acute febrile neutrophilic d.
    bullous d.
    neutrophilic d.
    radiation d.
    vulvar d.

migraine
    abdominal m.
    acute confusional m.
    basilar artery m.
    Bickerstaff m.
    classic m.

(2) An *adjective* main entry-subentry organization, which lists words and phrases as you hear them. The main entries are the adjectives or modifiers in a multiword term. The subentries are the nouns around which the terms are constructed and to which the adjectives or modifiers pertain:

congenital
    c. absence of pericardium
    c. adrenal hyperplasia
    c. adrenocortical hyperplasia
    c. agranulocytosis

nonspecific
    n. arthralgia
    n. effector cell
    n. interstitial pneumonia
    n. stomatitis

This format provides the user with more than one way to locate and identify a multiword term. For example:

cycling
    c. dialysis

dialysis
    cycling d.

disease
    Dutton d.

Dutton
    D. disease

It also allows the user to see together all terms that contain a particular descriptor, as well as all types, kinds, or variations of a noun entity. For example:

cough
    aneurysmal c.
    bronchospastic reflect c.
    c. fracture
    c. suppressant

phosphate
    p. depletion
    oral p.
    p. supplementation
    tubular reabsorption p. (TRP)

Wherever possible, abbreviations are separately defined and cross-referenced. For example:

FUO
    fever of unknown origin

fever
    f. of unknown origin (FUO)

origin
    fever of unknown o. (FUO)

References

In addition to the manufacturers' literature we gather at various medical meetings, scientific reports from hospitals, and the lists of our MT Editorial Advisory Board members (from their daily transcription work), we used the following sources for terms and appendices for *Stedman's Internal Medicine and Geriatric Words:*

Books

Ahya SN, Flood K, Paranjothi S. Washington Manual of Medical Therapeutics, 30th Edition. Philadelphia: Lippincott Williams & Wilkins, 2001.

Balch JF, Balch PA. Prescription for Nutritional Healing, 2nd Edition. Garden City Park, NY: Avery Publishing Group, 1997.

Blumenthal M, Goldberg A, Brinckmann J. Herbal Medicine: Expanded Commission E Monographs. Newton, MA: Integrative Medicine Communications, 2000.

Cassileth BR. The Alternative Medicine Handbook: The Complete Reference Guide to Alternative and Complementary Therapies. New York: W. W. Norton & Company, 1998.

Clinical Laboratory Tests: Values and Implications, 3rd Edition. Springhouse, PA: Springhouse, 2001.

Dambro MR. Griffith's 5-Minute Clinical Consult 2001. Philadelphia: Lippincott Williams & Wilkins, 2001.

Danna M. Internal Medicine Words. Windsor, CA: Rayve Productions, 1997.

Drake E. Sloane's Medical Word Book, 4th Edition. Philadelphia: Saunders, 2001.

Fauci AS, Braunwald E, Isselbacher KJ, et al. Harrison's Principles of Internal Medicine, 14th Edition. New York: McGraw-Hill, 1998.

Fischbach FT. Nurses' Quick Reference to Common Laboratory and Diagnostic Tests, 3rd Edition. Philadelphia: Lippincott Williams & Wilkins, 2002.

Gallo JJ, Busby-Whitehead J, Rabins PV, et al. Reichel's Care of the Elderly, 5th Edition. Philadelphia: Lippincott Williams & Wilkins, 1999.

Goldman L, Bennett JC. Cecil Textbook of Medicine, 21st Edition. Philadelphia: Saunders, 2000.

Goroll AH, Mulley AJ, Jr. Primary Care Medicine, 4th Edition. Philadelphia, Lippincott Williams & Wilkins, 2000.

Hazzard WR, Blass JP, Ettinger WH, Jr., et al. Principles of Geriatric Medicine and Gerontology, 4th Edition. New York: McGraw-Hill, 1999.

Humes HD, DuPont HL, Garnder LB, et al. Kelley's Textbook of Internal Medicine, 4th Edition. Philadelphia: Lippincott Williams & Wilkins, 2000.

Jacobs DS, DeMott WR, Oxley DK. Laboratory Test Handbook, Concise 2nd edition. Hudson, OH: Lexi-Comp, 2002.

Lance LL. Quick Look Drug Book 2002. Baltimore: Lippincott Williams & Wilkins, 2002.

Lorenzini JA, Ley LL. Medical Phrase Index, 4th Edition. Los Angeles: Practice Management Information Corporation, 2001.

Michota FA. Diagnostic Procedures Handbook, 2nd Edition. Hudson, OH: Lexi-Comp, 2001.

Robbers JE, Tyler VE. Tyler's Herbs of Choice. New York: Haworth Herbal Press, 1999.

Schrier, RW. The Internal Medicine Casebook, 2nd Edition. Philadelphia: Lippincott Williams & Wilkins, 2000.

Stedman's Concise Medical Dictionary, 4th Edition. Baltimore: Lippincott Williams & Wilkins, 2001.

Stedman's Medical Dictionary, 27th Edition. Baltimore: Lippincott Williams & Wilkins, 2000.

Stoller JK, Ahmad M, Longworth DL. The Cleveland Clinic Intensive Review of Internal Medicine, 2nd Edition. Philadelphia: Lippincott Williams & Wilkins, 2000.

Wilson DD. Nurses' Guide to Understanding Laboratory and Diagnostic Tests. Philadelphia: Lippincott Williams & Wilkins, 1999.

Journals

Annals of Internal Medicine. Philadelphia: American College of Physicians, 2001.

Internal Medicine Alert. Atlanta: American Health Consultants, 2000–2001.

Journal of General Internal Medicine. Malden, MA: Blackwell Publishing, Inc., 2000–2001.

New England Journal of Medicine. Boston: Massachusetts Medical Society, 2001.

Patient Care. Montvale, NJ: Medical Economics Company, 2000–2001.

Primary Care Reports. Atlanta: American Health Consultants, 2001.

Websites

http://www.ama-assn.org

http://www.elsevier.com/locate/archger

http://www.geri.com/geriatrics

http://www.lwwmedicine.com

http://www.medscape.com

http://www.nih.gov/nia

A

> A bile
> A wave

2A

> 5-hydroxytryptamine 2A (5-HT$_{2A}$)

A$_2$

> aortic second sound
> hemoglobin A$_2$

a

> a torus palatinus

A$_{1c}$

> hemoglobin A$_{1c}$ (HbA$_{1c}$)

AA

> Alcoholics Anonymous

AAA

> abdominal aortic aneurysm

aaa disease

AACD

> abdominal aortic counterpulsation device
> age-associated cognitive decline

AACN

> American Association of Critical-Care Nurses

AACVPR

> American Association of Cardiovascular and Pulmonary Rehabilitation

AAD

> American Academy of Dermatology

AAFP

> American Academy of Family Physicians

AAGP

> American Association for Geriatric Psychiatry

AAHSA

> American Association of Homes and Services for the Aging

AAI

> acute adrenal insufficiency

AAMC

> Association of American Medical Colleges

AAMFT

> American Association for Marriage and Family

AAMI

> age-associated memory impairment

AAN

> American Academy of Neurology

AAO

> American Academy of Ophthalmology

AAO-HNS

> American Academy of Otolaryngology-Head and Neck Surgery

AAPMR

> American Academy of Physical Medicine and Rehabilitation

Aaron sign

AARP

> American Association of Retired Persons

Aarskog syndrome

A$_1$AT

> alpha-1-antitrypsin

AB, Ab

> abortion
> > early missed AB

ABA

> allergic bronchopulmonary aspergillosis
> American Bar Association

abacavir sulfate

abacterial pyuria

Abadie sign

abarticular gout

abasia

ABC

> Activities-Specific Balance Confidence Scale

abciximab

ABD

> abdomen

Abderhalden dialysis

abdomen (ABD)

> acute a.
> doughy a.
> left lower quadrant (of a.)
> left upper quadrant (of a.)
> pendulous a.
> right lower quadrant (of a.)
> right upper quadrant (of a.)
> surgical a.
> tympanitic a.

abdominal

> a. adiposity
> a. angina
> a. aorta
> a. aortic aneurysm (AAA)
> a. aortic counterpulsation device (AACD)
> a. apoplexy
> a. ballottement
> a. binder
> a. distress
> a. epilepsy
> a. guarding
> a. infection
> a. left ventricular assist device (ALVAD)
> a. mass
> a. migraine

abdominal *(continued)*
    a. pain
    a. pain in pregnancy
    a. paradox
    a. pool
    a. pulse
    a. typhoid
    a. ultrasonography
    a. ultrasound
abdominalis
    angina a.
    ectopia cordis a.
    pulsus a.
    purpura a.
abdominocardiac reflex
abdominojugular reflux
abdominopelvic zygomycosis
abduction
ABE
    acute bacterial endocarditis
abenteric
Abercrombie
    A. degeneration
    A. syndrome
aberrans
    vasculum a.
aberrant
    a. motor behavior
    a. pancreas
    a. thyroid
A-beta
abetalipoproteinemia
abeyance
ABG
    arterial blood gas
ABI
    ankle-brachial index
ability
    decisional a.
    learning a.
    olfactorial a.
    postural a.
ABIM
    American Board of Internal Medicine
abiotic
abiotrophy
    retinal a.
abirritation
ablate
ablation
    cardiac a.
    a. therapy
    transurethral needle a. (TUNA)
ablution
abnormal
    a. behavior
    a. left axis deviation (ALAD)
    a. liver chemistry
    a. Pap smear

    a. right axis deviation (ARAD)
    a. screening test
    a. tubular myelin (ATM)
    a. uterine bleeding
abnormality
    congenital chest wall a.
    electrolyte a.
    hereditary renal a.
    intraretinal microvascular a. (IRMA)
    neurohormonal a.
    ST-T a.
    T-wave a.
    vestibulocerebellar a.
ABO
    ABO antibody
    ABO antigen
abort
abortion (AB, Ab)
    first-trimester a.
    nonsurgical therapeutic a.
    second-trimester a.
    surgical a.
    therapeutic a.
abortive
above-knee amputation (AKA)
ABP
    arterial blood pressure
ABPM
    ambulatory blood pressure monitor
ABR
abraded skin
Abrahams sign
Abrams disease
abrasion
    corneal a.
abridged ocular chart (AOC)
abrupt
    a. attack
    a. attack of vertigo
abscess
    acquired a.
    amebic liver a.
    Bezold a.
    brain a.
    breast a.
    Brodie a.
    caseous a.
    cheesy a.
    cholangitic a.
    cranial epidural a.
    diverticular a.
    Dubois a.
    embolic a.
    eosinophilic a.
    epidural a.
    gangrenous a.
    glandular a.
    hepatic a.
    intraabdominal a.

labial a.
lung a.
lymphatic a.
pancreatic a.
Pautrier a.
perinephric a.
perivalvular a.
postoperative intraabdominal a.
pyogenic liver a.
subphrenic a.
subungual toe a.
tooth a.
abscission
corneal a.
Absidia
absolute
a. agraphia
a. cardiac dullness (ACD)
a. hemianopia
a. neutrophil count
a. refractory period (ARP)
a. scotoma
Absorbine, Jr.
absorptiometry
dual-energy a.
dual-energy x-ray a. (DEXA)
single dual-beam photon a.
single-photon a.
absorption
fat a.
intestinal a.
iron a.
absorptive hypercalciuria
abstinence symptoms
abstract
abstraction
impaired a.
ABTA
American Brain Tumor Association
Abt-Letterer-Siwe syndrome
abulia
abuse
alcohol a.
drug a.
elder a.
ethanol a.
familial a.
laxative a.
National Center on Elder A.
(NCEA)
National Institute on Drug A.
(NIDA)

spousal a.
substance a.
tobacco a.
abuser
intravenous drug a.
IV drug a.
A-C
Robitussin A-C
AC
acromioclavicular
a.c.
before meals [L. *ante cibum*]
ACA
American Chiropractic Association
American Counseling Association
acacia
acalculia
acalculous cholecystitis
Acanthamoeba **infection**
acanthocyte
acanthocytosis
acquired a.
acantholytic
acanthosis
acapnia
acapnial alkalosis
acapnic
acarbia
acarbose
ACAT
automated computerized axial
tomography
acathectic
acathexia
ACB
American Council of the Blind
accelerated
a. hypertension
a. idioventricular rhythm
a. rate
a. silicosis
acceleration
defective a.
accentuation
accès pernicieux
accessorium
pancreas a.
accessory
a. cell
a. pancreas
a. sign
a. spleen

NOTES

3

accessory *(continued)*
    a. symptom
    a. thyroid
accident
    cardiovascular a. (CVA)
    cerebrovascular a. (CVA)
    motor vehicle a. (MVA)
    serum a.
accidental
    a. hypothermia
    a. symptom
accident-prone
ACCLA
    anticardiolipin lupus anticoagulant
acclimating fever
Accolate
accommodation
    pupils equal and reactive to light
       and a. (PERLA)
    pupils equal, round and reactive to
       light and a. (PERRLA)
accommodative asthenopia
accretio cordis
Accu-Chek
    A.-C. II
    A.-C. Comfort Curve test strips
    A.-C. II glucometer
accumulation disease
Accupril
Accutane
ACD
    absolute cardiac dullness
ACE
    acute care for the elderly
    angiotensin-converting enzyme
       ACE inhibitor
acebutolol
ACEI
    angiotensin-converting enzyme inhibitor
acellular pertussis vaccine
acetabuli
    protrusio a.
acetabulum, pl. acetabula
acetaldehyde syndrome
acetaminophen
    a. poisoning
    a. toxicity
acetate
    depomedroxyprogesterone a.
    desmopressin a.
    glatiramer a.
acetazolamide
acetohexamide
acetonemic
acetonide
    triamcinolone a.
acetonuria
acetowhite test

acetylcholine
    a. receptor antibody level
acetylcholinesterase (AchE)
    a. inhibitor (AChEI)
acetylcysteine
acetyltransferase
    choline a.
Ace wrap
achalasia
Achard-Thiers syndrome
AchE
    acetylcholinesterase
ache
    bone a.
    stomach a.
AChEI
    acetylcholinesterase inhibitor
Achilles
    A. bursitis
    A. tendinitis
    A. tendon
Achillis
    tendo A.
achlorhydria
    watery diarrhea, hypokalemia, a.
       (WDHA)
achlorhydric anemia
Acholeplasma
acholia
acholic
acholuric
    a. hemolytic icterus
    a. jaundice
achondroplasia
achondroplastic
achoresis
achrestic anemia
achromasia
Achromobacter
Achromycin
achylia
    a. gastrica
    a. pancreatica
achylic anemia
achylous
ACI
    asymptomatic cardiac ischemia
acid
    alpha-linolenic a.
    alpha-lipoic a. (ALA)
    amino a.
    aminocaproic a.
    aminolevulinic a. (ALA)
    aspartic a.
    azelaic a.
    bile a.
    branched chain a.
    a. clearance
    deoxyribonucleic a. (DNA)

dihydroxy bile a.
diisopropyliminodiacetic a. (DISIDA)
dimercaptosuccinic a.
docosahexaenoic a.
a. dyspepsia
eicosapentaenoic a.
ethacrynic a.
fibric a.
gamma-aminobutyric a. (GABA)
a. hemolysin
hepatic 2,6-dimethyliminodiacetic a. (HIDA)
hepatoiminodiacetic a. (HIDA)
hyaluronic a.
hydrobromic a. (HBr)
5-hydroxyindoleacetic a. (5-HIAA)
a. indigestion
a. intoxication
isoleucine a.
lactic a.
leucine amino a.
lipoteichoic a.
methylmalonic a.
modified a.
monounsaturated fatty a.
omega-3 polyunsaturated fatty a.
p-aminohippuric a. (PAHA)
para-aminosalicylic a. (PASA)
a. perfusion test
a. phosphatase
polyunsaturated fatty a. (PUFA)
a. reflux
a. reflux test
a. regurgitation
ribonucleic a. (RNA)
salicylic a.
serum methylmalonic a.
teichoic a.
ticarcillin-clavulanic a.
a. toxicity
trans fatty a.
trihydroxy bile a.
ursodeoxycholic a.
valine a.
valproic a.
w-3 polyunsaturated fatty a.
xanthurenic a.
acid-ash diet
acid-base
  a.-b. disorder
  a.-b. disturbance

acidemia
  isovaleric a.
  methylmalonic a.
  propionic a.
acid-fast
  a.-f. bacillus (AFB)
  a.-f. culture
  a.-f. stain
acid-induced pain
acidism
acid-labile prodrug
acid-maltase deficiency
acidophilus
  a. milk
acidosis
  anion gap a.
  carbon dioxide a.
  compensated respiratory a.
  concomitant metabolic a.
  diabetic a.
  dilutional a.
  hypercapnic a.
  hyperchloremic metabolic a.
  lactic a.
  metabolic a.
  nonanion gap a.
  nonrespiratory a.
  nonunion gap metabolic a.
  primary renal tubular a.
  renal tubular a. (RTA)
  respiratory a.
  secondary renal tubular a.
  starvation a.
  uncompensated a.
  uremic a.
acidotic
acid-suppressive agent
aciduria
  beta-aminoisobutyric a.
  glutamic a.
  l-glyceric a.
  glycolic a.
  methylmalonic a.
  orotic a.
  paradoxical a.
  xanthurenic a.
aciduric
Aci-jel
Acinetobacter
acinic
  a. cell adenocarcinoma
  a. cell carcinoma

NOTES

acinous
    a. cancer
    a. carcinoma
Aciphex
acitretin
ackee poisoning
aclasia
aclasis
    diaphyseal a.
Aclovate
ACLS
    advanced cardiac life support
acne
    a. aestivalis
    a. arthritis
    a. conglobata
    conglobate a.
    a. excoriée
    a. fulminans
    a. mechanica
    propionibacterium a.
    a. rosacea
    a. vulgaris
acneiform eruption
ACOG
    American College of Obstetricians and
    Gynecologists
Acosta disease
acoustic neuroma
acoustogram study
ACOVE
    Assessing Care of Vulnerable Elders
ACP-ASIM
    American College of Physicians-
    American Society of Internal Medicine
ACPE
    acute cardiogenic pulmonary edema
acquired
    a. abscess
    a. acanthocytosis
    a. atelectasis
    a. bleeding diathesis
    a. coagulation disorder
    a. hemolytic anemia
    a. hemolytic icterus
    a. hypercoagulability
    a. hyperlipoproteinemia
    a. immune deficiency syndrome
    (AIDS)
    a. immunodeficiency syndrome
    (AIDS)
    a. long QT syndrome
    a. megacolon
    a. methemoglobinemia
    a. neutrophilia
    a. sensitivity
    a. sideroblastic anemia
    a. stomatocytosis
    a. toxoplasmosis

acquisition
    multiple gaited a. (MUGA)
    nuclear multiple gaited a.
acral lentiginous melanoma
9-acridinamine
acrid poison
acrimonia
acritical
acroarthritis
acrochordon
acrocyanosis
acrocyanotic
acrodermatitis
    a. chronica atrophicans
    chronic atrophicans a.
    a. enteropathica
    Hallopeau a.
acrodynia
acrodynic erythema
acrohyperhidrosis
acrohypothermy
acrokeratosis
    paraneoplastic a.
acromegalia
acromegalic
    a. arthralgia
    a. arthropathy
    a. facies
    a. gigantism
    a. heart disease
acromegalogigantism
acromegaloidism
acromegaly
acromelalgia
acromelic dysplasia
acrometagenesis
acromial
acromicria
acromioclavicular (AC)
    a. joint disease
acromion
acropachy
acropachyderma
acroparesthesia
    Nothnagel-type a.
    Schultze a.
    Schultze-type a.
acrosclerosis
acrotic
acrotrophodynia
acrotrophoneurosis
ACS
    American Cancer Society
    American College of Surgeons
ACSM
    American College of Sports Medicine
act
    Dietary Supplement Health and
    Education A.

Health Insurance Portability and
Accountability A. (HIPAA)
1974 Privacy A.
ACTH
adrenocorticotropic hormone
big ACTH
ACTH stimulation test
Acthar
ACTH-RF
adrenocorticotropic hormone-releasing
factor
Actifed
Actigall
actinic
a. cheilitis
a. keratosis (AK)
Actinomyces
actinomycetoma
actinomycin D
actinomycosis
actinomycotica
perityphlitis a.
actinomycotic appendicitis
action
cumulative a.
DES A.
a. tremor
ACTIS
AIDS Clinical Trials Information Service
Activa
A. Parkinson's Control Therapy
A. Parkinson's Control Therapy
System
**activated partial thromboplastin time
(APTT, aPTT)**
activation
defective a.
activator
recombinant plasminogen a. (r-PA)
recombinant tissue plasminogen a.
tissue plasminogen a. (TPA, tPA,
t-PA)
active
a. core rewarming
a. electrode
a. external rewarming
a. hepatitis
a. life expectancy (ALE)
a. liver disease
a. treatment
a. tuberculosis

**Activities-Specific Balance Confidence
Scale (ABC)**
activity, pl. **activities**
anticholinergic a.
beta 1, 2 a.
compromised a.
activities of daily living (ADL)
functional a.
physical a.
QEEG a.
quantitative
electroencephalographic a.
relaxing a.
seizure a.
theta a.
Actonel
Actos
ACU
ambulatory care unit
acuity
high-frequency a.
visual a.
Acular
acuminatum, pl. **acuminata**
condyloma acuminata
acupressure
acupuncture
acupuncturist
acusis
acuta
polyarthritis rheumatica a.
acute
a. abdomen
a. abdomen in pregnancy
a. acalculous cholecystitis
a. adrenal insufficiency (AAI)
a. adrenocortical insufficiency
a. African sleeping sickness
a. alcoholism
a. angle-closure glaucoma
a. appendicitis
a. arterial occlusion
a. aseptic meningitis
a. bacterial endocarditis (ABE)
a. bacterial meningitis
a. bacterial myocarditis
a. bacterial prostatitis
a. beryllium disease
a. blood loss
a. bone marrow transplant-
associated nephropathy
a. bronchitis

NOTES

acute *(continued)*
a. cardiogenic pulmonary edema (ACPE)
a. care for the elderly (ACE)
a. chest syndrome
a. confusional migraine
a. coronary syndrome
a. decompensated diabetes
a. delirium
a. demyelinating disease
a. diarrhea
a. dissecting aneurysm
a. disseminated encephalomyelitis
a. eosinophilic pneumonia
a. febrile neutrophilic dermatosis
a. febrile polyneuritis
a. febrile respiratory illness (AFRI)
a. follicular conjunctiva
a. fulminating meningococcal septicemia
a. fulminating meningococcemia
a. gonococcal arthritis (AGA)
a. gouty arthritis
a. hematogenous osteomyelitis
a. herpetic gingivostomatitis
a. herpetic vulvovaginitis
a. HIV infection syndrome
a. hypertension
a. idiopathic polyneuritis
a. incontinence
a. infectious nonbacterial gastroenteritis
a. infective endocarditis (AIE)
a. infective polyneuritis
a. inflammation
a. insomnia
a. intermittent porphyria
a. interstitial pneumonia
a. interstitial pneumonitis
a. isolated myocarditis
a. labyrinthitis
a. laryngitis
a. lower gastrointestinal bleeding
a. lung injury
a. lymphoblastic leukemia (ALL)
a. malaria
a. mesenteric ischemia
a. mitral regurgitation
a. monocytic leukemia (AML)
a. myeloblastic leukemia (AML)
a. myelocytic leukemia (AML)
a. myelogenous leukemia (AML)
a. myeloid leukemia
a. myelomonoblastic leukemia (AMMOL)
a. myelomonocytic leukemia (AMML)
a. myocardial infarction (AMI)
a. necrotizing stomatitis
a. nephrosis
a. nonlymphocytic leukemia (ANLL)
a. nonlymphoid leukemia (ANLL)
a. obstruction
a. obstruction of small intestine
a. on chronic symptom
a. organ dysfunction
a. organ rejection
a. otitis media
a. pancreatitis
a. parathyroidectomy (APTX)
a. parenchymatous hepatitis
a. pelvic pain
a. pericarditis
a. peritonitis
a. pharyngoconjunctival (APC)
a. pharyngoconjunctival reaction
a. physiology and chronic health evaluation (APACHE)
a. physiology and chronic health evaluation score
a. postinfectious polyneuritis
a. poststreptococcal glomerulonephritis
a. promyelocytic leukemia (APL)
a. pulmonary alveolitis
a. recurrent rhabdomyolysis
a. renal failure (ARF)
a. respiratory disease (ARD)
a. respiratory distress syndrome (ARDS)
a. respiratory failure (ARF)
a. respiratory injury
a. respiratory insufficiency
a. rheumatic arthritis
a. rheumatic fever
a. rickets
a. silicosis
a. sinusitis
a. suppurative sialadenitis
a. systemic lupus erythematosus
a. thromboembolism
a. thyrotoxicosis
a. trypanosomiasis
a. uncomplicated cystitis
a. upper gastrointestinal bleeding
a. urethral syndrome
a. urticaria
a. viral hepatitis
a. yellow atrophy
a. yellow atrophy of liver
acutely decompensated congestive heart failure (ADCHF)
acute-phase reactant
ACVD
 autoimmune collagen vascular disease
acyanotic
acyclovir

acylated plasminogen streptokinase
    activated complex
acylcarnitine
acyltransferase
    lecithin-cholesterol a. (LCAT)
AD
    Alzheimer disease
a.d.
    as desired
        a.d. lib
ADA
    American Dental Association
    American Diabetes Association
    American Dietetic Association
        ADA diet
Adalat
Adamantiades-Behçet syndrome
Adamkiewicz test
Adams-Stokes
    A.-S. attack
    A.-S. disease
    A.-S. syndrome
Adapin
adaptation
    cardiovascular a.
    dark a.
    a. disease
    musculoskeletal a.
adapted
adaptic
adaptive
    a. equipment
    a. immune system
    a. scale
ADAS
    Alzheimer Disease Assessment Scale
ADAS-cog
    Alzheimer Disease Assessment Scale-
        Cognitive Subscale
ADCHF
    acutely decompensated congestive heart
        failure
ADD
    attention deficit disorder
addict
addiction
    heroin a.
    methamphetamine a.
    opioid a.
Addis count
Addison
    A. anemia

A. crisis
A. disease
Addison-Biermer disease
addisonian
    a. anemia
    a. cachexia
    a. crisis
    a. syndrome
addisonii
    melasma a.
addisonism
additive effect
adduct
adduction
adductor
    a. hallucis
    a. longus
    a. lurch
adductus primus varus
ADEAR
    Alzheimer's Disease Education and
        Referral
adenalgia
adenasthenia gastrica
adenectopia
adenemphraxis
Aden fever
adenia
    leukemic a.
adenine
    a. phosphoribosyl transferase
        (APRT)
    a. phosphoribosyl transferase
        deficiency
adenitis
    mesenteric a.
    phlegmonous a.
adenocarcinoma
    acinic cell a.
    alveolar a.
    esophageal a.
    renal cell a.
Adenocard
adenocele
adenocellulitis
adenocystoma
adenodynia
adenofibroma
    pseudomucinous a.
    serous a.
adenofibrosis
adenogenous

NOTES

adenohypophysial
adenoidectomy
    tonsillectomy and a. (T&A)
adenolymphitis
adenolymphocele
adenolymphoma
adenoma
    adrenal a.
    aldosterone-producing a. (APA)
    benign a.
    corticotroph a.
    Hürthle cell a.
    parathyroid a.
    Pick a.
    pituitary a.
    rectosigmoid villous a.
    secretory a.
    thyroid a.
    tubular a.
    villous a.
adenomalacia
adenomatosis
    familial multiple endocrine a.
    fibrosing a.
    multiple endocrine a. (MEA)
    pancreatic islet a.
    polyendocrine a.
    pulmonary a.
adenomatous goiter
adenomegaly
adenomyomatous
adenomyosis
adenoncus
adenopathy
    anterior cervical chain a.
    axillary a.
    cervical chain a.
    generalized a.
    hilar a.
    inguinal a.
    localized a.
adenophlegmon
adenose
adenosine
    a. deaminase deficiency
    a. thallium study
adenosis
    florid a.
adenosquamous
adenous
adenovillous
adenoviral pneumonia
adenovirus
    a. infection
    a. serotype
adenylate kinase deficiency
adequacy

ADH
    alcohol dehydrogenase
    antidiuretic hormone
ADHD
    attention deficit hyperactivity disorder
adherence
adherent
adhesin
adhesion
    defective a.
    a. dyspepsia
    intercellular a.
    platelet a.
adhesive
    a. capsulitis
    a. inflammation
    a. serositis
adiadochokinesia
adiaspiromycosis
Adie
    A. tonic pupil
adipocyte
adipokinetic hormone
adipokinin
adiposalgia
adipose tissue
adiposis
    a. cerebralis
    a. dolorosa
    a. hepatica
    a. orchica
    a. tuberosa simplex
    a. universalis
adiposity
    abdominal a.
adiposogenital
    a. degeneration
    a. dystrophy
    a. syndrome
adiposogenitalis
    dystrophia a.
adiposuria
adipsia
adipsous
adjunct
adjustment
    a. disorder
    lifestyle a.
adjuvant chemotherapy
ADL
    activities of daily living
administered
administration
    enteral a.
    Food and Drug A. (FDA)
    Health Care Finance A. (HCFA)
    Occupational Safety and Health A. (OSHA)
    A. on Aging (AoA)

oral a.
Pension and Welfare Benefits A. (PWBA)
Social Security A. (SSA)
Substance Abuse and Mental Health Services A. (SAMSHA)
Veterans Health A. (VHA)
admission
hospital a.
adnexa
adnexal mass
adolescence
adolescent
a. health
a. medicine
adoption
adoptive cellular therapy
ADR
allergic drug reaction
adrenal
a. adenoma
a. androgen
a. apoplexy
a. computerized tomography
a. cortex
a. cortex injection
a. cortical syndrome
a. crisis
a. failure
a. gland
a. hermaphroditism
a. hyperplasia
a. hypofunction
a. hypoplasia
a. infarction
a. insufficiency
Marchand a.'s
a. mass
a. medulla
a. medullary disorder
a. neoplasm
a. nodule
a. steroid
a. suppression
a. virilism
a. virilizing syndrome
adrenalectomy
Adrenalin
adrenalinemia
adrenalinogenesis
adrenalism
adrenalopathy

adrenarche
adrenergic
a. agonist
a. blockade
a. blocking agent
a. paraganglion
a. receptor
adrenoceptive
adrenocortical
a. cancer
a. crisis
a. hyperplasia
a. insufficiency
a. obesity
a. steroid
adrenocorticohyperplasia
adrenocorticomimetic
adrenocorticotropic
a. hormone (ACTH)
a. hormone deficiency
a. hormone level
a. hormone-releasing factor (ACTH-RF)
a. hormone-secreting tumor
a. hormone stimulation test
adrenocorticotropic-releasing factor
adrenocorticotropin
adrenogenic
adrenogenital syndrome (AGS)
adrenoleukodystrophy
adrenomedullary hormone
adrenomegaly
adrenopathy
adrenopause
adrenoprival
adrenoreceptor
adrenosterone
adrenotropic hormone
adrenotropin
Adriamycin
Adson maneuver
adult
a. day-care center
a. immunization
a. lactase deficiency
a. life span
a. polycystic kidney disease (APKD)
a. respiratory distress syndrome (ARDS)
a. rickets

NOTES

adult *(continued)*
    a. T-cell leukemia
    a. tuberculosis
adult-onset
    a.-o. asthma
    a.-o. diabetes
    a.-o. diabetes mellitus
    a.-o. obesity
Advair
advance
    a. directive
    a. directive continuity
advanced
    a. age
    a. cardiac life support (ACLS)
    a. glycosylation end products
    a. life support
    a. renal failure
    a. sleep phase disorder
Advantage glucometer
adventitia
adventitious
adverse
    a. drug event
    a. drug reaction
    a. effect
advice
    against medical a. (AMA)
Advil
adynamia episodica hereditaria
adynamic
    a. bone lesion
    a. ileus
AECG
    ambulatory electrocardiography
    AECG monitoring
AEF
    amyloid-enhancing factor
aerial sickness
aerobe
aerobic
AeroBid
Aerochamber
aerodigestive tract
aerodontalgia
aerogastria
    blocked a.
aerogenic tuberculosis
aerogenosum
    sputum a.
aeromedicine
Aeromonas
    A. *hydrophila*
    A. infection
    A. *shigelloides*
aeropathy
aerophagia
aeropiesotherapy

aerosis
aerosol
    manganese dioxide a.
    QVAR Inhalation A.
    a. therapy
aerosolized
    a. microdroplet
    a. pentamidine
aerospace medicine
aerotherapeutic
aeruginosa
    Pseudomonas a.
Aesculapius
    staff of A.
aestival
aestivalis
    acne a.
aestivoautumnal fever
AET
    atrial ectopic tachycardia
AF
    Arthritis Foundation
    atrial fibrillation
AFAR
    American Federation of Aging Research
AFB
    acid-fast bacillus
    American Foundation for the Blind
afbrinogenemia
afebrile
affair
    Department of Veterans A.'s (VA)
affect
    flat a.
affection
affective sphere
affectivity
afferent
    a. loop syndrome
    a. nociceptor
    primary sensory a.
affusion
afibrinogenemia
aflatoxin
AFO
    ankle-foot orthosis
AFRI
    acute febrile respiratory illness
African
    A. Burkitt lymphoma
    A. hemorrhagic fever
    A. plum tree bark extract
    A. sleeping sickness
    A. tick fever
    A. trypanosomiasis
africanum
    Pygeum a.
Afrin

after
    a. depolarization
    a. a meal [L. *post cibum*] (p.c.)
aftercare
    a. plan
    a. treatment
afterload
AFUD
    American Foundation for Urologic
      Diseases
AG
    albumin-globulin ratio
AGA
    acute gonococcal arthritis
against medical advice (AMA)
agalactiae
    Streptococcus a.
agammaglobulinemia (AGG)
    Bruton a.
aganglionic
aganglionosis
age
    advanced a.
    anatomical a.
    basal a.
    Catholic Golden A. (CGA)
    chronological a.
    a. correlation
    a. dependent
    healthy old a.
    mental a. (MA)
    physical a.
    a. specific
age-associated
    a.-a. cognitive decline (AACD)
    a.-a. memory impairment (AAMI)
aged
    National Caucus and Center on
      Black A., Inc. (NCBA)
agency
    Environmental Protection A. (EPA)
    A. for Healthcare Research &
      Quality (AHRQ)
agenesis
agent
    acid-suppressive a.
    adrenergic blocking a.
    alpha-1 adrenergic blocking a.
    antianginal a.
    antianxiety a.
    antibacterial a.
    anticholinergic a.

    antidiabetic a.
    antidiarrheal a.
    antiemetic a.
    antifungal a.
    antiherpetic a.
    antihyperlipidemic a.
    antihypertensive a.
    antinociceptic a.
    antiproliferative a.
    antipsychotic a.
    antituberculous a.
    anxiolytic a.
    azole antifungal a.
    beta-blocking a.
    bulking a.
    chelating a.
    chemopreventive a.
    chemotherapeutic a.
    dopaminergic a.
    emulsifying a.
    etiologic a.
    exogenous pressor a.
    fibrinolytic a.
    hormonal a.
    hypocholesterolemia a.
    infectious a.
    inotropic a.
    keratinolytic a.
    lipid-lowering a.
    nonglycoside inotropic a.
    oral antidiabetic a.
    over-the-counter a.
    parenteral antihypertensive a.
    platinum-containing a.
    progestational a.
    prokinetic a.
    promotility a.
    psychotherapeutic a.
    sulfonylurea a.
    sympatholytic a.
    sympathomimetic a.
    thrombolytic a.
    vasoactive a.
agerasia
age-related
    a.-r. cataract
    a.-r. change
    a.-r. diastolic dysfunction
    a.-r. disease
    a.-r. factor
    a.-r. macular degeneration (AMD,
      ARMD)

NOTES

ageusia
    central a.
    conduction a.
    peripheral a.
AGG
    agammaglobulinemia
agglutination assay
agglutinin
    cold a.
    conduction a.
    peripheral a.
    tularensis a.
Aggrastat
aggrecan
aggregate
aggregation
    defective platelet a.
    familial a.
    platelet a.
aggregometer
aggression
aggressive
    a. care
    a. hepatitis
AGH
    amenorrhea, galactorrhea,
    hypothyroidism
AGHE
    Association for Gerontology in Higher
    Education
aging
    Administration on A. (AoA)
    American Association of Homes
    and Services for the A.
    (AAHSA)
    American Society on A. (ASA)
    amyloidosis of a.
    Brookdale Center on A. (BCOA)
    demographic a.
    Lighthouse National Center for
    Vision and A. (LNCVA)
    National Asian Pacific Center
    on A. (NAPCA)
    National Association of Area
    Agencies on A. (N4A)
    National Association of State Units
    on A. (NASUA)
    National Council on A., Inc.
    (NCOA)
    National Hispanic Council on A.
    (NHCoA)
    National Indian Council on A.
    (NICOA)
    National Institute on A. (NIA)
    National Interfaith Coalition on A.
    (NICA)
    National Policy and Resource
    Center on Nutrition and A.

    National Policy and Resource
    Center on Women and A.
    (NPRCWA)
    National Resource Center on
    Native American A. (NRCNAA)
    Oxford Project to Investigate
    Memory and A. (OPTIMA)
    premature a.
    primary a.
    a. process
    secondary a.
    successful a.
    tertiary a.
Agiolax
agitans
    paralysis a.
agitation
agitation/retardation
    psychomotor a/r.
agitator caudae
aglycosuric
agnea
agnogenic
agnosia
agonadal
agonadism
agonal
    a. gasp
    a. infection
    a. respiration
    a. rhythm
    a. thrombosis
agonist
    adrenergic a.
    alpha-adrenergic a.
    beta a.
    beta-2 adrenergic a.
    cholinergic a.
    dopamine a.
    dopamine-receptor a.
    gonadotropin a.
    gonadotropin-releasing hormone a.
    long-acting beta a.
    muscarinic a.
    serotonin receptor a.
    short-acting beta a.
agony
agoraphobia
agrammatism
agranulocytica
    mucositis necroticans a.
agranulocytosis
    congenital a.
agraphesthesia
agraphia
    absolute a.
agreement
agrypnotic

AGS
adrenogenital syndrome
American Geriatrics Society
ague
brass founder's a.
AHA
American Heart Association
American Hospital Association
AHAF
American Health Assistance Foundation
AHCA
American Health Care Association
AHF
American Health Foundation
AHI
apnea-hypopnea index
AHM
ambulatory Holter monitor
ambulatory Holter monitoring
AHRQ
Agency for Healthcare Research &
Quality
AHTA
American Horticultural Therapy
Association
Ahumada-Del Castillo syndrome
AI
aortic insufficiency
Aicardi syndrome
AICD
automatic implantable cardioverter-
defibrillator
aid
first a.
hearing a.
mobility a.
walking a.
AIDS
acquired immune deficiency syndrome
acquired immunodeficiency syndrome
AIDS cholangiopathy
AIDS Clinical Trials Information
Service (ACTIS)
AIDS-associated retrovirus (ARV)
AIDS-related
A.-r. complex (ARC)
A.-r. non-Hodgkin lymphoma
A.-r. tumor
AIE
acute infective endocarditis
AIL
angiocentric immunoproliferative lesion

AILD
angioimmunoblastic lymphadenopathy
with dysproteinemia
ainhumoides
sclerodactylia annularis a.
air
a. bed
a. curtain
a. embolism
a. hunger
a. mattress
room a. (RA)
a. sickness
a. splint
A. stirrup brace
a. trapping
airborne
a. droplet
a. precaution
Aircast
air-conditioner lung
air-contrast barium enema
air-fluidized bed
airplane travel
airsickness
airway
a. management
a. obstruction
a. obstruction in conscious patient
a. obstruction in unconscious
patient
a. suctioning
AK
actinic keratosis
AKA
above-knee amputation
akamushi
a. disease
Leptotrombidium a.
Trombicula a.
akari
Rickettsia a.
akathisia
tardive a.
Akcoline
akembe
akinesia
akinetic mutism
akiyami
ALA
alpha-lipoic acid

NOTES

ALA *(continued)*
    American Lung Association
    aminolevulinic acid
alactasia
ALAD
    abnormal left axis deviation
Alagille syndrome
Alajouanine
    A. disease
    A. syndrome
ala nasi
alanine aminotransferase (ALT)
alastrim
alba
       pityriasis a.
Albalon
Albarran test
albendazole
Albers-Schönberg disease
albicans
       Candida a.
albiduria *(var. of* albinuria)
Albini nodule
albinism
       oculocutaneous a.
albinuria, albiduria
Albright
    A. disease
    A. hereditary osteodystrophy
    A. syndrome
albuginea
       tunica a.
albumin
       radioiodinated serum a. (RISA)
       serum a.
albumin-globulin ratio (AG)
albuminoptysis
albuminoreaction
albuminorrhea
albuminuretic
albuminuria
albuminuric amaurosis
albuterol
alcohol
    a. abuse
    a. dehydrogenase (ADH)
    a. dependence scale
    a. diuresis
    ethyl a. (ETOH)
    a. overdose
    a. screening test
    a. use disorders inventory
    a. withdrawal
    a. withdrawal syndrome (AWS)
alcoholemia
alcoholic
    A.'s Anonymous (AA)
    a. apoptosis
    a. blackout

    a. cardiomyopathy
    a. cerebellar degeneration
    a. cirrhosis
    a. foamy degeneration
    a. hepatitis
    a. ketoacidosis
    a. liver disease
    a. paralysis
    a. pneumonia
    a. polyneuritis
    a. steatohepatitis
alcohol-induced hypertension
alcoholism
    acute a.
    chronic a.
    National Institute on Alcohol
      Abuse and A. (NIAAA)
Aldactazide
Aldactone
aldehyde dehydrogenase
aldesleukin
aldocorten
aldolase level
Aldomet
Aldoril
aldose reductase pathway
aldosterone
    a. antagonist
aldosterone-producing adenoma (APA)
aldosteronism
    idiopathic a.
    juvenile a.
    primary a.
    pseudoprimary a.
    secondary a.
aldosteronogenesis
aldosteronoma
aldosteronopenia
aldosteronuria
Aldrich-Mees line
Aldrich syndrome
Aldrich-Wiskott syndrome
ALE
    active life expectancy
alendronate
aleukemic
    a. leukemia
    a. myelosis
aleukia hemorrhagica
aleukocythemic leukemia
aleukocytic
Aleve
alexic
ALFA
    Assisted Living Federation of America
alfa
       dornase a.
alfa-2a
       interferon a.-2a

alfa-2b
    interferon a.-2b
alfacon
    interferon a.-1
algid
    a. malaria
    a. pernicious fever
    a. stage
alginolyticus
algorithm
    CAM Diagnostic A.
alible
Alice in Wonderland syndrome
Aliento
    Project A.
aliment
alimentary
    a. apparatus
    a. diabetes
    a. glycosuria
    a. hyperinsulinism
    a. hypoglycemia
    a. lipemia
    a. obesity
    a. osteopathy
alimentation
    forced a.
    parenteral a.
    rectal a.
aliquot
alkaline
    a. diuresis
    a. phosphatase
    a. toxicity
alkaline-ash diet
alkalinization
alkalitherapy
alkaloid
    plant a.
alkalosis
    acapnial a.
    altitude a.
    carbon dioxide a.
    compensated metabolic a.
    compensated respiratory a.
    congenital gastrointestinal a.
    hypochloremic a.
    hypokalemic metabolic a.
    metabolic a.
    respiratory a.
    tetany of a.
alkalotic

alkaluria
alkaptonuria
alkaptonuric
Alka-Seltzer
Alkeran
alkylate
alkylation
ALL
    acute lymphoblastic leukemia
all-cause mortality
Allegra
Allegra-D
allele
Allen
    A. paradoxical law
    A. test
    A. treatment
allergen challenge testing
allergic
    a. bowel disease
    a. bronchopulmonary aspergillosis
     (ABA)
    a. drug reaction (ADR)
    a. granulomatosis
    a. granulomatous angiitis
    a. purpura
    a. reaction
    a. rhinitis
    a. stomatitis
allergies (*pl. of* allergy)
allergology
allergosorbent
allergy, pl. **allergies**
    atopic a.
    cold a.
    environmental a.
    IgE-mediated food a.
    insulin a.
    intestinal a.
    milk protein a.
    no known allergies (NKA)
    no known drug allergies (NKDA)
    physical a.
All-Flex
    Ortho A.-F.
Alliance for Aging Research
allied health professional
all-inclusive care
allocation
    resource a.
allodynia

NOTES

allogeneic, allogenic
  a. marrow transplantation
  a. stem cell transplant
allograft
  a. nephropathy
alloimmunization
  platelet a.
allopath
allopathic
allopathist
allopathy
allopregnane
allopurinol
allotriogeustia
allotriophagy
allotrophic
allowance
  recommended dietary a. (RDA)
alloxan diabetes
Almeida disease
almotriptan
aloe
alopecia
  androgenic a.
  a. areata
Alora
Alpers disease
alpha
  a. antagonist
  a. blocker
  a. chain disease
  a. fetoprotein
  a. interferon
  interferon a.
  tumor necrosis factor-a. (TNF-
    alpha)
alpha-1
  a. adrenergic blocking agent
  a. antichymotrypsin
  a. protease inhibitor replacement
alpha-adrenergic
  a.-a. agonist
  a.-a. antagonist
  a.-a. blocker
  a.-a. receptor antagonist
alpha-allocortol
alpha-allopregnanediol
alpha-1-antitrypsin (A_1AT)
  a.-1-a. deficiency
alpha-cortol
alpha-cortolone
alpha-fetoprotein
  a.-f. test
alpha-glucosidase inhibitor
alpha granule
alpha-hemolytic streptococcus
17-alpha-hydroxyprogesterone
alpha-linolenic acid
alpha-lipoic acid (ALA)

alpha-methyldopa
alpha-thalassemia
alphavirus
Alpine scurvy
Alport syndrome
alprazolam
alprostadil
ALS
  amyotrophic lateral sclerosis
Alström
  A. disease
  A. syndrome
ALT
  alanine aminotransferase
Altace
ALTE
  apparent life-threatening event
alteplase
alteration
  a. in consciousness
  functional a.
  sleep architecture a.
  structural a.
altered
  a. eating habit
  a. level of consciousness
  a. mental status
  a. pharmacodynamics
ALternaGEL
alternans
  diabetes a.
  pulsus a.
Alternaria
alternative
  a. cancer therapy
  a. drug
  a. medicine
  a. practitioner
altitude
  a. alkalosis
  a. disease
  a. erythremia
  a. illness
  a. sickness
aluminosis
ALVAD
  abdominal left ventricular assist device
alveolar
  a. adenocarcinoma
  a. duct emphysema
  a. hypoventilation
  a. proteinosis of lung
alveolar-arterial oxygen gradient
alveoli (*pl. of* alveolus)
alveolitis
  acute pulmonary a.
  cryptogenic fibrosing a.
  extrinsic allergic a.

alveolocapillary block
alveolus, pl. **alveoli**
alymphia
Alzheimer
 A. Association
 A. dementia
 A. disease (AD)
 A. Disease Assessment Scale
  (ADAS)
 A. Disease Assessment Scale-
  Cognitive Subscale (ADAS-cog)
 A. Disease Education and Referral
  (ADEAR)
 A. Disease Education and Referral
  Center
 A. neurofibrillary change
AMA
 against medical advice
 American Medical Association
amalgam tattoo
amantadine HCl
Amaryl
amastia
amatol
amaurosis
 albuminuric a.
 diabetic a.
 a. fugax
 uremic a.
amazia
Ambien
ambiguous
ambilateral
amblyopia
 toxic a.
 uremic a.
ambulance
ambulans
 pestis a.
ambulant
 a. edema
 a. plague
ambulation
ambulator
 community a.
 household a.
ambulatory
 a. blood pressure monitor (ABPM)
 a. care
 a. care unit (ACU)
 a. electrocardiography (AECG)
 a. electrocardiography monitoring

 a. Holter monitor (AHM)
 a. Holter monitoring (AHM)
 a. surgery
 a. typhoid
 a. visit
AMD
 age-related macular degeneration
 atrophic AMD
 dry AMD
 exudative AMD
 wet AMD
AMDA
 American Medical Directors Association
amebiasis
 a. disorder
 hepatic a.
 pulmonary a.
amebic
 a. colitis
 a. disease
 a. dysentery
 a. granuloma
 a. liver abscess
 a. pneumonia
amebicide
 intestinal luminal a.
amebiosis
amebism
ameboma
ameliorate
amelioration
amenable
amenia
amenorrhea
 dietary a.
 exercise-induced a.
 a., galactorrhea, hypothyroidism
  (AGH)
 hypophysial a.
 hypothalamic a.
 lactation a.
 ovarian a.
 pathologic a.
 postpartum a.
 primary a.
 secondary a.
 traumatic a.
amenorrheal
America
 Assisted Living Federation of A.
  (ALFA)

NOTES

America *(continued)*
  Community Transportation
    Association of A. (CTAA)
  Gerontological Society of A.
    (GSA)
  Health Insurance Association of A.
    (HIAA)
  Huntington's Disease Society of A.
    (HDSA)
  Lupus Foundation of A. (LFA)
  Meals on Wheels Association
    of A. (MOWAA)
  Opticians Association of A. (OAA)
  Prevent Blindness A. (PBA)
  United Way of A.
  Visiting Nurse Association of A.
    (VNAA)
  Volunteers of A.
American
  A. Academy of Dermatology
    (AAD)
  A. Academy of Family Physicians
    (AAFP)
  A. Academy of Neurology (AAN)
  A. Academy of Ophthalmology
    (AAO)
  A. Academy of Orthopedic
    Surgeons
  A. Academy of Otolaryngology-
    Head and Neck Surgery (AAO-
    HNS)
  A. Academy of Physical Medicine
    and Rehabilitation (AAPMR)
  A. Association of Cardiovascular
    and Pulmonary Rehabilitation
    (AACVPR)
  A. Association of Critical-Care
    Nurses (AACN)
  A. Association for Geriatric
    Psychiatry (AAGP)
  A. Association of Homes and
    Services for the Aging (AAHSA)
  A. Association for Marriage and
    Family (AAMFT)
  A. Association of Retired Persons
    (AARP)
  A. Bar Association (ABA)
  A. Board of Internal Medicine
    (ABIM)
  A. Brain Tumor Association
    (ABTA)
  A. Cancer Society (ACS)
  A. Chiropractic Association (ACA)
  A. College of Obstetricians and
    Gynecologists (ACOG)
  A. College of Physicians-American
    Society of Internal Medicine
    (ACP-ASIM)

  A. College of Sports Medicine
    (ACSM)
  A. College of Surgeons (ACS)
  A. Council of the Blind (ACB)
  A. Counseling Association (ACA)
  A. Dental Association (ADA)
  A. Diabetes Association (ADA)
  A. Diabetes Association diet
  A. Dietetic Association (ADA)
  A. Federation of Aging Research
    (AFAR)
  A. Foundation for the Blind
    (AFB)
  A. Foundation for Urologic
    Diseases (AFUD)
  A. Geriatrics Society (AGS)
  A. Health Assistance Foundation
    (AHAF)
  A. Health Care Association
    (AHCA)
  A. Health Foundation (AHF)
  A. Heart Association (AHA)
  A. Horticultural Therapy
    Association (AHTA)
  A. Hospital Association (AHA)
  A. Lung Association (ALA)
  A. Medical Association (AMA)
  A. Medical Directors Association
    (AMDA)
  A. Menopause Foundation (AMF)
  A. Music Therapy Association
    (AMTA)
  A. Nurses Association (ANA)
  A. Occupational Therapy
    Association, Inc. (AOTA)
  A. Optometric Association (AOA)
  Organization of Chinese A.'s
    (OCA)
  A. Osteopathic Association (AOA)
  A. Parkinson's Disease Association
    (APDA)
  A. Pharmaceutical Association
    (APhA)
  A. Physical Therapy Association
    (APTA)
  A. Podiatric Medical Association
    (APMA)
  A. Psychiatric Association (APA)
  A. Psychological Association (APA)
  A. Red Cross
  A. Society of Internal Medicine
    (ASIM)
  A. Society on Aging (ASA)
  A. Speech-Language-Hearing
    Association (ASHA)
  A. Stroke Association (ASA)
  A. Tinnitus Association (ATA)
  A. trypanosomiasis
ametropia

A

AMF
American Menopause Foundation
AMI
acute myocardial infarction
Amicar
amikacin
amiloride
amine
sympathomimetic a.
amino
a. acid
a. acid metabolism disorder
aminoacidemia
aminoacidopathy
aminoaciduria
aminocaproic acid
aminoglutethimide
aminoglycoside
a. antibiotic
a. nephrotoxicity
a. therapy
aminoguanidine
aminolevulinic acid (ALA)
aminophylline
5-aminosalicylate
aminotransferase
alanine a. (ALT)
aspartate a. (AST)
asymptomatic elevated a.
a. level
serum a.
amiodarone
amitriptyline
AML
acute monocytic leukemia
acute myeloblastic leukemia
acute myelocytic leukemia
acute myelogenous leukemia
amlodipine
AMML
acute myelomonocytic leukemia
AMMOL
acute myelomonoblastic leukemia
ammonemia
ammonia
a. excretion
a. inhalation
serum a.
amnesia
Broca a.
amnion
amorphous

amoxapine
amoxicillin
Amoxil
amphetamine toxicity
Amphojel
amphoric
a. rale
a. resonance
a. respiration
a. voice
a. voice sound
amphoriloquy
amphorophony
amphotericin
a. B
a. B colloidal dispersion
a. B deoxycholate
a. B lipid complex
liposomal a. B
ampicillin
ampicillin-sulbactam
amplitude
ampule
ampulla, pl. **ampullae**
a. of Vater
ampullitis
amputation
above-knee a. (AKA)
Beclard a.
below-knee a. (BKA)
Bunge a.
Callander a.
Camden a.
Chopart a.
Farabeuf a.
Gritti a.
Gritti-Stokes a.
Guyon a.
Hancock a.
Hey a.
Jaboulay a.
Kirk a.
Langenbeck a.
Mackenzie a.
Maisonneuve a.
pedicle tip a.
Pirogoff a.
a. rehabilitation
Ricard a.
Stokes a.
Syme a.
Teale a.

NOTES

amputation *(continued)*
    Tripier a.
    Wladimiroff-Mikulicz a.
amrinone
AMTA
    American Music Therapy Association
amylase
amyloid
    cardiac a.
    a. degeneration
    a. liver
    a. nephrosis
    a. neuropathy
    a. plaque
    a. precursor protein (APP)
    a. precursor protein gene
    a. tongue
amyloid-enhancing factor (AEF)
amyloidogenesis
amyloidosis
    a. of aging
    Andrade-type a.
    cutaneous a.
    a. cutis
    dialysis-associated a.
    familial a.
    hemodialysis a.
    hepatic a.
    Indiana-type a.
    Iowa-type a.
    kidney a.
    a. of larynx
    light chain-related a.
    a. of multiple myeloma
    Portuguese-type a.
    primary a.
    renal a.
    secondary a.
    senile systemic a.
amylopectinosis
amylorrhea
amylosuria
amyopathic dermatomyositis
amyotrophic
    a. cachexia
    a. lateral sclerosis (ALS)
amyotrophy
    diabetic a.
amyxorrhea
AN-1792 vaccine
ANA
    American Nurses Association
    antinuclear antibody
        positive ANA
anabiosis
anabiotic
anabolic
anacidity
anadenia

anadipsia
anadrenalism
Anadrol
anaerobic
    a. cellulitis
    a. infection
    a. myonecrosis
anaerobic-cavitary pneumonia syndrome
Anaerococcus
anaeroplasty
Anafranil
anagen arrest
anagrelide hydrochloride
anal
    a. cancer
    a. function
    a. verge
analeptic enema
analgesia
    intrathecal a.
    parenteral-controlled a. (PCA)
    patient-controlled a. (PCA)
analgesic
    narcotic a.
    nonnarcotic a.
    opioid a.
analog
    short-acting insulin a.
analphalipoproteinemia
Analpram-HC
analysis, pl. **analyses**
    bioelectric impedance a.
    bivariate a.
    cerebrospinal fluid a.
    direct mutation a.
    gastric acid a.
    life-table a.
    quantitative a.
    semen a.
    sequential multiple a.-20 (SMA-20)
    Southern blot a.
anamnesis
anamnestic
anaphylactic
anaphylactogen
anaphylactogenesis
anaphylactogenic
anaphylactoid
    a. phenomenon
    a. purpura
    a. reaction
anaphylatoxin
anaphylaxis
    heterocytotropic a.
    homocytotropic a.
    idiopathic a.
    recurrent a.
anaplasia

anaplastic
    a. anemia
    a. thyroid carcinoma
Anaprox
anarthritic rheumatoid disease
anasarca
Anaspaz
anastomosis, pl. **anastomoses**
    biliary-enteric a.
    ileal pouch-anal a.
    Martin-Gruber a.
    Potts a.
    Roux-en-Y a.
anastomotic stenosis
anatomic
anatomical age
anatomicomedical
anatomy
    applied a.
    medical a.
anatripsis
anatriptic
ANCA
    antineutrophil cytoplasmic antibody
Ancef
ancillary
    a. dialysis
    a. measures
    a. therapy
anconeus
ancylostome anemia
ancylostomiasis
Anders disease
Andersen
    A. disease
    A. syndrome
    A. triad
Anderson-Collip test
Anderson-Fabry disease
Andes virus
Andrade
    A. indicator
    A. syndrome
Andrade-type amyloidosis
Andral decubitus
andrenosterone
andriatrics
Androgel
androgen
    adrenal a.
    a. receptor antagonist
    a. resistance

androgen-deprivation therapy
androgenic
    a. alopecia
    a. hormone
androgenous
Android-10
android
andrology
andromorphous
andropathy
andropause
androstanediol
androstanedione
androstenol
androstenolone
androsterone
anecdotal
anejaculation
anemia
    achlorhydric a.
    achrestic a.
    achylic a.
    acquired hemolytic a.
    acquired sideroblastic a.
    Addison a.
    addisonian a.
    anaplastic a.
    ancylostome a.
    aplastic a.
    arctic a.
    aregenerative a.
    asiderotic a.
    atrophic a.
    autoimmune hemolytic a.
    Baghdad Spring a.
    Banti splenic a.
    Bartonella a.
    Belgian Congo a.
    Biermer a.
    Biermer-Ehrlich a.
    Blackfan-Diamond a.
    breast a.
    brickmaker's a.
    cameloid a.
    cancer-associated a.
    cerebral a.
    chlorotic a.
    chronic disease a.
    a. of chronic disease
    chronic hemolytic a. (CHA)
    chronic myelocytic a.
    chronic myelomonocytic a.

NOTES

anemia *(continued)*
    chronic refractory a.
    Chvostek a.
    cold antibody autoimmune
      hemolytic a.
    combined cold and warm antibody
      autoimmune hemolytic a.
    congenital aplastic a.
    congenital dyserythropoietic a.
    congenital nonspherocytic
      hemolytic a.
    constitutional aplastic a.
    Cooley a.
    Coombs-negative immune
      hemolytic a.
    cow's milk a.
    crescent cell a.
    cytogenic a.
    Czerny a.
    deficiency a.
    Diamond-Blackfan a.
    dilution a.
    dimorphic a.
    diphyllobothrium a.
    drepanocytic a.
    Dresbach a.
    drug-induced hemolytic a.
    Edelmann a.
    elliptocytary a.
    elliptocytotic a.
    enzyme deficiency a.
    enzyme deficiency hemolytic a.
    erythroblastic a.
    erythronormoblastic a.
    essential a.
    Faber a.
    false a.
    familial erythroblastic a.
    familial microcytic a.
    Fanconi a.
    febrile pleiochromic a.
    fish tapeworm a.
    folic acid deficiency a.
    fragmentation hemolytic a.
    globe cell a.
    glucose-6-phosphate dehydrogenase
      deficiency a.
    goat's milk a.
    ground itch a.
    hemoglobin hemolytic a.
    hemolytic a.
    Herrick a.
    hookworm a.
    hyperchromic a.
    hyperproliferative a.
    a. hypochromica siderochestica
      hereditaria
    hypochromic microcytic a.
    hypoferric a.

    hypoplastic a.
    hypoproliferative a.
    icterohemolytic a.
    immunohemolytic a.
    infectious a.
    iron-deficiency a.
    isochromic a.
    Israels-Wilkinson a.
    Jaksch a.
    Larzel a.
    lead a.
    Lederer a.
    Leishman a.
    leukoerythroblastic a.
    lysolecithin hemolytic a.
    macrocytic achylic a.
    malignant a.
    Marchiafava-Micheli a.
    Mediterranean a.
    megaloblastic a.
    megalocytic a.
    meniscocytic a.
    metaplastic a.
    microangiopathic hemolytic a.
    microcytic a.
    microdrepanocytic a.
    microelliptopoikilocytic a.
    milk a.
    miner's a.
    mountain a.
    myelophthisic a.
    myelosclerotic a.
    nonmegaloblastic macrocytic a.
    normochromic normocytic a.
    normocytic a.
    nutritional macrocytic a.
    ovalocytary a.
    pernicious a.
    physiologic a.
    polar a.
    preoperative a.
    primary erythroblastic a.
    primary refractory a.
    profound a.
    pyridoxine-responsive a.
    pyruvate kinase deficiency a.
    radiation a.
    refractory a.
    renal failure a.
    Rundles-Falls a.
    Runeberg a.
    scorbutic a.
    secondary refractory a.
    severe aplastic a. (SAA)
    sickle cell a.
    sideremic a.
    sideroblastic a.
    sideropenic a.
    slaty a.

spherocytic a.
splenic a.
spur cell a.
target cell a.
thrombopenic a.
thrombotic microangiopathic
  hemolytic a.
toxic paralytic a.
traumatic hemolytic a.
triose-phosphate isomerase
  deficiency a.
tropical a.
tunnel a.
unstable hemoglobin hemolytic a.
von Jaksch a.
warm antibody autoimmune
  hemolytic a.
Wills a.
Witts a.
x-ray a.

anemic polyneuritis
anenzymia
anergia
anergic stupor
anergy
antigen-specific a.
T-cell a.
aneroid
a. device
a. sphygmomanometer
anesthesia
saddle a.
therapeutic a.
anesthesiologist
anesthesiology
anesthetic
local a.
anesthetist
certified registered nurse a.
  (CRNA)
anestrum
aneurysm
abdominal aortic a. (AAA)
acute dissecting a.
Bérard a.
berry a.
celiac artery a.
Charcot-Bouchard a.
colonic artery a.
Crisp a.
dissecting a.
gastric artery a.

gastroduodenal artery a.
gastroepiploic artery a.
hepatic artery a.
jejunal artery a.
mesenteric artery a.
pancreatic artery a.
pancreaticoduodenal artery a.
Park a.
popliteal artery a.
Pott a.
Rasmussen a.
Richet a.
Rodrigues a.
saccular a.
Shekelton a.
sinus of Valsalva a.
splanchnic artery a.
splenic artery a.
aneurysmal cough
ANF
antinuclear factor
Angelman syndrome
angiitis, angitis
allergic granulomatous a.
visceral a.
angina
abdominal a.
a. abdominalis
a. angina
atypical a.
Bretonneau a.
classic a.
cold a.
a. cordis
a. diphtheritica
a. equivalent
Heberden a.
intestinal a.
Ludwig a.
monocytic a.
a. nervosa
a. pectoris
Plaut a.
Prinzmetal a.
pseudomembranous a.
Schultz a.
stable a.
stress-induced a.
toilet-seat a.
ulceromembranous a.
unstable a.

NOTES

angina *(continued)*
    vasomotor a.
    Vincent a.
anginal
anginiform
anginoid
anginose scarlatina
angiocentric immunoproliferative lesion (AIL)
angiocholitis
angioedema
    hereditary a. (HAE)
    Quincke a.
angioendothelioma
angioendotheliomatosis
    a. proliferans
    systemic proliferating a.
angiofollicular mediastinal lymph node hyperplasia
angiogram
    exercise multigated a.
    multigated a. (MUGA)
angiogranuloma
angiography
    coronary a.
    equilibrium radionuclide a. (ERNA)
    four-vessel a.
    iodine contrast a.
    magnetic resonance a. (MRA)
    pulmonary a.
    selective renal a.
    stenotic renal a.
    systolic/diastolic a.
angioimmunoblastic
    a. lymphadenopathy
    a. lymphadenopathy with dysproteinemia (AILD)
angiokeratoma
    diffuse a.
angiolupoid
angioma
    cavernous a.
    cherry a.
    spider a.
    tuberous a.
angiomatoid
angiomatosis
    bacillary a. (BA)
    familial a.
    hemorrhagic familial a.
angiomyolipoma
angioneurotic
    a. anuria
    a. edema
angiopathy
    cerebral amyloid a.
    congophilic a.
angiophacomatosis

angioplasty
    balloon a.
    excimer laser coronary a. (ELCA)
    percutaneous transluminal coronary a. (PTCA)
angiosa
    syncope a.
angiosarcoma
    cardiac a.
angiostatin
angiostrongyliasis
angiotensin
    a. I–III
angiotensin-converting
    a.-c. enzyme (ACE)
    a.-c. enzyme inhibitor (ACEI)
    a.-c. enzyme inhibitor cough
angiotensinogen
angitis *(var. of* angiitis)
angle
    Bohler a.
    cardiohepatic a.
    costophrenic a.
    costovertebral a. (CVA)
    Lovibond a.
    a. of mandible
    rectoanal a.
    Virchow a.
anglicus
    sudor a.
angor
angular
    a. cheilitis
    a. stomatitis
ANH
    atrial natriuretic hormone
anhedonia
anhepatogenous jaundice
anhidrotics
anhydrase
anhydrosis
anhydrous
    theophylline a.
ani (*pl. of* anus)
aniacinamidosis
aniacinosis
anicteric
    a. leptospirosis
    sclerae a.
    a. virus hepatitis
anilinism
anilism
animal-naming test
animation
    suspended a.
anion
    a. gap
    a. gap acidosis
anisakiasis

A

anismus
anisocoria
anisocytosis
anisometropia
anisopoikilo
anisotropic conduction
anisoylated plasminogen streptokinase
  activator complex (APSAC)
ankle
    a. arthrocentesis
    a. edema
    a. mortise
    a. sprain
ankle-brachial index (ABI)
ankle-foot orthosis (AFO)
ankylobrachial
ankyloglossia
ankylosing
    a. hyperostosis
    a. spondylitis
ankylostomiasis
ANLL
  acute nonlymphocytic leukemia
  acute nonlymphoid leukemia
ANN
  artificial neural network
annular
    a. calcification
    a. pancreas
annulare
    erythema a.
    granuloma a.
annuloplasty
    mitral a.
annulus
    calcified mitral a.
ano
    fissura in a.
Anodynos
anomalotrophy
anomaly
    Chédiak-Higashi a.
    Chédiak-Steinbrinck-Higashi a.
    Chiari a.
    Ebstein a.
    Hegglin a.
    Huët-Pelger nuclear a.
    Jordan a.
    May-Hegglin a.
    Pelger-Huët nuclear a.
    right-side Ebstein a.
    Steinbrinck a.

    Undritz a.
    vascular rings a.
anomia
anonymous
    Alcoholics A. (AA)
anopsia
anorectal
    a. disorder
    a. examination
    a. manometry
    a. syndrome
anorectic drug
anorexia
    a. nervosa
anorexiant
anorexic
anorexigenic
anorgasmy
anoscopy
anosmia
    hypogonadism with a.
anosognosia
anovulation
anovulatory
    a. bleeding
anoxia
    cerebral a.
    diffusion a.
    global a.
    histotoxic a.
    myocardial a.
    stagnant a.
anoxic
    a. brain damage
    a. encephalopathy
Ansaid
anserina
    Podospora a.
anserine
anserinus
    pes a.
Anspor
Antabuse
antacid
antagonism
antagonist
    aldosterone a.
    alpha a.
    alpha-adrenergic a.
    alpha-adrenergic receptor a.
    androgen receptor a.
    angiotensin II receptor a.

NOTES

27

antagonist (continued)
    beta-adrenergic a.
    calcium channel a.
    dopamine a.
    glycoprotein IIb-IIIa receptor a.
    histamine receptor a.
    histamine-2 receptor a.
    H_2 receptor a.
    5-HT-receptor a.
    leukotriene receptor a.
    metabolic a.
    neurokinin-1 receptor a.
    serotonin receptor a.
antalgesia
antalgic gait
antarthritic
antasthmatic
antebrachial
antecedent
    a. sign
    a. streptococcal infection
ante cibum
antecubital
antedate
antefebrile
anteflexed
antegrade flow
antepyretic
anterior
    a. cervical chain adenopathy
    a. cervical lymph node
    a. chest wall syndrome
    a. cruciate ligament
    a. cruciate ligament tear
    a. descent
    a. horn cell disease
    a. infarction
    a. interosseous nerve entrapment
    a. pituitary gonadotropin
    a. pituitary hormone
    a. pituitary insufficiency
    a. and posterior (A&P)
    a. superior iliac spine (ASIS)
    a. wall infarction (AWI)
    a. wall myocardial infarction
      (AWMI)
anteroapical
anterograde
anteroinferior myocardial infarction
anterolateral myocardial infarction
anteroposterior and lateral
anteroseptal myocardial infarction
anthelone
    a. E, U
    a. U
anthracic
anthraconecrosis
anthracosilicosis
anthracosis

anthracotic tuberculosis
anthracycline
    a. antibiotic
    a. cardiomyopathy
anthraquinone
anthrax
    a. bacillus
    cerebral a.
    cutaneous a.
    gastrointestinal a.
    inhalation a.
    intestinal a.
    a. pneumonia
    pulmonary a.
anthropometric
    a. measurement
    a. value
anthropometry
antiadrenergic effect
antiandrogen
antianginal agent
antianxiety agent
antiarrhythmic drug
antiarthritic
antiasthmatic
antibacterial agent
antibiotic
    aminoglycoside a.
    anthracycline a.
    antitumor a.
    bactericidal a.
    bacteriostatic a.
    beta-lactam a.
    broad-spectrum a.
    carbapenem a.
    cephalosporin a.
    a. course
    a. diarrhea
    empiric a.
    a. enterocolitis
    fluoroquinolone a.
    glycopeptide a.
    lincosamide a.
    macrolide a.
    oral a.
    polyene a.
    a. prophylaxis
    sulfonamide a.
    tetracycline a.
    a. tongue
    topical a.
antibiotic-associated colitis
antibiotic-resistant
    a.-r. bacteria
    a.-r. bacterial infection
antiblennorrhagic
antibody
    ABO a.
    anticapsular a.

anticardiolipin a.
anti-double-stranded DNA a.
antiglomerular basement
  membrane a.
antimitochondrial a.
antineural a.
antineutrophil cytoplasmic a.
  (ANCA)
antinuclear a. (ANA)
antiphospholipid a.
antiplatelet a.
antistriational a.
antithrombocyte a.
antithyroid a.
core a.
a. deficiency disease
a. deficiency syndrome
equimolar a.
insulin a.
a. level
monoclonal anti-IgE a.
pneumolysin a.
radiofluorescent a. (RFA)
ribonucleoprotein a.
RNP a.
thyroglobulin a.
thyroid microsomal a.
TSH-displacing a.
wheat product a.
anticapsular antibody
anticardiolipin
  a. antibody
  a. lupus anticoagulant (ACCLA)
anticentromere
anticholagogue
anticholinergic
  a. activity
  a. agent
anticholinesterase drug
antichymotrypsin
  alpha-1 a.
anticipation
anticoagulant
  anticardiolipin lupus a. (ACCLA)
  circulating a.
anticoagulate
anticoagulation
anticollagen
anticonvulsant
  parenteral a.
  a. property
anticrotalus serum

anticus
antidepressant
  a. medication
  a. toxicity
  tricyclic a. (TCA)
antidiabetic
  a. agent
antidiarrheal agent
antidiphosphopyridine nucleotide
antidiuresis
antidiuretic
  a. hormone (ADH)
antidopaminergic
antidote
anti-double-stranded DNA antibody
antidromic tachycardia
antidysenteric
antidysuric
antiemetic agent
antiepileptic
antiestrogen
antifebrile
antifolate
antifungal agent
antigen
  ABO a.
  capsid a.
  carcinoembryonic a. (CEA)
  exogenous a.
  human leukocyte a. (HLA)
  prostate-specific a. (PSA)
antigen-antibody
  pneumolysin a.-a.
antigen-specific anergy
antiglobulin
antiglomerular
  a. basement membrane antibody
  a. basement membrane antibody
    disease
antigonorrheic
antiherpetic agent
antihistamine
  oral a.
antihydropic
antihyperlipidemic agent
antihypertensive
  a. agent
  a. medication
antiicteric
antiinflammatory drug
antiinsulin
antilipemic

NOTES

antimalarial drug
antimicrobial
    a. chemoprophylaxis
    a. therapy
    a. treatment
antimicrosomal
antimitochondrial
    a. antibody
antimony
antimuscarinic
    GI a.
    urinary a.
antinauseant
antineoplastic
antineural antibody
antineutrophil
    a. cytoplasmic antibody (ANCA)
    a. cytoplasmic autoantibody
antinociceptic agent
antinuclear
    a. antibody (ANA)
    a. factor (ANF)
antioxidant
antiparasitic
antiparkinsonian
antiperiodic
antiperistalsis
antiperistaltic
antiphagocytic factor
antiphlogistic
antiphospholipid
    a. antibody
    a. antibody syndrome
antiplatelet
    a. antibody
    a. therapy
antiprogestin
antiproliferative agent
antipsychotic
    a. agent
antipyresis
antipyretic therapy
antipyrotic
antirabies serum
antirachitic
antireflux
    a. surgery
    a. therapy
antiretroviral
    a. chemotherapy
    a. regimen
    a. therapy
antirheumatic
antiruminant
antiscorbutic
antisecretory
antiseptic
    urinary a.

antiserum
    C-reactive protein a. (CRPA)
antispasmodic
antistreptolysin-O (ASO)
    a.-O. titer
antistriational antibody
antisympathetic
antithrombin III
antithrombocyte
    a. antibody
antithymocyte globulin
antithyroid
    a. antibody
    a. drug
antitoxic serum
antitoxin
    botulinum a.
antitragicus
antitrypsin
antitumor antibiotic
antitussive
antivenereal
antivenom
    Crotalinae polyvalent immune
    Fab a.
Antivert
antiviral
    a. drug
    a. therapy
antra (*pl. of* antrum)
antral gastritis
antrectomy
antritis
antrum, pl. **antra**
    Willis a.
Anturane
anucleated
anuria
    angioneurotic a.
anuric
anus, pl. **ani**
    pruritus ani
Anusol-HC
anxiety
    a. attack
    chronic a.
    a. disorder
    a. state
anxiolytic
AOA
    American Optometric Association
    American Osteopathic Association
AoA
    Administration on Aging
AOC
    abridged ocular chart
aorta, pl. **aortae**
    abdominal a.
    coarctation of a.

aortic
- a. coarctation
- a. dissection
- a. dwarfism
- a. insufficiency (AI)
- a. leaflet
- a. paraganglion
- a. regurgitation (AR)
- a. root
- a. sclerosis
- a. second sound (A₂)
- a. systolic ejection murmur
- a. valve
- a. valve disease
- a. valve replacement
- a. valvular stenosis

aortitis
- syphilitic a.

aortocoronary bypass

aortoenteric fistula

aortoiliac

AO screw

AOTA
- American Occupational Therapy Association, Inc.

A&P
- anterior and posterior

APA
- aldosterone-producing adenoma
- American Psychiatric Association
- American Psychological Association

APACHE
- acute physiology and chronic health evaluation
  - APACHE II score

apancreatic

aparathyreosis

aparathyroidism

apareunia

apathetic
- a. hyperthyroidism
- a. thyrotoxicosis

apathy

apatite
- a. deposition disease

APC
- acute pharyngoconjunctival
  - APC reaction

APDA
- American Parkinson's Disease Association

apenteric

apepsinia

aperiodic

aperistalsis

aperitive

Apert hirsutism

apex pneumonia

APhA
- American Pharmaceutical Association

aphagia

aphakia

aphasia
- Broca a.
- expressive a.
- global a.
- Wernicke a.

aphemia

apheresis
- low-density lipoprotein a.

aphrophilus
- *Haemophilus a.*

aphtha, pl. **aphthae**

aphthobullous stomatitis

aphthosa
- cachexia a.
- stomatitis a.

aphthous
- a. stomatitis
- a. ulcer

aphylactic

aphylaxls

apical
- a. bleb
- a. middiastolic
- a. murmur
- a. myocardial infarction
- a. pneumonia
- a. systolic

apinealism

apituitarism

APKD
- adult polycystic kidney disease

APL
- acute promyelocytic leukemia

aplasia
- congenital a.
- germinal a.
- red cell a.

aplastic
- a. anemia
- a. crisis
- a. leukemia
- a. myelosis

NOTES

APMA
American Podiatric Medical Association
apnea
a. attack
central sleep a.
deglutition a.
a. index
obstructive sleep a. (OSA)
sleep a.
a. test
apnea-hypopnea index (AHI)
apneic
a. oxygenation
a. spell
a. spell associated with loud
snoring
apodia
ApoE
apolipoprotein E
ApoE4
apolipoprotein E epsilon 4
ApoE4 gene
apogee
apolipoprotein
a. E epsilon 4 gene
a. E epsilon 4 gene on
chromosome 19
familial defective a. b-100
apolipoprotein E (ApoE)
apomorphine
sublingual a.
aponeurosis
aponeurotica
apophyseal
apophysis
apoplexia
Raymond a.
apoplexy
abdominal a.
adrenal a.
Broadbent a.
heat a.
Raymond a.
apoptosis
alcoholic a.
apostaxis
apothanasia
APP
amyloid precursor protein
APP gene
apparatus
alimentary a.
digestive a.
a. digestorius
inhalation therapy a.
Tiselius a.
apparent
appearance
cushingoid a.

jelly belly a.
toxic a.
appendalgia
appendiceal
appendicectasis
appendices (*pl. of* appendix)
appendicism
appendicitis
actinomycotic a.
acute a.
bilharzial a.
focal a.
foreign-body a.
left-sided a.
perforating a.
recurrent a.
relapsing a.
stercoral a.
verminous a.
appendix, pl. appendices
perforated retrocecal a.
apperception
apperceptive
appetite
application
topical a.
applicator
applied anatomy
approach
brachial a.
directed a.
percutaneous femoral a.
step-down a.
step-up a.
appropriateness
apraxia
ideational a.
ideomotor a.
limb a.
limb-kinetic a.
oculomotor a.
apraxic
Apresazide
Apresoline
aprosopia
APRT
adenine phosphoribosyl transferase
APRT deficiency
APSAC
anisoylated plasminogen streptokinase
activator complex
APTA
American Physical Therapy Association
APTT, aPTT
activated partial thromboplastin time
APTX
acute parathyroidectomy
apyretic
apyrexia

apyrexial
AQ
    Nasacort AQ
AquaMEPHYTON
aquapuncture
aqueductal stenosis
aquiparous
aquosa
    cachexia a.
AR
  aortic regurgitation
arabinoside
    cytosine a. (Ara-C, ara-C)
arabinosis
arabinosylcytosine (Ara-C, ara-C)
Ara-C, ara-C
  arabinosylcytosine
  cytarabine
  cytosine arabinoside
arachnidism
arachnodactyly
arachnoid
arachnoiditis
arachnophobia
ARAD
  abnormal right axis deviation
araneism
ARB
  angiotensin II receptor blocker
arbovirus-associated arthritis
ARC
  AIDS-related complex
arc
    xenon a.
arch
    right aortic a.
    Treitz a.
arctic anemia
arcus
ARD
  acute respiratory disease
ardent fever
ardor
ARDS
  acute respiratory distress syndrome
  adult respiratory distress syndrome
area
    calcaneal a.
    calcaneus a.
    glans a.
    infraumbilical a.
    Kiesselbach a.

    pudendal a.
    surface a.
areata
    alopecia a.
arecoline
Aredia IV
areflexia
    detrusor a.
aregenerative anemia
areola, pl. **areolae**
areolitis
ARF
  acute renal failure
  acute respiratory failure
argatroban
Argentinean hemorrhagic fever
Argentine hemorrhagic fever
arginine
    a. test
    a. vasopressin (AVP)
argininosuccinicaciduria
argon laser photocoagulation
Argyll Robertson pupil
argyria
argyric
argyrism
ariboflavinosis
Aricept
Aristocort
Aristospan
armamentarium
Armanni-Ebstein
    A.-E. change
    A.-E. kidney
    A.-E. lesion
Armanni-Ehrlich degeneration
armarium
ARMD
    age-related macular degeneration
Armour Thyroid
Armstrong disease
arnica
Arnold-Chiari malformation
Arnold nerve reflex cough syndrome
aromatase inhibitor
arousal
ARP
    absolute refractory period
arrectores pilorum
arrest
    anagen a.

NOTES

arrested
    a. growth and development
    a. tuberculosis
arrhythmia
    atrial a.
    cardiac a.
    Mönckeberg a.
    a. in pregnancy
    ventricular a.
    ventriculophasic sinus a.
    Wenckebach a.
arrhythmogenic
    a. right ventricular cardiomyopathy
arrival
    dead on a. (DOA)
arseniasis
arsenicalism
arsenical paralysis
arsenic tremor
arsenotherapy
artefact
artem
    secundum a.
arterial
    a. arteriolar resistance
    a. baroreceptor
    a. blood gas (ABG)
    a. blood pressure (ABP)
    a. disease
    a. embolus
    a. hypertension
    a. insufficiency
    a. oxygenation
    a. oxygen pressure (PAO_2)
    a. oxygen saturation (SaO_2)
    a. pressure
    a. pyemia
    a. stiffening
    a. switch operation
    a. thrombosis
arteries (*pl. of* artery)
arteriogram
    pulmonary a.
arteriography
    percutaneous transluminal
      coronary a. (PTCA)
arteriohepatic dysplasia
arteriolar
arteriolar atherosclerosis
arteriole
    pancreatic a.
    systemic a.
arterionephrosclerosis
arteriopathy
    autosomal dominant a.
    calcific uremic a.
    cerebral autosomal dominant a.

arteriosclerosis
    coronary a.
    a. obliterans (ASO)
arteriosclerotic
    a. cardiovascular disease (ASCVD)
    a. dementia
    a. dementia with delirium
    a. heart disease (ASHD)
    a. mesenteric vascular occlusive
      disease
    a. vertigo
arteriosus
    patent ductus a. (PDA)
    truncus a.
arteriovenous (AV)
    a. fistula (AVF)
    a. malformation (AVM)
    a. shunt
    a. shunting
arteritis
    brachiocephalic a.
    giant cell a. (GCA)
    Horton a.
    Takayasu a.
    temporal a.
artery, pl. **arteries**
    carotid a.
    cervicocerebral a.
    cilioretinal a.
    coronary a.
    dextrotransposition of great arteries
    a. disease
    external carotid a.
    femoral a.
    internal carotid a.
    left gastric a. (LGA)
    levotransposition of great arteries
    pial a.
    profundus femoral a.
    pulmonary a. (Ppa)
    right coronary a. (RCA)
    a. stenosis
    stenotic renal a.
    superficial femoral a.
    tibial a.
arthralgia
    acromegalic a.
    nonspecific a.
    periodic a.
    a. saturnine
arthritic
arthriticus
    status a.
arthritis, pl. **arthritides**
    acne a.
    acute gonococcal a. (AGA)
    acute gouty a.
    acute rheumatic a.
    arbovirus-associated a.

bacterial a.
chronic gouty a.
chylous a.
crystal a.
crystal-induced a.
a. deformans
degenerative a. (DA)
enteropathic a.
erosive a.
filarial a.
A. Foundation (AF)
fungal a.
gonococcal a.
gonorrheal a.
gouty a.
hemophilic a.
hepatitis-associated a.
a. hiemalis
hip a.
HIV-associated a.
hypertrophic a.
idiopathic blennorrheal a.
infectious a.
inflammatory bowel disease a.
Jaccoud a.
juvenile chronic a.
juvenile-onset rheumatoid a.
juvenile rheumatoid a. (JRA)
Lyme a.
Marie-Strümpell a.
metastatic a.
monoarticular a.
a. mutilans
a. nodosa
nonbacterial infectious a.
nondeforming a.
nongonococcal septic a.
ochronotic a.
parvovirus-associated a.
peripheral a.
polyarticular a.
primary gouty a.
progressive inflammatory a.
proliferative a.
psoriatic a.
pyogenic sterile a.
rheumatic a.
rheumatoid a. (RA)
rubella-associated a.
sarcoid a.
self-limited inflammatory a.
septic a.

seronegative a.
shoulder a.
subtalar a.
suppurative a.
tuberculous a.
a. urethritica
viral a.
arthrocentesis
ankle a.
hand a.
knee a.
wrist a.
arthrodesis
arthrogram
arthrogryposis
arthrokatadysis
arthrolithiasis
arthropathy
acromegalic a.
Charcot a.
diabetic a.
hemophilic a.
Jaccoud a.
myxedematous a.
neuropathic a.
arthroplasty
arthropod-borne viral fever
arthroscopy
arthrosia
exanthesis a.
arthrotyphoid
Arthus response
articular
a. chondrocalcinosis
a. gout
a. rheumatism
a. syndrome
articularis cubiti
artifact
artifactitious
artifactual
artificial
a. fever
a. neural network (ANN)
a. sphincter
a. tear
ARV
AIDS-associated retrovirus
aryepiglottic fold
arytenoid
as
as desired (a.d. lib, a.d.)

NOTES

as *(continued)*
    as much as needed (q.l.)
    as needed (p.r.n.)
    as soon as possible (ASAP)
ASA
    American Society on Aging
    American Stroke Association
Asacol
ASAP
    as soon as possible
asbestosis pneumoconiosis
ascariasis disorder
Ascaris lumbricoides
ascending
    a. cholangitis
    a. colon
    a. flaccid paralysis
    a. pathway
    a. polyneuritis
Ascher syndrome
Aschoff
    A. cell
    A. nodule
Ascholl syndrome
ascites
    chyliform a.
    a. chylosus
    chylous a.
    dialysis a.
    gelatinous a.
    malignant a.
    mucinous a.
    nephrogenic a.
    refractory a.
    transudative a.
    yellow-brown serous a.
ascitic fluid
Ascriptin
ASCUS
    atypical squamous cell of undetermined
        significance
ASCVD
    arteriosclerotic cardiovascular disease
ASD
    atrial septal defect
asecretory
Asendin
aseptic
    a. fever
    a. meningitis
asexual dwarfism
ASH
    asymmetric septal hypertrophy
ASHA
    American Speech-Language-Hearing
        Association
ASHD
    arteriosclerotic heart disease
ashen gray color

Asherman syndrome
Ashkenazi Jew
Asian influenza
Asiatic
    A. cholera
    A. schistosomiasis
asiderotic anemia
ASIM
    American Society of Internal Medicine
ASIS
    anterior superior iliac spine
asitia
ASO
    antistreptolysin-O
    arteriosclerosis obliterans
        ASO titer
aspart
    insulin a.
aspartate aminotransferase (AST)
aspartic acid
aspartylglycosaminuria
aspect
    buccal a.
    palmar and dorsal a.'s
Aspercreme
Asperger disorder
aspergilloma
    pulmonary a.
aspergillosis
    allergic bronchopulmonary a.
        (ABA)
    bronchopulmonary a.
    disseminated a.
    miliary pulmonary a.
    nosocomial a.
    pulmonary a.
Aspergillus
    A. *flavus*
    A. *niger*
aspermatogenic sterility
aspermia
aspersion
asphyxia
    autoerotic a.
    sexual a.
    symmetric a.
asphyxiation
aspiration
    fine-needle a. (FNA)
    irrigation and a. (I&A)
    needle a.
    oropharyngeal a.
    tracheobronchial a.
    transbronchial needle a.
    transthoracic needle a.
    transtracheal a.
aspirin
    enteric-coated a.
    warfarin and a.

asplenia
    functional a.
    a. syndrome
asplenic
asplenism
Assam fever
assaultive episode
assay
    agglutination a.
    D-dimer a.
    direct fluorescent a. (DFA)
    enzyme-linked immunosorbent a.
      (ELISA)
    estrogen receptor a. (ERA)
    plasma thyroid-stimulating
      hormone a.
    recombinant immunoblot a. (RIBA)
    serum thyroid-stimulating
      hormone a.
    sulfonylurea a.
    Western blot a.
Assessing Care of Vulnerable Elders
    (ACOVE)
assessment
    Berg Balance A.
    comprehensive a.
    comprehensive geriatric a. (CGA)
    Duke Mobility A.
    echocardiographic a.
    Fugl-Meyer Sensory-Motor A.
    Geriatric Pain A.
    health risk a. (HRA)
    home safety a.
    preoperative a.
assident
    a. sign
    a. symptom
assiduous
assistance
    National Organization of Victim A.
      (NOVA)
assistant
    certified medical a. (CMA)
    personal digital a. (PDA)
    physician a. (PA)
assisted
    a. living facility
    A. Living Federation of America
      (ALFA)
    a. living setting
    a. suicide
assistive device

association
    Alzheimer's A.
    American Bar A. (ABA)
    American Brain Tumor A. (ABTA)
    American Chiropractic A. (ACA)
    American Counseling A. (ACA)
    American Dental A. (ADA)
    American Diabetes A. (ADA)
    American Dietetic A. (ADA)
    American Health Care A. (AHCA)
    American Heart A. (AHA)
    American Horticultural Therapy A.
      (AHTA)
    American Hospital A. (AHA)
    American Lung A. (ALA)
    American Medical A. (AMA)
    A. of American Medical Colleges
      (AAMC)
    American Medical Directors A.
      (AMDA)
    American Music Therapy A.
      (AMTA)
    American Nurses A. (ANA)
    American Occupational Therapy A.,
      Inc. (AOTA)
    American Optometric A. (AOA)
    American Osteopathic A. (AOA)
    American Parkinson's Disease A.
      (APDA)
    American Pharmaceutical A.
      (APhA)
    American Physical Therapy A.
      (APTA)
    American Podiatric Medical A.
      (APMA)
    American Psychiatric A. (APA)
    American Psychological A. (APA)
    American Speech-Language-
      Hearing A. (ASHA)
    American Stroke A. (ASA)
    American Tinnitus A. (ATA)
    National Bar A. (NBA)
    National Family Caregivers A.
      (NFCA)
    National Gerontological Nursing A.
      (NGNA)
    National Medical A. (NMA)
    National Mental Health A.
      (NMHA)
    National Rural Health A. (NRHA)
    National Senior Games A. (NSGA)
    National Stroke A. (NSA)

NOTES

association *(continued)*
>Vestibular Disorders A. (VEDA)
>Young Men's Christian A. (YMCA)
>Young Women's Christian A. (YWCA)

assuage

assurance
>quality a.

AST
>aspartate aminotransferase

astasia

astasia-abasia

asteatosis

astemizole

astereognosis

asterion

asterixis

asthenia
>a. gravis hypophyseogenea
>muscle a.

asthenic orthophoria

asthenopia
>accommodative a.

asthma
>adult-onset a.
>atopic a.
>bronchial a.
>bronchitic a.
>cardiac a.
>catarrhal a.
>cotton-dust a.
>cough-variant a.
>dust a.
>exercise-induced a.
>extrinsic a.
>food a.
>hay a.
>Heberden a.
>intermittent a.
>intrinsic a.
>mild intermittent a.
>mild persistent a.
>miller's a.
>miner's a.
>moderate persistent a.
>nervous a.
>occupational a.
>persistent a.
>postexertional a.
>a. and pregnancy
>reflex a.
>severe persistent a.
>spasmodic a.
>steam-fitter's a.
>stripper's a.
>summer a.

asthmatic
>a. bronchitis

>a. inflammatory airway disease
>a. response

asthmaticus
>status a.

asthmatoid wheeze

asthmogenic

astigmatism

astragaloscaphoid joint

astragalus

astrocytoma

asylum

asymmetric septal hypertrophy (ASH)

asymmetry

asymptomatic
>a. bacteriuria
>a. cardiac ischemia (ACI)
>a. carotid bruit
>a. cholelithiasis
>a. elevated aminotransferase
>a. gallstone
>a. hyperuricemia
>a. hypotonicity
>a. inflammatory prostatitis

asynchronous breathing

asystematic

asystole
>ventricular a.

at
>at bedtime (hora somni)
>at once (stat., STAT)

ATA
>American Tinnitus Association

Atacand HCT

Atarax

ataxia
>autosomal dominant cerebellar a.
>cerebellar a.
>Friedreich a.
>gait a.
>gluten a.
>mitochondrial a.
>optic a.
>paroxysmal a.
>spinocerebellar a.

ataxia-telangiectasis

ataxic
>a. breathing
>cerebellar a.

atelectasis
>acquired a.
>patchy a.
>segmental a.

atelectatic rale

ateliotic dwarfism

atenolol

atherectomy
>directional coronary a.

atheroembolism

atheroembolus, pl. **atheroemboli**

atherogenesis
atherogenic low-density lipoprotein
  pattern B phenotype
atheroma
atheromatous
atherosclerosis
      arteriolar a.
      premature a.
      A. Risk in Communities Study
atherosclerotic
      a. heart disease
      a. plaque
      a. stroke
atherothrombic stroke
atherothrombosis
atherothrombotic
athetosis
athetotic
athlete's heart
athrepsia
athymia
athymism
athyrea
athyroidism
athyrosis
athyrotic
ATIS
      HIV/AIDS Treatment Information
      Service
Ativan
atlantoaxial subluxaton
atlantooccipital
ATM
      abnormal tubular myelin
atonic
      a. bladder
      a. dyspepsia
atopic
      a. allergy
      a. asthma
      a. dermatitis
atopy
atorvastatin calcium
atovaquone
atovaquone/proguanil
atresia
      biliary a.
      pulmonary a.
      tricuspid a.
atrial
      a. arrhythmia
      a. contraction

a. ectopic beat
a. ectopic tachycardia (AET)
a. fibrillation (AF)
a. flutter
a. hypertrophy
a. infarction
a. myxoma
a. natriuretic factor
a. natriuretic hormone (ANH)
a. septal defect (ASD)
a. septostomy
a. tachycardia
atriopeptin
atrioventricular (AV)
      a. block
      a. canal septal defect
      a. dissociation
      a. fistula
      a. junctional escape beat
      a. junctional tachycardia
      a. nodal reentrant tachycardia
      a. Wenckebach block
atriplicism
atrium
Atrohist L.A.
Atromid-S
atrophia
atrophic
      a. anemia
      a. cirrhosis
      a. gastric mucosa
      a. glossitis
      a. thrombosis
      a. vaginitis
atrophicans
      acrodermatitis chronica a.
      chronica a.
atrophicus
      lichen sclerosus et a.
atrophied
atrophoderma of Pasini and Pierini
atrophy
      acute yellow a.
      cerebral a.
      cyanotic a.
      dentatorubral-pallidoluysian a.
      disuse a.
      fat replacement a.
      gastric a.
      idiopathic adrenal a.
      inactivity a.
      lobar a.

NOTES

atrophy *(continued)*
>marantic a.
>multiple system a. (MSA)
>multisystem a.
>olivopontocerebellar a.
>Pick a.
>posterior cortical a.
>senile a.
>Sudeck a.
>tubular a.
>yellow a.
>Zimmerlin a.

atropine
atropinism
Atrovent inhaler
attack
>abrupt a.
>Adams-Stokes a.
>anxiety a.
>apnea a.
>brain a.
>cataplectic a.
>cluster a.
>drop a.
>ischemic a.
>a. rate
>Stokes-Adams a.
>syncopal a.
>transient ischemic a. (TIA)

attending
>a. physician
>a. staff

attention
>a. deficit disorder (ADD)
>a. deficit hyperactivity disorder (ADHD)

attenuated
>a. mumps virus
>a. tuberculosis

attenuation
>rest a.

attitude
attorney
>National Academy of Elder Law A.'s, Inc. (NAELA)
>power of a.

attractin
attrition
atypia
atypical
>a. angina
>a. lymphocyte
>a. measles
>a. mycobacterial infection
>a. pneumonia
>a. sensory modality
>a. squamous cell of undetermined significance (ASCUS)
>a. tuberculosis

audiogram
audiologic evaluation
audiometer
>AudioScope 3 a.

audiometry
>Békésy a.

AudioScope 3 audiometer
auditory brainstem-evoked response
Auerbach plexus
Auerbrugger sign
Aufranc-Turner hip prosthesis
Aufrecht
>A. disease
>A. sign

augmentation
augmented
>a. voltage unipolar left arm lead (aVL)
>a. voltage unipolar left foot lead (aVF)
>a. voltage unipolar right arm lead (aVR)

Augmentin ES-600
aura
>migraine with a.
>migraine without a.

Auralgan drops
aural glomus
aureus
>methicillin-resistant *Staphylococcus a.* (MRSA)
>*Staphylococcus a.*

auricular
aurium
>tinnitus a.

auromercaptoacetanilid
aurotherapy
aurothioglucose
aurothioglycanide
Aurum Analgesic Cream
auscultate
auscultation
>immediate a.
>mediate a.
>percussion and a. (P&A)

auscultatory
>a. percussion
>a. sound

Austin-Flint murmur
Austin Moore prosthesis
Australian
>A. Q fever
>A. tick typhus
>A. X disease

australis
>*Rickettsia a.*

autacoid (*var. of* autocoid)
autemesia
autism

autoantibody
  antineutrophil cytoplasmic a.
autochthonous malaria
autocoid, autacoid
  a. substance
autoerotic asphyxia
autogenic training
autogenous cartilage implantation
autoimmune
  a. cholangitis
  a. collagen vascular disease
    (ACVD)
  a. disease
  a. hemolytic anemia
  a. hepatitis
  a. hypophysitis
  a. polyglandular failure
  a. thyroiditis
autoinoculable
autoinoculation
autointoxicant
autointoxication
autologous
  a. stem cell transplant
  a. thrombin
  a. transfusion
autolytic debridement
automated computerized axial
  tomography (ACAT)
automatic
  a. implantable cardioverter-
    defibrillator (AICD)
  a. internal cardioverter-defibrillator
autonomic
  a. function test
  a. insufficiency
  a. neuropathy
autonomous breathing
autonomy
  functional a.
  patient a.
autopathic
autopepsia
autopoisonous
autopositive end-expiratory pressure
autopsy
autoreactivity
autoregulation
  cerebral a.
  a. filtration
autosomal
  a. dominant arteriopathy

  a. dominant cardiomyopathy
  a. dominant cerebellar ataxia
  a. dominant disorder
  a. recessive disorder
autosufficiency
autotherapy
autotoxemia
autotoxic
autotoxicosis
autotoxin
autotransfusion
autumn fever
auxodrome
AV
  arteriovenous
  atrioventricular
    AV block
    AV dissociation
    AV fistula
    AV nodal reentrant tachycardia
Avandia
Avapro
avascular necrosis
AVC cream
Aveeno
Avelox
avenae
Aventyl
AVF
  arteriovenous fistula
aVF
  augmented voltage unipolar left foot lead
    aVF lead
aviation medicine
aviator's disease
avitaminosis
  conditioned a.
avium
  Enterococcus a.
  Mycobacterium a.
avium-intracellulare
  mycobacterium a.-i.
aVL
  augmented voltage unipolar left arm lead
    aVL lead
AVM
  arteriovenous malformation
avoidance reflex
AVP
  arginine vasopressin

NOTES

41

aVR
    augmented voltage unipolar right arm
    lead
        aVR lead
A/V ratio
avulsion
AWI
    anterior wall infarction
AWMI
    anterior wall myocardial infarction
AWS
    alcohol withdrawal syndrome
Axert
axes (*pl. of* axis)
axial
Axid
axillary
    a. adenopathy
    hidradenitis a.'s
    a. hyperhidrosis
    a. temperature
    a. thermometer
axilla thermometer
axillofemoral
axis, pl. **axes**
    hypothalamic-pituitary a. (HPA)
    hypothalamic-pituitary-adrenal a.
    (HPAA)
    QRS a.
    superior a.
    a. X

axon
    tract a.
axonal
Axsain Cream
Ayerza
    A. disease
    A. syndrome
Aygestin
8-azaguanine
azar
    kala a.
azathioprine
azelaic acid
azithromycin
Azlin
Azmacort inhaler
Azo Gantrisin
azole antifungal agent
Azo-Standard
azotemia
    prerenal a.
azotemic
azothermia
azotorrhea
aztreonam
Azulfidine
azurophil
azygous

B-100
B₁₂

B$_{12}$ deficiency
serum vitamin B$_{12}$
vitamin B$_{12}$

2b
BA

bacillary angiomatosis
Baastrup syndrome
Baber syndrome
babesiosis

human b.
Babinski

B. reflex
B. sign
B. syndrome
Babinski-Fröhlich syndrome
baby

b. boomer
b. boomer era
b. boomer population
BAC

blood alcohol content
Baccelli sign
bacillary

b. angiomatosis (BA)
b. diarrhea
b. dysentery
b. meningitis
b. peliosis (BP)
b. pneumonia
bacille

b. Calmette-Guérin (BCG)
b. Calmette-Guérin vaccine
Bacillus

B. cereus infection
B. subtilis
bacillus, pl. bacilli

acid-fast b. (AFB)
anthrax b.
Bang b.
Boas-Oppler b.
b. Calmette-Guérin vaccine
Chauveau b.
Döderlein b.
Ducrey b.
Fick b.
Flexner b.
Flexner-Strong b.
Friedländer b.
Gärtner b.
Ghon-Sachs b.
Hansen b.
Hofmann b.
Johne b.

Klebs-Löffler b.
Klein b.
Koch-Weeks b.
Morax-Axenfeld b.
Morgan b.
Newcastle-Manchester b.
Nocard b.
Pfeiffer b.
Preisz-Nocard b.
Schmitz b.
Schmorl b.
Shiga b.
Sonne-Duval b.
Strong b.
Whitmore b.
bacitracin
back

b. pain
b. sprain
b. strain
background

b. diabetic retinopathy (BDR)
b. noise
backwash ileitis
baclofen
bacteremia

Bartonella quintana b.
clostridial b.
community-acquired b.
gonococcal b.
transient b.
bacteria (*pl. of* bacterium)
bacterial

b. arthritis
b. cholangitis
b. conjunctivitis
b. endocarditis
b. endocarditis in pregnancy
b. endophthalmitis
b. food poisoning
b. infection
b. meningitis
b. myocarditis
b. peliosis
b. pneumonia
b. prostatitis
b. synergism
b. vaginosis (BV)
b. vulvovaginitis
bactericidal antibiotic
bacteriostatic antibiotic
bacterium, pl. bacteria

antibiotic-resistant bacteria
multiresistant bacteria

B

43

bacteriuria
  asymptomatic b.
  catheter-associated b.
  polymicrobial b.
Bacteroides fragilis
bacteroidosis
bacteruria
Bactrim
Bactroban
Baelz syndrome
BAER
  brainstem auditory evoked response
Baer nystagmus
bagassosis
Baggenstoss change
Baghdad Spring anemia
baja patella
baked tongue
Baker cyst
Bakwin-Elger syndrome
BAL
  bronchoalveolar lavage
balance
  calcium b.
  Clinical Test of Sensory Interaction
   & B. (CTSIB)
  magnesium b.
  potassium b.
  sodium b.
  water b.
balance-and-gait training
balanced diet
balanitis
  circinate b.
  b. diabetica
balanoposthitis
balantidial dysentery
balantidiasis
balantidosis
baldness
  female-pattern b.
  male-pattern b.
bald tongue
Balint syndrome
Balkan nephropathy
Balke-Ware test
Ballance sign
Ballantyne-Runge syndrome
Ballet sign
ballistic exercise jerking
balloon
  b. angioplasty
  b. catheter
  b. dilation
  Nasostat hemostatic nasal b.
  b. sickness
  b. tamponade
ballottable

ballottement
  abdominal b.
  renal b.
balm
  Carmex lip b.
Balneol
balneotherapeutics
Baló disease
balsalazide disodium
Bamberger disease
Bamberger-Marie disease
bananas
  b., rice, applesauce, tea, toast diet
  b., rice, applesauce, toast (BRAT)
  b., rice, applesauce, toast, tea
   (BRATT)
  b., rice cereal, applesauce, toast
   (BRAT)
  b., rice cereal, applesauce, toast
   diet
Bancroft
band
  creatine kinase myocardial b.
   (CKMB)
  iliotibial b. (ITB)
  intervertebral iliotibial b.
Band-Aid
bandbox resonance
bandlike
bandwidth
  EEG b.
  electroencephalogram b.
Bang bacillus
banging
  head b.
bank
  Senior Job B.
Bannister disease
Bannwarth syndrome
Banti
  B. disease
  B. splenic anemia
  B. syndrome
bar
  cricopharyngeal b.
  grab b.
  B. syndrome
Bárány
  B. maneuver
  B. syndrome
barbae
  chronic sycosis b.
  pili incarnati b.
  pseudofolliculitis b.
  tinea b.
barber's itch
barbiturate toxicity
barbiturism
Barcoo vomit

Bardex
bariatric
baritosis
barium
    b. enema (BE)
    b. swallow
bark
    cramp b.
    white willow b.
    willow b.
Barkman reflex
Barlow
    B. disease
    B. syndrome
baroreceptor
    arterial b.
    b. sensitivity
baroreflex response
barotitis media
barotrauma
barrel chest
barrel-shaped thorax
Barré sign
Barrett
    B. esophagus
    B. syndrome
    B. ulcer
Bàrsony-Polgàr syndrome
Barter-Schwartz syndrome
Barthel Index
Bart hemoglobin
Barth hernia
Bartholin cyst
Bartonella
    B. anemia
    B. infection
    B. quintana bacteremia
bartonellosis
Bartter syndrome
Baruch law
basal
    b. age
    b. body temperature
    b. cell carcinoma
    b. diet
    b. forebrain
    b. ganglion
    b. insulin
    b. metabolic rate (BMR)
    b. metabolism
    b. middiastolic

    b. ration
    b. tuberculosis
basalis
    nucleus b.
Basaljel
based
    empirically b.
basedoid
Basedow
    B. disease
    B. goiter
    B. pseudoparaplegia
    B. syndrome
    B. triad
basedowian
basedowificata
    struma b.
base hospital
baseline value
basic
    b. calcium phosphate crystal
      deposition disease
    b. diet
    b. fibroblast growth factor (bFGF)
    b. life support
    b. metabolic profile (BMP)
    b. multicellular unit (BMU)
basilar
    b. artery migraine
    b. crackle
    b. interstitial infiltrate
    b. skull fracture
basilic vein
basiliximab
basin
    emesis b.
    pus b.
basket
    Stokes b.
basophil
basophilia
    pituitary b.
    punctate b.
basophilic
    b. cell
    b. hyperpituitarism
    b. leukemia
basophilism
    Cushing b.
    Cushing pituitary b.
    pituitary b.
Bassen-Kornzweig syndrome

NOTES

Bassler sign
Bastedo sign
bastokinin
bath
    colloid b.
    contrast b.
    douche b.
    dousing b.
    electric b.
    Greville b.
    hafussi b.
    hydroelectric b.
    immersion b.
    light b.
    Nauheim b.
    needle b.
    paraffin b.
    sitz b.
    whirlpool b.
Batten disease
Batten-Mayou disease
battered
    b. child syndrome
    b. spouse syndrome
battery
    dizziness simulation b.
    Halstead-Reitan b.
    7-minute neurocognitive b.
    neuropsychological test b.
    NHANES B.
    Solomon 7-Minute Mental
       Status B.
Battey avian swine
bauxite pneumoconiosis
Baycol
Bayer syndrome
Bayesian outlook
B bile
B-cell
    lymphoid precursor B-c.
    B-c. lymphoma
BCG
    bacille Calmette-Guérin
    BCG vaccine
BCNU
    bischloroethylnitrosourea
    carmustine
BCOA
    Brookdale Center on Aging
BDI
    Beck Depression Inventory
BDR
    background diabetic retinopathy
BE
    barium enema
beaded hair
Beale
    sacculi of B.
Beano

beard dermatophytosis
Bearn-Kunkel-Slater syndrome
Bearn-Kunkel syndrome
beat
    atrial ectopic b.
    atrioventricular junctional escape b.
    b.'s of clonus
    ventricular ectopic b.
    ventricular premature b. (VPB)
Beau
    B. disease
    B. syndrome
Beauvais disease
Beck
    B. Depression Inventory (BDI)
    B. triad
Becker
    B. muscular dystrophy (BMD)
    B. phenomenon
    B. sign
Beckwith syndrome
Beckwith-Wiedemann syndrome
Beclard amputation
beclomethasone
    b. dipropionate
    b. nasal inhaler
    b. with CFC propellant
    b. with HFA propellant
Beclovent oral inhaler
Beconase
bed
    air b.
    air-fluidized b.
    Gatch b.
    low air-loss b.
    mud b.
    b. rest
    Roho b.
    b. sore
    water b.
bedridden
bedside cystometry
bedtime
    at b. (hora somni)
    b. insulin, daytime sulfonylurea
    (BIDS)
bedwetting
Beelith
beet-tongue
beeturia
before-after comparison
before meals [L. *ante cibum*] (a.c.)
Begbie disease
behavior
    aberrant motor b.
    abnormal b.
    bizarre b.
    b. change
    disturbed b.

B

problematic b.
risk b.
risk-taking b.
behavioral
  b. means
  b. medicine
  b. problem
  B. Risk Factor Surveillance System (BRFSS)
  b. symptom
  b. technique
  b. therapy
Behçet
  Behçet triple symptom complex
  B. disease
  B. syndrome
Bèhier-Hardy sign
Behr
  B. disease
  B. syndrome
BEI
  butanol-extractable iodine
  BEI test
bejel
Békésy
  B. audiometry
  B. test
Bekhterev-Strümpell spondylitis
belching
Belgian Congo anemia
Belgium Netherlands stent (BENESTENT)
bell
  B. palsy
  B. paralysis
  b. sound
belladonna
Bellergal-S
Bell-Horn knee sleeve
bellmetal resonance
bellyache
below-knee amputation (BKA)
Bel-Phen-Ergot
belt
  rib b.
  b. test
beltlike distribution
bemetizide
Benadryl
benazepril hydrochloride
Bence
  B. Jones body

  B. Jones myeloma
  B. Jones protein
  B. Jones proteinemia
  B. Jones proteinuria
benchmark
bends
Benedikt syndrome
beneficiary, pl. **beneficiaries**
benefit
benefited
Benemid
BENESTENT
  Belgium Netherlands stent
  BENESTENT Study Group Trial
benign
  b. adenoma
  b. brachial plexopathy
  b. dry pleurisy
  b. familial icterus
  b. forgetfulness
  b. glycosuria
  b. hepatic neoplasm
  b. hypertension
  b. inoculation lymphoreticulosis
  b. inoculation reticulosis
  b. mediastinal lymph node hyperplasia
  b. monoclonal gammopathy (BMG)
  b. myalgic encephalomyelitis
  b. paroxysmal peritonitis
  b. paroxysmal positional vertigo (BPPV)
  b. paroxysmal postural vertigo
  b. positional vertigo (BPV)
  b. prostatic hyperplasia (BPH)
  b. prostatic hypertrophy (BPH)
  b. proteinuria
  b. recurrent intrahepatic cholestasis
  b. senescence
  b. senescent forgetfulness
  b. stupor
  b. syphilis
  b. tertian malaria
benigna
  variola b.
benignancy
  humoral hypercalcemia of b.
Bennett
  B. disease
  B. leukemia
Benson disease
Bentyl

NOTES

Benzagel
Benzamycin
benzathine
    penicillin b.
    b. penicillin
benzimidazole
benzodiazepine toxicity
benzothiazepine
benzoylecgonine
benzoyl peroxide
benztropine
bepridil
Beradinelli syndrome
Bérard aneurysm
bereaved
bereavement
Berg
    B. Balance Assessment
    B. balance test
Berger
    B. disease
    B. focal glomerulonephritis
beriberi
    infantile b.
    ship b.
Berkow formula
Bernard-Homer syndrome
Bernard-Sergent syndrome
Bernard-Soulier syndrome
Bernoulli law
Bernstein test
Berocca Plus tabs
berry aneurysm
berylliosis
beryllium
    b. disease
    b. granulomatosis
    b. sarcoidosis
Besnier-Boeck disease
beta
    b. 1, 2 activity
    b. agonist
    b. blockade
    b. blocker
    b. cell dysfunction
    b. hCG screen
    b. islet cell
    recombinant interferon b.
    b. thalassemia minor
    transforming growth factor b.
      (TGF-beta)
beta-2
    B.-2 adrenergic agonist
    B.-2 antagonist bronchodilator
beta-adrenergic
    b.-a. antagonist
    b.-a. antagonist toxicity
    b.-a. blocker
    b.-a. stimulation

beta-agonist
    long-acting inhaled b.-a.
beta-allopregnanediol
beta-aminoisobutyric aciduria
beta-amyloid precursor protein gene on
    chromosome 21
beta-blocker
beta-blocking agent
beta-cell
beta-corticotropin
beta-cortol
beta-cortolone
betacyaninuria
Betadine
Betagen Liquifilm
beta-hemolytic streptococcal infection
beta-human chorionic gonadotropin
    subunit
beta-lactam
    b.-l. antibiotic
    b.-l. monotherapy
    b.-l. sensitivity
beta-lactamase inhibitor
betamethasone valerate cream
Betapace
beta-thalassemia
betaxolol
bethanechol
Bethesda guidelines
Betoptic
better
    B. Hearing Institute
    B. Vision Institute (BVI)
Beverly Foundation
bezoar
Bezold abscess
bFGF
    basic fibroblast growth factor
bias
    lead-time b.
    length b.
    potential b.
    referral filter b.
    selection b.
Biaxin
bibasilar
    b. dullness
    b. rale
bibrachial paresis
bicarbonate
    b. therapy
biceps
bicho
Bicillin IM
bicipital
Bickerstaff migraine
bicornuate
bicuspid aortic valve

b.i.d.
    bis in die
    twice a day [L. *bis in die*]
bidet
bidirectional Glenn shunt
BIDS
    bedtime insulin, daytime sulfonylurea
    brittle hair, impaired intelligence,
      decreased fertility, short stature
biduous
Biederman sign
Bielschowsky disease
Biermer
    B. anemia
    B. disease
Biermer-Ehrlich anemia
Biernacki sign
Bier passive hyperemia
bifascicular block
bifid
bifida
    spina b.
bifrontal
bifurcation
big ACTH
bigeminy
biguanide
biiliac bypass
bilateral
    b. ankle edema
    b. foraminal stenosis
    b. Glenn shunt
    b. infiltrates
    b. lateral
    b. leg edema
    b. lung transplant
    b. pleurisy
    b. salpingo-oophorectomy (BSO)
    b., symmetrical, equal (BSE)
    b. tubal ligation (BTL)
    b. vestibular loss
bilayered
    b. membrane
    b. micelle
bile
    A b.
    b. acid
    b. acid deficiency
    b. acid secretory diarrhea
    b. acid sequestrant
    b. acid sequestrant resin
    B b.

C b.
    b. duct obstruction
    b. salt
    b. sequestrant
    white b.
bilevel positive airway pressure (BiPAP)
bilharzial
    b. dysentery
bilharzial appendicitis
bilharziasis
bilharzioma
bilharziosis
biliary
    b. atresia
    b. cirrhosis
    b. colic
    b. fistula
    b. leak
    b. pancreatitis
    b. radicle
    b. sludge
    b. steatorrhea
    b. stricture
    b. tract disease
    b. tree
    b. xanthomatosis
biliary-enteric anastomosis
bilifaction
biliferous
biligenesis
biligenic
bilingual
bilious
    b. cholera
    b. pneumonia
    b. remittent fever
    b. remittent malaria
    b. typhoid
    b. typhoid of Griesinger
    b. vomit
biliousness
biliptysis
bilirachia
bilirubin
    conjugated b.
    b. icterus
    minimum concentration of b.
      (MCBR)
    total b.
bilitherapy
biliuria

B

NOTES

Billroth
  B. disease
  B. II gastrojejunostomy
biloba
  Ginkgo b.
bilobar transplant
biloculare
  core b.
bimanual
  b. palpation
  b. percussion
binaural stethoscope
binder
  abdominal b.
binge eating disorder
bingeing and purging
Bing-Neel syndrome
binocular diplopia
Binswanger
  B. dementia
  B. disease
bioavailability
biochemistry
bioecology
bioelectric impedance analysis
bioengineering
biofeedback
biogerontology
bioimmunotherapy
biological function
biology
  vascular b.
biomarker
biomass
biome
biomechanics
biomedical engineering
biomolecular mechanism
bion
bionomics
bionomy
Bion Tears
biopsy
  bone marrow b.
  closed pleural b.
  CT-guided b.
  endomyocardial b.
  excisional b.
  fine-needle b.
  gastrointestinal b.
  guided needle b.
  liver b.
  lung b.
  lymph node b.
  needle aspiration lung b.
  open lung b.
  percutaneous liver b.
  percutaneous needle aspiration b.
    (PNAB)

  pleural b.
  renal b.
  shave excisional b.
  thoracoscopic b.
  transthoracic needle b.
  upper gastrointestinal b.
  video-assisted thoracoscopic b.
biopsychosocial
biopsy-proven diagnosis
Bioptic
  B. spectacle-mounted telescope for
    driving
  B. telescope
bioptome
biosis
biosphere
biostatistics
biosystem
Biot
  B. breathing
  B. breathing sign
biotic
biotics
biotinidase
biotransformation
Biotronik pacemaker
BiPAP
  bilevel positive airway pressure
bipartite
bipolar
bird
  B. sign
  thermal b.
bird-breeder's
  b.-b. disease
  b.-b. lung
bird-fancier's lung
birminghamensis
  Legionella b.
birth
  b. control pill
  date of b. (DOB)
  zero stool since b. (ZSB)
birthmark
  port-wine stain b.
bisacodyl
bisalbuminemia
bischloroethylnitrosourea (BCNU)
bis in die (b.i.d.)
  twice a day [L. *bis in die*]
bisferiens
bishop's nod
Biskra boil
bismuth
  b. line
  milk of b.
  b. stomatitis
bisoprolol
bisphosphonate

bite
> cat b.
> crotaline snake b.
> dog b.
> groundhog b.
> human b.
> insect b.
> lizard b.
> snake b.
> spider b.
> tick b.

bitemporal
Bitot spot
bitter
> b. melon
> b. tonic

Bittorf reaction
bivariate analysis
bizarre behavior
Bjerrum scotoma
Bjork-Shiley valve
BKA
> below-knee amputation

black
> b. death
> b. fever
> b. hairy tongue
> b. lung
> b. measles
> b. pigment gallstone
> b. plague
> b. sickness
> b. stone
> b., tarry stool
> b. vomit

Blackfan-Diamond
> B.-D. anemia
> B.-D. syndrome

blackout
> alcoholic b.

blackwater fever
bladder
> atonic b.
> b. cancer
> b. capacity
> b. exstrophy
> b. infection
> kidneys, ureters, b. (KUB)
> malignant neoplasm of b.
> neurogenic b.
> b. outlet obstruction
> overactive b.

> poorly contractile b.
> b. relaxant therapy
> b. schistosomiasis
> b. training
> urinary b.

Blalock-Taussig
> classic B.-T.
> modified B.-T.
> B.-T. procedure

bland
> b. diet
> b. necrosis

blanket
> hypothermic b.

blast
> b. cell
> b. cell leukemia
> b. chest
> b. crisis
> b. effect
> lung b.

blastic leukemia
blastocyst
Blastocystis hominis
Blastomyces dermatitidis **infection**
blastomycosis
> Brazilian b.
> cutaneous b.
> North American b.
> South American b.
> systemic b.

Blatin syndrome
bleb
> apical b.
> emphysematous b.

bleeder
bleeding
> abnormal uterine b.
> acute lower gastrointestinal b.
> acute upper gastrointestinal b.
> anovulatory b.
> b. disorder
> diverticular b.
> dysfunctional uterine b. (DUB)
> gastrointestinal b.
> lower gastrointestinal b.
> nonvariceal b.
> occult gastrointestinal b.
> ovulatory b.
> postmenopausal b.
> puberty and anovulatory b.
> upper gastrointestinal b.

NOTES

B

bleeding *(continued)*
    uremic b.
    uterine b.
    vaginal b.
    variceal b.
blennemesis
blennorrhagic
blennorrhagicum, pl. **blennorrhagica**
    keratoderma blennorrhagica
    keratosis blennorrhagica
blennorrhea
blennorrheal
blennostasis
blennostatic
bleomycin
Blephamide
blepharitis
    seborrheic b.
blepharophimosis
blepharoplasty
blepharoptosis
blepharospasm
Blessed Dementia Rating Scale
blind
    American Council of the B.
      (ACB)
    American Foundation for the B.
      (AFB)
    b. enema
    b. loop syndrome
blindness
    night b.
    transient monocular b.
blink test reflex
blister
    burn b.
    fever b.
bloat
bloater
    blue b.
bloating
Blocadren
block
    alveolocapillary b.
    atrioventricular b.
    atrioventricular Wenckebach b.
    AV b.
    bifascicular b.
    bundle-branch b.
    b. dissection
    first-degree atrioventricular b.
    heart b.
    incomplete bundle-branch b.
    left anterior divisional b.
    left bundle-branch b. (LBBB)
    left posterior divisional b.
    Mobitz type I, II b.
    nerve b.
    b. resection

    right bundle-branch b. (RBBB)
    SA exit b.
    second-degree atrioventricular b.
    sinoatrial exit b.
    sympathetic b.
    third-degree atrioventricular b.
    Wenckebach b.
    Wolff-Chaikoff b.
blockade
    adrenergic b.
    beta b.
    lumbar sympathetic b.
    neuromuscular b.
    stellate ganglion b.
blocked aerogastria
blocker
    alpha b.
    alpha-adrenergic b.
    alpha-adrenoceptor b.
    angiotensin II receptor b. (ARB)
    beta b.
    beta-adrenergic b.
    calcium channel b. (CCB)
    H_2 b.
    histamine-2 b.
    nondihydropyridine calcium
      channel b.
    slow-channel b.
    starch b.
    t-type calcium channel b.
blood
    b. acetylcholine receptor antibody
      level
    b. alcohol content (BAC)
    b. chemistry profile
    b. component therapy
    b. culture
    b. dyscrasia
    b. ethanol level
    b. flow
    b. flow obstruction
    b. flux
    b. gas
    b. glucose
    b. glucose meter
    b. glucose monitor
    b. glucose monitoring system
    b. infection
    b. loss
    lysed horse b.
    occult b.
    b. oxygen content
    b. poisoning
    b. pressure (BP)
    b. pressure dysregulation syndrome
    b. pressure monitor
    b. sugar (BS)
    b. test

trace occult b.
b. urea nitrogen (BUN)
blood-borne virus
bloodstream infection (BSI)
bloody diarrhea
blot
Western b.
blotting
Southern b.
Blount disease
blowing
b. diastolic murmur
b. respiration
b. systolic ejection murmur
blue
b. bloater
b. disease
b. dome cyst
eosin methylene b. (EMB)
b. fever
methylene b.
b. nevus
Pantene B.
Selsun B.
b. toe syndrome
Blumberg sign
Blumenthal
B. disease
B. lesion
blurring
visual b.
blurry vision
B-lymphocyte
BM
bowel movement
BMD
Becker muscular dystrophy
bone mineral density
BMG
benign monoclonal gammopathy
BMI
body mass index
BMP
basic metabolic profile
BMR
basal metabolic rate
BMU
basic multicellular unit
BNMSE
Brief Neuropsychological Mental Status
Examination
board certified

Boas-Oppler bacillus
bobbing
ocular b.
Bock
B. ganglion
B. nerve
Bodian-Schwachman syndrome
body
b. adipose tissue
Bence Jones b.
b. fat
b. fluid
Heinz b.
b. image
Jaworski b.
ketone b. (KB)
Lewy b.
loose b.
Mallory b.
b. mass
b. mass index (BMI)
Pick b.
Purkinje cell b.
Schaumann b.
b. sway
vertebral b.
b. weight
Boeck
B. sarcoid
B. sarcoid disease
B. sarcoidosis
Boerhaave syndrome
Bohler angle
Bohn nodule
Bohr
B. effect
B. equation
boil
Biskra b.
bois
bruit de b.
Bolivian
B. hemorrhagic fever
B. hemorrhagic fever virus
Bolognini symptom
bolus
intravenous b.
bone
b. ache
cortical b.
b. cyst
b. disease

NOTES

bone *(continued)*
    b. island
    jugal b.
    b. lesion
    lunate b.
    malignant neoplasm of b.
    b. marrow biopsy
    b. marrow metastasis
    b. marrow suppression
    b. marrow transplant
    b. marrow transplant-associated
      nephropathy
    b. marrow transplantation
    b. mass measurement
    b. mineral densitometry
    b. mineral density (BMD)
    b. mineral density study
    b. necrosis
    Paget disease of b.
    b. pain
    b. remodeling
    b. resorption
    b. scan
    subchondral b.
    trabecular b.
    b. turnover
    wormian b.
bone-specific protein
Bonfiglio graft
Bonnevie-Ullrich syndrome
Bonnot gland
bony deformity
boomer
    baby b.
Boost
booster
    b. dose
    Td b.
boot
    Gibney b.
    Unna b.
borage
borborygmus, pl. **borborygmi**
border
    sternal heart b.
borderline case
Bordetella
    B. infection
    B. pertussis
borism
Börjeson-Forssman-Lehmann syndrome
Bornholm disease
Borrelia burgdorferi
bosselated
Boston sign
both eyes
Botox
botryoid

botulinum
    b. a
    b. antitoxin
    b. toxin
    b. toxin injection
botulism
boubas
Bouchard
    B. disease
    B. node
    B. nodule
    B. sign
bougie
Bouillaud
    B. disease
    B. syndrome
boulimia (*var. of* bulimia)
boundary
    tracing b.
bouquet fever
bouton en chemise
boutonneuse
    b. fever
    fièvre b.
Bovie cautery
bovine pericardial strip reinforcement
bovis
    Streptococcus b.
bowel
    b. bypass syndrome
    b. disease
    b. irrigation
    irritable b.
    b. movement (BM)
    b. obstruction
    b. resection
    b. sound
Bowen disease
Bowles type stethoscope
Bowman
    capsule of B.
    B. membrane
bowstring sign
Boyd communicating perforation vein
Boyden meal
Bozzolo sign
BP
    bacillary peliosis
    blood pressure
BPH
    benign prostatic hyperplasia
    benign prostatic hypertrophy
    clinical BPH
    macroscopic BPH
    microscopic BPH
BPPV
    benign paroxysmal positional vertigo
BpTRU blood pressure monitor

B

BPV
benign positional vertigo
brace
Air stirrup b.
Cheetah ankle b.
neoprene b.
polypropylene b.
brachial
b. approach
b. plexopathy
b. plexus
b. plexus neuritis
brachiocephalic
b. arteritis
b. vein
brachioplexus
brachioradialis
brachium
brachycephalic
brachyolmia
brachytherapy
Bradburn Affect Balance Scale
Bradley disease
bradyarrhythmia
bradycardia
postinfectious b.
sinus b.
bradykinesia
bradykinetic
bradykinin
bradypepsia
bradyphagia
bradypnea
bradyspermatism
bradystalsis
bradyuria
Brailsford-Morquio disease
brain
b. abscess
b. attack
b. damage
b. death
b. herniation
b. injury
b. metastasis
b. tumor
brainstem
b. auditory evoked response (BAER)
b. evoked response (BSER)
b. stroke

branch
b. retinal artery occlusion (BRAO)
b. retinal vein occlusion (BRVO)
branched
b. chain acid
b. chain ketoaciduria
b. chain ketonuria
brancher
b. deficiency glycogenosis
b. glycogen storage disease
Branhamella catarrhalis
BRAO
branch retinal artery occlusion
brash
water b.
brass
b. founder's ague
b. founder's fever
BRAT
bananas, rice, applesauce, toast
bananas, rice cereal, applesauce, toast
BRAT diet
BRATT
bananas, rice, applesauce, toast, tea
BRATT diet
brawny
b. edema
b. induration
Braxen
Brazilian
B. blastomycosis
B. hemorrhagic fever
B. purpuric fever
B. spotted fever
breakaway
breakbone fever
breakdown
nervous b.
breast
b. abscess
b. anemia
b. cancer
b. cancer and pregnancy
b. mass
b. self-examination (BSE)
b. thickening
breast-conserving surgery
breastfeeding
b. and seizure
breath
liver b.
shortness of b. (SOB)

NOTES

breath *(continued)*
    b. testing
    uremic b.
breathe
breathing
    apneustic b.
    asynchronous b.
    ataxic b.
    autonomous b.
    Biot b.
    bronchial b.
    b. cessation
    Cheyne-Stokes b.
    diaphragmatic b.
    b. exercise
    frog b.
    glossopharyngeal b.
    intermittent positive-pressure b. (IPPB)
    Kussmaul b.
    labored b.
    pursed-lip b.
    shallow b.
    sleep-disordered b.
    stertorous b.
    suppressed b.
    vesicular b.
Breda disease
Brehmer
    B. method
    B. treatment
Brennemann syndrome
Brescio-Cimino arteriovenous fistula
Breslow thickness
Brethaire inhaler
Brethine
Bretonneau
    B. disease
Bretonneau angina
brevicollis
    dystrophia b.
Brevicon
brevis
    peroneus b.
    pollicis longus b.
BRFSS
    Behavioral Risk Factor Surveillance System
Bricanyl
brickmaker's anemia
Brief Neuropsychological Mental Status Examination (BNMSE)
Brill disease
Brill-Symmers disease
Brill-Zinsser disease
brimstone liver
Brinton disease
Brion-Kayser disease

Briquet hysteria
brisk capillary refill
Brissaud infantilism
Bristow procedure
brittle
    b. diabetes
    b. hair, impaired intelligence, decreased fertility, short stature (BIDS)
Broadbent apoplexy
broad-beta proteinemia
broad-spectrum antibiotic
Broca
    B. aphasia
Brock syndrome
Brodie abscess
Bromfed
bromide
    ipratropium b.
    propantheline b.
    rocuronium b.
bromism
bromocriptine
    b. mesylate
    b. suppression test
brompheniramine
bromsulfophthalein (BSP)
bromsulphalein test
bronchi *(pl. of* bronchus)
bronchial
    b. asthma
    b. breathing
    b. fremitus
    b. obstruction
    b. pneumonia
    b. respiration
    b. voice
bronchiectasis
    nodular b.
bronchiloquy
bronchiolitis
    exudative b.
    b. fibrosa obliterans
    b. obliterans organizing pneumonia
    obliterative b.
    proliferative b.
bronchitic asthma
bronchitis
    acute b.
    asthmatic b.
    Castellani b.
    chronic b.
    croupous b.
    fibrinous b.
    hemorrhagic b.
    industrial b.
    obliterative b.
    plastic b.

B

pseudomembranous b.
putrid b.
bronchoalveolar lavage (BAL)
bronchocentric granulomatosis
bronchodilator
beta-2 antagonist b.
broncholithiasis
bronchomycosis
bronchophony
whispered b.
bronchopleural fistula
bronchopneumonia
postoperative b.
tuberculous b.
bronchoprovocation
bronchopulmonary
b. aspergillosis
b. spirochetosis
bronchorrhea
bronchoscope
bronchoscopy
fiberoptic b.
fluorescent b.
bronchospasm
bronchospastic
b. disease
b. reflex cough
bronchospirochetosis
bronchovesicular respiration
bronchus, pl. **bronchi**
malignant neoplasm of b.
mucoid impaction of b.
pig b.
Bronkaid mist
Bronkosol
Brontex
bronzed
b. disease
b. skin
bronze diabetes
Brookdale
B. Center on Aging (BCOA)
B. Center on Aging of Hunter
College
broth
B. dilution test
b. microdilution
brown
b. lung
b. pigment gallstone
b. stone
Brown-Seéquard syndrome

Brucella
B. melitensis
B. suis
brucellosis
Bruce protocol
Brudzinski sign
Brugada syndrome
Brug filariasis
Brugia
B. malayi
B. malayi infection
B. timori infection
bruisability
bruissement
bruit
asymptomatic carotid b.
carotid b.
cranial b.
b. d'airain
b. de bois
b. de canon
b. de choc
b. de clapotement
b. de claquement
b. de cuir neuf
b. de diable
b. de drapeau
b. de froissement
b. de frôlement
b. de frottement
b. de galop
b. de grelot
b. de la roue de moulin
b. de Leudet
b. de lime
b. de parchemin
b. de piaulement
b. de pot fété
b. de rappel
b. de Roger
b. de scie
b. de scie ou de rape
b. de soufflet
b. de tabourka
b. de tambour
b. de triolet
epigastric b.
full and equal without b.'s
intracranial b.
Leudet b.
musical b.
Roger b.

NOTES

bruit *(continued)*
    seagull b.
    b. skodique
    thyroid b.
    Traube b.
    Verstraeten b.
Brunner gland
brush
    b. burn
    protected specimen b. (PSB)
Bruton
    B. agammaglobulinemia
    B. disease
bruxism
BRVO
    branch retinal vein occlusion
BS
    blood sugar
BSE
    bilateral, symmetrical, equal
    breast self-examination
BSER
    brainstem evoked response
BSI
    bloodstream infection
BSO
    bilateral salpingo-oophorectomy
BSP
    bromsulfophthalein
BTL
    bilateral tubal ligation
buaki
buba madre
bubas
bubbling rale
bubo
    bullet b.
    chancroidal b.
    indolent b.
    malignant b.
    parotid b.
    primary b.
    tropical b.
    venereal b.
    virulent b.
bubonalgia
bubonica
    pestis b.
bubonic plague
buccal
    b. aspect
    b. mucosa
buccofacial
Budd
    B. cirrhosis
    B. syndrome
Budd-Chiari
    B.-C. disease
    B.-C. syndrome

buddy taped
budesonide
Buerger
    B. disease
    B. exercise
    B. symptom
buffalo
    b. hump
    b. type
buffering
    meal-related b.
buffy coat
buflomedil
Buf-puf
building-related illness
bulb
    duodenal b.
    b. ulceration
bulbar poliomyelitis
bulbocavernosus
    b. muscle
    b. reflex
bulimia, boulimia
    b. nervosa
bulimic
bulking agent
bulk laxative
bulla, pl. **bullae**
bullet bubo
bull neck
bullosa
    epidermolysis b.
bullosis diabeticorum
bullous
    b. dermatosis
    b. pemphigoid
bumetanide
Bumex
bump
    pump b.
    razor b.'s
BUN
    blood urea nitrogen
bundle
    b.-branch block
    b.-branch reentrant ventricular
    tachycardia
    b. of His
Bunge amputation
bungpagga
bunion deformity
bunionette
Bunyamwera fever
bunyavirus
Buprenex
buprenorphine
bupropion
burden
    pill b.

selenium b.'s
tumor b.
Burdwan fever
bureau
    Census B.
    Council of Better Business B.'s
    (CBBB)
burgdorferi
    Borrelia b.
Bürger-Grütz
    B.-G. disease
    B.-G. syndrome
Burkitt
    B. lymphoma
    B. tumor
Burkitt-type acute lymphoblastic leukemia
burn
    b. blister
    brush b.
    chemical b.
    first-degree b.
    flash b.
    fourth-degree b.
    full-thickness b.
    high-tension b.
    immersion b.
    b. infection
    ocular chemical b.
    partial-thickness b.
    powder b.
    radiation b.
    second-degree b.
    b. shock
    thermal b.
    third-degree b.
Burnett syndrome
burning drops sign
burnout
bursitis
    Achilles b.
    deep b.
    iliopsoas b.
    b. infrapatellar
    intracalcaneal b.

ischiogluteal b.
pes anserinus b.
prepatellar b.
retrocalcaneal b.
septic b.
subcutaneous b.
trochanteric b.
burst
    prednisone b.
    b. of therapy
Burton sign
Buschke disease
BuSpar
buspirone HCl
Busse-Buschke disease
busulfan
butalbital
butanol-extractable
    b.-e. iodine (BEI)
    b.-e. iodine test
Butazolidin
Butisol
butschlii
    Iodamoeba b.
butterfly rash
butter stool
button
    Jaboulay b.
    Pudenz b.
buttonholer
BV
    bacterial vaginosis
BVI
    Better Vision Institute
Bwamba fever
Byler disease
bypass
    aortocoronary b.
    biiliac b.
    femoral-femoral b.
    ileojejunal b.
    iliofemoral b.
byssinosis
bystander killing

NOTES

C
Celsius
    C bile
    C peptide
    C peptide level
    C peptide suppression test
CA
    cancer
        scirrhous CA
CA-125
cabbage goiter
cabergoline
CABG
    coronary artery bypass graft
    coronary artery bypass grafting
        CABG surgery
CAC
    coronary artery calcification
cachectic
        c. diarrhea
        c. edema
        c. fever
        c. pallor
cachectica
        purpura c.
cachexia
        addisonian c.
        amyotrophic c.
        c. aphthosa
        cancer c.
        cardiac c.
        exophthalmica c.
        fluoric c.
        Grawitz c.
        hypophyseal c.
        c. hypophyseopriva
        hypophysial c.
        hypothalamic pituitary c.
        malarial c.
        neurogenic c.
        pituitary c.
        c. strumipriva
        c. thyroidea
        c. thyropriva
cacoethes
cacosmia
CAD
    coronary artery disease
        CAD mortality
CADASIL
    cerebral autosomal dominant arteriopathy
        with subcortical infarct
cadaver
cadaveric
cadaverous

cadmium exposure
caduceus
café
        c. au lait spot
        c. coronary
Cafergot
caffeine
        c., alcohol, pepper, spicy foods
            (CAPS)
        c., alcohol, pepper, spicy foods-free
            diet
        nocturnal c.
        c. use
caffeinism
CAGE
        cut down (on drinking), annoyance, guilt
            (about drinking), (need for) eyeopener
        CAGE test
CAH
        chronic active hepatitis
CAHC
        chronic active hepatitis with cirrhosis
Cairns stupor
caisson
        c. disease
        c. sickness
Caladryl lotion
calamine lotion
Calan SR
calcaneal area
calcaneus area
calcar
calcareous pancreatitis
calcemia
calcifames
        status c.
Calciferol tablets
calcific
        c. pancreatitis
        c. tendinitis
        c. uremic arteriopathy
calcific aortic stenosis
calcification
        annular c.
        cardiac c.
        coronary artery c. (CAC)
        mitral annular c.
        mitral annulus c. (MAC)
        perihilar c.
        pineal c.
        subcutaneous c.
calcifying pancreatitis
Calcijex
Calcimar
calcineurin inhibitor

C

calcinosis
    c. cutis, Raynaud phenomenon,
       esophageal
       dysfunction/hypermotility,
       sclerodactyly, telangiectasia
       syndrome
    c. interstitialis
    c., Raynaud phenomenon,
       esophageal motility disorders,
       sclerodactyly, telangiectasia
       (CREST)
    reversible c.
    c. universalis
calcinuric diabetes
calciostat
calcipectic
calcipenia
calcipenic
calciphylaxis
calcipotriene
calciprivia
calciprivic
calcis
    os c.
calcitonin
    intranasal c.
calcitriol
calcium
    c. apatite stone
    atorvastatin c.
    c. balance
    c. carbonate
    c. channel antagonist
    c. channel antagonist toxicity
    c. channel blocker (CCB)
    c. citrate
    c. deficiency
    flecks of c.
    c. gout
    ionized PTH c.
    c. oxalate
    c. polycarbophil
    c. pyrophosphate dehydrate
       deposition disease
    c. pyrophosphate deposition disease
       (CPPDD)
    c. pyrophosphate dihydrate (CPPD)
    c. salt
    c. supplementation
calculus, pl. calculi
    metabolic c.
    renal c.
    salivary gland c.
    staghorn c.
calefacient
calf vein thrombosis
calibrated aneroid manometer
calicectasis
calices (*pl. of* calix)

California flea rickettsiosis
caliper
    skin c.
calisthenics
calix, pl. **calices**
Callander amputation
callosity
callus
Calmette-Guérin
    bacille C.-G. (BCG)
    C.-G. vaccine
Calm-X
calor
    c. febrilis
    c. fervens
    c. innatus
    c. internus
caloric
    c. intake
    c. restriction
calorie
Caltrate
calvaria
calvarium
calyceal
CAM
    Confusion Assessment Method
    CAM Diagnostic Algorithm
cambogia
    Garcinia c.
Camden amputation
cameloid anemia
Cameron
    C. erosion
    C. lesion
Camitz transfer
CAMP
    Christie-Atkins-Munch-Petersen
    CAMP test
camp
    c. fever
    c. hospital
campath
camptodactyly
Campylobacter
    C. enteritis
    C. fetus infection
    C. infection
    C. jejuni
canal
    complete atrioventricular c.
    Hunter c.
    neural foraminal c.
    c. paresis
    Stensen c.
canalicular membrane
canalization
cancer (CA)
    acinous c.

adrenocortical c.
anal c.
bladder c.
breast c.
c. cachexia
C-cell c.
cervical c.
colon c.
colorectal c.
c. diagnosis
early-stage breast c.
endometrial c.
esophageal c.
follicular c.
gallbladder c.
gastric c.
gastrointestinal c.
genital tract c.
genitourinary c.
head and neck c.
hereditary medullary thyroid c.
hereditary nonpolyposis colorectal c.
  (HNPCC)
inflammatory breast c.
lower urinary tract c.
lung c.
male breast c.
medullary thyroid c.
metastatic breast c.
metastatic colon c.
metastatic lung c.
metastatic prostate c.
nasopharyngeal c.
nonpolyposis colorectal c.
non-small-cell lung c. (NSCLC)
oral c.
ovarian c.
c. pain
pancreatic c.
prostate c.
rectal c.
regional c.
c. registry
renal cell c.
skin c.
small-cell lung c. (SCLC)
sporadic medullary thyroid c.
stage III lung c.
stage I–IV breast c.
c. staging
terminal c.
testicular c.

c. therapy
thyroid c.
ureter c.
urinary tract c.
uterine c.
vagina c.
villous duct c.
vulva c.
c. with unknown primary site
cancer-associated anemia
cancrum oris
candesartan cilexetil
Candida
    C. albicans
    C. esophagitis
candidal
    c. endocarditis
    c. pharyngitis
    c. pneumonia
    c. vulvovaginitis
***Candida*-related complex**
candidemia
    catheter-related c.
candidiasis
    cerebral c.
    disseminated c.
    esophageal c.
    gastrointestinal c.
    hepatosplenic c.
    mucocutaneous c.
    oral c.
    oropharyngeal c.
    perineal c.
    pharyngeal c.
    vulvovaginal c.
candidosis
CANE
    Clearinghouse on Abuse and Neglect of
    the Elderly
cane
    quad c.
    straight c.
canicola fever
canis
    Toxocara c.
canker
    water c.
cannabinoid
cannabism
cannabis sativa
Cannon
    C. law

NOTES

Cannon *(continued)*
    C. syndrome
    C. theory
cannula
cannulation
    cricothyroid needle c.
canon
    bruit de c.
Cantelli sign
cantharidin
Cantil
CAP
    community-acquired pneumonia
cap
    cradle c.
    phrygian c.
capacity
    bladder c.
    cognitive c.
    decision-making c.
    exercise c.
    forced vital c. (FVC)
    functional c.
    iron-binding c. (IBC)
    proliferative c.
    reduced c.
    total iron-binding c. (TIBC)
    total lung c. (TLC)
    vital c.
CAPD
    continuous ambulatory peritoneal dialysis
Capener splint
capillariasis
    intestinal c.
capillaritis
capillaropathy
capillary
    c. fragility test
    c. refill
    c. refill time
    c. resistance test
capita (*pl. of* caput)
capitated health plan
capitation
capitellum
capitis
    tinea c.
Capitrol shampoo
Caplan
    C. nodule
    C. syndrome
Capoten
Capozide
Capps reflex
capriloquism
CAPS
    caffeine, alcohol, pepper, spicy foods
    carbamoyl phosphate synthetase

    Children of Aging Parents
    CAPS deficiency
    CAPS diet
caps
    Pavabid c.
capsaicin
CAPS-free diet
capsid antigen
capsomere
capsular
    c. cirrhosis
    c. cirrhosis of liver
    c. distention
capsule
    c. of Bowman
    Carey c.
    Glisson c.
    radiotelemetering c.
capsulitis
    adhesive c.
captioned media program (CMP)
captopril
    C. Prevention Project
caput, pl. **capita**
    c. medusae
    c. quadratum
Carafate
carbachol
carbamazepine
carbamide peroxide
carbamoyl
    c. phosphate synthetase (CAPS)
    c. phosphate synthetase deficiency
carbapenem antibiotic
carbenicillin indanyl sodium
Carbex
carbidopa
Carbocaine
carbohydrate-induced hyperlipemia
carbohydrate metabolism disorder
carbon
    c. dioxide (CO_2)
    c. dioxide acidosis
    c. dioxide alkalosis
    c. dioxide laser treatment
    c. disulfide poisoning
    c. monoxide inhalation
    c. monoxide poisoning
    c. monoxide pressure
    c. monoxide tension
carbonate
    calcium c.
    lithium c.
carbonic
    c. anhydrase II deficiency
    c. anhydrase inhibitor
carboplatin
carboxyhemoglobin

carbuncle
    renal c.
carcinoembryonic antigen (CEA)
carcinogenesis
carcinoid
    c. flush
    c. syndrome
carcinoma
    acinic cell c.
    acinous c.
    anaplastic thyroid c.
    basal cell c.
    cervical c.
    ductal c.
    esophageal c.
    follicular thyroid c.
    hepatocellular c.
    Hürthle cell c.
    infiltrating c.
    infiltrative ductal c.
    laryngeal c.
    lobular c.
    medullary thyroid c.
    oat cell c.
    papillary thyroid c.
    c. in situ (CIS)
    squamous cell c. (SCC)
    undifferentiated large-cell c.
carcinomatous
    c. meningitis
    c. neuropathy
Cardene
cardia
    gastric c.
    c. malposition
cardiac
    c. ablation
    c. amyloid
    c. angiosarcoma
    c. arrhythmia
    c. asthma
    c. cachexia
    c. calcification
    c. catheterization
    c. chest pain
    c. complication
    c. conduction effect
    c. conduction prolongation
    c. denervation syndrome
    c. dropsy
    c. dyspnea
    c. enzyme

    c. evaluation
    c. fibroma
    c. fibrosarcoma
    c. hemangioma
    c. hormone
    c. index (CI)
    c. infarction
    c. ischemia
    c. leiomyosarcoma
    c. lipoma
    c. myxoma
    c. output (CO)
    c. paraganglion
    c. pump failure
    c. pump function
    c. rehabilitation
    c. rhabdomyoma
    c. rhabdomyosarcoma
    c. risk factor (CRF)
    c. rupture
    c. shock
    c. surgery
    c. tamponade
    c. thrombosis
    c. toxicity
    c. transplantation
    c. tumor
    c. valve
    c. vegetation
    c. vertigo
cardiac-specific troponin
cardialgia
cardinal
    c. sign
    c. sign of inflammation
    c. symptom
CardioBeeper CB-12L cardiac monitor
cardioembolic
    c. event
    c. stroke
cardioesophageal relaxation
cardiofacial syndrome
cardiogenic
    c. embolus
    c. pulmonary edema
    c. shock
cardiography
    echo-Doppler c.
cardiohepatic
    c. angle
    c. triangle
cardiolipin

C

NOTES

Cardiolite
cardiologist
cardiology
  interventional c.
cardiomegaly
  glycogen c.
  glycogenic c.
cardiomyopathy
  alcoholic c.
  anthracycline c.
  arrhythmogenic right ventricular c.
  autosomal dominant c.
  dilated c.
  familial dilated c.
  hypertensive hypertrophic c.
  hypertrophic obstructive c.
  hypotrophic c.
  idiopathic dilated c.
  mitochondrial c.
  obstructive c.
  postinfarction c.
  restrictive c.
  right ventricular c.
  ventricular c.
  X-linked c.
cardiomyoplasty
cardiopaludism
cardioprotective effect
cardiopulmonary resuscitation (CPR)
Cardioquin
cardiorespiratory
cardiospasm
cardiothyrotoxicosis
cardiotoxica
  myolysis c.
cardiotoxicity
cardiovascular
  c. accident (CVA)
  c. adaptation
  c. autonomic neuropathy
  c. disease
  c. drug
  c. failure
  c. faintness
  c. morbidity
  c. mortality
  c. organ transplant complication
  c. rehabilitation
  c. risk status
  c. syphilis
  c. system
  c. toxicity
  c. vertigo
cardiovasculorenal
cardioversion
cardioverter
cardioverter-defibrillator
  automatic implantable c.-d. (AICD)

  automatic internal c.-d.
  implantable c.-d. (ICD)
Cardizem
Cardura
CARE
  Cholesterol and Recurrent Events
  CARE trial
care
  aggressive c.
  all-inclusive c.
  ambulatory c.
  collaborative c.
  complex c.
  comprehensive medical c.
  critical c.
  cure-oriented c.
  custodial c.
  daily nursing c.
  end-of-life c.
  extended c.
  geriatric acute c.
  health c.
  hospice c.
  intensive therapeutic c.
  long-term c.
  managed c.
  medical c.
  National Association for Home C.
    (NAHC)
  National Resource Center Diversity
    and Long-Term C. (NRCDLTC)
  nursing c.
  oral health c.
  palliative c.
  c. planning
  post acute c.
  post resuscitation c.
  post resuscitative c.
  primary medical c.
  psychosocial c.
  residential c.
  respite c.
  restorative c.
  secondary medical c.
  c. services
  short-term institutional respite c.
  skilled c.
  step c.
  step-down c.
  stratified c.
  subacute c.
  tertiary medical c.
  urgent c.
caregiver
  designated c.
  in-home c.
  primary c.
Carey capsule
caribi

caries
>dental c.
carina, pl. carinae
caring
>Partnership for C. (PFC)
carinii
>*Pneumocystis c.*
carious
carisoprodol
carmelization
Carmex lip balm
carminative
Carmol HC
carmustine (BCNU)
Carnett sign
carnosity
Caroli disease
carotene
>serum c.
carotenemia
carotid
>c. artery
>c. bruit
>c. Doppler study
>c. endarterectomy (CEA)
>c. sinus hypersensitivity
>c. sinus syncope
>c. sinus syndrome
>c. stenosis
>c. ultrasonography
>c. ultrasound
carotodynia
carpal
>c. navicular
>c. tunnel syndrome (CTS)
Carpenter syndrome
carphologia
carphology
carpometacarpal joint
carpopedal
carpoptosis
carriage
>organism c.
carrier screening
Carrington pad
Carrión disease
CARS
>Childhood Autism Rating Scale
>Children's Affective Rating Scale
car sickness
cart
>crash c.

carteolol
cartilage
>cricoid c.
>hyaline c.
>shark c.
cartridge
>insulin c.
>Novolin PenFill c.
>PenFill insulin c.
Cartrol
caruncula, pl. carunculae
Carvallo sign
carvedilol
CAS
>chronic alcohol syndrome
Casal
>C. collar
>C. necklace
cascara
CASCSP
>Center for the Advancement of State
>Community Services Programs
case
>borderline c.
>c. control study
>c. fatality rate
>c. fatality ratio
caseous
>c. abscess
>c. lymphadenitis
>c. pneumonia
Casoni
>C. intradermal test
>C. skin test
caspase-3
casseliflavus
>*Enterococcus c.*
cassette
>susceptibility c.
Cassidy-Scholte syndrome
Cassidy syndrome
cast
>gel c.
>granular c.
>long-leg c.
>Muenster c.
>c. nephropathy
>Scotch short arm c.
>short leg c.
Castellani
>C. bronchitis
>C. disease

NOTES

C

67

Castle intrinsic factor
castration
functional c.
medical c.
casualty
CAT
computed axial tomography
catabolic state
catabolism
lean-mass c.
catabolized
Cataflam
catalyst
catamenial epilepsy
catamnesis
catamnestic
cataplectic attack
cataplexy
Catapres
Catapres TTS
cataract
age-related c.
dense c.
c. spectacle
catarmal pneumonia
catarrh
catarrhal
c. asthma
c. cholangitis
c. fever
c. gastritis
c. stomatitis
catarrhalis
Branhamella c.
herpes c.
icterus c.
catastasis
catatonia
catatonic stupor
cat-bite
c.-b. disease
c.-b. fever
cat bite
catechol
c. methyltransferase (COMT)
c. methyltransferase inhibitor
catecholamine
category
moderate c.
catharsis
cathartic salt
cathepsin-G
catheter
balloon c.
central venous c.
Cournand cardiac c.
c. fever
Fogarty c.
Foley c.

indwelling urinary c.
intraaortic balloon c. (IABC)
intraarterial c.
Nélaton c.
peripherally inserted c. (PIC)
peripherally inserted central c.
(PICC)
pigtail c.
Raaf c.
Raimondi spring c.
red rubber c.
Sheldon c.
Slinky balloon c.
spinal c.
Swan-Ganz c.
Tenckhoff c.
urinary c.
vascular c.
catheter-associated
c.-a. bacteriuria
c.-a. infection
c.-a. nosocomial septicemia
c.-a. urosepsis
catheter-directed thrombolytic therapy
catheterization
cardiac c.
celiac c.
pulmonary artery c.
self-intermittent c.
catheterize
catheter-related
c.-r. candidemia
c.-r. infection
Catholic
C. Charities USA (CCUSA)
C. Golden Age (CGA)
catholicon
cation exchange resin
cat-scratch disease (CSD)
cauda, pl. **caudae**
agitator caudae
c. equina
c. equina syndrome
caudal lobe
caudate
c. lobe
c. putamen receptor
causalgia
causal treatment
cause
chronic persistent cough of
unknown c.
constitutional c.
exciting c.
noncoronary c.
precipitating c.
predisposing c.
proximate c.

specific c.
unknown c.
cauterization
cautery
Bovie c.
CAV
croup-associated virus
cava (*pl. of* cavum)
caveat
Caverject
caverniloquy
cavernosa
corpora c.
cavernous
c. angioma
c. rale
c. resonance
c. respiration
c. rhonchus
c. sinus thrombophlebitis
c. voice
c. voice sound
cave sickness
cavitary
c. lung lesion
c. space
cavitis
cavity
nasal c.
peritoneal c.
cavum, pl. cava
inferior vena cava (IVC)
superior vena cava
vena cava
c. vergae
cavus
pes c.
Cawthorne
C. exercise
C. maneuver
CBBB
Council of Better Business Bureaus
CBC
complete blood count
CBE
clinical breast examination
CC
chief complaint
CCAC
Continuing Care Accreditation
Commission

CCB
calcium channel blocker
CCC
chronic calculous cholecystitis
C-cell
C-c. cancer
C-c. hyperplasia
CCNU
chloroethylcyclohexylnitrosourea
CCP
chronic calcifying pancreatitis
Cooperative Cardiovascular Project
CCPD
crystalline calcium pyrophosphate
dihydrate
CC-RC
continuing care retirement community
CCS
central cord syndrome
CCU
coronary care unit
critical care unit
CCUSA
Catholic Charities USA
CD4
CD4 cell
CD4 cell count
CD4 T cell
C/D
conjunctiva diagonalis
C/D ratio
CD4+ cell
CD8+ cell
CD8 T cell
CDC
Centers for Disease Control and
Prevention
CDP
computerized dynamic posturography
CEA
carcinoembryonic antigen
carotid endarterectomy
CEBV
chronic Epstein-Barr virus
Ceclor
cecum
Cedax
Ceelen-Gellerstedt syndrome
cefaclor
cefadroxil
cefazolin
cefepime

NOTES

C

Cefobid
cefoperazone
cefotaxime
cefotetan
cefoxitin
cefpodoxime proxetil
cefprozil
cefsulodin
ceftazidime
ceftibuten
Ceftin
ceftriaxone
cefuroxime
CEI
    continuous extravascular infusion
Celebrex
celecoxib
Celestone
Celexa
celiac
    c. artery aneurysm
    c. catheterization
    c. disease
    c. rickets
    c. sprue
    c. syndrome
celiagra
celiomyalgia
celiopathy
cell
    accessory c.
    Aschoff c.
    basophilic c.
    beta islet c.
    blast c.
    CD4+ c.
    CD4 c.
    CD8+ c.
    CD4 T c.
    CD8 T c.
    ciliated c.
    clue c.
    cumulus c.
    foam c.
    c. function
    c. function deficiency
    giant c.
    c. growth
    hyaline c.
    islet c.
    Leydig c.
    lymphocyte c.
    mesenchymal c.
    mesothelial c.
    microcytic red c.
    morpheaform basal c.
    mucus-secreting c.
    natural killer c.
    neuronal c.

    nondifferentiated c. (NDC)
    nonspecific effector c.
    c. number deficiency
    packed red blood c.'s (PRBC)
    Pick c.
    plasma c.
    polymorphonuclear c.
    Purkinje c.
    red blood c. (RBC)
    Reed-Sternberg c.
    c. senescence
    Sertoli c.
    sickle c.
    signet ring c.
    small c.
    spur c.
    Sternberg giant c.
    Sternberg-Reed c.
    trabecular meshwork c.
    tumor c.
    Tzanck c.
    c. volume
    white blood c. (WBC)
cell-aging theory
cell-mediated immunity
cellophane
    c. maculopathy
    c. tape test
cell-to-cell transfer
cellular
    c. differentiation
    c. humoral immunological function
    c. immunity deficiency syndrome
    c. immunodeficiency
cellulites
cellulitis
    anaerobic c.
    clostridial c.
    facial c.
    gangrenous c.
    gaseous c.
    Haemophilus influenzae type b c.
    necrotizing c.
    postadenectomy c.
    postvenectomy c.
    preseptal c.
    Pseudomonas c.
cellulose
    sodium c.
Celsius (C)
cement
    polymethylmethacrylate bone c.
Census Bureau
centenarian
center
    adult day-care c.
    C. for the Advancement of State Community Services Programs (CASCSP)

Alzheimer's Disease Education and
   Referral C.
child-care c.
day-care c.
C.'s for Disease Control and
   Prevention (CDC)
C. for Epidemiologic Studies
   Depression Scale (CES-D)
Federal Consumer Information C.
   (FCIC)
Food and Nutrition Information C.
   (FNIC)
health c.
Kansas Geriatric Education C. (KS-
   GEC)
Medicare Rights C. (MRC)
multidisciplinary pain
   management c.
National Association of Community
   Health C.'s (NACHC)
National Health Information C.
   (NHIC)
National Heart, Lungs, and Blood
   Institute Information C.
National Information and Referral
   Support C. (NIRSC)
National Long-Term Care
   Ombudsman Research C.
   (NLTCORC)
National Long-Term Care
   Research C. (NLTCRC)
National Rehabilitation
   Information C. (NARIC)
National Resource and
   Information C. (NRIC)
National Senior Citizens' Education
   and Research C. (NSCERC)
National Senior Citizens' Law C.
   (NSCLC)
National Women's Health
   Information C. (NWHIC)
Native Elder Health Care
   Resource C. (NEHCRC)
NIH Osteoporosis and Related
   Bone Diseases National
   Resource C. (NIH-ORBD-NRC)
pain management c.
Pension Rights C. (PRC)
rehabilitation c.
sacral micturition c.
sleep c.

c. for the Study of
   Aging/International Association of
   Physical Activity, Aging, and
   Sports (IAPAAS)
The C.'s for Medicare and
   Medicaid Services
The C. for Social Gerontology
   (TCSG)
centesis
centigray (cGy)
centimeter (cm)
centimeter-gram-second (CGS)
   c.-g.-s. unit
central
   c. ageusia
   c. alveolar hypoventilation
   c. cord syndrome (CCS)
   c. core disease
   c. diabetes insipidus
   c. enchondroma
   c. hypothalamic neurochemical
      pathway
   c. hypothyroidism
   c. nervous system (CNS)
   c. nervous system dysfunction
   c. nervous system infection
   c. nervous system lymphoma
   c. nervous system poisoning
   c. nervous system stimulant
   c. nervous system tumor
   c. parenteral nutrition
   c. pneumonia
   c. retinal artery occlusion (CRAO)
   c. retinal vein occlusion (CRVO)
   c. sleep apnea
   c. thecal sac
   c. venous catheter
centrally acting sympatholytic
Centrax
centriacinar emphysema
centripetal
centrocytic lymphoma
centromere
centronuclear myopathy
Centrum Silver
Cepastat
cephalad
cephalalgia, cephalgia
   Horton c.
cephalexin
cephalic
cephalization

C

NOTES

cephalopathy
cephalosporin antibiotic
cephradine
ceramidase deficiency
Ceratophyllus punjatensis
cerclage
    Shirodkar procedure c.
cerebellar
    c. ataxia
    c. ataxic
    c. degeneration
    c. disease
    c. function
    c. hemorrhage
cerebellopontine
cerebral
    c. amyloid angiopathy
    c. anemia
    c. anoxia
    c. anthrax
    c. artery occlusion
    c. atrophy
    c. autoregulation
    c. autosomal dominant arteriopathy
    c. autosomal dominant arteriopathy
      with subcortical infarct
      (CADASIL)
    c. blood flow
    c. candidiasis
    c. cortex receptor
    c. cortical dysplasia
    c. gigantism
    c. herniation
    c. lipidosis
    c. malaria
    c. palsy
    c. pneumonia
    c. rheumatism
    c. sphingolipidosis
    c. vasospasm
    c. vomiting
cerebralis
    adiposis c.
cerebri
    falx c.
    pseudotumor c.
cerebrooocular-dysplasia muscular
  dystrophy
cerebroside
    c. lipidosis
    c. lipoidosis
cerebrosidosis
cerebrospinal
    c. fluid (CSF)
    c. fluid analysis
cerebrotendinous xanthomatosis
cerebrovascular
    c. accident (CVA)
    c. disease (CVD)

cerevisiae
    Saccharomyces c.
cerivastatin sodium
ceroid lipofuscinosis
ceroma
certifiable
certification
certified
    board c.
    c. medical assistant (CMA)
    c. medical transcriptionist (CMT)
    c. nurse-midwife (CNM)
    c. registered nurse anesthetist
      (CRNA)
certify
ceruloplasmin
cerumen
Cerumenex
cervical
    c. cancer
    c. carcinoma
    c. chain adenopathy
    c. collar
    c. dysplasia
    c. hyperextension
    c. incompetence
    c. intraepithelial neoplasia, grade 2
      (CIN II)
    c. lymphadenopathy
    c. magnetic resonance imaging
    c. malignancy
    c. mediastinoscopy
    c. MRI
    c. polyp
    c. radiculopathy
    c. rib syndrome
    c. root compression
    c. root syndrome
    c. spinal stenosis
    c. spine disease
    c. spondylosis
    c. sympathetic syndrome
    c. venous hum
cervices (*pl. of* cervix)
cervicitis
    mucopurulent c.
cervicocerebral artery
cervicofacial
cervicogenic headache
cervix, pl. cervices
    os c.
    c. uteri
cesarean section
CES-D
    Center for Epidemiologic Studies
    Depression Scale
cesium
cessation
    breathing c.

smoking c.
transient period of breathing c.
cestodiasis
cetirizine
CF
cystic fibrosis
CFIDS
chronic fatigue immune deficiency
syndrome
CFP
cystic fibrosis of pancreas
CFS
chronic fatigue syndrome
CGA
Catholic Golden Age
comprehensive geriatric assessment
CGI-S
Clinical Global Impression-Severity of
Illness Scale
CGS
centimeter-gram-second
CGS unit
cGy
centigray
CHA
chronic hemolytic anemia
Chagas-Cruz disease
Chagas disease
chagoma
chain
light c.
chair
computer-drive rotational c.
geri c.
c. rise
chalazion, pl. **chalazia**
chalcitis (*var. of* chalkitis)
chalcosis
chalicosis
chalkitis, chalcitis
chalky gout
challenge diet
chalone
chamomile tea
chancre
chancriform syndrome
chancroidal bubo
Chandipura virus
change
age-related c.
Alzheimer neurofibrillary c.
Armanni-Ebstein c.

Baggenstoss c.
behavior c.
Charcot c.
contrast sensitivity c.
Crooke hyaline c.
E to A c.
fibrocystic c.
granulomatous c.
hormone c.
mental status c.
neuroanatomic c.
neurophysiologic c.
neurotransmitter c.
nonspecific ST c.
osteoarthritic c.
pharmacodynamic c.
pharmacokinetic c.
polyneuropathy, organomegaly,
endocrinopathy, monoclonal
gammopathy, skin c. (POEMS)
shift c.
ST-T wave c.
venous stasis c.
chaos
dietary c.
chappa
characteristic
functional c.
individual c.
nutritional c.
pathological c.
primary sex c.'s
secondary sex c.'s
Charcot
C. arthropathy
C. change
C. cirrhosis
C. intermittent fever
C. joint
C. joint disease
C. triad
C. triad of symptoms
Charcot-Bouchard aneurysm
Charcot-Leyden crystal protein
Charcot-Marie-Tooth disease
Chardack pacemaker
charge nurse
charlatan
charlatanism
Charlson comorbidity index
Charnley clamp

C

NOTES

chart
 abridged ocular c. (AOC)
 Snellen eye c.
 Tanner growth c.
charting
Chauffard-Still syndrome
Chauffard syndrome
Chauveau bacillus
CHD
 coronary heart disease
Cheadle disease
checklist
 Symptom C. 90 (SLC-90)
Chédiak-Higashi
 C.-H. anomaly
 C.-H. disease
 C.-H. syndrome
Chédiak-Steinbrinck-Higashi anomaly
cheese-worker's lung
cheesy abscess
Cheetah ankle brace
cheilitis
 actinic c.
 angular c.
cheilosis
cheirarthropathy
chelate
chelating agent
chelation therapy
Chem-7, -20
chemical
 c. burn
 c. diabetes
 c. esophagitis
 c. peel
 c. peritonitis
 c. pneumonia
 c. pneumonitis
 c. thyroidectomy
chemically
chemise
 bouton en c.
chemistry
 abnormal liver c.
 clinical c.
chemo
 chemotherapy
chemokine
chemoprevention
chemopreventive agent
chemoprophylaxis
 antimicrobial c.
chemoradiotherapy
chemoreceptor
chemoserotherapy
chemotaxis

chemotherapeutic
 c. agent
 c. drug
chemotherapy (chemo)
 adjuvant c.
 antiretroviral c.
 combination c.
 consolidation c.
 FAC c.
 5-FU, Adriamycin, Cytoxan c.
 induction c.
 intensification c.
 intraarterial c.
 intrathecal c.
 maintenance c.
 multiagent c.
 neoadjuvant c.
 postoperative adjuvant c.
 salvage c.
Chenix
chenodeoxycholic
cherry angioma
cherry-red spot
cherubic facies
chest
 barrel c.
 blast c.
 c. discomfort
 pigeon c.
 c. radiography
 c. thump
 c. wall disease
 c. wall pain
 c. wall tumor
 c. wall vibration
 c. x-ray (CXR)
Cheyne-Stokes
 C.-S. breathing
 C.-S. respiration
CHF
 congestive heart failure
chi
 tai c.
Chiari
 C. anomaly
 C. disease
 C. osteotomy
 C. syndrome
Chiari-Arnold syndrome
Chiari-Budd syndrome
Chiba needle
Chicago disease
chickenpox
chiclero ulcer
chief complaint (CC)
chigger
chikungunya
Chilaiditi sign

chilblain
    c. lupus
    c. lupus erythematosus
child-care center
childhood
    C. Autism Rating Scale (CARS)
    erythroblastic anemia of c.
    c. type tuberculosis
Children
    C. Affective Rating Scale (CARS)
    C. of Aging Parents (CAPS)
Child-Turcotte-Pugh classification
chill
    smelter's c.'s
chilling sensation
chimerism
Chinese
    C. liver fluke
    C. restaurant syndrome (CRS)
chiropractic
    Doctor of C. (DC)
chiropractor
chiufa
Chlamydia
    C. pneumoniae
    C. psittaci
    C. trachomatis
chlamydial
    c. conjunctivitis
    c. pneumonia
chlamydiosis
chloasma
chloral hydrate
chloralism
chlorambucil
chloramiphene
chloramphenicol
Chloraseptic
chlordiazepoxide
chloremia
chlorhydria
chloride
    oxybutynin c.
    potassium c. (KCl)
    sodium c. (NaCl)
    vinyl c.
chloridorrhea
chlorine
    c. gas inhalation
    c. reabsorption
chloroanemia
chloroethylcyclohexylnitrosourea (CCNU)

chloroformism
chloroma
Chloromycetin
chloroquine
chlorosis
chlorothiazide
chlorotic anemia
chlorpheniramine
chlorpromazine
chlorpropamide
chlorthalidone
Chlor-Trimeton
chlorzoxazone
choanal
choc
    bruit de c.
chokes
cholagogic
cholagogue
cholaneresis
cholangeitis
cholangiocarcinoma
cholangiogram
    intraoperative c.
cholangiography
    percutaneous c.
cholangiohepatitis
cholangiolitic hepatitis
cholangiopancreatogram
    endoscopic retrograde c. (ERCP)
cholangiopancreatography
    endoscopic retrograde c. (ERCP)
    magnetic resonance c.
cholangiopathy
    AIDS c.
cholangitic abscess
cholangitis
    ascending c.
    autoimmune c.
    bacterial c.
    catarrhal c.
    c. lenta
    sclerosing c.
    secondary sclerosis c.
cholascos
cholecystagogic
cholecystagogue
cholecystatony
cholecystectomy
    laparoscopic c. (LC)
cholecystitis
    acalculous c.

C

NOTES

cholecystitis *(continued)*
    acute acalculous c.
    chronic calculous c. (CCC)
cholecystogram
cholecystokinetic
cholecystokinin
cholecystopathy
choledochal
choledochoduodenostomy
choledocholithiasis
choledochoscopy
choledochostomy
Choledyl
cholelithiasis
    asymptomatic c.
    symptomatic c.
cholemesis
cholemia
    familial c.
    Gilbert c.
cholemic
cholepathia spastica
cholera
    Asiatic c.
    bilious c.
    c. infantum
    c. morbus
    c. nostras
    pancreatic c.
    c. sicca
    typhoid c.
choleraesuis
    Salmonella enterica choleraesuis
choleragen
choleraica
    vox c.
choleraic diarrhea
choleraicus
    status c.
choleresis
choleretic
cholerheic
choleric
choleriform
cholerigenic
cholerine
choleroid
cholerrhagia
cholerrhagic
cholestasia
cholestasis
    benign recurrent intrahepatic c.
    drug-induced intrahepatic c.
    extrahepatic c.
    familial intrahepatic c.
    intrahepatic c.
    total parenteral nutrition c.
cholestatic
    c. hepatitis

    c. liver disease
    c. pattern
cholesteatoma
cholesterinosis
cholesterol
    c. ester storage disease
    c. gallstone
    HDL c.
    high-density lipoprotein c. (HDL-C)
    LDL c.
    c. level
    low-density lipoprotein c. (LDL-C)
    C. and Recurrent Events (CARE)
    C. and Recurrent Events trial
    c. solubilization
cholesterolemia
cholesterolosis
cholesterosis
cholesteryl ester transfer protein
    deficiency
Cholestin
cholestyramine
choliformis
    mycetism c.
choline
    c. acetyltransferase
    c. magnesium trisalicylate
cholinergic
    c. agonist
    c. deficit
    c. paraganglion
    c. release enhancer
    c. urticaria
cholinesterase inhibitor
cholorrhea
choluric
    c. hemolytic icterus
    c. hemolytic icterus with
        splenomegaly
chondritis
chondroblastoma
chondrocalcinosis
    articular c.
chondrodynia
    parasternal c.
chondrodysplasia
chondroitin sulfate
chondroma
chondromalacia patellae
chondromatosis
chondromatous hamartoma
chondromyxoid
chondroplasty
chondrosarcoma
chondrosarcomatosis
chondrosarcomatous
chondrosternal

CHOP
cyclophosphamide, hydroxydaunomycin,
Oncovin, prednisone
Chopart amputation
chordae rupture
chordee
chordoma
chorea
Huntington c.
Morvan c.
Sydenham c.
choreal
choreic tongue
choreiform
choreoathetotic gait
chorioamnionitis
choriocarcinoma
chorioepithelioma malignum
choriogonadotropin
choriomammotropin
choriomeningitis
lymphocytic c.
pseudolymphocytic c.
chorionic
c. gonadotropic hormone
c. gonadotropin
c. growth hormone-prolactin
chorioretinitis
chorioretinopathy
choroidal nevus
choroideremia
choroidopathy
choroid plexus
Christian
C. disease
C. syndrome
Christie-Atkins-Munch-Petersen (CAMP)
C.-A.-M.-P. test
Christmas
C. disease
C. factor
chromatin stain
chromium picolinate
chromomycosis
chromophototherapy
chromosomal
c. disorder
c. rearrangement
chromosome
apolipoprotein E epsilon 4 gene
on c. 19

beta-amyloid precursor protein gene
on c. 21
Philadelphia c.
presenilin-1 gene on c. 1, 14
chromotherapy
chronic
c. acholuric jaundice
c. active hepatitis (CAH)
c. active hepatitis with cirrhosis
(CAHC)
c. active liver disease
c. adrenal insufficiency
c. adrenocortical insufficiency
c. African sleeping sickness
c. alcoholism
c. alcohol syndrome (CAS)
c. altitude illness
c. anxiety
c. arteriosclerotic mesenteric
vascular occlusive disease
c. aspiration pneumonitis
c. asymptomatic hypotonicity
c. atrophicans acrodermatitis
c. autoimmune thyroiditis
c. bacillary diarrhea
c. bacterial prostatitis
c. beryllium disease
c. bone marrow transplant-
associated nephropathy
c. bronchitis
c. calcifying pancreatitis (CCP)
c. calculous cholecystitis (CCC)
c. cicatrizing enteritis
c. coronary artery disease
c. cough
c. dermatitis
c. ductopenic rejection
c. dyspnea
c. eosinophilic pneumonia
c. Epstein-Barr virus (CEBV)
c. familial icterus
c. familial nonhemolytic jaundice
c. fatigue immune deficiency
syndrome (CFIDS)
c. fatigue syndrome (CFS)
c. fibrosing thyroiditis
c. fibrous thyroiditis
c. functional abdominal pain
c. gouty arthritis
c. granulocytic leukemia
c. hemolysis
c. hemolytic anemia (CHA)

NOTES

chronic (continued)
  c. hypertension in pregnancy
  c. hyperventilation syndrome
  c. hypoplastic neutropenia
  c. idiopathic neutropenia
  c. idiopathic orthostatic hypotension
  c. idiopathic xanthomatosis
  c. incontinence
  c. inflammation
  c. inflammatory bowel disease
    (CIBD)
  c. insomnia
  c. intermittent abdominal pain
  c. interstitial cystitis
  c. interstitial nephritis
  c. intestinal ischemia
  c. liver failure
  c. low back pain (CLBP)
  c. lung disease
  c. lymphadenoid thyroiditis
  c. lymphocytic leukemia (CLL)
  c. lymphocytic thyroiditis
  c. malaria
  c. mediastinitis
  c. mesenteric ischemia
  c. mitral regurgitation
  c. moniliasis
  c. mountain sickness
  c. myelocytic anemia
  c. myelocytic leukemia
  c. myelogenous leukemia (CML)
  c. myeloid leukemia
  c. myelomonocytic anemia
  c. myelomonocytic leukemia (CML,
    CMMoL)
  c. myocarditis
  c. neutrophilia
  c. nonleukemic myelosis
  c. obstructive pulmonary disease
    (COPD)
  c. organ rejection
  c. osteomyelitis
  c. otitis media
  c. paroxysmal hemicrania
  c. passive congestion (CPC)
  c. pelvic pain
  c. pelvic pain syndrome
  c. peritoneal dialysis (CPD)
  c. persistent abdominal pain
  c. persistent cough of unknown
    cause
  c. persistent hepatitis
  c. persisting hepatitis
  c. pleurisy
  c. progressive pulmonary
    histoplasmosis
  c. refractory anemia
  c. relapsing pancreatitis
  c. renal failure

  c. renal insufficiency
  c. silicosis
  c. sinusitis
  c. soroche
  c. steroid use
  c. stress
  c. subdural hematoma
  c. sycosis barbae
  c. systemic lupus erythematosus
  c. tension-type headache
  c. thromboembolic pulmonary
    hypertension
  c. trypanosomiasis
  c. ulcerative proctitis
  c. venous insufficiency
  c. viral hepatitis
  c. vulvar vestibulitis
chronica
    polyarthritis c.
chronicity
chronobiologic rhythm
chronological age
chronotropic
Chronulac
Chrysosporium parvum
chrysotherapy
chuan
    tai chi c.
chubby puffer syndrome
Churg-Strauss
    C.-S. disease
    C.-S. syndrome
Chvostek anemia
Chvostek and Trousseau signs
chylemia
chylifaction
chylifactive
chyliferous
chylification
chyliform
    c. ascites
    c. pleural effusion
    c. pleurisy
chylomicron
chylomicronemia syndrome
chylophoric
chylopoiesis
chylopoietic
chylorrhea
chylosa
    diarrhea c.
chylosis
chylosus
    ascites c.
chylous
    c. arthritis
    c. ascites
    c. hydrothorax
chymase

Chymex test
chymification
chymopapain
chymopoiesis
chymorrhea
CI
  cardiac index
    CI therapy
CIBD
  chronic inflammatory bowel disease
cibum
    ante c.
    post c. (after a meal [L. *post cibum*],
      p.c.)
cicatricial pemphigus
cicatrix
CID
  combined immunodeficiency disease
  cytomegalic inclusion disease
cidofovir
CIDS
  continuous insulin delivery system
Ciel
    Kay C.
ciguatera
cilexetil
    candesartan c.
cilia
ciliated cell
cilioretinal artery
cilostazol
cimetidine
cimicosis
cimino
cinchonism
cine
cineangiocardiography
cineangiography
cineplasty
cineradiography
cingulate gyrus
CIN II
  cervical intraepithelial neoplasia, grade 2
cinnarizine
Cinobac
Cipro
ciprofloxacin
circadian
    c. pattern
    c. rhythm
    c. rhythm-based sleep disorder
    c. rhythm disorder

circinate balanitis
circle
    defensive c.
    vicious c.
    c. of Willis
circuit
    pulmonary c.
circulating anticoagulant
circulation
    splenic c.
circulatory failure
circumcised
circumduction
circumference
    waist c.
circumferential
circumoral paresthesia
circumstantial
cirrhogenous
cirrhosis
    alcoholic c.
    atrophic c.
    biliary c.
    Budd c.
    capsular c.
    Charcot c.
    chronic active hepatitis with c.
      (CAHC)
    congenital hepatic c.
    Cruveilhier-Baumgarten c.
    cryptogenic c.
    fatty c.
    Glisson c.
    Hanot c.
    juvenile c.
    Laënnec c.
    macronodular c.
    Maixner c.
    micronodular c.
    necrotic c.
    nutritional c.
    obstructive c.
    pericholangiolitic c.
    periportal c.
    pigment c.
    pigmentary c.
    pipe stem c.
    portal c.
    posthepatitic c.
    postnecrotic c.
    primary biliary c. (PBC)
    pulmonary c.

C

NOTES

cirrhosis *(continued)*
    syphilitic c.
    Todd c.
    toxic c.
cirrhotic
    c. hydrothorax
    c. liver
cirrus
cirsomphalos
CIS
    carcinoma in situ
cisapride
cisplatin
    methotrexate, vinblastine,
      Adriamycin, c. (M-VAC)
cis-**retinoic acid study**
cisterna
    Pecquet c.
    c. pontis
cisternogram
    radioiodinated serum albumin c.
    RISA c.
citalopram HBr
citizen
    senior c.
Citracal
citrate
    calcium c.
    clomiphene c.
Citrobacter paracolon
Citrucel
citrullinemia
Civatte
CJD
    Creutzfeldt-Jakob disease
CK
    creatine kinase
      CK isoenzyme
      CK test
CKMB
    creatine kinase myocardial band
      CKMB level
Clado point
cladosporiosis
cladribine
Claforan
Clagett procedure
claim settlement
clamp
    Charnley c.
clapotage
clapotement
    bruit de c.
claquement
    bruit de c.
clarithromycin
Claritin

Clark
    C. sign
    C. weight rule
Clarke-Hadfield syndrome
clasmatocyte
class
    c. A diabetes
    c. III Pap
classic
    c. angina
    c. Blalock-Taussig
    c. Glenn shunt
    c. heat stroke
    c. migraine
classification
    Child-Turcotte-Pugh c.
    van Heuven anatomical c.
    Waterlow c.
claudication
    intermittent c. (IC)
    venous c.
claustrophobia
claustrum receptor
clavi (*pl. of* clavus)
clavicle
clavicular percussion
clavulanate potassium
clavus, pl. **clavi**
clawtoe deformity
Claybrook sign
CLBP
    chronic low back pain
clean-catch
    c.-c. urinalysis
    c.-c. urine
clearance
    acid c.
    creatinine paraaminohippurate c.
    drug c.
    hepatic drug c.
    impaired drug c.
    renal drug c.
    thyroxine c.
clearing
    throat c.
clearinghouse
    National Arthritis and
      Musculoskeletal and Skin Diseases
      Information C.
    National Center for Complementary
      and Alternative Medicine C.
      (NCCAM)
    National Diabetes Information C.
      (NDIC)
    National Digestive Diseases
      Information C. (NDDIC)
    National Institute of Child Health
      and Human Development
      Information C.

National Kidney and Urological Diseases Information C. (NKUDIC)

National Self-Help C. (NSHC)

C. on Abuse and Neglect of the Elderly (CANE)

clear liquid diet

clecoxib

cleft

    c. lip

    c. palate

cleidagra

cleidocranial

cleidomastoid

clemastine fumarate

clenched-fist injury

Cleocin T gel

click

    hip c.

    Mulder c.

clicking

    c. rale

    c. tinnitus

climacteric

climacterium

Climara

climatology

climatotherapy

climax

climograph

clindamycin

Clindex

clinic

    urgent care c.

    walk-in c.

clinical

    c. BPH

    c. breast examination (CBE)

    c. chemistry

    c. constipation

    c. diagnosis

    c. epidemiology

    c. evaluation

    c. fitness

    C. Global Impression-Severity of Illness Scale (CGI-S)

    c. lethal

    c. medicine

    c. practice guideline (CPG)

    c. recording

C. Test of Sensory Interaction & Balance (CTSIB)

    c. thermometer

clinician

clinicopathologic

clinodactyly

clinography

Clinoril

Clinoxide

clitoral surgery

clival meningioma

CLL

    chronic lymphocytic leukemia

cloaca

clobetasol ointment

clock

    c. completion test

    c. drawing test

Clomid

clomiphene citrate

clomipramine

clonal

clonazepam

clonic

    c. jerk

    c. seizure

clonidine patch

cloning

clonorchiasis disorder

Clonorchis sinensis

clonus

    beats of c.

clopidogrel

clorazepate

closed

    c. hospital

    c. pleural biopsy

    c. reduction

clostridial

    c. bacteremia

    c. cellulitis

    c. infection

    c. myonecrosis

Clostridium

    C. *difficile*

    C. *difficile* colitis

    C. *difficile* infection

    C. *difficile*-related diarrhea

    C. *difficile* toxin

    C. *perfringens*

    C. *perfringens* infection

    C. *septicum*

NOTES

clot
>fibrinous c.
>vegetatious c.

clotrimazole

clotting
>c. factor
>c. factor problem

cloudy cornea

clover
>sweet c.
>white c.

cloxacillin

clozapine toxicity

Clozaril

clubbed
>c. digit
>c. fingers

clubbing

clue cell

cluster
>c. attack
>c. headache

clustering
>familial c.

clysis

clyster

cm
>centimeter

CMA
>certified medical assistant

CMAP
>compound muscle action potential

CML
>chronic myelogenous leukemia
>chronic myelomonocytic leukemia

CMMoL
>chronic myelomonocytic leukemia

CMP
>captioned media program

CMT
>certified medical transcriptionist

CMV
>cytomegalic inclusion virus
>cytomegalovirus
>>CMV titer

CNM
>certified nurse-midwife

CNS
>central nervous system
>Corporation for National Service

CO
>cardiac output

C/O
>complains of

CO$_2$
>carbon dioxide

Co2smo Plus! respiratory monitor

coagulable

coagulase

coagulation
>c. disorder
>disseminated intravascular c. (DIC)
>c. factor

coagulopathy

coal
>c. miner's lung
>c. tar shampoo
>c. worker's pneumoconiosis (CWP)

coalesce

coalescence

coapt

coarctation
>c. of aorta
>aortic c.
>congenital aortic c.

CoA reductase

coarse tremor

coat
>buffy c.

coated tongue

cobalamin deficiency

Coban dressing

cobblestoning

cocaine
>c. toxicity
>c. withdrawal

cocci (*pl. of* coccus)

coccidioidal granuloma

Coccidioides immitis

coccidioidomycosis
>disseminated c.
>extrapulmonary c.
>primary extrapulmonary c.
>secondary c.
>subclinical c.

coccidiomycosis

coccus, pl. **cocci**
>gram-negative cocci
>gram-positive cocci

coccyalgia

coccygeal joint

coccyodynia

coccyx, pl. **coccyges**

Cochin China diarrhea

cochlear
>c. degeneration
>c. implant
>c. otosclerosis
>c. transduction

Cochliomyia hominivorax

Cockett communicating perforating vein

cocktail
>gastrointestinal c.
>GI c.
>IV c.
>c. purpura

cock-up wrist splint

Codamine

codeine
    Phenergan with c.
coding
    ICD-9 c.
codominant
coenurosis
coenzyme Q
coexisting disease
coffeeground
    c. emesis
    c. vomit
    c. vomitus
Cogan-Reese syndrome
Cogan syndrome
Cogentin
Cognex
cognition
    social c.
cognitive
    c. behavior therapy
    c. capacity
    c. coping skill
    c. decline
    c. dysfunction
    c. impairment
    c. performance
    c. status
    c. testing
cogwheel
    c. respiration
    c. rigidity
    c. sign
Cohen syndrome
cohort study
coil embolization
coin test
coital
    c. headache
coition
coitus
    c. interruptus
    c. reservatus
Cola
Colabid
Colace
Colazal
ColBenemid
colchicine
cold
    c. agglutinin
    c. agglutinin disease
    c. allergy

    c. angina
    c. antibody autoimmune hemolytic
      anemia
    c. erythema
    c. hemagglutinin disease
    c. intolerance
    c. lesion
    c. nodule
    c. pack
    c. pressor test
    c. stage
    c. urticaria
cold-induced
    c.-i. illness
    c.-i. necrosis
    c.-i. vasospasm
colectomy
    subtotal c.
colesevelam hydrochloride
Colestid
colestipol
coli
    diverticulosis c.
    E. c.
      Escherichia coli
    Entamoeba c.
    enterohemorrhagic *Escherichia c.*
      (EHEC)
    enteroinvasive *Escherichia c.*
      (EIEC)
    enteropathogenic *Escherichia c.*
      (EPEC)
    enterotoxigenic *Escherichia c.*
      (ETEC)
    Escherichia c. (E. coli)
    juvenile polyposis c.
    melanosis c.
colibacillosis
colic
    appendicular c.
    biliary c.
    copper c.
    Devonshire c.
    gallstone c.
    gastric c.
    hepatic c.
    infantile c.
    lead c.
    painter's c.
    pancreatic c.
    Poitou c.
    renal c.

C

NOTES

colic (*continued*)
    saturnine c.
    stercoral c.
    ureteral c.
    uterine c.
    vermicular c.
    zinc c.
colicky pain
colicoplegia
colistimethate
colitis
    amebic c.
    antibiotic-associated c.
    Clostridium difficile c.
    collagenous c.
    c. cystica profunda
    c. cystica superficialis
    diversion c.
    fulminant c.
    granulomatous c.
    hemorrhagic c.
    ischemic c.
    juvenile ulcerative c.
    microscopic c.
    mucous c.
    myxomembranous c.
    pseudomembranous c. (PMC)
    regional c.
    ulcerative c. (UC)
    uremic c.
collaboration
collaborative care
collagen
    c. injection
    c. vascular disease
collagenolytic
collagenosis
collagenous
    c. colitis
    c. pneumoconiosis
    c. sprue
collapse
    c. delirium
    postural c.
collapsing pulse
collar
    Casal c.
    cervical c.
    Madelung c.
    Stokes c.
    Stryker c.
college
    Association of American
      Medical C.'s (AAMC)
    Brookdale Center on Aging of
      Hunter C.
Colles fracture
collier lung
colliquation

colliquative diarrhea
colloid
    c. bath
    c. goiter
    c. nodule
colloidal dispersion
coloenteritis
colon
    ascending c.
    c. cancer
    descending c.
    diverticula of c.
    irritable c.
    sigmoid c.
    transverse c.
colonalgia
colonic
    c. artery aneurysm
    c. diverticulum
    c. perforation
    c. polyposis syndrome
    c. transit
    c. transit testing
colonization
colonopathy
    fibrosing c.
colonorrhagia
colonorrhea
colonoscopy
colopathy
color
    ashen gray c.
    c. duplex imaging
    c. flow
    c. flow Doppler
    stool c.
    c. triangle
Colorado tick fever
colorectal
    c. cancer
    c. dysmotility
    c. neoplasm
    c. polyp
colorrhagia
colorrhea
colovesical
colporrhaphy
colposcopy
Colton blood group
coltsfoot
columella
columnar epithelium
Coly-Mycin Otic
colypeptic
coma
    diabetic c.
    hepatic c.
    hyperglycemic nonketotic c.

hyperosmolar hyperglycemic nonketotic c.
hypoglycemic c.
Kussmaul c.
myxedema c.
thyrotoxic c.

comalike syndrome
comatosa
malaria c.
comatose
combination chemotherapy
combined
c. aortic and mitral disease
c. cold and warm antibody autoimmune hemolytic anemia
c. fat- and carbohydrate-induced hyperlipemia
c. immunodeficiency disease (CID)
Combipres
Combivent
Comby sign
comedo, pl. **comedones, comedos**
comedocarcinoma
comfort measures
comfrey
Comhist LA
commemorative sign
comminuted fracture
commission
Continuing Care Accreditation C. (CCAC)
Equal Employment Opportunity C. (EEOC)
Federal Trade C. (FTC)
commissurotomy
mitral c.
common
c. bile duct
c. duct obstruction
c. migraine
c. peroneal compression
c. variable hypogammaglobulinemia
communicable disease
community
c. ambulator
continuing care retirement c. (CC-RC)
c. health nurse
therapeutic c.
C. Transportation Association of America (CTAA)

community-acquired
c.-a. bacteremia
c.-a. bladder infection
c.-a. pneumonia (CAP)
c.-a. sepsis
community-dwelling patient
community-residing person
comorbidity
cumulative c.'s
comparative medicine
comparison
before-after c.
compartment syndrome
Compazine
compensated
c. erythrocytosis
c. metabolic alkalosis
c. respiratory acidosis
c. respiratory alkalosis
compensatory polycythemia
complains of (C/O)
complaint
chief c. (CC)
semantic c.
somatic c.
complement
complementary medicine
complete
c. atrioventricular canal
c. blood cell count
c. blood count (CBC)
complex
acylated plasminogen streptokinase activated c.
AIDS-related c. (ARC)
amphotericin B lipid c.
anisoylated plasminogen streptokinase activator c. (APSAC)
Behçet triple symptom c.
Candida-related c.
c. care
disseminated *Mycobacterium avium* c.
EAHF c.
eczema, asthma, hay fever c.
Eisenmenger c.
Ghon c.
heteromodal association c.
interdigestive migratory motor c.
membrane attack c. (MAC)
Mycobacterium avium c. (MAC)
Parkinson c.

NOTES

complex *(continued)*
    Parkinson dementia c.
    premature atrial c.
    premature atrioventricular
      junctional c.
    premature ventricular c.
    QRS c.
    sicca c.
    symptom c.
    triple symptom c.
    c. ventricular ectopy
compliance
    medication c.
    patient c.
    respiratory c.
complicated migraine
complication
    cardiac c.
    cardiovascular organ transplant c.
    endocrine organ transplant c.
    iatrogenic c.
    metabolic organ transplant c.
    perioperative cardiac c.
    postoperative pulmonary c.
    postradiation c.
component
    medial c.
composition
compos mentis
compound
    c. muscle action potential (CMAP)
    c. nevus
comprehension
comprehensive
    c. assessment
    c. directive
    c. geriatric assessment (CGA)
    c. medical care
compression
    cervical root c.
    common peroneal c.
    c. cyanosis
    metastatic epidural spinal cord c.
    nerve c.
    nerve root c.
    peripheral root c.
    sciatic nerve c.
    spinal cord c.
    vertebral c.
compromised
    c. activity
    c. renal function
compulsive vesiculoprostatitis
computed
    c. axial tomography (CAT)
    c. tomography (CT)
    c. tomography scan

computer
    Sequential Multiple Analyzer C.
    (SMAC)
computer-drive rotational chair
computerized
    c. dynamic posturography (CDP)
    c. patient record
COMT
    catechol methyltransferase
    COMT inhibitor
Concato disease
concentration
    hepatic iron c.
    hydrogen ion c. (pH)
    intraluminal conjugated bile acid c.
    maximum urinary c. (MUC)
    mean corpuscular hemoglobin c.
    (MCHC)
    plasma leptin c.
    serum sodium c.
    tissue tin c.
    urinary c.
    urine c.
concentric left ventricular hypertrophy
Concerta
concoction
    herbal c.
concomitant
    c. cardiovascular disease
    c. esophageal spasm
    c. medical problem
    c. metabolic acidosis
    c. symptom
concordance
concretion
condensans
    osteitis c.
condition
    conventional c.
    cormorbid c.
    hypertonic c.
    inflammatory musculoskeletal c.
    medical c.
    metabolic c.
    physiological c.
conditioned avitaminosis
condom
    female c.
conductance vessel
conduction
    c. ageusia
    c. agglutinin
    anisotropic c.
    c. disturbance
    nerve c.
    spinal cord c.
    sural nerve c.
    c. velocity
conductive hearing loss

condyle
condyloma acuminata
Condylox
cone
    vaginal c.
coned-down view
confabulation
confidentiality
confined
    organ c.
confinement
    estimated date of c. (EDC)
conflict
    extrapsychic c.
    c.'s of interest
confluent
    c. smallpox
conformationis
    vitium c.
confusion
    C. Assessment Method (CAM)
    right-left c.
confusional migraine
congenita
    dyskeratosis c.
    macrosomatia adiposa c.
    myatonia c.
    osteogenesis imperfecta c.
    paramyotonia c.
congenital
    c. absence of pericardium
    c. adrenal hyperplasia
    c. adrenocortical hyperplasia
    c. agranulocytosis
    c. aortic coarctation
    c. aplasia
    c. aplasia of thymus
    c. aplastic anemia
    c. cardiovascular disease
    c. chest wall abnormality
    c. deficiency
    c. deficiency of testosterone
      production
    c. diarrhea
    c. disorder
    c. dyserythropoietic anemia
    c. erythropoietic porphyria
    c. gastrointestinal alkalosis
    c. hemolytic icterus
    c. hemolytic jaundice
    c. hepatic cirrhosis
    c. hyperbilirubinemia

    c. immunodeficiency
    c. long QT syndrome
    c. melanocytic nevus
    c. methemoglobinemia
    c. myxedema
    c. neutropenia
    c. nonspherocytic hemolytic anemia
    c. pancytopenia
    c. pneumonia
    c. pulmonary valve stenosis
    c. rubella
    c. structural heart disease
    c. syphilis
    c. total lipodystrophy
    c. valvular aortic stenosis
    c. valvular disease
    c. valvular incompetence
    c. virilizing adrenal hyperplasia
congenitally corrected transposition
congestion
    chronic passive c. (CPC)
    nasal c.
    pulmonary c.
congestive heart failure (CHF)
conglobata
    acne c.
conglobate acne
conglutinating complement absorption
    test
Congo-Crimean hemorrhagic fever
Congolian red fever
congophilic angiopathy
congregate housing
coniosis
conization
conjugated
    c. bilirubin
    c. equine estrogen
    c. hyperbilirubinemia
conjunctiva, pl. conjunctivae
    acute follicular c.
    c. diagonalis (C/D)
conjunctivitis
    bacterial c.
    chlamydial c.
    hypersensitive c.
    viral c.
connective
    c. tissue disease
    c. tissue disorder
Conn syndrome

NOTES

C

conorii
    Rickettsia c.
conotruncal defect
consciousness
    alteration in c.
    altered level of c.
    content of c.
    control of c.
    level of c.
conscious patient
consecutive symptom
consensually
consensus
consent
    informed c.
    parental c.
consequence
conservative treatment
conservatrix
    vis c.
consideration
consistency
    doughy c.
consolidation chemotherapy
consonating rale
constellation of symptoms
constellatus
    Streptococcus c.
constipation
    clinical c.
    idiopathic c.
    self-report of c.
    slow-transit c.
constitution
constitutional
    c. aplastic anemia
    c. cause
    c. hepatic dysfunction
    c. hirsutism
    c. hyperbilirubinemia
    c. symptom
    c. thrombopathy
constraint
    financial c.
constraint-induced
    c.-i. movement
    c.-i. movement therapy
constriction hyperemia
consultant
consultation
consulting staff
consumption
consumptive
contact
    c. precaution
    c. stomatitis
contagiosum
    molluscum c.
contagious disease

content
    blood alcohol c. (BAC)
    blood oxygen c.
    c. of consciousness
contiguous gene syndrome
Contin
    MS C.
continence
    fecal c.
    National Association for C.
      (NAFC)
    Simon Foundation for C.
    urinary c.
continent
continued fever
continuing
    C. Care Accreditation Commission
      (CCAC)
    c. care retirement community (CC-
      RC)
continuity
    advance directive c.
continuous
    c. ambulatory peritoneal dialysis
      (CAPD)
    c. extravascular infusion (CEI)
    c. hypersomnia
    c. insulin delivery system (CIDS)
    c. positive airway pressure (CPAP)
    c. positive airway pressure device
    c. quality improvement
    c. subcutaneous insulin infusion
      (CSII)
    c. venovenous hemofiltration
continuous-infusion opioid
contraceptive
    oral c. (OC)
contractile
    c. state
    c. state of myocardium
    c. velocity
contractility
    detrusor hyperactivity with
      impaired c. (DHIC)
contraction
    atrial c.
    frequent premature ventricular c.
    myocardial c.
    postoperative premature
      ventricular c.
    premature ventricular c. (PVC)
contract for safety
contracture
    Dupuytren c.
    Volkmann c.
contraindicant
contraindicated
contraindication
    exercise c.

contrast
- c. agent-enhanced spiral computed tomography
- c. agent-enhanced spiral CT
- c. bath
- c. sensitivity change

contrecoup
contribution
contributor
control
- c. of consciousness
- glycemic c.
- postprandial glycemic c.
- sphincter c.

controlled-release formulation
controversial
convalescence
convalescent
conventional condition
convergence
- ocular c.

convergent
conversation
conversion
- lysogenic c.

convulsion
- hypoglycemic c.

Cook-Medley questionnaire
Cooley
- C. anemia
- C. disease

cool mist humidifier
Coombs-negative immune hemolytic anemia
Coombs test
Cooper
- C. disease
- C. ligament

Cooperative Cardiovascular Project (CCP)
coordination
- motor c.

COPD
- chronic obstructive pulmonary disease

Cope sign
coping skill
copper
- c. colic
- c. storage disease

copremesis
coprolalia
- mental c.

coprophilic
coproporphyrin
coptosis
copulation
copulines
cor
- c. pulmonale
- c. triatriatum

coracoacromial
coracoid process
cord
- hard c.
- spinal c.
- vocal c.

Cordarone
cordis
- accretio c.
- angina c.
- diastasis c.

Cordis Checkmate System
cordotomy
Cordran
core
- c. antibody
- c. biloculare
- c. body temperature
- c. pneumonia
- c. rewarming

Coreg
Corgard
Coricidin D
Cori disease
corkscrew
- c. esophagus
- c. hair

Cormax
cormorbid condition
corn
- soft c.

cornea
- arcus c.
- cloudy c.

corneal
- c. abrasion
- c. abscission
- c. reflex
- c. ulcer
- c. ulceration

corneum
- stratum c.

cornified squamous epithelium
corona radiata

NOTES

89

coronary
    c. allograft vasculopathy
    c. angiography
    c. arteriosclerosis
    c. artery
    c. artery bypass graft (CABG)
    c. artery bypass grafting (CABG)
    c. artery bypass graft surgery
    c. artery calcification (CAC)
    c. artery disease (CAD)
    c. artery disease mortality
    c. artery embolism
    café c.
    c. care unit (CCU)
    c. heart disease (CHD)
    c. microvascular dysfunction
    c. reperfusion
    c. stenosis
    c. syndrome
    c. vasospasm
coronavirus
coroner
corpora cavernosa
Corporation for National Service (CNS)
corporis
    tinea c.
corps
    Medical C. (MC)
corpse
corpulence
corpulent
corpuscular
corpus hemorrhagicum
corpus-predominant gastritis
correctable
corrected
    QT c.
corrective
Correctol
correlate
correlation
    age c.
    negative c.
Corrigan sign
corrigent
corrodens
    Eikenella c.
corrosive injury
corset
    Warm and Form c.
Cortef
cortex, pl. **cortices**
    adrenal c.
    somatosensory c.
cortical
    c. bone
    c. hormone
    c. layer
    c. shot

corticobasal ganglionic degeneration
corticobulbar neuron
corticoid
    exogenous mineral c.
corticomotor excitability
corticoreticular
corticospinal motor
corticosteroid
    inhaled c.
    oral c.
    systemic c.
    topical c.
    trifluorinated c.
corticosteroid-resistant dermatomyositis
corticotroph adenoma
corticotropic hormone
corticotropin
    c. deficiency
    c. excess
    c. stimulation test
corticotropin-releasing
    c.-r. factor (CRF)
    c.-r. hormone (CRH)
    c.-r. hormone test
Cortifoam
cortisol
    24-hour urine c.
    c. level
    plasma c.
    urinary free c. (UFC)
cortisone
Cortisporin Otic Solution
Cortrosyn stimulation test
coruscation
Corvisart
    C. disease
    C. facies
corynebacteria
corynebacterial infection
Corynebacterium
coryneform
    erythrasma c.
coryza
Corzide
cosmesis
cost
    health care c.
costalgia
cost-effectiveness
Costen syndrome
costive
costiveness
costochondral
costochondritis syndrome
costoclavicular syndrome
costogenic
costophrenic angle

costovertebral
  c. angle (CVA)
  c. angle tenderness
cosyntropin
cot death
Cotrel traction
cotton-dust asthma
cotton-mill fever
cottonpox
cotton wool spot
cotyledon
cough
  aneurysmal c.
  angiotensin-converting enzyme
    inhibitor c.
  bronchospastic reflex c.
  chronic c.
  c. fracture
  c. headache
  ineffective c.
  nonproductive c.
  psychogenic c.
  c. suppressant
  c. syncope
  c. test
  c. test for stress incontinence
  weaver's c.
  whooping c.
cough-variant asthma
Coumadin
coumarin
council
  C. of Better Business Bureaus
    (CBBB)
  United Seniors Health C. (USHC)
Councilman lesion
counseling
  dietary c.
  smoking cessation c.
count
  absolute neutrophil c.
  Addis c.
  CD4 cell c.
  complete blood c. (CBC)
  complete blood cell c.
  platelet c.
  reticulocyte c.
  too numerous to c. (TNTC)
  white blood cell c.
counter
  over the c. (OTC)
counteract

counting
  manual c.
coup de sabre
couplet
coupling defect
Cournand cardiac catheter
course
  antibiotic c.
Courvoisier
  C. gallbladder
  C. law
  C. sign
Covera HS
Cowden
  C. disease
  C. syndrome
Cowen sign
Cowling rule
cowpox
cow's milk anemia
COX
  cyclooxygenase
COX-1
  cyclooxygenase-1
COX-2
  cyclooxygenase-2
  COX-2 inhibitor
coxa
  c. magna
  c. valga
  c. vara luxans
Coxiella **infection**
coxodynia
Coxsackievirus
Cozaar
CPAP
  continuous positive airway pressure
CPC
  chronic passive congestion
CPD
  chronic peritoneal dialysis
C-peptide
CPG
  clinical practice guideline
CPK
  creatine phosphokinase
CPPD
  calcium pyrophosphate dihydrate
CPPDD
  calcium pyrophosphate deposition disease
CPR
  cardiopulmonary resuscitation

C

NOTES

cracked-pot
  c.-p. resonance
  c.-p. sound
crackle
  basilar c.
  end-respiratory c.
  pleural c.
crackling rale
cradle cap
craftsmen
  Elder C. (EC)
cramp
  c. bark
  heat c.
  intermittent c.
  muscle c.
cramping
Crandall syndrome
cranial
  c. bruit
  c. epidural abscess
  c. nerve
  c. nerve palsy
  c. neuralgia
  c. polyneuritis
craniocaudal
craniopathy
  metabolic c.
craniopharyngioma
craniosynostosis
CRAO
  central retinal artery occlusion
crapulent
craquelé
  eczema c.
crash cart
C-reactive
  C-r. protein (CRP)
cream
  Aurum Analgesic C.
  AVC c.
  Axsain C.
  betamethasone valerate c.
  Epilyt C.
  5-fluorouracil c.
  Halog c.
  lindane 1% c.
  liniment c.
  Locoid c.
  Loprox c.
  Mytrex c.
  Oxistat c.
  Temovate C.
  Tinactin c.
  Tridesilon c.
  vaginal c.
crease
  Sydney c.
  volar wrist flexion c.

creatine
  c. kinase (CK)
  c. kinase isoenzyme
  c. kinase myocardial
  c. kinase myocardial band (CKMB)
  c. kinase myocardial band level
  c. kinase test
  c. phosphokinase (CPK)
creatinine paraaminohippurate clearance
Creative diabetic socks
creeping thrombosis
creepy-craze crawly syndrome of legs
cremaster
Creon
crepitant rale
crepitation
crepitus
crescendo
crescendo-decrescendo murmur
crescent cell anemia
crescentic glomerulonephritis
CREST
  calcinosis, Raynaud phenomenon,
    esophageal motility disorders,
    sclerodactyly, telangiectasia
  CREST syndrome
crest
  iliac c.
cretin
cretinism
cretinistic
cretinoid
cretinous
Creutzfeldt-Jakob disease (CJD)
CRF
  cardiac risk factor
  corticotropin-releasing factor
CRH
  corticotropin-releasing hormone
crib death
cricoarytenoid
cricoid cartilage
cricopharyngeal bar
cricopharyngeous
cricopharyngeus muscle
cricothyroid needle cannulation
cri-du-chat syndrome
Crigler-Najjar
  C.-N. disease
  C.-N. syndrome
Crimean-Congo hemorrhagic fever
Crimean fever
crinogenic
crisis, pl. **crises**
  Addison c.
  addisonian c.
  adrenal c.
  adrenocortical c.
  aplastic c.

blast c.
Dietl c.
febrile c.
gastric c.
hypertensive c.
myasthenic c.
Parkinson c.
renal c.
salt-depletion c.
sickle cell c.
splenic sequestration c.
thyroid c.
thyrotoxic c.
vasoocclusive pain c.
Crisp aneurysm
criterion, pl. **criteria**
Manning criteria
Ranson criteria
Rome criteria
critical
c. care
c. care unit (CCU)
CRNA
certified registered nurse anesthetist
Crocq disease
Crohn
C. disease
C. ileitis
C. ileocolitis
cromoglycate
sodium c.
cromolyn sodium
cromone
Crooke
C. hyaline change
C. hyaline degeneration
cross
American Red C.
International Committee of the Red C.
Maltese c.
Red C.
c. tolerance
crosslink
deoxypyridinoline c.
cross-section
cross-sectional study
Crotalidae
Crotalinae polyvalent immune Fab antivenom
crotaline snake bite
croup-associated virus (CAV)

croupous
c. bronchitis
c. pneumonia
Crouzon
C. disease
C. syndrome
CRP
C-reactive protein
CRPA
C-reactive protein antiserum
CRS
Chinese restaurant syndrome
CRST
cyanosis, redness, scleroderma, telangiectasia
cruciate
cruciferous
cruentes
vomitus c.
crunching sound
crural
c. fold
c. triangle
cruris
tinea c.
crush kidney
Cruveilhier-Baumgarten
C.-B. cirrhosis
C.-B. sign
C.-B. syndrome
Cruveilhier sign
Cruz trypanosomiasis
CRVO
central retinal vein occlusion
cryoablation
cryocautery
cryocrit
cryofibrinogen
cryofibrinogenemia
cryogenic
cryoglobulin
c. disease
c. syndrome
cryoglobulinemia
cryopathy
cryoprecipitate
cryoretinopexy
cryosurgery
cryothalamectomy
cryotherapy
crypt
tonsillar c.

C

NOTES

cryptic
cryptococcal meningitis
cryptococcosis
    disseminated c.
Cryptococcus neoformans
cryptogenic
    c. chronic hepatitis
    c. cirrhosis
    c. fibrosing alveolitis
    c. hemoptysis
    c. organizing pneumonitis
    c. pyemia
cryptopodia
cryptopyic
cryptorchidism
cryptosporidiosis
Cryptosporidium infection
cryptotoxic
crystal
    c. arthritis
    Polycitra-K c.
    pyrophosphate c.
    urinary c.
    c. violet
crystal-induced
    c.-i. synovitis
crystal-induced arthritis
crystallina
    uridrosis c.
crystalline calcium pyrophosphate
  dihydrate (CCPD)
crystalluria
C&S
    culture and sensitivity
CSD
    cat-scratch disease
CSF
    cerebrospinal fluid
CSII
    continuous subcutaneous insulin infusion
CT
    computed tomography
      contrast agent-enhanced spiral CT
      CT scan
CTAA
    Community Transportation Association
      of America
CTCL
    cutaneous T-cell lymphoma
CT-guided biopsy
CTS
    carpal tunnel syndrome
CTSIB
    Clinical Test of Sensory Interaction &
      Balance
Cuban itch
cube pessary

cubital
    c. fossa
    c. joint
cubitus, pl. cubiti
    articularis cubiti
cucurbita
cuff
    rotator c.
cuirass
cul-de-sac
culdocentesis
Cullen sign
culture
    acid-fast c.
    blood c.
    c. and sensitivity (C&S)
    sinus c.
    throat c.
    wound c.
cumulative
    c. action
    c. comorbidities
    c. effect
    C. Index Medicus
    c. injury
cumulus cell
cuneiform
cup
    MF heel c.
cup-to-disk ratio
curantur
    similia similibus c.
Curasol gel wound dressing
curative dose
cure
cure-oriented care
curettage
    dilatation and c. (D&C)
    electrodesiccation and c. (ED&C)
curette, curet
curettement
Curling ulcer
currant jelly sputum
current
Curretab
curriculum, pl. curricula
Curschmann disease
curse
    Ondine c.
curtain
    air c.
Curtius syndrome
curve
    force-velocity c.
    growth c.
curvilinear incision
Curvularia lunata
Cushing
    C. basophilism

C. disease
C. disease myopathy
C. disease of omentum
C. phenomenon
C. pituitary basophilism
C. reaction
C. response
C. syndrome
C. syndrome medicamentosus
cushingoid
c. facies
cushion
Viscoheel c.
custodial care
cutaneomucouveal syndrome
cutaneous
c. amyloidosis
c. anthrax
c. blastomycosis
c. herpes
c. horn
c. lupus erythematosus
c. mastocytosis
c. paraneoplastic syndrome
c. *Schistosoma japonica*
c. schistosomiasis
c. T-cell lymphoma (CTCL)
c. ulcer
c. vasculitis
c. zygomycosis
cut down (on drinking), annoyance, guilt (about drinking), (need for) eyeopener (CAGE)
cutis
amyloidosis c.
leukemia c.
c. marmorata
c. vertices gyrata
cutlery
thick-handled c.
CVA
cardiovascular accident
cerebrovascular accident
costovertebral angle
CVA tenderness
CVD
cerebrovascular disease
CWP
coal worker's pneumoconiosis
CXR
chest x-ray
cyanide intoxication

cyanochroic
cyanosed
cyanosis
compression c.
enterogenous c.
false c.
hereditary methemoglobinemic c.
c., redness, scleroderma, telangiectasia (CRST)
c. retinae
toxic c.
cyanotic
c. atrophy
c. congenital heart disease
cyclandelate
cycle
feeding-fasting c.
growth c.
Krebs-Henseleit urea c.
life c.
light-dark c.
sexual response c.
sleep-wake c.
cyclic
c. antidepressant toxicity
c. neutropenia
c. vomiting
cycling
c. dialysis
rapid c.
weight c.
cyclobenzaprine
Cyclogyl
cyclooxygenase (COX)
cyclooxygenase-1 (COX-1)
cyclooxygenase-2 (COX-2)
c. inhibitor
cyclophosphamide
c., hydroxydaunomycin, Oncovin, prednisone (CHOP)
Platinol, Adriamycin, c. (PAC)
cycloserine
cyclosporin
cyclosporine
c. A
c. effect
cyclosporosis
cyclothymia
Cycrin
Cylert
CYP1A2 enzyme isoform
CYP2C enzyme isoform

NOTES

C

CYP2D6 enzyme isoform
CYP3A enzyme isoform
cypionate
cyst
    Baker c.
    Bartholin c.
    blue dome c.
    bone c.
    epididymal c.
    ganglion c.
    hydatid c.
    infected pilonidal c.
    myxoid c.
    nabothian c.
    pericardial c.
    pilonidal c.
    popliteal c.
    renal c.
    Tarlov c.
    thin-walled c.
cystalgia
cystathioninuria
cystic
    c. acne syndrome
    c. disease
    c. duct obstruction
    c. fibrosis (CF)
    c. fibrosis of pancreas (CFP)
    c. goiter
    c. myxoma
cystica
    osteitis fibrosa c.
    osteogenesis imperfecta c.
cysticercosis
    ocular c.
    spinal c.
cysticercus disease
cystine
    c. stone
    c. storage disease
cystinemia
cystinosis
cystinuria
cystitis
    acute uncomplicated c.
    chronic interstitial c.
    interstitial c.
    recurrent c.
    uncomplicated c.
cystocele
cystocytoma
cystoid macular edema
cystometric
cystometrogram
    multichannel c.
cystometry
    bedside c.
    multichannel c.
    simple c.

cystomyoma
cystomyxoadenoma
cystomyxoma
cystonuria
cystopathy
    diabetic c.
cystosarcoma phyllode
cystoscopy
Cystospaz
cystourethrography
cystourethroscopy
cytarabine (Ara-C, ara-C)
cythemolytic icterus
cytobrush
cytochemical
cytochrome
    c. oxidase
    c. P450
cytogenetic
cytogenic anemia
cytoid
cytokine
    c. growth factor
    pyrogenic c.
cytology
    exfoliative c.
    fine-needle aspiration c.
cytolytic vaginosis
cytomegalic
    c. inclusion disease (CID)
    c. inclusion virus (CMV)
cytomegalovirus (CMV)
    c. esophagitis
    c. immune globulin
    c. inclusion disease
    c. infection
    c. pneumonia
    c. retinitis
    c. titer
Cytomel
cytometric
cytopathic effect
cytopathologist
cytopathy
cytoprotective effect
cytoreductive
    c. surgery
    c. therapy
Cytosar-U
Cytotec
cytotoxic
    c. T-cell (Tc)
    c. T-cell responsive
    c. therapy
Cytoxan
    5-FU, Adriamycin, C. (FAC)
Czerny anemia

DA
   degenerative arthritis
Daae disease
daclizumab
Dacomed snap gauge
dacryocystitis
dacryocystography
dactinomycin
dactylitis
   sickle cell d.
dactylolysis spontanea
daily
   d. dose
   d. nursing care
d'airain
   bruit d.
Dalmane
Dalrymple
   D. disease
   D. sign
damage
   anoxic brain d.
   brain d.
   ischemic-anoxic brain d.
   myocardial d.
DAN
   diabetic autonomic neuropathy
Dana
   The D. Alliance for Brain
   Initiative
danaparoid sodium
danazol
Danbolt-Closs syndrome
dance
   D. sign
   St. Vitus d.
dandy fever
Dandy-Walker syndrome
Danocrine
Danubian endemic familial nephropathy
Danysz phenomenon
dapsone
daptomycin
Darco shoe
Darier disease
Darier-Roussy sarcoid
dark adaptation
Darling disease
Darvocet-N 100
Darvon
DASH
   Dietary Approaches to Stop Hypertension
   DASH combination diet

date
   d. of birth (DOB)
   d. fever
daunomycin
daunorubicin
DAV
   Disabled American Veterans
David disease
Davol PermCath
dawn
   d. effect
   d. phenomenon
Dawson inclusion
day
   every d. [L. *quaque die*] (q.d.)
   every other d. [L. *quaque altera
   die*] (q.o.d.)
   four times a d. (q.i.d.)
   d. hospital
   three times a d. (t.i.d.)
   twice a d. [L. *bis in die*] (b.i.d.,
   bis in die)
day-care center
Daypro
DayQuil
daytime
   d. sleepiness
   d. sulfonylurea
DC
   discontinue
   Doctor of Chiropractic
D&C
   dilatation and curettage
DCBE
   dual-contrast barium enema
DCIS
   ductal carcinoma in situ
D-dimer
   D-d. assay
   D-d. testing
DE
   dobutamine echocardiogram
   dobutamine echocardiography
de
   de Morsier-Gauthier syndrome
   de Morsier syndrome
   de Musset sign
   de Mussy point
   de Mussy sign
   de novo
   de Quervain disease
   de Quervain syndrome
   de Quervain tenosynovitis
   de Quervain thyroiditis

D

dead
> d. labyrinth
> d. on arrival (DOA)

dead-in-bed syndrome

deaf
> National Association of the D. (NAD)

deafness
> diabetes insipidus, diabetes mellitus, optic atrophy, d. (DIMOAD)
> lentigines, electrocardiographic abnormalities, ocular hypertelorism, pulmonary stenosis, abnormalities of genitalia, retardation of growth, d. (LEOPARD)
> sensorineural d.

dearth
> d. of evidence
> d. of findings
> d. of symptoms

death
> apoptotic cell d.
> black d.
> brain d.
> cot d.
> crib d.
> local d.
> maternal d.
> necrotic cell d.
> d. rate
> selective neuronal d.
> somatic d.
> sudden cardiac d.
> d. trance

debilitate

debilitating

debilitation

debilitative disease

debility

Debove disease

debrancher deficiency

debranching deficiency limit dextrinosis

Debré-Sémélaigne syndrome

debridement
> autolytic d.
> enzymatic d.
> surgical d.

Debrox

debulking

Decadron

Deca-Durabolin injection

decay
> tone d.
> tooth d.

decerebrate rigidity

dechloridation, dechlorination

decholesterolization

deciliter (dL)

> grams per d. (g/dL)
> milligram per d. (mg/dL)

decision
> end-of-life d.

decisional ability

decision-maker
> medical d.-m.
> surrogate d.-m.

decision-making
> d.-m. capacity
> ethical d.-m.
> surrogate d.-m.

decision-support tools

decline
> age-associated cognitive d. (AACD)
> cognitive d.
> functional d.

Declomycin

decompensated erythrocytosis

decompression
> d. disease
> d. sickness

Deconamine

deconditioned

deconditioning

decongestant

decorticate rigidity

decreased
> d. functionality
> d. pinprick

decrement

decrudescence

decubital necrosis

decubitus
> Andral d.
> d. ulcer
> ventral d.

decussate

deep
> d. bursitis
> d. cerebral hemorrhage
> d. frostbite
> d. muscle relaxation
> d. neck infection
> d. palpation
> d. percussion
> d. tendon reflex (DTR)
> d. vein thrombophlebitis
> d. vein thrombosis (DVT)
> d. venous thrombosis (DVT)

DEEP-IN
> delirium, dementia, depression, drugs; eyes and ears; physical performance and "phalls" (falls); incontinence; nutrition

deer-fly
> d.-f. disease
> d.-f. fever

deer tick

defecation syncope
defecography
defect
    atrial septal d. (ASD)
    atrioventricular canal septal d.
    conotruncal d.
    coupling d.
    extrinsic pathway d.
    fibrinolytic system d.
    filling d.
    glycogenolysis d.
    intrinsic pathway d.
    iodide transport d.
    iodotyrosine deiodinase d.
    luteal phase d.
    membrane transport d.
    neutrophil d.
    organification d.
    perfusion d.
    platelet activation d.
    quantitative platelet d.
    renal tubular d.
    salt-losing d.
    sinus venous d.
    vascular d.
    vascular septal d. (VSD)
    ventricular septal d. (VSD)
defective
    d. acceleration
    d. activation
    d. adhesion
    d. platelet aggregation
    d. regulation of intestinal water
      and electrolytes
defemination
defensive
    d. circle
    d. medicine
deferens
    vas d.
deferoxamine
defervescence
defervescent stage
defibrillator
    external d.
    implantable d.
deficiency
    acid-maltase d.
    adenine phosphoribosyl
      transferase d.
    adenosine deaminase d.
    adenylate kinase d.

    adrenocorticotropic hormone d.
    adult lactase d.
    alpha-1-antitrypsin d.
    d. anemia
    apolipoprotein C-II d.
    APRT d.
    B_{12} d.
    bile acid d.
    calcium d.
    CAPS d.
    carbamoyl phosphate synthetase d.
    carbonic anhydrase II d.
    cell function d.
    cell number d.
    ceramidase d.
    cholesteryl ester transfer protein d.
    cobalamin d.
    congenital d.
    corticotropin d.
    debrancher d.
    d. disease
    erythropoietin d.
    factor XI, XIII d.
    familial high-density lipoprotein d.
    familial lecithin:cholesterol
      acyltransferase d.
    fat-soluble vitamin d.
    folic acid d.
    galactokinase d.
    glucocorticoid d.
    glucose-6-phosphate
      dehydrogenase d.
    gonadotropin d.
    growth hormone d. (GHD)
    hepatic lipase d.
    hereditary sucrase-alpha-
      dextrinase d.
    high-molecular-weight kininogen d.
    homozygous C2 d.
    hormone d.
    humoral immune d.
    11-hydroxylase d.
    21-hydroxylase d.
    hypoxanthine guanine
      phosphoribosyltransferase d.
    immunoglobulin A d.
    inherited complement d.
    inherited immunoglobulin d.
    integrin alpha$_2$beta$_1$ d.
    intrinsic factor d.
    intrinsic sphincter d.
    iron d.

D

NOTES

deficiency *(continued)*
  lactase d.
  LCAT d.
  lecithin-cholesterol acyltransferase d.
  lipoprotein lipase d.
  luteal phase d.
  lysly hydroxylase d.
  mineral d.
  muscle phosphorylase d.
  myoadenylate deaminase d.
  ornithine transcarbamylase d.
  Owren d.
  prolactin d.
  protein d.
  protein C, S d.
  pseudocholinesterase d.
  pyruvate kinase d.
  qualitative d.
  r binder d.
  riboflavin d.
  selective IgA d.
  d. symptom
  taste d.
  thiamine d.
  thyroid d.
  thyroid-stimulating hormone d.
  transcobalamin II d.
  vitamin d.
  vitamin A d.
  vitamin B_{12} d.
  vitamin D d.
  vitamin K d.
  zinc d.
deficient
deficit
  cholinergic d.
  intrinsic d.
  multiple sensory d.
  neurobehavioral d.
  perceptual-spatial d.
  potassium d.
  prolonged reversible ischemic
    neurologic d. (PRIND)
  sensory d.
deformans
  arthritis d.
  osteitis d.
  osteoarthritis d.
  osteochondrodystrophia d.
  peritonitis d.
deformity
  bony d.
  bunion d.
  clawtoe d.
  equinus d.
  Haglund d.
  mallet d.
  saddle bump d.
  silver fork d.

  Sprengel d.
  Velpeau d.
degeneration
  Abercrombie d.
  adiposogenital d.
  age-related macular d. (AMD,
    ARMD)
  alcoholic cerebellar d.
  alcoholic foamy d.
  amyloid d.
  Armanni-Ehrlich d.
  cerebellar d.
  cochlear d.
  corticobasal ganglionic d.
  Crooke hyaline d.
  disk d.
  hepatolenticular d.
  hyaline d.
  macular d.
  myxomatous d.
  popliteal cystic d.
  striatonigral d.
  subacute cerebellar d.
  subacute cortical cerebellar d.
    (SCCD)
  wet age-related macular d.
degenerative
  d. arthritis (DA)
  d. joint disease (DJD)
  d. process
degenerativus
  status d.
deglutition
  d. apnea
  d. pneumonia
  d. syncope
Degos
  D. disease
  D. syndrome
degradation
  mental d.
dehiscence
dehydration fever
11-dehydrocorticosterone
dehydroepiandrosterone (DHEA)
  d. sulfate (DHEAS)
dehydro-3-epiandrosterone
dehydrogenase
  alcohol d. (ADH)
  aldehyde d.
  glucose-6-phosphate d. (G6PD)
  lactate d. (LDH)
  lactic d. (LDH)
dehydroisoandrosterone
dejecta
dejection
delavirdine mesylate
delay
  rectal-outlet d.

delayed
    d. emesis
    d. gastric emptying
    d. hemolytic transfusion reaction
    d. hypersensitivity (DH)
    d. puberty
    d. sleep phase disorder
    D. Word Recall Test
delayed-type hypersensitivity (DTH)
Del Castillo syndrome
de-lead
Delestrogen
deleterious
Delhi sore
delicate
deliensis
    Trombicula d.
delimitation
delirio
    delirium sine d.
delirium, pl. **deliria**
    acute d.
    arteriosclerotic dementia with d.
    collapse d.
    d., dementia, depression, drugs;
      eyes and ears; physical
      performance and "phalls" (falls);
      incontinence; nutrition (DEEP-IN)
    febrile d.
    d. grave
    d., infection, atrophic urethritis and
      vaginitis, pharmaceuticals,
      psychological disorders, excessive
      urine output, restricted mobility,
      stool impaction (DIAPPERS)
    low d.
    multiinfarct dementia with d.
    d. mussitans
    oneiric d.
    organic d.
    postcardiotomy d.
    postoperative d.
    primary degenerative dementia of
      Alzheimer type, presenile onset,
      with d.
    senile d.
    d. sine delirio
    substance-induced d.
    substance-intoxication d.
    substance withdrawal d.
    d. syndrome
    toxic d.

    traumatic d.
    d. tremens (DT)
delitescence
delivery
    insulin d.
    oxygen d.
    subcutaneous insulin d.
delouse
Delphian node
Delsym
delta
    D. Society
    d. virus
    d. wave
Deltasone
delusion
    persecutory d.
    primary degenerative dementia of
      Alzheimer type, presenile onset,
      with d.'s
    primary degenerative dementia of
      Alzheimer type, senile onset,
      with d.'s
delusional disorder
Demadex
demand
    oxygen d.
    d. pacemaker
demarcation
    fibrin d.
demasculinizing
d'emblée
    syphilis d.
demeclocycline
dementia
    Alzheimer d.
    arteriosclerotic d.
    Binswanger d.
    dialysis d.
    diffuse Lewy body d.
    existing d.
    frontotemporal d.
    irreversible d.
    Lewy body d.
    metabolic d.
    multiinfarct d. (MID)
    myxedematous d.
    presenile d.
    primary degenerative d.
    d. progression
    d. pugilistica

D

NOTES

dementia *(continued)*
    senile d.
    vascular d.
Demerol
demise
demographic
    d. aging
    d. information
demography
    dynamic d.
demorphinization
Demulen 1/35
demyelinating disease
demyelination
dendrite
denervation
dengue
    hemorrhagic d.
    d. hemorrhagic fever
    d. shock syndrome
Dennie-Marfan syndrome
dense cataract
densitometry
    bone mineral d.
density
    bone mineral d. (BMD)
    prostate-specific antigen transition
     zone d.
    PSA-TZ d.
    reticulonodular pulmonary d.
dental caries
dentatorubral-pallidoluysian atrophy
dentition
denture stomatitis
denudation
deontology
deoxycholate
    amphotericin B d.
2′ deoxycoformycin
deoxycorticosterone
deoxycorticosterone-producing tumor
deoxycortone
deoxypyridinoline crosslink
deoxyribonuclease
    d. A–D
deoxyribonucleic acid (DNA)
deoxyribose
Depakene
Depakote
department
    emergency d. (ED)
    D. of Justice (DOJ)
    D. of Labor (DOL)
    D. of Public Health (DPH)
    D. of Transportation (DOT)
    D. of Veterans Affairs (VA)
dependence
    drug d.

    National Council on Alcoholism
     and Drug D. (NCADD)
dependent
    age d.
    d. edema
    d. nonthrombocytopenic purpura
    d. personality disorder
    d. zone
depigmentation
depigmented
    d. rash
    d. rash of tinea versicolor
depilatory
depletion
    extracellular fluid volume d.
    phosphate d.
    potassium d.
    d. response
    sodium d.
    volume d.
depletional hyponatremia
Depo-Estradiol
depolarization
    after d.
Depo-Medrol
depomedroxyprogesterone acetate
Deponit Patch
Depo-Provera
depot
    d. injection
    d. leuprolide
    Lupron D.
    d. medroxyprogesterone (DMPA)
    d. therapy
Depo-Testosterone
deprenyl
depressant
    sedating version tricyclic d.
depressing
depression
    d. and the elderly
    endogenous d.
    Hamilton Rating Scale for D.
     (HAMD)
    late-life d.
    pacchionian d.
    psychotic d.
    ST-segment d.
depressive
    d. disorder
    d. illness
    d. symptom
deprivation
    sleep d.
deranged water and electrolyte
  transport
Dercum disease
derivative
    purified protein d. (PPD)

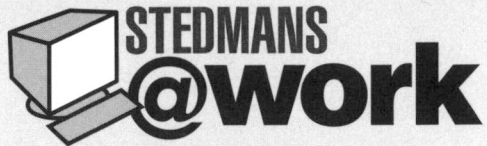

BUSINESS REPLY MAIL
FIRST CLASS   PERMIT NO. 724   BALTIMORE, MD

POSTAGE WILL BE PAID BY ADDRESSEE

ATTN: JULIE K. STEGMAN
LIPPINCOTT WILLIAMS & WILKINS
351 WEST CAMDEN STREET
BALTIMORE MD 21201-2436

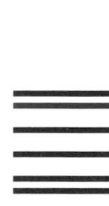

Got a Good Word for STEDMAN'S?

Help us keep STEDMAN'S products fresh and up-to-date with new words and new ideas! How can we make your STEDMAN'S product the best medical word reference possible for you?

Do we need to add or revise any items? Is there a better way to organize the content?

Be specific! Fill in the lines below with your thoughts and recommendations and FAX the page to **ATTENTION STEDMANS, 410.528.4153**.

You are our most important contributor, and we want to know what's on your mind. Thanks!

Please tell us a little bit about yourself:

Name/Title: _____

Company: _____

Address: _____

City/State/Zip: _____

Day Telephone No.: (_____) _____

E-mail Address: _____

TERMS YOU BELIEVE ARE INCORRECT:

Appears as: Suggested revision:

_____   _____

_____   _____

_____   _____

NEW TERMS/WORDS YOU WOULD LIKE US TO ADD:

_____

_____

Other comments:

_____

_____

_____

May we quote you?   ☐ Yes   ☐ No

All done? Great, just FAX this page to the attention of STEDMAN'S at 410.528.4153 or MAIL the page to us at:

ATTN: STEDMAN'S
Lippincott Williams & Wilkins
P.O. Box 17344
Baltimore, MD 21298-9595

OR enter your information
ONLINE at **www.stedmans.com**

Thanks again!

IM 738326

BUSINESS REPLY MAIL

FIRST CLASS   PERMIT NO. 724   BALTIMORE, MD

POSTAGE WILL BE PAID BY ADDRESSEE

LIPPINCOTT WILLIAMS & WILKINS
ATTN: STEDMAN'S MARKETING
351 WEST CAMDEN ST.
BALTIMORE MD. 21201-2436

dermal
>d. lymphocytic
>d. nevus

dermatitis
>atopic d.
>chronic d.
>lichenoid d.
>livedoid d.
>perioral d.
>seborrheic d.
>xerotic d.

dermatitis-arthritis syndrome
dermatitis-arthritis-tenosynovitis syndrome
dermatobiasis
dermatochalasis
dermatofibroma
dermatographism
dermatoheliosis
dermatologic
dermatology
>American Academy of D. (AAD)

dermatomal pattern
dermatome
dermatomycosis
dermatomyositis
>amyopathic d.
>corticosteroid-resistant d.
>juvenile d.

dermatopathic lymphadenopathy
dermatophyte
dermatophytid
dermatophytosis
>beard d.

dermatopolyneuritis
dermatosis, pl. **dermatoses**
>acute febrile neutrophilic d.
>bullous d.
>neutrophilic d.
>radiation d.
>vulvar d.

dermenchysis
dermoepidermal junction
dermoid
derotative osteotomy
DES
>diethylstilbestrol
>DES Action

Descemet membrane
descending
>d. colon
>left anterior d. (LAD)

d. motor pathway
>d. pathway

descensus
descent
>anterior d.
>laryngeal d.

Desenex
desensitization
desert fever
desferrioxamine
desiccated thyroid
designated caregiver
desipramine HCl
desired
>as d. (a.d. lib, a.d.)

Desitin
Desjardins point
desmoid tumor
desmopathy
desmopressin acetate
Desogen
Desonide
DesOwen
desoxycortone
Desoxyn
d'Espine sign
Desquam
desquamation
desquamative
>d. interstitial pneumonia (DIP)
>d. pneumonia

destruction
>platelet d.

desynchronization
Desyrel
detachment
>posterior vitreous d. (PVD)
>retinal d.
>rhegmatogenous retinal d. (RRD)

detection
>direct d.

deterioration
>functional d.
>senile d.

deteriorization
determinant
>disease d.

determination
>postvoid residual d.
>sweat chloride d.

determining
deterministic

D

NOTES

detoxification
Detrol
Detrol-LA
Detrusitol
detrusor
    d. areflexia
    d. hyperactivity
    d. hyperactivity with impaired
      contractility (DHIC)
    d. hyperreflexia
    d. hyporeflexia
    d. motor instability
    d. overactivity
    d. underactivity
detumescence
deuterated water
deuteropathic
deuteropathy
devastation
    senile cortical d.
development
    arrested growth and d.
    National Association for Human D.
      (NAHD)
    National Institute of Child Health
      and Human D. (NICHD)
    psychosocial d.
developmental disability
deviation
    abnormal left axis d. (ALAD)
    abnormal right axis d. (ARAD)
    standard d.
device
    abdominal aortic counterpulsation d.
      (AACD)
    abdominal left ventricular assist d.
      (ALVAD)
    aneroid d.
    assistive d.
    continuous positive airway
      pressure d.
    Diskus inhalation d.
    external vacuum d.
    fixation d.
    glucose monitoring d.
    GlucoWatch glucose monitoring d.
    Innovo Dial-a-Dose insulin
      delivery d.
    insulin delivery d.
    intrauterine d. (IUD)
    Tacticon d.
    thrombin activation d. (TAD)
    vacuum constriction d.
devil grip
devitalization
devitalize
devitalized tissue
Devonshire colic

DEXA
    dual-energy x-ray absorptiometry
    DEXA scan
dexamethasone-suppressible
  hyperaldosteronism
dexamethasone suppression test (DST)
Dexedrine
dexfenfluramine
dexterity
    manual d.
dextranomer
dextrinosis
    debranching deficiency limit d.
dextroamphetamine
dextrocardia
dextromethorphan
dextroscoliosis
dextrose
DFA
    direct fluorescent assay
DH
    delayed hypersensitivity
DHEA
    dehydroepiandrosterone
DHEAS
    dehydroepiandrosterone sulfate
DHIC
    detrusor hyperactivity with impaired
      contractility
DHT
    dihydrotestosterone
DHy
    Doctor of Hygiene
DiaBeta
diabetes
    acute decompensated d.
    adult-onset d.
    alimentary d.
    alloxan d.
    d. alternans
    brittle d.
    bronze d.
    calcinuric d.
    chemical d.
    class A d.
    d. control system
    d. education
    galactose d.
    gestational d.
    growth-onset d.
    d. innocens
    d. insipidus
    insulin-dependent d. (IDD)
    insulinopenic d.
    d. intermittens
    juvenile d.
    juvenile-onset d. (JOD)
    ketosis-prone d.
    ketosis-resistant d.

Lancereaux d.
latent d.
lipoatrophic d.
lipogenous d.
maturity-onset d.
d. mellitus (DM)
metahypophysial d.
Mosler d.
non–insulin-dependent d. (NIDD)
obesity-associated d.
overt d.
pancreatic d.
phlorizin d.
phosphate d.
piqûre d.
pregnancy d.
d. of pregnancy
puncture d.
renal d.
secondary d.
D. Self-Help Handbook
starvation d.
steroid d.
steroidogenic d.
subclinical d.
d. test
thiazide d.
type 1, 2 d.
vasopressin-resistant d.

diabetic
d. acidosis
d. amaurosis
d. amyotrophy
d. arthropathy
d. autonomic neuropathy (DAN)
d. coma
d. cystopathy
d. diarrhea
d. diet
d. enteropathy
d. foot ulcer
d. gastroenteropathy
d. glomerulosclerosis
d. iritis
d. ketoacidosis (DKA)
d. lipemia
d. mononeuropathy
d. myelopathy
d. nephropathy
d. neuropathic osteoarthropathy
   (DNOA)
d. neuropathy

d. ophthalmoplegia
d. phthisis
d. polyneuritis
d. retinopathy (DR)
d. tabes
d. xanthoma

diabetica
balanitis d.
rubeosis iridis d.
xanthosis d.

diabeticorum
bullosis d.
gastroparesis d.
xanthoma d.
xanthosis d.

diabetogenic
diabetogenous
diabetology
Diabinese
diable
bruit de d.

diabrosis
diabrotic
diachronic study
diacrisis
diacritic
diadochokinesia
diagnose
over d.

diagnosed
not yet d. (NYD)

diagnosis, pl. **diagnoses**
biopsy-proven d.
cancer d.
clinical d.
differential d.
d. by exclusion
laboratory d.
pathologic d.
physical d.

diagnosis-related group (DRG)
diagnostic
d. paracentesis
d. radiology
D. and Statistical Manual of
   Mental Disorders, Revised Third
   Edition (DSM-III-R)
d. test

diagnostician
diagonalis
conjunctiva d. (C/D)

dialysis, pl. **dialyses**

NOTES

D

dialysis *(continued)*
    Abderhalden d.
    ancillary d.
    d. ascites
    chronic peritoneal d. (CPD)
    continuous ambulatory peritoneal d.
      (CAPD)
    cycling d.
    d. dementia
    d. disequilibrium
    d. disequilibrium syndrome
    d. encephalopathy syndrome
dialysis-associated amyloidosis
dialyze
diameter
    increased colorectal d.
Diamond-Blackfan
    D.-B. anemia
    D.-B. syndrome
Diamox
Dianeal
diapedesis
diaphoresis
diaphoretic
diaphragm
    flattening of d.
diaphragmalgia
diaphragmatic
    d. breathing
    d. hernia
    d. infarction
    d. pleurisy
    d. spasm
diaphragmodynia
diaphyseal
    d. aclasis
    d. dysplasia
diaphysis, pl. **diaphyses**
diapiresis
DIAPPERS
    delirium, infection, atrophic urethritis and
    vaginitis, pharmaceuticals,
    psychological disorders, excessive urine
    output, restricted mobility, stool
    impaction
diarrhea
    acute d.
    antibiotic d.
    bacillary d.
    bile acid secretory d.
    bloody d.
    cachectic d.
    choleraic d.
    chronic bacillary d.
    d. chylosa
    Clostridium difficile-related d.
    Cochin China d.
    colliquative d.
    congenital d.

    diabetic d.
    dientamoeba d.
    drug-induced d.
    dysenteric d.
    fatty d.
    flagellate d.
    gastrogenous d.
    HIV-associated d.
    iatrogenic d.
    inflammatory d.
    lienteric d.
    morning d.
    mucous d.
    nausea, vomiting, d. (NVD)
    nocturnal d.
    osmotic d.
    pancreatic d.
    d. pancreatica
    pancreatogenous d.
    pancreatogenous fatty d.
    secretory d.
    serous d.
    summer d.
    traveler's d.
    tropical d.
    viral d.
diarrheal disease
diarrhetic
diary
    sleep d.
diastasis cordis
diastematomyelia
diastole
diastolic
    d. dysfunction
    d. hypertension
    d. murmur
diathermy
    medical d.
    shortwave d.
    ultrashortwave d.
diathesis, pl. **diatheses**
    acquired bleeding d.
    gouty d.
diathetic
diazepam
DIC
    disseminated intravascular coagulation
diclofenac
    d. gel
    d. potassium
dicloxacillin
dicyclomine
didactic
didanosine
Didronel
diem
    per d.
dienestrol

dientamoeba diarrhea
diet
    acid-ash d.
    ADA d.
    alkaline-ash d.
    American Diabetes Association d.
    balanced d.
    bananas, rice, applesauce, tea,
      toast d.
    bananas, rice cereal, applesauce,
      toast d.
    basal d.
    basic d.
    bland d.
    BRAT d.
    BRATT d.
    caffeine, alcohol, pepper, spicy
      foods-free d.
    CAPS d.
    CAPS-free d.
    challenge d.
    clear liquid d.
    DASH combination d.
    diabetic d.
    Dietary Approaches to Stop
      Hypertension d.
    Dr. Atkin's D.
    Ebstein d.
    elimination d.
    Feingold d.
    full liquid d.
    gastric II d.
    Giordano-Giovannetti d.
    Giovannetti d.
    gluten-free d.
    gout d.
    high-calorie d.
    high-fat d.
    high-fiber d.
    Kempner d.
    ketogenic d.
    lactovegetarian d.
    low-calorie d.
    low-fat d.
    low-purine d.
    low-residue d.
    low-salt d.
    low-sodium d.
    macrobiotic d.
    medically restricted d.
    Meulengracht d.
    Minot-Murphy d.

    NAS d.
    no added salt d.
    novel d.
    prudent heart d.
    puréed d.
    purine-free d.
    purine-restricted d.
    d. quality index
    rachitic d.
    reducing d.
    Schmidt d.
    Schmidt-Strassburger d.
    Sippy d.
    smooth d.
    soft mechanical d.
    subsistence d.
    vegan d.
    vegetarian d.
    Wilder d.
dietary
    d. amenorrhea
    D. Approaches to Stop
      Hypertension (DASH)
    D. Approaches to Stop
      Hypertension diet
    d. chaos
    d. counseling
    d. fiber
    d. guideline
    d. protein
    d. regulation
    d. supplement
    D. Supplement Health and
      Education Act
dietetic
    d. neuritis
    d. treatment
dietetics
diethylamide
    d-lysergic acid d.
diethylcarbamazine
diethylene glycol toxicity
diethylstilbestrol (DES)
    d. diphosphate
    d. diphosphate exposure
dieting
    yo-yo d.
dietitian
    registered d. (RD)
Dietl crisis
Dieulafoy
    D. erosion

D

NOTES

Dieulafoy *(continued)*
    D. lesion
    D. syndrome
differential
    d. diagnosis
    d. stethoscope
differentiation
    cellular d.
difficile
    Clostridium d.
difficulty
    eating d.
diffusa
    encephalitis periaxialis d.
diffuse
    d. angiokeratoma
    d. connective tissue disease
    d. cutaneous mastocytosis
    d. esophageal spasm
    d. fasciitis
    d. glandularity
    d. idiopathic skeletal hyperostosis
    (DISH)
    d. Lewy body dementia
    d. lumbosacral tenderness
    d. mastocytosis
    d. scleroderma
diffusing
    d. capacity of carbon monoxide
    d. capacity of lung for carbon
    monoxide (DLCO)
diffusion
    d. anoxia
    d. imaging
    d. impairment
    lateral d.
    d. respiration
Diflucan
diflunisal
DiGeorge syndrome
digestive
    d. apparatus
    d. fever
    d. glycosuria
digestorius
    apparatus d.
digit
    clubbed d.
    D. Symbol Subtest
digital
    d. dilatation
    d. rectal examination (DRE)
digitalis
    d. intoxication
    d. toxicity
digitalism
digitalization
digitus, pl. **digiti**
    digiti hippocratici

digoxin
    d. toxicity
Di Guglielmo syndrome
dihydrate
    calcium pyrophosphate d. (CPPD)
    crystalline calcium pyrophosphate d.
    (CCPD)
4,5-dihydrocortisol
dihydrocortisone
dihydroergotamine mesylate
dihydropteridine
dihydropyridine
dihydrotestosterone (DHT)
dihydroxy bile acid
diiodohydroxyquinoline
diisopropyliminodiacetic
    d. acid (DISIDA)
    d. acid scan
Dilacor
Dilantin
dilatation
    d. and curettage (D&C)
    digital d.
    RV d.
dilate
dilated
    d. cardiomyopathy
    d. common bile duct
    d. intrahepatic bile duct
dilation
    balloon d.
    esophageal d.
    pneumatic d.
dilator
Dilatrate-SR
Dilaudid
diltiazem hydrochloride
dilution
    d. anemia
    gas d.
    indicator d.
dilutional
    d. acidosis
    d. hyponatremia
dimercaprol
dimercaptopropanesulfonate
dimercaptosuccinic acid
Dimetane
Dimetapp
dimethyltryptamine
diminuta
    hymenolepiasis d.
diminution
dim light melatonin onset (DMLO)
DIMOAD
    diabetes insipidus, diabetes mellitus,
    optic atrophy, deafness
    DIMOAD syndrome

dimorphic
   d. anemia
   d. fungal infection
dimorphism
   sexual d.
DIMS
   disturbance in maintaining sleep
dinitrate
   isosorbide d.
Diogenes syndrome
Diovan
dioxide
   carbon d. (CO_2)
   partial pressure of carbon d.
      (PCO_2)
DIP
   desquamative interstitial pneumonia
      DIP joint
Dipentum
diphenhydramine
diphenoxylate
diphosphate
   diethylstilbestrol d.
diphosphate-glucuronosyltransferase
   uridine d.-g.
diphosphonate
diphtheria
   false d.
   faucial d.
   laryngeal d.
   laryngotracheal d.
   d., pertussis, tetanus (DPT)
   d.-tetanus toxoid (dT)
   d., tetanus toxoids, and acellular
      pertussis (DTaP)
diphtherial
diphtheric
diphtheritic
   d. enteritis
   d. myocarditis
   d. paralysis
diphtheritica
   angina d.
diphtheroid
diphyllobothriasis
diphyllobothrium anemia
diplegia
diplococcemia
Diplococcus
Diploma of Public Health (DPH)
diplomelituria

diplopia
   binocular d.
dipper
   extreme d.
dipping
   extreme d.
   ocular d.
Diprivan
Diprolene
dipropionate
   beclomethasone d.
Diprosone
dipsesis, dipsosis
dipsotherapy
dipstick
   urine d.
dipstick-positive proteinuria
dipylidiasis
dipyridamole
dipyridamole-thallium scintigraphy
direct
   d. detection
   d. diuretic
   d. fluorescent assay (DFA)
   d. mutation analysis
   d. percussion
   d. symptom
direct-acting vasodilator
direct-current shock
directed approach
direction
directional coronary atherectomy
directive
   advance d.
   comprehensive d.
director
dirithromycin
dirt-eating
disability
   developmental d.
   functional d.
disabled
   D. American Veterans (DAV)
   moderately d.
   severely d.
disabling positional vertigo
Disalcid
disarticulation
disc (*var. of* disk)
discharge
   home d.
   hospital d.

D

NOTES

discharge *(continued)*
    nipple d.
    vaginal d.
disclose
disclosure
discogenic
discoid lupus
discomfiture
discomfort
    chest d.
    respirophasic chest d.
discontinuation test
discontinue (DC)
discrete
    d. smallpox
    d. thyromegaly
discriminate
discrimination
    two-point d.
disease
    aaa d.
    Abrams d.
    accumulation d.
    Acosta d.
    acromegalic heart d.
    acromioclavicular joint d.
    active liver d.
    acute beryllium d.
    acute demyelinating d.
    acute respiratory d. (ARD)
    Adams-Stokes d.
    adaptation d.
    Addison d.
    Addison-Biermer d.
    adult polycystic kidney d. (APKD)
    age-related d.
    akamushi d.
    Alajouanine d.
    Albers-Schönberg d.
    Albright d.
    alcoholic liver d.
    allergic bowel d.
    Almeida d.
    Alpers d.
    alpha chain d.
    Alström d.
    altitude d.
    Alzheimer d. (AD)
    amebic d.
    American Foundation for
      Urologic D.'s (AFUD)
    anarthritic rheumatoid d.
    Anders d.
    Andersen d.
    Anderson-Fabry d.
    anemia of chronic d.
    anterior horn cell d.
    antibody deficiency d.

    antiglomerular basement membrane
      antibody d.
    aortic valve d.
    apatite deposition d.
    Armstrong d.
    arterial d.
    arteriosclerotic cardiovascular d.
      (ASCVD)
    arteriosclerotic heart d. (ASHD)
    arteriosclerotic mesenteric vascular
      occlusive d.
    artery d.
    asthmatic inflammatory airway d.
    atheroembolic renal d.
    atherosclerotic heart d.
    Aufrecht d.
    Australian X d.
    autoimmune d.
    autoimmune collagen vascular d.
      (ACVD)
    aviator's d.
    Ayerza d.
    Baló d.
    Bamberger d.
    Bamberger-Marie d.
    Bannister d.
    Banti d.
    Barlow d.
    Basedow d.
    basic calcium phosphate crystal
      deposition d.
    Batten d.
    Batten-Mayou d.
    Beau d.
    Beauvais d.
    Begbie d.
    Behçet d.
    Behr d.
    Bennett d.
    Benson d.
    Berger d.
    beryllium d.
    Besnier-Boeck d.
    Bielschowsky d.
    Biermer d.
    biliary tract d.
    Billroth d.
    Binswanger d.
    bird-breeder's d.
    Blount d.
    blue d.
    Blumenthal d.
    Boeck sarcoid d.
    bone d.
    Bornholm d.
    Bouchard d.
    Bouillaud d.
    bowel d.
    Bowen d.

Bradley d.
Brailsford-Morquio d.
brancher glycogen storage d.
Breda d.
Bretonneau d.
Brill d.
Brill-Symmers d.
Brill-Zinsser d.
Brinton d.
Brion-Kayser d.
bronchospastic d.
bronzed d.
Bruton d.
Budd-Chiari d.
Buerger d.
Bürger-Grütz d.
Buschke d.
Busse-Buschke d.
Byler d.
caisson d.
calcium pyrophosphate dehydrate
  deposition d.
calcium pyrophosphate deposition d.
  (CPPDD)
cardiovascular d.
Caroli d.
Carrión d.
Castellani d.
cat-bite d.
cat-scratch d. (CSD)
celiac d.
central core d.
cerebellar d.
cerebrovascular d. (CVD)
cervical spine d.
Chagas d.
Chagas-Cruz d.
Charcot joint d.
Charcot-Marie-Tooth d.
Cheadle d.
Chédiak-Higashi d.
chest wall d.
Chiari d.
Chicago d.
cholestatic liver d.
cholesterol ester storage d.
Christian d.
Christmas d.
chronic active liver d.
chronic arteriosclerotic mesenteric
  vascular occlusive d.
chronic beryllium d.

chronic coronary artery d.
chronic inflammatory bowel d.
  (CIBD)
chronic lung d.
chronic obstructive pulmonary d.
  (COPD)
Churg-Strauss d.
coexisting d.
cold agglutinin d.
cold hemagglutinin d.
collagen vascular d.
combined aortic and mitral d.
combined immunodeficiency d.
  (CID)
communicable d.
Concato d.
concomitant cardiovascular d.
congenital cardiovascular d.
congenital structural heart d.
congenital valvular d.
connective tissue d.
contagious d.
Cooley d.
Cooper d.
copper storage d.
Cori d.
coronary artery d. (CAD)
coronary heart d. (CHD)
Corvisart d.
Cowden d.
Creutzfeldt-Jakob d. (CJD)
Crigler-Najjar d.
Crocq d.
Crohn d.
Crouzon d.
cryoglobulin d.
Curschmann d.
Cushing d.
cyanotic congenital heart d.
cystic d.
cysticercus d.
cystine storage d.
cytomegalic inclusion d. (CID)
cytomegalovirus inclusion d.
Daae d.
Dalrymple d.
Darier d.
Darling d.
David d.
debilitative d.
Debove d.
decompression d.

D

NOTES

disease *(continued)*
   deer-fly d.
   deficiency d.
   degenerative joint d. (DJD)
   Degos d.
   demyelinating d.
   de Quervain d.
   Dercum d.
   d. determinant
   diarrheal d.
   diffuse connective tissue d.
   diverticular d.
   dog d.
   dominantly inherited Lévi d.
   Dressler d.
   drug-induced d.
   drug-related liver d.
   drunken rose gardener's d.
   Dubois d.
   Dukes d.
   Duncan d.
   Durand d.
   Dutton d.
   Ebstein d.
   echinococcus d.
   Ehlers-Danlos d.
   Eisenmenger d.
   elevator d.
   endemic d.
   endocrine d.
   end-stage liver d.
   end-stage renal d. (ESRD)
   English sweating d.
   epidemic d.
   Epstein d.
   Erdheim d.
   esophageal d.
   eye d.
   Fabry d.
   familial Alzheimer d. (FAD)
   Fanconi d.
   Farber d.
   Favre-Durand-Nicholas d.
   febrile d.
   Fenwick d.
   fibrocystic d.
   fibrocystic breast d.
   fifth d.
   Filatov d.
   Filatov-Dukes d.
   first d.
   Flajani d.
   flax-dresser's d.
   flint d.
   focal metastatic d.
   Fölling d.
   Forbes d.
   Forestier d.
   Fothergill d.

   fourth d.
   Francis d.
   Friedländer d.
   functional bowel d.
   Gaisböck d.
   gallbladder d.
   gallstone d.
   Gamna d.
   Gamstorp d.
   Gandy-Gamna d.
   Gandy-Nanta d.
   garapata d.
   Garré d.
   gastroesophageal reflux d. (GERD)
   gastrointestinal d.
   Gaucher d.
   genital ulcer d.
   Gerhardt-Mitchell d.
   Gierke d.
   Gilbert d.
   Gilchrist d.
   Glénard d.
   Glisson d.
   glycogen storage d.
   graft-versus-host d. (GVHD)
   Graves d.
   Greenfield d.
   Gull d.
   gum d.
   gynecologic d.
   Haff d.
   Hallervorden-Spatz d.
   Hand d.
   hand-foot-mouth d.
   Hand-Schüller-Christian d.
   Hanot d.
   Harada d.
   hard-metal lung d.
   Hartnup d.
   Hashimoto d.
   HBH d.
   heart d.
   heavy chain deposition d.
   Heberden d.
   Heerfordt d.
   hemolytic d.
   hepatocellular d.
   herring-worm d.
   Hers d.
   Herter d.
   high bone turnover d.
   Hirschsprung d.
   HIV-associated lung d.
   HIV-associated neurologic d.
   Hodgkin d.
   hookworm d.
   Horton d.
   host d.
   Huchard d.

Huntington d.
Hurler d.
Hutinel d.
hydatid d.
hydroxyapatite deposition d.
Iceland d.
I-cell d.
idiopathic d.
immune complex d.
inborn lysosomal d.
inclusion cell d.
industrial d.
infantile celiac d.
infectious d.
inflammatory airway d.
inflammatory bowel d. (IBD)
intercurrent d.
International Classification of D.'s (ICD)
interstitial d.
interstitial lung d. (ILD)
iron storage d.
ischemic coronary d. (ICD)
ischemic heart d.
island d.
Itai-Itai d.
Itsenko d.
Jakob-Creutzfeldt d.
Jansky-Bielschowsky d.
Jod-Basedow d.
juvenile Crohn d.
juvenile inflammatory bowel d.
Kahler d.
Kaposi d.
Katayama d.
Kawasaki d.
Keshan d.
Kikuchi d.
Kimmelstiel-Wilson d.
kinky-hair d.
Kirkland d.
Klemperer d.
Klippel d.
Krabbe d.
Krishaber d.
Kufs d.
Kussmaul d.
Kussmaul-Maier d.
Kyasanur Forest d.
Kyrle d.
Laënnec d.
Lafora d.

Lancereaux-Mathieu d.
Landouzy d.
Larrey-Weil d.
late-onset familial Alzheimer d.
Legal d.
Legg-Calvé-Perthes d.
Legionnaires d.
Leriche d.
Letterer-Siwe d.
Lévi d.
Lewy body d.
light chain deposition d.
Lignac d.
Lignac-Fanconi d.
lipid storage d.
liver d.
local d.
Lorain d.
Lou Gehrig d.
low bone turnover d.
Luft d.
lumbar root d.
lung fluke d.
Lutz-Splendore-Almeida d.
Lyme d.
lymphatic d.
lysosomal d.
Mackenzie d.
macrovascular d.
macular d.
mad cow d.
Madelung d.
malignant spinal d.
Manson d.
maple bark d.
maple syrup urine d.
Marburg d.
Marburg virus d.
Marchiafava-Micheli d.
Marek d.
Marie d.
Marie-Strümpell d.
Maroteaux-Lamy d.
Marsh d.
mast cell d.
Mathieu d.
McArdle d.
McArdle-Schmid-Pearson d.
mediastinal d.
medullary cystic d.
Meige d.
Meleda d.

D

NOTES

disease *(continued)*
  Menetrier d.
  Ménière d.
  meningococcal d.
  Menkes d.
  mesenteric vascular occlusive d.
  metabolic bone d.
  metabolic liver d.
  Meyer-Betz d.
  Mibelli d.
  microcrystalline d.
  microvascular d.
  Mikulicz d.
  Milroy d.
  Milton d.
  miner's d.
  mitral valve d.
  mixed aortic valve d.
  mixed connective tissue d.
    (MCTD)
  mixed mitral d.
  Möbius d.
  molecular d.
  Mondor d.
  Monge d.
  Morel d.
  Morquio d.
  Morquio-Ullrich d.
  Moschcowitz d.
  motor neuron d.
  mountain d.
  multifactorial d.
  multiinfarct d.
  multisystem d.
  multivessel d.
  muscle d.
  Myà d.
  myeloproliferative d.
  myocardial d.
  National Institute of Allergy and
    Infectious D. (NIAID)
  neoplastic d.
  neurodegenerative d.
  neurologic d.
  neuromuscular d.
  neuropsychiatric d.
  neutral lipid storage d.
  Newcastle d.
  Nicolas-Favre d.
  Niemann d.
  Niemann-Pick C d.
  Niemann-Pick C1 d.
  no appreciable d. (NAD)
  no evidence of d. (NED)
  no evidence of pulmonary d.
    (NEPD)
  no evidence of recurrent d.
    (NERD)
  noninfectious diarrheal d.

  Nonne-Milroy d.
  nontuberculin mycobacterial d.
  notifiable d.
  oasthouse urine d.
  obstructive airflow d.
  obstructive airway d. (OAD)
  obstructive lung d.
  occlusive d.
  occupational airway d.
  occupational lung d.
  occupational parenchymal d.
  Ohara d.
  Ollier d.
  ophthalmic Graves d.
  Opitz d.
  optic nerve d.
  oral d.
  organic d.
  Ormond d.
  Osgood-Schlatter d.
  Osler d.
  Osler-Vaquez d.
  Osler-Weber-Rendu d.
  Otto d.
  Owren d.
  Paget d.
  paper mill worker's d.
  parainfluenza viral d.
  parasitic d.
  parenchymal d.
  parenchymatous d.
  Parkinson d.
  Parrot d.
  Parry d.
  Parsons d.
  Pavy d.
  Payr d.
  Pel-Ebstein d.
  Pelizaeus-Merzbacher d.
  Pellegrini-Stieda d.
  pelvic inflammatory d. (PID)
  Pendred d.
  peptic ulcer d. (PUD)
  perianal d.
  pericardial d.
  periodic d.
  periodontal d.
  peripheral arterial d. (PAD)
  peripheral vascular d.
  peripheral venous d.
  Perthes d.
  Peyronie d.
  Pfeiffer d.
  Pick d.
  pineal d.
  pink d.
  pleural d.
  pleuropulmonary d.
  Plummer d.

polycystic kidney d.
polycystic ovary d.
Pompe d.
Poncet d.
Posadas d.
Posadas-Wernicke d.
Pott d.
Poulet d.
poultry handler's d.
preulcer d.
primary d.
d. process
d. progression
pseudo-Hurler d.
pulmonary d.
Quincke d.
ragpicker's d.
ragsorter's d.
rat-bite d.
Rayer d.
Raynaud d.
reactive airway d. (RAD)
Reclus d.
Reed-Hodgkin d.
reemergence of controlled d.
Refsum d.
Reichmann d.
Reiter d.
renal tubulointerstitial d.
Rendu-Osler-Weber d.
reportable d.
respiratory bronchiolitis-associated
  interstitial lung d.
respiratory muscle d.
restrictive obstructive lung d.
rheumatic aortic valve d.
rheumatic heart d.
rheumatoid d.
Ribas-Torres d.
rice d.
Riedel d.
Roger d.
Rokitansky d.
rose gardener's d.
Roth d.
Runeberg d.
Rust d.
Sach d.
salivary gland d.
Sandhoff d.
Sanfilippo d.
San Joaquin Valley d.

Saunders d.
Schamberg d.
Schaumann d.
Schenck d.
Scheuermann d.
Schilder d.
Scholz d.
Schottmüller d.
Schüller d.
Schüller-Christian d.
sclerocystic d.
screening for Alzheimer d.
secondary liver d.
self-limited d.
Senear-Usher d.
serum d.
sexually transmitted d. (STD)
Shaver d.
Sheehan d.
shimamushi d.
Shoshin d.
SH renal d.
Sichel d.
sickle cell C d.
sickle cell-thalassemia d.
silent coronary artery d.
silent coronary heart d.
silo-filler's d.
Simmonds d.
Simon d.
sixth d.
Sjögren d.
slow virus d.
Smith-Strang d.
specific d.
Spielmeyer-Sjögren d.
Spielmeyer-Vogt d.
sporadic Alzheimer d.
stage I–IV Hodgkin d.
St. Anthony d.
Steinert d.
Sternberg d.
Still d.
stonemason's d.
storage pool d.
structural heart d.
Strümpell d.
Stuart-Bras d.
Stühmer d.
Sturge d.
Sturge-Weber-Dimitri d.
Sudeck d.

D

NOTES

disease *(continued)*
- Swift d.
- swineherd's d.
- Sylvest d.
- Symmers d.
- systemic autoimmune d.
- systemic febrile d.
- Takahara d.
- Takayasu pulseless d.
- Talma d.
- Tangier d.
- Tay-Sachs d.
- tertiary d.
- Thaysen d.
- Thiemann d.
- thin basement membrane d.
- third d.
- thromboembolic d. (TED)
- thyroid d.
- Tietze d.
- Tommaselli d.
- toxic liver d.
- transfusion-associated graft-versus-host d.
- d. triad
- tricuspid valve d.
- tsutsugamushi d.
- tubulointerstitial d.
- tubulointestinal d.
- tunnel d.
- type II, III, IV, VI, VII glycogen storage d.
- ulcerative d.
- underlying d.
- Underwood d.
- undifferentiated connective tissue d.
- upper airway d.
- Urbach-Wiethe d.
- uremic small artery d.
- uterine d.
- Valsuani d.
- valvular heart d.
- vascular hepatic d.
- venereal d. (VD)
- venoocclusive d.
- venous d.
- vestibular d.
- Vogt-Spielmeyer d.
- von Gierke d.
- von Mikulicz d.
- von Recklinghausen d.
- von Willebrand d.
- Wartenberg d.
- Weber-Christian d.
- Wegener d.
- Weil d.
- Weir Mitchell d.
- Werdnig-Hoffman d.
- Werlhof d.
- Wermer d.
- Wernicke d.
- Wesselsbron d.
- Westphal-Strümpell d.
- Whipple d.
- Wilkie d.
- Wilkins d.
- Willebrand d.
- Willis d.
- Wilson d.
- Winkler d.
- Woillez d.
- Wolman d.
- woolsorter's d.
- zymotic d.

disease-modifying antirheumatic drug (DMARD)
disenrollment
disequilibrium
- dialysis d.

DISH
- diffuse idiopathic skeletal hyperostosis

DISIDA
- diisopropyliminodiacetic acid
- DISIDA scan

disimpaction
- physical d.

disinhibition
- social d.

disk, disc
- d. degeneration
- fibrovascular tissue on d. (FVD)
- herniated d.
- neovascularization of d. (NVD)

diskectomy
diskitis
Diskus inhalation device
dislocated shoulder
dislocation
disodium
- balsalazide d.

disomic disorder
disomy
disorder
- acid-base d.
- acquired coagulation d.
- adjustment d.
- adrenal medullary d.
- advanced sleep phase d.
- amebiasis d.
- amino acid metabolism d.
- anorectal d.
- antisocial personality d.
- anxiety d.
- appetite d.
- ascariasis d.
- Asperger d.
- attention deficit d. (ADD)

attention deficit hyperactivity d.
 (ADHD)
autosomal dominant d.
autosomal recessive d.
binge eating d.
bleeding d.
carbohydrate metabolism d.
chromosomal d.
circadian rhythm d.
circadian rhythm-based sleep d.
clonorchiasis d.
coagulation d.
congenital d.
connective tissue d.
delayed sleep phase d.
delusional d.
dependent personality d.
depressive d.
disomic d.
dysthymic d.
eating d.
echinococcosis d.
electrolyte d.
esophageal motility d.
esophageal motor d.
extrapyramidal d.
fascioliasis d.
female sexual arousal d.
functional gastrointestinal d.
gait d.
gastrointestinal d.
generalized anxiety d. (GAD)
genetic d.
Haglund d.
hemostatic d.
hepatic infiltrative d.
heredogenerative d.
histrionic personality d.
hypoactive sexual desire d.
immune complex d.
inherited bleeding d.
inherited connective tissue d.
inherited thromboembolic d.
intestinal myopathic d.
lacrimal d.
late luteal phase dysphoric d.
 (LLPDD)
LDL receptor d.
loss-of-function d.
low-density lipoprotein receptor d.
mendelian d.
metabolic d.

metabolism d.
mitochondrial d.
mixed acid-base d.
mood d.
motility d.
movement d.
multifactorial d.
myeloproliferative d.
National Institute on Deafness and
 Other Communication D.'s
 (NIDCD)
National Organization of Rare D.'s
 (NORD)
neuronal migration d.
obsessive-compulsive d. (OCD)
obsessive-compulsive personality d.
Paget Foundation for Paget's
 Disease of Bone and
 Related D.'s
pancreaticobiliary d.
panic d.
periodic limb movement d.
 (PLMD)
peripheral nervous system d.
personality d.
pituitary d.
plasma iodoprotein d.
platelet d.
posttraumatic stress d.
premenstrual dysphoric d. (PMDD)
primary sleep d.
psychiatric d.
qualitative platelet d.
schistosomiasis d.
schizoaffective d.
schizophreniform d.
seasonal affective d. (SAD)
sensory d.
sexual aversion d.
sexual desire d.
simple acid-base d.
sleep phase d.
smell d.
somatoform d.
spastic motility d.
spinal d.
storage d.
stress-related d.
strongyloidiasis d.
taste d.
testicular d.
thromboembolic d.

D

NOTES

disorder *(continued)*
    toxocariasis d.
    ventilatory control d.
    X-linked d.
disorganization
disparity
    National Center on Minority Health
      and Health D.'s (NCMHD)
dispensary
dispensatory
dispense
dispersion
    amphotericin B colloidal d.
    colloidal d.
disproportionately
disruption
    sleep d.
dissecans
    osteochondritis d.
    pneumonia d.
dissecting aneurysm
dissection
    aortic d.
    block d.
    lymph node d.
disseminate
disseminated
    d. aspergillosis
    d. candidiasis
    d. coccidioidomycosis
    d. cryptococcosis
    d. fungal infection
    d. gonococcal infection
    d. herpes simplex virus infection
    d. intravascular coagulation (DIC)
    d. lipogranulomatosis
    d. lupus erythematosus (DLE)
    d. MAC
    d. *Mycobacterium avium* complex
dissemination
    hematogenous d.
disseminatus
    lupus erythematosus d. (LED)
dissociated sensation
dissociation
    atrioventricular d.
    AV d.
    electromechanical d. (EMD)
distal
    d. chevron osteotomy
    d. flow rate
    d. ileitis
    d. interphalangeal joint
    d. intestinal obstructive syndrome
    d. to proximal
    d. pulse
distance
    shuttle-walking d.

distention, distension
    capsular d.
    jugular venous d. (JVD)
    sudden d.
distinguishing
distomiasis
    hemic d.
    hepatic d.
    pulmonary d.
distortion
    visuospatial d.
distraction
    d. injury
    d. technique
distress
    abdominal d.
    psychological d.
distribution
    beltlike d.
    stocking d.
    volume of d.
distributive shock
disturbance
    acid-base d.
    conduction d.
    electrolyte d.
    gait d.
    intraventricular conduction d.
    d. in maintaining sleep (DIMS)
    psychiatric d.
    visual d.
disturbed behavior
disuse
    d. atrophy
    d. syndrome
dithiocarbamate
Ditropan XL
Diulo
diurese
diuresis
    alcohol d.
    alkaline d.
    forced alkaline d.
    osmotic d.
    saline d.
    water d.
diuretic
    direct d.
    indirect d.
    loop d.
    non-potassium-sparing d.
    potassium-sparing d.
    d. therapy
    thiazide d.
diuretic-induced
    d.-i. hyponatremia
Diuril
diurnal blood pressure

diver's
> d. palsy
> d. paralysis

diversion colitis

diverticula (*pl. of* diverticulum)

diverticular
> d. abscess
> d. bleeding
> d. disease

diverticulitis

diverticulosis coli

diverticulum, pl. **diverticula**
> diverticula of colon
> colonic d.
> duodenal d.
> esophageal d.
> Meckel d.
> pharyngoesophageal d.
> Rokitansky d.
> urethral d.
> Zenker d.

divided
> d. dose
> d. pancreas

divisum
> pancreas d.

Dix-Hallpike maneuver

Dixon Mann sign

dizygotic twin

dizziness
> multiple sensory defect d.
> psychogenic d.
> d. simulation battery

DJD
> degenerative joint disease

djenkol poisoning

DKA
> diabetic ketoacidosis

dL
> deciliter

DLCO
> diffusing capacity of lung for carbon
> monoxide

DLE
> disseminated lupus erythematosus

d-lysergic acid diethylamide

DM
> diabetes mellitus

DMARD
> disease-modifying antirheumatic drug

DMLO
> dim light melatonin onset

DMPA
> depot medroxyprogesterone

DNA
> deoxyribonucleic acid
> hepatitis B DNA
> DNA synthesis

DNH
> do not hospitalize
> DNH order
> DNH status

DNOA
> diabetic neuropathic osteoarthropathy

DNR
> do not resuscitate
> DNR order
> DNR status

DO
> Doctor of Osteopathy

do
> do not hospitalize (DNH)
> do not resuscitate (DNR)

DOA
> dead on arrival

DOB
> date of birth

Dobbhoff tube

dobutamine
> d. echocardiogram (DE)
> d. echocardiography (DE)
> d. hydrochloride
> d. spiff
> d. stress echocardiography

Dobutrex

docetaxel

docosahexaenoic acid

doctor
> D. of Chiropractic (DC)
> D. of Hygiene (DHy)
> D. of Medicine (MD)
> D. of Osteopathy (DO)
> D. of Public Health (DPH, DrPH)

doctor-patient relationship

doctrine
> humoral d.

docusate

Döderlein bacillus

DOE
> dyspnea on exertion

dofetilide

dog
> d. bite
> d. disease

NOTES

D

DOJ
Department of Justice
DOL
Department of Labor
doll's
d. eyes
d. eye sign
d. eye test
d. head maneuver
Dolobid
dolor
dolorosa
adiposis d.
facies d.
domain
recognition d.
Domeboro soak
domestic violence
domiciliated
dominant
left-hand d.
right-hand d.
dominantly inherited Lévi disease
domperidone study
Donath-Landsteiner syndrome
donepezil hydrochloride
Donnagel
Donnatal Extentabs
donner
long-handled sock d.
donor
living d.
lung d.
d. selection
do-not-hospitalize
d.-n.-h. order
d.-n.-h. status
do-not-resuscitate
d.-n.-r. order
d.-n.-r. status
donovanosis
dopamine
d. agonist
d. antagonist
d. precursor
dopamine-receptor agonist
dopaminergic agent
dope
Doppler
color flow D.
D. probe
pulsed D.
D. study
D. ultrasound
Doral
d'orange
peau d.
Dorcol
Dorfman-Chanarin syndrome

dornase alfa
dorsa (*pl. of* dorsum)
dorsal
d. column neurostimulation
d. column stimulator
d. horn
d. raphe
d. recumbent
d. root ganglion (DRG)
dorsalgia
dorsalis
d. pedis (DP)
tabes d.
dorsi
elastofibroma d.
longissimus d.
dorsiflexion
dorsiflexor
dorsum, pl. **dorsa**
Doryx
dosage
trough of d.
dose
booster d.
curative d.
daily d.
divided d.
effective d. (ED)
fractional d.
initial d.
d. intensification
lethal d. (LD)
loading d.
maintenance d.
maximal permissible d.
minimal d.
optimum d.
pediatric d. (PD)
preventive d.
tolerance d.
Dosepak
Medrol D.
doser
insulin d.
dose-response effect
dosimetry
dosing
d. regimen
d. schedule
Dospan
Tenuate D.
Dostinex
DOT
Department of Transportation
dot
Schüffner d.
dot-and-blot hemorrhage
double
d. blind study

d. pleurisy
d. pneumonia
d. quartan
d. quotidian fever
d. tertian
d. tertian malaria
douche bath
doughnut pessary
doughy
d. abdomen
d. consistency
douloureux
tic d.
dousing bath
Dovonex
dowager's hump
downbeat nystagmus
Down syndrome
doxazosin
doxepin HCl
Doxidan
doxorubicin
liposomal d.
doxycycline
doxylamine
DP
dorsalis pedis
D-penicillamine
DPH
Department of Public Health
Diploma of Public Health
Doctor of Public Health
DPT
diphtheria, pertussis, tetanus
DR
diabetic retinopathy
Dr.
Dr. Atkin's Diet
Dr. Scholl
dracunculiasis
drain
Jackson-Pratt d.
Penrose d.
drainage
incision and d. (I&D)
draining sinus
Dramamine
drape
drapeau
bruit de d.
drawback
potential d.

drawer sign
drawing
DRE
digital rectal examination
drepanocytic anemia
Dresbach
D. anemia
D. syndrome
dressing
Coban d.
Curasol gel wound d.
DuoDerm d.
hydrocolloid d.
hydrogel d.
Silon Dual-Dress wound d.
silver sulfadizine d.
Telfa d.
wet-to-dry d.
wound d.
Dressler
D. disease
D. syndrome
DRG
diagnosis-related group
dorsal root ganglion
dribble
dribbling
terminal d.
drift
pronator d.
drinking
problem d.
drip phleboclysis
Drisdol
driving
Bioptic spectacle-mounted telescope
for d.
Drixoral
dronabinol
drop
d. attack
Auralgan d.'s
d. hand
OcuHist antihistamine decongestant
eye d.'s
polymyxin B-neomycin-cortisone d.
droplet
airborne d.
d. precaution
dropper

D

NOTES

dropsical
>d. nephritis
>d. nephropathy

dropsy
>cardiac d.
>epidemic d.
>famine d.
>nutritional d.
>d. of pericardium

drowning
>secondary d.

drowsiness

DrPH
>Doctor of Public Health

drug
>d. abuse
>alternative d.
>anorectic d.
>antiarrhythmic d.
>anticholinesterase d.
>antiinflammatory d.
>antimalarial d.
>antithyroid d.
>antiviral d.
>cardiovascular d.
>chemotherapeutic d.
>d. clearance
>d. dependence
>disease-modifying antirheumatic d. (DMARD)
>d. fever
>generic d.
>d. half-life
>high-hepatic clearance d.
>immunomodulatory d.
>d. interaction
>lipid-lowering d.
>low-hepatic clearance d.
>d. metabolism
>neuroleptic antipsychotic d.
>neuroprotective d.
>neutropic d.
>nonsteroidal antiinflammatory d. (NSAID)
>over-the-counter d.
>prokinetic d.
>psychoactive d.
>d. reaction
>d. study
>supergeneric d.
>d. tolerance
>d. toxicity
>uricosuric d.
>vestibulotoxic d.
>d. withdrawal

drug-drug interaction

drug-induced
>d.-i. diarrhea
>d.-i. disease
>d.-i. dyspepsia
>d.-i. fever
>d.-i. hemolytic anemia
>d.-i. hepatitis
>d.-i. immune thrombocytopenia
>d.-i. intrahepatic cholestasis
>d.-i. lupus
>d.-i. lupus erythematosus
>d.-i. neutropenia
>d.-i. parkinsonism
>d.-i. platelet dysfunction
>d.-i. steatosis
>d.-i. vascular purpura

drug-related liver disease

drunkenness

drunken rose gardener's disease

drusen

dry
>d. AMD
>d. eye
>d. eye syndrome
>d. heaves
>d. mouth
>d. nurse
>d. pack
>d. rale
>d. skin
>d. vomiting
>d. weight

Drysol

DS
>Septra DS
>Tolectin DS

DSC
>Parafon Forte DSC

DSM-III-R
>Diagnostic and Statistical Manual of Mental Disorders, Revised Third Edition

DST
>dexamethasone suppression test

DT
>delirium tremens

dT
>diphtheria-tetanus toxoid

DTaP
>diphtheria, tetanus toxoids, and acellular pertussis
>>Infanrix DTaP

DTH
>delayed-type hypersensitivity

DTIC-Dome

DTR
>deep tendon reflex

D-TRON insulin pump

dual-contrast barium enema (DCBE)

dual-energy
>d.-e. absorptiometry

d.-e. x-ray absorptiometry (DEXA)
d.-e. x-ray absorptiometry scan
duality of pain
dual pacing
Dual-Pak
Monistat D.-P.
DUB
dysfunctional uterine bleeding
Dubin-Johnson syndrome
Dubois
D. abscess
D. disease
DuBois formula
Dubowitz
Duchenne
D. muscular dystrophy
D. sign
Duckworth sign
Ducrey bacillus
duct
common bile d.
dilated common bile d.
dilated intrahepatic bile d.
intrahepatic bile d.
müllerian d.
Pecquet d.
Wharton d.
Wirsung d.
wolffian d.
ductal
d. carcinoma
d. carcinoma in situ (DCIS)
ductopenic rejection
ductus
patent d.
Duke Mobility Assessment
Dukes disease
Dulcolax
dullness
absolute cardiac d. (ACD)
bibasilar d.
shifting d.
Dumdum fever
dumping syndrome
Duncan
D. disease
D. syndrome
duocrinin
duodenal
d. bulb
d. diverticulum

d. gastrinoma
d. ulcer
duodenitis
duodenogastric reflux
duodenum
DuoDerm dressing
DuoFilm
DuoNeb
DuoPlant
duplication
ureteral d.
Dupuytren
D. contracture
D. fascia
D. hydrocele
D. suture
Duragesic
Durand disease
durans
Enterococcus d.
duration
QRS d.
Duratuss
Dura-Vent
Duricef
Durkan sign
durum
heloma d.
dust asthma
Dutton
D. disease
D. relapsing fever
DVT
deep vein thrombosis
deep venous thrombosis
dwarf
achondroplastic d.
hypophysial d.
hypopituitary d.
hypothyroid d.
Laron d.
Paltauf d.
pituitary d.
dwarfism
aortic d.
asexual d.
ateliotic d.
Fröhlich d.
hypothyroid d.
infantile d.
Laron d.
Laron-type d.

D

NOTES

123

dwarfism *(continued)*
    Lorain-Lévi d.
    physiologic d.
    pituitary d.
    primordial d.
    sexual d.
    snub-nose d.
    true d.
    tryptophanuria with d.
D-xylose
Dyazide
Dymelor
DynaCirc
dynamic
    d. demography
    d. ileus
dynamometer
    Jamar d.
Dynapen
dynorphin
Dyrenium
dysarthria
dysautonomia
    familial d. (FD)
    Riley-Day d.
dysbetalipoproteinemia
    familial d.
dysbolism
dyschezia
    rectal d.
dyschondroplasia
dyscrasia
    blood d.
    lymphatic d.
dysdiadochokinesia
dysenteric
    d. algid malaria
    d. diarrhea
dysentery
    amebic d.
    bacillary d.
    balantidial d.
    bilharzial d.
    fulminating d.
    helminthic d.
    institutional d.
    malignant d.
    viral d.
dysequilibrium
dysesthesia
dysfibrinogenemia
dysfunction
    acute organ d.
    age-related diastolic d.
    beta cell d.
    central nervous system d.
    cognitive d.
    constitutional hepatic d.
    coronary microvascular d.

    diastolic d.
    drug-induced platelet d.
    erectile d. (ED)
    female sexual d.
    gastric motor d.
    gastrointestinal d.
    generalized distal nephron d.
    gonadal d.
    hematologic d.
    hepatobiliary d.
    hypothalamic d.
    hypothalamic-pituitary d.
    left ventricular systolic d. (LVSD)
    liver d.
    orgasmic d.
    ovarian d.
    parietooccipital d.
    proximal renal tubule d.
    renal allograft d.
    renal tubule d.
    senile sinus node d.
    spinal cord d.
    sudomotor d.
    systolic d.
    thyroid d.
dysfunctional
    d. pulmonary vascular endothelium
    d. uterine bleeding (DUB)
dysgenesis
    gonadal d.
    seminiferous tubule d.
    testicular d.
dysgerminoma
dysgeusia
dysgraphia
dyshidrosis
dyshidrotic eczema
dyskeratosis congenita
dyskinesia
    paroxysmal d.
    poststatic d.
    tardive d.
dyskinetic
dyslipidemia
dyslipidosis
dyslipoproteinemia
dysmenorrhea
dysmetria
dysmorphic
dysmotility
    colorectal d.
dysmyelopoietic syndrome
dysorexia
dysosmia
dysostosis multiplex
dyspareunia
dyspepsia
    acid d.
    adhesion d.

atonic d.
drug-induced d.
fermentative d.
flatulent d.
functional d.
nervous d.
nonulcer d.
reflex d.
dyspeptic
dysphagia
esophageal d.
oropharyngeal d.
dysphagic stroke
dysphasia
dysphonia
dysphoria
dysphoric manic episode
dyspigmentation
dyspinealism
dyspituitarism
dysplasia
acromelic d.
arteriohepatic d.
cerebral cortical d.
cervical d.
diaphyseal d.
ectodermal d.
fibromuscular d.
fibrous d.
histologic benign prostatic d.
keratinocytic d.
olfactogenital d.
septooptic d.
spondyloepiphysial d.
squamous d.
dysplastic
d. Barrett epithelium
d. kidney
d. nevus
dyspnea
cardiac d.
chronic d.
exertional d.
expiratory d.
functional d.
nocturnal d.
d. on exertion (DOE)
paroxysmal nocturnal d. (PND)
Traube d.

dyspneic
dysponderal
dyspragia
dyspraxia
dysproteinemia
angioimmunoblastic
lymphadenopathy with d. (AILD)
dysproteinemic
dysraphism
dysrhythmia
esophageal d.
dysspermatogenic sterility
dyssynergia
pelvic floor d.
dysthymia
dysthymic
d. disorder
d. disorder dystonia
dysthyroidal infantilism
dysthyroid myopathy
dystonia
dysthymic disorder d.
nocturnal paroxysmal d.
tardive d.
dystrophia
d. adiposogenitalis
d. brevicollis
dystrophic
dystrophy
adiposogenital d.
Becker muscular d. (BMD)
cerebroocular-dysplasia muscular d.
Duchenne muscular d.
facioscapulohumeral muscular d.
Fuchs d.
hyperplastic d.
hypertrophic d.
Landouzy d.
Landouzy-Déjèrine d.
limb-girdle d.
muscular d. (MD)
myotonic d.
oculopharyngeal d.
reflex sympathetic d. (RSD)
thoracic asphyxiant d. (TAD)
vulval d.
dysuria
dysuric
dysury

D

NOTES

E_1
    prostaglandin E_1
E1A protein
each (q.)
E to A change
EAHF
    eczema, asthma, hay fever
    EAHF complex
ear
    e. loop
    swimmer's e.
early
    e. asthmatic response
    e. latent syphilis
    e. missed AB
    e. morning surge
    e. reinfarction
    e. syphilis
    E. versus Later L-DOPA
      (ELLDOPA)
    E. versus Later L-DOPA study
    e. wakening
early-stage breast cancer
earplug
ears, nose, throat (ENT)
east
    E. African sleeping sickness
    E. African trypanosomiasis
eating
    e. difficulty
    e. disorder
Eaton-Lambert
    myasthenic syndrome of E.-L.
      (MSEL)
    E.-L. syndrome
EBCT
    electron beam computed tomography
Ebola
    E. hemorrhagic fever
    E. virus
EBRT
    external beam radiation therapy
Ebstein
    E. anomaly
    E. diet
    E. disease
    E. lesion
EBV
    Epstein-Barr virus
    EBV titer
EC
    Elder Craftsmen
ecchymosis, pl. **ecchymoses**
ecchymotic purpura
ecdemic

ECG, EKG
    electrocardiogram
    electrocardiograph
    electrocardiography
ecgonine methyl ester
echinacea
    E. purpura
echinococciasis
echinococcosis disorder
echinococcus disease
echinocytosis
echinostomiasis
echocardiogram
    dobutamine e. (DE)
    transesophageal e. (TEE)
    transthoracic e.
    two-dimensional e.
echocardiographic assessment
echocardiography
    dobutamine e. (DE)
    dobutamine stress e.
    transesophageal e. (TEE)
    transthoracic e. (TTE)
    transthoracic two-dimensional e.
    two-dimensional transthoracic e.
echo-Doppler cardiography
echogenic
echoic memory
echolalia
echophony
echovirus
eclampsia
eclectic
E. coli
    Escherichia coli
ecology
    human e.
econazole nitrate
economic status
ECT
    electroconvulsive therapy
ectasia
ectatic emphysema
ecthyma
ectocrine
ectodermal dysplasia
ectopia
    e. cordis abdominalis
    thyrotoxicosis e.
ectopic
    e. ACTH syndrome
    e. adrenocorticotropic hormone
    syndrome
    e. atrial tachycardia
    e. hormone

E

ectopic *(continued)*
    e. RNA
    e. schistosomiasis
    e. thyroid
ectopy
    complex ventricular e.
    ureteral e.
    ventricular e.
ectoscopy
ectrocheiry
ectropion
eczema
    e., asthma, hay fever (EAHF)
    e., asthma, hay fever complex
    e. craquelé
    dyshidrotic e.
    nummular e.
eczematoid
ED
    effective dose
    emergency department
    erectile dysfunction
EDC
    estimated date of confinement
ED&C
    electrodesiccation and curettage
Edecrin
Edelmann anemia
edema
    acute cardiogenic pulmonary e.
     (ACPE)
    ambulant e.
    angioneurotic e.
    ankle e.
    bilateral ankle e.
    bilateral leg e.
    brawny e.
    cachectic e.
    cardiogenic pulmonary e.
    cystoid macular e.
    dependent e.
    high-altitude cerebral e.
    hydremic e.
    hydrostatic pulmonary e.
    idiopathic leg e.
    laryngeal e.
    leg e.
    marantic e.
    Milroy e.
    Milton e.
    nonhydrostatic pulmonary e.
    nonpitting e.
    nutritional e.
    pedal e.
    peripheral e.
    Pirogoff e.
    pitting e.
    prehepatic e.
    pulmonary e.

    Quincke e.
    reentry pulmonary e.
    refeeding e.
    Reinke e.
    salt e.
    Stellwag brawny e.
    trace ankle e.
    unilateral leg e.
edematous
edentulous
edition
    Diagnostic and Statistical Manual
     of Mental Disorders, Revised
     Third E. (DSM-III-R)
edrophonium test
education
    Association for Gerontology in
     Higher E. (AGHE)
    diabetes e.
    National Council on Patient
     Information and E. (NCPIE)
EDVI
    end-diastolic volume index
EEG
    electroencephalogram
    EEG bandwidth
EEOC
    Equal Employment Opportunity
     Commission
E.E.S. 400 Filmtab
EF
    ejection fraction
efavirenz
effect
    additive e.
    adverse e.
    antiadrenergic e.
    blast e.
    Bohr e.
    cardiac conduction e.
    cardioprotective e.
    cumulative e.
    cyclosporine e.
    cytopathic e.
    cytoprotective e.
    dawn e.
    dose-response e.
    extrapyramidal side e.
    Haldane e.
    hemodynamic e.
    hepatotoxic e.
    inoculum e.
    inotropic e.
    placebo e.
    pressure e.
    side e.
    Somogyi e.
    Staub-Traugott e.
    synergistic e.

thermic e.
Wolff-Chaikoff e.
effective dose (ED)
effectiveness
effemination
efferent
Effexor XR
efficacious
efficacy
efficiency
sleep e.
effluvium
efflux
effort
e. syncope
unsustained e.
effusion
chyliform pleural e.
exudative pleural e.
ipsilateral pleural e.
joint e.
loculated pleural e.
malignant pericardial e.
malignant pleural e.
neoplastic pericardial e.
pericardial e.
pleural e.
transudative pleural e.
undiagnosed pleural e.
Efudex
EGD
esophagogastroduodenoscopy
egesta
egg crate foam mattress
egg-white
e.-w. injury
e.-w. syndrome
egophony
Egyptian hematuria
EHC
essential hypercholesterolemia
EHEC
enterohemorrhagic *Escherichia coli*
EHL
endogenous hyperlipidemia
Ehlers-Danlos
E.-D. disease
E.-D. syndrome
Ehrlichia
E. infection
E. phagocytophilia

ehrlichiosis
human granulocytic e. (HGE)
EICL
Eldercare Initiative in Consumer Law
eicosapentaenoic acid
EIEC
enteroinvasive *Escherichia coli*
Eikenella corrodens
Eisenmenger
E. complex
E. disease
E. physiology
E. syndrome
ejaculate
ejaculation
premature e.
retarded e.
ejecta
ejection
e. fraction (EF)
e. fraction of heart
EKC
epidemic keratoconjunctivitis
EKG (*var. of* ECG)
electrocardiogram
electrocardiograph
electrocardiography (*See also* ECG)
ekiri
elastic
e. skin
e. stocking
elasticum
pseudoxanthoma e.
elastin fibril
elastofibroma dorsi
Elastoplast wrap
elastosis
solar e.
Elavil
elbow
golfer's e.
e. pain
tennis e.
ELCA
excimer laser coronary angioplasty
Eldepryl
elder
e. abuse
Assessing Care of Vulnerable E.'s
(ACOVE)
E. Craftsmen (EC)

E

NOTES

Eldercare
> E. Initiative in Consumer Law (EICL)
> E. Locator

Elderhostel

elderly
> acute care for the e. (ACE)
> Clearinghouse on Abuse and Neglect of the E. (CANE)
> depression and the e.
> epilepsy and the e.
> frail e.
> Hearing-Handicap Inventory for the E.
> inflammatory bowel disease and the e.
> innocent murmur of e.
> insomnia and the e.
> Legal Counsel for the E. (LCE)
> Legal Services for the E. (LSE)
> National Association for Hispanic E.
> Program of All-Inclusive Care for the E. (PACE)

Elderweb

electric
> e. bath
> e. shock
> e. shock-like

electrical stimulation

electrobioscopy

electrocardiogram (ECG, EKG)
> exercise e.
> 12-lead e.
> resting e.

electrocardiograph (ECG, EKG)

electrocardiography (ECG, EKG)
> ambulatory e. (AECG)
> exercise e.
> resting e.

electrocoagulation

electroconvulsive therapy (ECT)

electrocute

electrocution

electrode
> active e.
> exciting e.
> localizing e.
> therapeutic e.

electrodesiccate

electrodesiccation and curettage (ED&C)

electrodiagnosis

electroencephalogram (EEG)
> e. bandwidth

electrogalvanic

electrogastrogram

electrogastrograph

electrogastrography

electrogustometry

electrolyte
> e. abnormality
> defective regulation of intestinal water and e.'s
> e. disorder
> e. disturbance
> e. imbalance
> e. therapy

electrolytes (*var. of* lytes)

electromechanical dissociation (EMD)

electromicturation

electromyogram (EMG)

electromyography (EMG)
> sphincter e.

electron
> e. beam computed tomography (EBCT)
> e. microscopy
> e. paramagnetic resonance (EPR)

electrooculogram (EOG)

electropharmacologic testing

electrophoresis
> serum protein e. (SPEP)

electrophysiologic testing

electrophysiology

electroretinogram (ERG)

electrostethograph

electrothanasia

electrotherapeutics

electrotherm

electrovaporization

eleotherapy

elephantoid fever

eletriptan

elevated
> e. lipoprotein
> e. prostate-specific antigen level

elevation
> jugular venous pressure e.
> liver enzyme e.
> rest, ice, compression, e. (RICE)
> serum transaminase level e.
> ST segment e.

elevator
> e. disease
> Goldman e.

elicit

elimination diet

Elimite

ELISA
> enzyme-linked immunoassay
> enzyme-linked immunosorbent assay

elixir
> Mycostatin e.
> Organidin e.

ELLDOPA
> Early versus Later L-DOPA
> ELLDOPA study

Ellipse compact spacer

elliptocytary anemia
elliptocyte
elliptocytosis
>hereditary e.
>spherocytic hereditary e.

elliptocytotic anemia
Ellsworth-Howard test
elm
>slippery e.

Elocon
Elspar
elucidate
elucidating
emaciation
EMB
>eosin methylene blue

embalm
emboli (*pl. of* embolus)
embolic
>e. abscess
>e. event
>e. mesenteric vascular occlusion
>e. stroke

embolism
>air e.
>coronary artery e.
>pulmonary e. (PE)

embolization
>coil e.
>systemic e.

embolus, pl. **emboli**
>arterial e.
>cardiogenic e.
>pulmonary e. (PE)

embryonal leukemia
EMD
>electromechanical dissociation

emebic infection
emergency
>e. department (ED)
>hypertensive e.
>medical e.
>oncologic e.
>e. RBC transfusion
>e. red blood cell transfusion
>treatment-related e.

emergent
emesis, pl. **emeses**
>e. basin
>coffeeground e.
>delayed e.
>refractory e.

emetic
emetocathartic
Emetrol
EMG
>electromyogram
>electromyography
>exomphalos, macroglossia, and gigantism
>>EMG syndrome

eminence
>thenar e.

emmetropia
emotion
emotional lability
emphysema
>alveolar duct e.
>centriacinar e.
>ectatic e.
>pulmonary interstitial e. (PIE)
>subcutaneous e.

emphysematous
>e. bleb
>e. pyelitis

empiric
>e. antibiotic
>e. risk
>e. treatment

empirical
empirically based
empiricism
emptying
>delayed gastric e.
>gastric e.
>incomplete e.

empty sella syndrome
empyema
>e. of gallbladder
>parapneumonic e.
>pneumococcal e.
>streptococcal e.
>subdural e.

emulsifying agent
emulsion
>fat e.

E-Mycin
enalapril maleate
enameloblastoma
enanthate
encainide HCl
encephalitis
>granulomatous amebic e.
>Japanese e.
>e. periaxialis diffusa

NOTES

encephalitis *(continued)*
    postinfluenzal e.
    Rasmussen e.
    tick-borne e. (TBE)
    toxic e.
    Venezuelan equine e.
    viral e.
    Wernicke-Korsakoff e.
    Western equine e. (WEE)
encephalomyelitis
    acute disseminated e.
    benign myalgic e.
    epidemic myalgic e.
encephalopathy
    anoxic e.
    hepatic e.
    hypernatremic e.
    hypertensive e.
    metabolic e.
    Wernicke e.
enchondroma
    central e.
enchondromatosis
encode
    genome e.
encopresis
encroachment
    foramen e.
end
    e. organ
    e. products
    e. stage
    e. systole
    e. terminal parathyroid hormone
Endal
endarterectomy
    carotid e. (CEA)
endarteritis
end diastole
end-diastolic volume index (EDVI)
endemic
    e. disease
    e. goiter
    e. hematuria
    e. hemoptysis
    e. influenza
    e. neuritis
    e. nonbacterial infantile
      gastroenteritis
    e. osteoarthritis
    e. polyneuritis
    e. stability
    e. syphilis
    e. typhus
endemica
    osteoarthritis deformans e.
Endep
endermic

end-expiratory
    e.-e. pressure
    e.-e. wheeze
endoauscultation
endocapillary
endocarditis
    acute bacterial e. (ABE)
    acute infective e. (AIE)
    bacterial e.
    candidal e.
    gonococcal e.
    infective e.
    Libman-Sacks e.
    native valve e.
    nonbacterial thrombotic e. (NBTE)
    prosthetic valve e. (PVE)
    subacute e.
    subacute bacterial e. (SBE)
endochondral osteogenesis
endocolitis
endocrine
    e. disease
    e. gland
    e. organ transplant complication
    e. system
    e. theory
    e. tumor
endocrinologist
endocrinology
endocrinopathic
endocrinopathy
endocrinotherapy
endocytosis
endodermal
endoenteritis
end-of-life
    e.-o.-l. care
    e.-o.-l. decision
    e.-o.-l. decision making
endogastritis
endogenic toxicosis
endogenous
    e. depression
    e. hyperglyceridemia
    e. hyperinsulinemic hypoglycemia
    e. hyperlipidemia (EHL)
    e. hypothermia
    e. obesity
    e. opioid peptide
    e. pattern
    e. pyrogen
Endolimax
endoluminal stenting
endolymphatic hydrops
endometrial
    e. cancer
    e. hyperplasia
endometrioma
endometriosis

endometritis
endomotorsonde
endomyocardial biopsy
endomyocardium
endoperimyocarditis
endophthalmitis
    bacterial e.
endorphin
endoscope
endoscopic
    e. band ligation
    e. hemostatic therapy
    e. injection sclerotherapy
    e. retrograde
      cholangiopancreatogram (ERCP)
    e. retrograde
      cholangiopancreatography (ERCP)
    e. ultrasonography
endoscopy
    peroral e.
    upper gastrointestinal e.
endostethoscope
endothelial
endothelioma
    Sidler-Huguenin e.
endothelium
    dysfunctional pulmonary vascular e.
endothelium dependent
endotoxin
endotracheal (ET)
    e. tube
endovaccination
endovascular therapy
endovenous
endplate
end-respiratory crackle
end-stage
    e.-s. acute leukemia
    e.-s. liver disease
    e.-s. renal disease (ESRD)
end-systolic
    e.-s. volume
    e.-s. volume index (ESVI)
Enduron
enema
    air-contrast barium e.
    analeptic e.
    barium e. (BE)
    blind e.
    dual-contrast barium e. (DCBE)
    flatus e.
    high e.

    nutrient e.
    oil retention e.
    soapsuds e.
    turpentine e.
enemator
enemiasis
energetic
energy
engineering
    biomedical e.
English sweating disease
engorgement
enhancer
    cholinergic release e.
enhancing ring lesion
Enkaid
enkephalin
enlargement
    pituitary e.
enophthalmos
enoxaparin
    e. sodium
    subcutaneous e.
en plaques
Enroth sign
Ensure
ENT
    ears, nose, throat
entamebiasis
Entamoeba
    E. coli
    E. histolytica
enteral
    e. administration
    e. feeding set
    e. nutrition
    e. nutritional therapy
enteralgia
enterdynia
enteric
    e. fever
    e. infection
    e. oxaluria
    e. tuberculosis
enteric-coated aspirin
entericoid fever
enteritidis
    Salmonella enterica e.
enteritis
    Campylobacter e.
    chronic cicatrizing e.
    diphtheritic e.

E

NOTES

enteritis *(continued)*
    granulomatous e.
    mucomembranous e.
    e. necroticans
    phlegmonous e.
    e. polyposa
    pseudomembranous e.
    radiation e.
    regional e.
    tuberculous e.
    viral e.
enteroanthelone
Enterobacter
Enterobacteriaceae
enterocele
enteroclysis
enterococcal
Enterococcus
    E. avium
    E. casseliflavus
    E. durans
    E. faecalis
    E. faecium
    E. gallinarum
    E. raffinosus
    vancomycin-resistant *E.* (VRE)
enterococcus, pl. **enterococci**
    glycopeptide-resistant enterococci
enterocolitica
    Yersinia e.
enterocolitis
    antibiotic e.
    necrotizing e.
    pseudomembranous e.
    regional e.
enterodynia
enterogastritis
enterogastrone
enterogenous cyanosis
enterograph
enterography
enterohemorrhagic *Escherichia coli*
    (EHEC)
enterohepatic
enteroidea
enteroinvasive *Escherichia coli* (EIEC)
enterology
enteromenia
enteromycosis
enteroparesis
enteropathic
    e. arthritis
    e. spondyloarthropathy
enteropathica
    acrodermatitis e.
enteropathogenic *Escherichia coli*
    (EPEC)
enteropathy
    diabetic e.

    gluten e.
    gluten-sensitive e. (GSE)
    protein-losing e.
enteroplegia
enteroscopy
enterospasm
enterostasis
enterostomal therapy (ET)
enterostomy
    tube e.
enterotoxication
enterotoxigenic *Escherichia coli* (ETEC)
enterotoxin
enterotoxism
enterotropic
enterovirus
Entex LA
enthesis
enthesopathy
entity
entomophthoramycosis
entrapment
    anterior interosseous nerve e.
    long thoracic nerve e.
    nerve e.
    ulnar nerve e.
ventriculi (*pl. of* ventriculus)
entropion
enucleate
enuresis
    nocturnal e.
    sleep e.
envelope
envenomation
    marine e.
    e. syndrome
environment
    home e.
environmental
    e. allergy
    e. hazard
    e. illness
    E. Protection Agency (EPA)
    e. risk factor
enzootic stability
enzymatic debridement
enzyme
    angiotensin-converting e. (ACE)
    cardiac e.
    e. deficiency anemia
    e. deficiency hemolytic anemia
    serum e.
    telomerase e.
enzyme-linked
    e.-l. immunoassay (ELISA)
    e.-l. immunosorbent assay (ELISA)
enzymolysis
enzymopathy

EOG
electrooculogram
EOM
external otitis media
EOMI
extraocular muscles intact
EORTC QLQ
European Organization for Research and
Treatment of Cancer Quality of Life
Questionnaire
eosin
e. methylene blue (EMB)
e. stain
eosinopenia
eosinopenic reaction
eosinophil
eosinophilia
Löffler e.
pleural fluid e.
simple pulmonary e.
tropical pulmonary e.
eosinophilic
e. abscess
e. fasciitis
e. gastritis
e. gastroenteritis
e. granuloma
e. hyperpituitarism
e. leukemia
e. pneumonia
e. pneumonopathy
EP
erythrocyte protoporphyrin
EPA
Environmental Protection Agency
eparterial
EPEC
enteropathogenic *Escherichia coli*
ependyma
ventricular e.
ependymoma
ephebic
ephebology
ephedra
ephedrine
ephelis
ephemeral fever
EPI
exocrine pancreatic insufficiency
epiandrosterone
epicanthal fold
epicondyle

epicondylectomy
epicondylitis
epicrisis
epidemic
e. benign dry pleurisy
e. diaphragmatic pleurisy
e. disease
e. dropsy
e. exanthema
e. gangrenous proctitis
e. hemorrhagic fever
e. hepatitis
e. keratoconjunctivitis (EKC)
e. myalgia
e. myalgic encephalomyelitis
e. myositis
c. nausea
e. neuromyasthenia
e. nonbacterial gastroenteritis
e. parotiditis
e. pleurodynia
point e.
e. polyarthritis
e. roseola
e. stomatitis
e. transient diaphragmatic spasm
e. typhus
e. vomiting
epidemica
nephropathia e.
panneuritis e.
epidemicity
epidemicum
erythema arthriticum e.
epidemiologic
epidemiologist
epidemiology
clinical e.
hospital e.
epidermal
e. growth factor
e. nevus syndrome
epidermidis
Staphylococcus e.
epidermoid
epidermolysis bullosa
epidermolytic hyperkeratosis
epididymal cyst
epididymis
epididymitis
epididymoorchitis

E

NOTES

epidural
  e. abscess
  e. hematoma
  e. lipomatosis
  e. steroid injection
epiestriol
epifascial
Epifoam
epigastralgia
epigastric
  e. bruit
  e. mass
  e. pain
  e. spot
epigastrium
epigenetic event
epiglottis
epiglottitis
epilepsy
  abdominal e.
  catamenial e.
  e. and the elderly
  E. Foundation
  gelastic e.
  e. and pregnancy
  primary generalized genetic e.
  progressive myoclonus e.
  symptomatic partial e.
  temporal lobe e.
epileptic migraine
epilepticus
  status e.
Epilyt Cream
epimastical fever
epinephrine
  racemic e.
EpiPen
epiphenomenon
epiphora
epiphysial, epiphyseal
epiphysiodesis
epiphysis
epiploic
epiretinal membrane
epirubicin
episcleritis
episiotomy
episode
  assaultive e.
  dysphoric manic e.
  lone e.
  presyncopal e.
episodic
  e. hypertension
  e. memory
epistasis
epistaxis
  Gull renal e.
  renal e.

17-epitestosterone
epithelia (*pl. of* epithelium)
epithelial
epithelioma
epithelium, pl. **epithelia**
  columnar e.
  cornified squamous e.
  dysplastic Barrett e.
  glandular e.
  stratified squamous e.
Epitol
epitope
  shared e.
epitrochlear
epituberculosis
epityphlitis
epizootic stomatitis
EPO
  erythropoiesis
  erythropoietin
Epogen
eponychial
epoprostenol pulmonary hypertension
EPR
  electron paramagnetic resonance
EPS
  exophthalmos-producing substance
Epsilometer test (E-test)
epsilon
  apolipoprotein E e. 4 (ApoE4)
Epstein-Barr
  E.-B. virus (EBV)
  E.-B. virus titer
Epstein disease
eptastigmine
eptifibatide
epulis
Equagesic
equal
  bilateral, symmetrical, e. (BSE)
  E. Employment Opportunity
    Commission (EEOC)
  present, active, e. (PA&E)
equation
  Bohr e.
  Fick e.
  Harris-Benedict e.
equi
  Rhodococcus e.
equilenin
equilibrium
  e. radionuclide angiography
    (ERNA)
  Starling e.
equilin
equimolar antibody
equina
  cauda e.
equinus deformity

equipment
adaptive e.
EquiTest
NeuroCom E.
equivalent
angina e.
equivocal symptom
ERA
estrogen receptor assay
era
baby boomer e.
Erb sign
Ercaf
ERCP
endoscopic retrograde
cholangiopancreatogram
endoscopic retrograde
cholangiopancreatography
Erdheim
E. disease
E. syndrome
ErecAid vacuum system
erectile dysfunction (ED)
erection
medicated urethral system for e.
(MUSE)
nocturnal e.
psychogenic e.
reflexogenic e.
erector spinae
erethism
ERG
electroretinogram
ergasthenia
ergocalciferol
ergoloid mesylate
ergometer
ergonomic
ergonovine
Ergostat
ergotamine
ERNA
equilibrium radionuclide angiography
erosion
Cameron e.
Dieulafoy e.
vaginal e.
erosive
e. arthritis
e. esophagitis
e. gastritis
e. inflammatory osteoarthritis

erratic
error
inborn e.
refractive e.
ERT
estrogen replacement therapy
eructation
eruption
acneiform e.
fixed drug e.'s
Kaposi varicelliform e.
maculopapular e.
serum e.
eruptione
variola sine e.
eruptive
e. stage
e. xanthoma
Erycette pledget
EryDerm
Erygel
EryPed
erysipelas
Erysipelothrix rhusiopathiae
Ery-Tab
erythema
acrodynic e.
e. annulare
e. arthriticum epidemicum
e. chronicum migrans
cold e.
e. marginatum
migratory necrolytic e.
mucosal e.
e. multiforme
e. nodosum
palmar e.
rectal e.
erythematopultaceous stomatitis
erythematosus
acute systemic lupus e.
chilblain lupus e.
chronic systemic lupus e.
cutaneous lupus e.
disseminated lupus e. (DLE)
drug-induced lupus e.
lupus e.
neuropsychiatric systemic lupus e.
pemphigus e.
pregnancy in systemic lupus e.
subacute cutaneous lupus e.
systemic lupus e. (SLE)

NOTES

E

erythematous pharynx
erythrasma coryneform
erythredema polyneuropathy
erythremia
    altitude e.
erythremic myelosis
erythrityl tetranitrate
erythroblastic
    e. anemia
    e. anemia of childhood
erythroblastosis fetalis
Erythrocin
erythrocyte
    e. protoporphyrin (EP)
    e. sedimentation rate (ESR)
erythrocytosis
    compensated e.
    decompensated e.
    leukemic e.
    e. megalosplenica
    pathologic secondary e.
    reactive e.
    relative e.
erythrogenesis imperfecta
erythroid
erythroleukemia
erythromelalgia
erythromycin
erythroplasia
    Queyrat e.
erythropoiesis (EPO)
erythropoietic
    e. porphyria
    e. protoporphyria
erythropoietin (EPO)
    e. deficiency
ES-600
    Augmentin ES-600
eschar
Escherichia
    E. coli (*E. coli*)
    E. coli infection
    E. histolytica
eschew
Esclim
esculent
escutcheon
Esgic
Esidrix
Eskalith
esmolol
esomeprazole magnesium
esophagalgia
esophageal
    e. adenocarcinoma
    e. cancer
    e. candidiasis
    e. carcinoma
    e. chest pain

e. dilation
e. disease
e. diverticulum
e. dysphagia
e. dysrhythmia
e. hernia
e. hyperalgesia
e. hypomotility
e. lead
e. manometry
e. manometry study
e. motility disorder
e. motility study
e. motor disorder
e. reflux
e. spasm
e. sphincter
e. tumor
e. varix
esophagi (*pl. of* esophagus)
esophagitis
    Candida e.
    chemical e.
    cytomegalovirus e.
    erosive e.
    herpes simplex virus e.
    herpetic e.
    infectious e.
    pill-induced e.
    reflux e.
esophagodynia
esophagogastrectomy
esophagogastric junction
esophagogastroduodenoscopy (EGD)
esophagogram (*var. of* esophagram)
esophagology
esophagospasm
esophagram, esophagogram
esophagus, pl. esophagi
    Barrett e.
    corkscrew e.
    nutcracker e.
esotropia
ESPRIT
    European/Australian Stroke Prevention in
    Reversible Ischaemia Trial
ESR
    erythrocyte sedimentation rate
ESRD
    end-stage renal disease
essential
    e. anemia
    e. fever
    e. fructosuria
    e. hypercholesterolemia (EHC)
    e. hypernatremia
    e. nutrients
    e. primary hypertension
    e. thrombocythemia

e. tremor
e. vertigo
estazolam
ester
ecgonine methyl e.
long-acting testosterone e.
esterase
esterified estrogen
esthesia
estimate
upper bound e.
estimated date of confinement (EDC)
estimating
estimation
Estinyl
estival
Estrace
Estraderm
estradiol transdermal
Estratab
Estratest H.S.
estrin (*See also* estrogen)
Estring
estriol
estrogen
conjugated equine e.
esterified e.
oral conjugated e.
e. receptor assay (ERA)
e. receptor assay test
e. receptor-positive tumor
e. replacement
e. replacement therapy (ERT)
topical e.
transdermal e.
estrogenic hormone
estrogen-induced hypertension
estrone
estropipate
Estrovis
ESVI
end-systolic volume index
ET
endotracheal
enterostomal therapy
etanercept
ETEC
enterotoxigenic *Escherichia coli*
E-test
Epsilometer test
ethacrynic acid
ethambutol

Ethamolin
ethanol
e. abuse
e. level
e. toxicity
ether
ethyl tert-butyl e.
methyl tert-butyl e.
ethical
e. decision-making
e. issue
ethics
medical e.
Ethiflex
Ethilon suture
ethmoid sinusitis
Ethmozine
ethnic predilection
ethyl
e. alcohol (ETOH)
e. tert-butyl ether
ethylene glycol toxicity
etidronate therapy
etiocholanolone fever
etiogenic
etiologic agent
etiological factor
etiology
polymicrobial e.
etiopathic
etiopathology
etiotropic
E to A change
ETOH
ethyl alcohol
etomidate
etoposide
Etrafon
ETT
exercise treadmill test
eubiotics
Eucerin
euchlorhydria
eucrasia
eudipsia
euglycemia
euglycemic
Eulexin
eumycetoma
eunuch
eunuchism
pituitary e.

E

NOTES

eunuchoid
  e. gigantism
  e. state
eunuchoidism
  hypergonadotropic e.
  hypogonadotropic e.
euphoria
European
  E. Organization for Research and
    Treatment of Cancer Quality of
    Life Questionnaire (EORTC QLQ)
  E. typhus
**European/Australian Stroke Prevention
  in Reversible Ischaemia Trial
  (ESPRIT)**
eustachian tube
eusthenia
euthanasia
euthenics
eutherapeutic
Euthroid
euthymic
euthyroid
  e. goiter
  e. hypometabolism
  e. sick syndrome
euthyroidism
euvolemic hyponatremia
evacuate
evacuation
  rectal e.
evaluation
  acute physiology and chronic
    health e. (APACHE)
  audiologic e.
  cardiac e.
  clinical e.
  health e.
  initial e.
  medical e.
  preoperative cardiac e.
  preoperative medical e.
  pretreatment e.
  swallowing e.
evanescent
Evans syndrome
event
  adverse drug e.
  apparent life-threatening e. (ALTE)
  cardioembolic e.
  Cholesterol and Recurrent E.'s
    (CARE)
  embolic e.
  epigenetic e.
  life-threatening e.
eventration
eversion
every (q.)
  e. day [L. *quaque die*] (q.d.)

  e. hour [L. *quaque hora*] (q.h.)
  e. morning [L. *quaque mane*]
    (q.a.m., q.m.)
  e. night [L. *quaque nocte*] (q.n.)
  e. other day [L. *quaque altera
    die*] (q.o.d.)
  e. other night [L. *quaaue altera
    nocte*]
evidence
  dearth of e.
evidence-based medicine
Evista
evolution
  stroke in e.
evulsed
Ewing sarcoma
exacerbate
exacerbation
Exaclesh blood glucose meter
examination
  anorectal e.
  Brief Neuropsychological Mental
    Status E. (BNMSE)
  clinical breast e. (CBE)
  digital rectal e. (DRE)
  Folstein Mini-Mental State E.
  funduscopic e.
  Lachman e.
  mental status e.
  Mini-Mental State E. (MMSE)
  Modified Mini-Mental State E.
    (3MSE)
  neuroophthalmologic e.
  physical e.
  pleural fluid cytologic e.
  postmortem e.
  short-colon e.
  slit-lamp e.
  sputum e.
  synovial fluid e.
  Woods light e.
examiner
  medical e.
examining table
exanthem
  roseoliform e.
exanthema
  epidemic e.
  e. subitum
exanthematica
  stomatitis e.
exanthematous
  e. fever
  e. typhus
exanthesis arthrosia
exanthrope
exanthropic
excavatum
  pectus e.

excellent functional status
excess
    apparent mineralocorticoid e.
    corticotropin e.
    extracellular fluid volume e.
    gonadotropin e.
excessive loading
exchange
    pulmonary gas e.
excimer laser coronary angioplasty (ELCA)
excision
    large loop e.
excisional biopsy
excitability
    corticomotor e.
excitant
exciting
    e. cause
    e. electrode
exclusion
    diagnosis by e.
excoriation
excoriée
    acne e.
excrement
excrementitious
excrescence
    warty e.
excreta
excrete
excretion
    ammonia e.
    renal potassium e.
excretory urography
excursion
    expiratory e.
executive function
exercise
    breathing e.
    Buerger e.
    e. capacity
    Cawthorne e.
    e. contraindication
    e. electrocardiogram
    e. electrocardiography
    habituation e.
    heel cord stretching e.
    Kegel e.
    e. MUGA
    e. multigated angiogram
    muscle-strengthening e.

    nonweightbearing e.
    peak e.
    pelvic muscle e.
    pendulum e.
    Rockwood e.
    e. stress test
    e. thallium
    Thera-Band e.
    thermic effect of e. (TEE)
    e. tolerance
    e. treadmill test (ETT)
    weightbearing e.
exercise-induced
    e.-i. amenorrhea
    e.-i. asthma
exertion
    dyspnea on e. (DOE)
exertional
    e. chest pain
    e. dyspnea
    e. headache
    e. heat stroke
    e. rhabdomyolysis
exfoliative cytology
exhaustion
    heat e.
existing dementia
exocrine
    e. gland
    e. pancreatic insufficiency (EPI)
exogenetic
exogenic toxicosis
exogenous
    e. antigen
    e. hormone
    e. hyperglyceridemia
    e. mineral corticoid
    e. obesity
    e. pressor agent
    e. pyrogen
exomphalos
    e., macroglossia, and gigantism (EMG)
    e., macroglossia, and gigantism syndrome
exophoria
exophthalmic
    e. goiter
    e. ophthalmoplegia
exophthalmica cachexia
exophthalmos
exophthalmos-producing substance (EPS)

E

NOTES

exophytic
exostosis, pl. **exostoses**
exotoxin
expansile
expectancy
    active life e. (ALE)
    life e.
    total life e. (TLE)
expectant treatment
expectation
expectoration
    prune-juice e.
expense
    out-of-pocket e.
expensive
experiential
experiment
    factorial e.
experimental medicine
expiratory
    e. dyspnea
    e. excursion
    e. phase
    e. sibilant
    e. wheeze
exploration
exploratory
explosive vomiting
exposure
    cadmium e.
    diethylstilbestrol diphosphate e.
    measurement of e.
    radiation e.
expression
expressive aphasia
exsanguinate
exsanguinating hemorrhage
exsiccation fever
exstrophy
    bladder e.
exstrophy
extended care
extension
    resisted hip e.
extensor
    e. digitorum longus
    e. hallucis longus
Extentabs
    Donnatal E.
    Quinidex E.
exteriorize
extern
externa
    malignant otitis e.
    otitis e.
external
    e. beam radiation therapy (EBRT)
    e. beam radiotherapy
    e. defibrillator

    e. hemorrhoid
    e. hernia
    e. otitis media (EOM)
    e. rewarming
    e. secretion
    e. vacuum device
exteroception
extrabuccal feeding
extracapillary
extracellular
    e. fluid volume depletion
    e. fluid volume excess
    e. matrix molecule
    e. proteins
    e. water
extracorporeal shock-wave lithotripsy
extract
    African plum tree bark e.
extrahepatic
    e. cholestasis
    e. obstruction
extraintestinal
extramedullary
extramural practice
extraocular
    e. muscle
    e. muscles intact (EOMI)
    e. palsy
extraovarian
extrapsychic conflict
extrapulmonary
    e. coccidioidomycosis
    e. tuberculosis
extrapyramidal
    e. disorder
    e. reaction
    e. rigidity
    e. side effect
    e. syndrome
Extra-Strength Tylenol
extrasystole
extrathoracic
extrathyroidal hypermetabolism
extravasate
extravasation
extravascular
extreme
    e. dipper
    e. dipping
extremis
    in e.
extrinsic
    e. allergic alveolitis
    e. asthma
    e. pathway defect
extrude
extubate
extubation
exudate

exudative
    e. AMD
    e. bronchiolitis
    e. pleural effusion
    e. tuberculosis
eye
    both e.'s
    e. disease
    doll's e.'s
    dry e.
    e. infection
    left e. (OS)

    e. movement
    e. pain
    red e.
    right e. (OD)
eyegrounds
eyelid
    lower e.
    upper e.
eyeopener
    cut down (on drinking), annoyance, guilt (about drinking), (need for) e. (CAGE)

NOTES

E

F
Fahrenheit
F wave
F7
factor VII
FAAN
Fellow of the American Academy of Nursing
Fab AV treatment
Faber
F. anemia
F. syndrome
fabere sign
Fabry
F. disease
F. syndrome
FAC
5-FU, Adriamycin, Cytoxan
FAC chemotherapy
FACCP
Fellow of the American College of Chest Physicians
face
hippocratic f.
mask f.
moon f.
moon-shaped f.
facet
f. hypertrophy
f. joint
f. joint injection
facial
f. cellulitis
f. nerve palsy
f. pain
faciale
pyoderma f.
faciei
tinea f.
facies
acromegalic f.
cherubic f.
Corvisart f.
cushingoid f.
f. dolorosa
f. hepatica
hippocratic f.
Hutchinson f.
masked f.
moon f.
myxedematous f.
Parkinson f.
parkinsonian f.
Parkinson-like f.
Potter f.

facility
assisted living f.
health care f.
long-term care f.
skilled nursing f. (SNF)
facioscapulohumeral
f. muscular dystrophy
FACP
Fellow of the American College of Physicians
factitia
thyrotoxicosis f.
factitious
f. hyperthyroidism
f. symptom
factor
f. VII (F7)
f. VIII
f. VIIIc
adrenocorticotropic hormone-releasing f. (ACTH-RF)
adrenocorticotropic-releasing f.
age-related f.
amyloid-enhancing f. (AEF)
antinuclear f. (ANF)
antiphagocytic f.
atrial natriuretic f.
basic fibroblast growth f. (bFGF)
cardiac risk f. (CRF)
Castle intrinsic f.
Christmas f.
clotting f.
coagulation f.
corticotropin-releasing f. (CRF)
cytokine growth f.
f. XI, XIII deficiency
environmental risk f.
epidermal growth f.
etiological f.
gonadotropin-releasing f. (GRF)
granulocyte colony-stimulating f. (G-CSF)
growth f.
growth hormone-releasing f. (GHRF, GH-RF)
hematopoietic growth f.
initiation f. (IF)
insulinlike growth f. (IGF)
intrinsic f. (IF)
f. V Leiden
luteinizing hormone/follicle-stimulating hormone-releasing f. (LH/FSH-RF)
luteinizing hormone-releasing f. (LH-RF, LRF)

F

factor *(continued)*
    mammotropic f.
    müllerian regression f.
    myocardial depressant f. (MDF)
    noninherited f.
    f. P
    platelet-derived growth f. (PDGF)
    platelet-stimulating f.
    precipitating f.
    prolactin-inhibiting f.
    releasing f.
    Rhesus f.
    rheumatoid f.
    risk f.
    seasonal f.
    socioeconomic f.
    somatotropin release-inhibiting f.
     (SRIF)
    somatotropin-releasing f. (SRF)
    stress f.
    Stuart f.
    sun protective f. (SPF)
    thyroid-stimulating hormone-
     releasing f. (TSH-RF)
    thyrotropin-releasing f. (TRF)
    tissue angiogenesis f. (TAF)
    tumor angiogenesis f. (TAF)
    tumor necrosis f.
    uterine relaxing f. (URF)
    virulence f.
    von Willebrand f.
    Willebrand f.
factor-alpha
    tumor necrosis f.-a. (TNF-alpha)
factorial experiment
FAD
    familial Alzheimer disease
faecalis
    Enterococcus f.
    Streptococcus f.
faecium
    Enterococcus f.
    Streptococcus f.
Faget sign
Fahrenheit (F)
failed back syndrome
failure
    acutely decompensated congestive
     heart f. (ADCHF)
    acute renal f. (ARF)
    acute respiratory f. (ARF)
    adrenal f.
    advanced renal f.
    autoimmune polyglandular f.
    cardiac pump f.
    cardiovascular f.
    chronic liver f.
    chronic renal f.

    circulatory f.
    congestive heart f. (CHF)
    fulminant hepatic f.
    graft f.
    heart f.
    hepatic f.
    high-output f.
    hypercapnic respiratory f.
    hypercarbic respiratory f.
    hypoxemic respiratory f.
    hypoxic respiratory f.
    intrarenal acute renal f.
    intrinsic renal f.
    ischemic heart f.
    left-sided heart f.
    left ventricular f.
    liver f.
    mixed respiratory f.
    myoglobinuric rhabdomyolytic acute
     renal f.
    ovarian f.
    postoperative heart f.
    postpartum renal f.
    postrenal acute renal f.
    posttraumatic acute renal f.
     (PTARF)
    prerenal acute renal f.
    primary adrenal f.
    primary graft f.
    refractory heart f.
    renal f.
    respiratory f.
    right-sided heart f.
    right ventricular f.
    secondary adrenal f.
    f. to thrive
    ventilatory f.
faint
fainting
    hysterical f.
faintness
    cardiovascular f.
faith-based rehabilitation
falciparum
    f. fever
    f. malaria
    Plasmodium f.
fall
    F.'s Efficacy Scale (FES)
    f. on outstretched hand (FOOSH)
    f. screen test
    sex-linked hypochromatic anemia of
     Rundles and F.'s
fall-and-rise phenomenon
falling
fallopian
    f. tube
    f. tube torsion

Fallot
>F. repair
>tetralogy of F.

false
>f. anemia
>f. cyanosis
>f. diphtheria
>f. thirst
>f. tympanites

false-negative
>f.-n. murmur
>f.-n. ratio

false-positive
>f.-p. murmur
>f.-p. result

false-reassurance ratio
Falta triad
falx cerebri
famciclovir
familial
>f. abuse
>f. aggregation
>f. Alzheimer disease (FAD)
>f. amyloidosis
>f. angiomatosis
>f. benign chronic neutropenia
>f. benign hypocalcemia
>f. cholemia
>f. clustering
>f. combined hyperlipidemia
>f. defective apolipoprotein b-100
>f. dilated cardiomyopathy
>f. dysautonomia (FD)
>f. dysbetalipoproteinemia
>f. erythroblastic anemia
>f. fat-induced hyperlipemia
>f. glycinuria
>f. goiter
>f. goitrous hypothyroidism
>f. hemiplegic migraine
>f. heterozygous hypercholesteremia
>f. high-density lipoprotein
> deficiency
>f. hyperbetalipoproteinemia
>f. hyperbetalipoproteinemia and
> hyperprebetalipoproteinemia
>f. hypercholesteremic xanthomatosis
>f. hypercholesterolemia (FH)
>f. hypercholesterolemia with
> hyperlipemia

>f. hyperchylomicronemia
>f. hyperchylomicronemia with
> hyperprebetalipoproteinemia
>f. hyperkalemic periodic paralysis
>f. hyperlipoproteinemia (type I–IV)
>f. hyperprolinemia
>f. hypertension
>f. hypertriglyceridemia
>f. hypocalciuric hypercalcemia
>f. hypogonadotropic hypogonadism
>f. hypokalemic periodic paralysis
>f. hypoparathyroidism
>f. icterus
>f. intrahepatic cholestasis
>f. lecithin:cholesterol acyltransferase
> deficiency
>f. Mediterranean fever
>f. microcytic anemia
>f. multiple endocrine adenomatosis
>f. nephropathy
>f. nephrosis
>f. osteochondrodystrophy
>f. paroxysmal polyserositis
>f. paroxysmal rhabdomyolysis
>f. screening

family
>American Association for Marriage
> and F. (AAMFT)
>f. medicine
>f. physician
>f. practice

famine dropsy
famotidine
Famvir
Fanconi
>F. anemia
>F. disease
>F. pancytopenia
>F. syndrome

Fansidar
Farabeuf amputation
faradization
faradotherapy
Farber
>F. disease
>F. syndrome

Far East hemorrhagic fever
farina tritici
farmer's lung
Farre tubercle

F

NOTES

FAS
  fetal alcohol syndrome
fascia, pl. **fasciae, fascias**
  Dupuytren f.
fascial herniation
fascicular
  f. lymphosarcoma
  f. twitching
fasciculata
  zona f.
fasciculation
fasciitis
  diffuse f.
  eosinophilic f.
  necrotizing f.
  plantar f.
fascioliasis disorder
fasciotomy incision
fashion
  rote f.
fast
  histamine f.
  prolonged f.
  Slim F.
  F. Take blood glucose monitoring
    system
fastigium
Fastin
fasting
  f. blood glucose
  f. blood sugar (FBS)
  f. hypoglycemia
  f. plasma glucose
  f. state
fat
  f. absorption
  body f.
  f. emulsion
  f. hernia
  f. indigestion
  f. malabsorption
  f. maldistribution
  f. pad sign
  qualitative stool f.
  f. replacement atrophy
fatal
fatality rate
fat-free mass (FFM)
fatigability
fatigue fever
fatiguing
fat-induced hyperlipemia
fat-soluble vitamin deficiency
fatty
  f. cirrhosis
  f. diarrhea
  f. metamorphosis
  f. stool

faucial diphtheria
favism
Favre-Durand-Nicholas disease
FBR
  Foundation for Biomedical Research
FBS
  fasting blood sugar
FCIC
  Federal Consumer Information Center
FD
  familial dysautonomia
FDA
  Food and Drug Administration
Fe
  iron
    Loestrin Fe
    Slow Fe
fear
febricant
febricula
febrifacient
febriferous
febrific
febrifugal
febrifuge
febrile
  f. crisis
  f. delirium
  f. disease
  f. illness
  f. panniculitis
  f. pleiochromic anemia
  f. polyneuritis
  f. reaction
  f. seizure
  f. urticaria
febrilis
  calor f.
febris
  f. melitensis
  f. undulans
fecal
  f. continence
  f. impaction
  f. incontinence
  f. occult blood test (FOBT)
  f. occult blood testing
  f. osmotic gap
  f. softener
  f. vomiting
fecalith
fecaloid
fecaluria
feces
  incontinence of f.
  scybalous f.
feculent
fecund

federal
    F. Consumer Information Center (FCIC)
    F. Trade Commission (FTC)
Federici sign
feeble
feedback
feeding
    extrabuccal f.
    Finkelstein f.
    forced f.
    gastric f.
    gavage f.
    nasal f.
    nasojejunal f.
    NJ f.
    tube f.
feeding-fasting cycle
FEES
    fiberoptic endoscopic examination of swallowing
feet (*pl. of* foot)
FEF
    forced expiratory flow
Feingold diet
felbamate
Feldene
fellow
    F. of the American Academy of Nursing (FAAN)
    F. of the American College of Chest Physicians (FACCP)
    F. of the American College of Physicians (FACP)
    F. of the Royal College of Physicians (Canada) (FRCP(C))
    F. of the Royal College of Physicians (Edinburgh) (FRCP(E))
    F. of the Royal College of Physicians (England) (FRCP)
    F. of the Royal College of Physicians (Ireland) (FRCP(I))
    F. of the Royal Society (Canada) (FRSC)
felodipine
Felty syndrome
female
    f. athlete triad
    f. condom
    f. infertility
    f. sexual arousal disorder
    f. sexual dysfunction
    well-nourished f. (WNF)
female-pattern baldness
feminization
    testicular f.
femoral
    f. head
    f. hernia
    f. neck
    f. neck fracture
    f. neuropathy
femoral-femoral bypass
femoropopliteal
femoxetine
FemPatch
Femstat
femur
Fenesin
fenfluramine and phentermine
fenoprofen
fenoterol
fentanyl
    transdermal f.
fenugreek
Fenwick disease
Feosol
Fergon
fermentans
    Mycoplasma f.
fermentative dyspepsia
ferritin
Ferro-Sequels
ferrotherapy
ferrous sulfate (FeSO)
fervens
    calor f.
fervescence
FES
    Falls Efficacy Scale
FeSO
    ferrous sulfate
fetal alcohol syndrome (FAS)
fetalis
    erythroblastosis f.
    hydrops f.
fété
    bruit de pot f.
fetid
fetoprotein
    alpha f.
fetor hepaticus

NOTES

F

FEV
    forced expiratory volume
FEV₁
    forced expiratory volume in one second
fever
    acclimating f.
    acute rheumatic f.
    Aden f.
    aestivoautumnal f.
    African hemorrhagic f.
    African tick f.
    algid pernicious f.
    ardent f.
    Argentinean hemorrhagic f.
    Argentine hemorrhagic f.
    arthropod-borne viral f.
    artificial f.
    aseptic f.
    Assam f.
    Australian Q f.
    autumn f.
    bilious remittent f.
    black f.
    blackwater f.
    f. blister
    blue f.
    Bolivian hemorrhagic f.
    bouquet f.
    boutonneuse f.
    brass founder's f.
    Brazilian hemorrhagic f.
    Brazilian purpuric f.
    Brazilian spotted f.
    breakbone f.
    Bunyamwera f.
    Burdwan f.
    Bwamba f.
    cachectic f.
    camp f.
    canicola f.
    catarrhal f.
    cat-bite f.
    catheter f.
    Charcot intermittent f.
    Colorado tick f.
    Congo-Crimean hemorrhagic f.
    Congolian red f.
    continued f.
    cotton-mill f.
    Crimean f.
    Crimean-Congo hemorrhagic f.
    dandy f.
    date f.
    deer-fly f.
    dehydration f.
    dengue hemorrhagic f.
    desert f.
    digestive f.
    double quotidian f.

drug f.
drug-induced f.
Dumdum f.
Dutton relapsing f.
Ebola hemorrhagic f.
eczema, asthma, hay f. (EAHF)
elephantoid f.
enteric f.
entericoid f.
ephemeral f.
epidemic hemorrhagic f.
epimastical f.
essential f.
etiocholanolone f.
exanthematous f.
exsiccation f.
falciparum f.
familial Mediterranean f.
Far East hemorrhagic f.
fatigue f.
field f.
five-day f.
flood f.
food f.
Fort Bragg f.
foundryman's f.
Gambian f.
Haverhill f.
hay f.
hemoglobinuric f.
hemorrhagic f.
hepatic intermittent f.
herpetic f.
hospital f.
icterohemorrhagic f.
Ilhéus f.
inanition f.
induced f.
intermittent malarial f.
inundation f.
island f.
Jaccoud f.
jail f.
Japanese river f.
jungle f.
Katayama f.
kedani f.
Kenya f.
Kew Gardens f.
Kinkiang f.
Korean hemorrhagic f.
Lassa hemorrhagic f.
malarial f.
malignant tertian f.
Malta f.
Manchurian hemorrhagic f.
Marburg hemorrhagic f.
marsh f.
Mediterranean erythematous f.

Mediterranean exanthematous f.
Mediterranean spotted f.
meningotyphoid f.
metal fume f.
Mexican spotted f.
miliary f.
milk f.
mill f.
miniature scarlet f.
monoleptic f.
Mossman f.
mumu f.
nanukayami f.
New World hemorrhagic f.
nodal f.
North Queensland tick f.
Omsk hemorrhagic f.
o'nyong-nyong f.
Oroya f.
Pahvant Valley f.
paludal f.
pappataci f.
paratyphoid f.
parenteric f.
parrot f.
Pel-Ebstein f.
periodic f.
Persian relapsing f.
pharyngoconjunctival f. (PCF)
Philippine hemorrhagic f.
phlebotomus f.
pinta f.
polka f.
polyleptic f.
polymer fume f.
pretibial f.
protein f.
Pym f.
pyogenic f.
Q f.
quartan f.
quintan f.
quotidian f.
rabbit f.
rat-bite f.
recrudescent typhus f.
recurrent f.
red f.
relapsing f.
remittent malarial f.
rheumatic f.
rice-field f.

Rocky Mountain spotted f.
Roman f.
Ross River f.
saddleback f.
sakushu f.
Salinem f.
salt f.
sandfly f.
San Joaquin Valley f.
São Paulo f.
scarlet f.
Schottmüller f.
septic f.
seven-day f.
shin bone f.
ship f.
shoddy f.
Sindbis f.
slime f.
slow f.
smelter's f.
snail f.
solar f.
Songo f.
South African tick-bite f.
spirillum f.
spotted f.
steroid f.
symptomatic f.
tertian f.
therapeutic f.
f. therapy
thermic f.
thirst f.
three-day f.
tick-bite f.
Tobia f.
traumatic f.
trench f.
trypanosome f.
tsutsugamushi f.
typhoid f.
typhus f.
f. of undetermined origin (FUO)
undifferentiated type f.
undulant f.
undulating f.
f. of unknown origin (FUO)
urethral f.
urinary f.
urticarial f.
Uzbekistan hemorrhagic f.

F

NOTES

151

fever *(continued)*
    valley f.
    viral hemorrhagic f.
    vivax f.
    Wesselsbron f.
    West African f.
    West Nile f.
    wound f.
    Yangtze Valley f.
    yellow f.
    zinc fume f.
feverfew
feverish
fexofenadine hydrochloride
FFDR
    full florid diabetic retinopathy
FFM
    fat-free mass
FFP
    fresh frozen plasma
FFS
    flexible fiberoptic sigmoidoscopy
FH
    familial hypercholesterolemia
fiber
    dietary f.
    f. supplement
    f. supplementation
Fiberall
FiberCon
fiberoptic
    f. bronchoscopy
    f. endoscopic examination of
      swallowing (FEES)
    f. gastroscope
    f. proctosigmoidoscopy
fiberscope
fibrate
fibric acid
fibril
    elastin f.
fibrillation
    atrial f. (AF)
    lone atrial f.
fibrin-bound plasminogen
fibrin demarcation
fibrinogen
fibrinolysis
fibrinolytic
    f. agent
    f. system defect
fibrinopeptide A
fibrinous
    f. bronchitis
    f. clot
fibroadenoma
fibroadenosis
fibroadipose

fibroblast
fibrochondroma
fibrocystic
    f. breast disease
    f. change
    f. disease
    f. disease of pancreas
fibroelastoma
    papillary f.
fibroid
    uterine f.
fibrolymphoangioblastoma
fibroma, pl. **fibromata**
    cardiac f.
    ossifying f.
fibromuscular dysplasia
fibromyalgia
    glucocorticoid reduction f.
    f. syndrome
fibromyoma
fibromyositis
fibromyxosarcoma
fibronectin-binding protein
fibroproliferative plaque
fibrosa
    osteitis f.
    renal osteitis f.
fibrosarcoma
    cardiac f.
fibrosing
    f. adenomatosis
    f. colonopathy
    f. thyroiditis
fibrosis
    cystic f. (CF)
    hepatic f.
    idiopathic pulmonary f. (IPF)
    interstitial f.
    papillary muscle f.
    progressive massive f.
    pulmonary f.
    retroperitoneal f.
    unilateral retroperitoneal f.
fibrositis
fibrosum
    myxoma f.
fibrotic streak
fibrous
    f. dysplasia
    f. goiter
    f. myocarditis
    f. plaque
    f. pneumonia
    f. thyroiditis
fibrovascular
    f. tissue
    f. tissue on disk (FVD)
fibula

Fick
    F. bacillus
    F. equation
fidgety
field
    f. fever
    high power f.
    lung f.
    visual f.
Fiessinger-Leroy-Reiter syndrome
fièvre boutonneuse
fifth disease
fifty
    National Association on HIV
      Over F. (NAHOE)
filarial arthritis
filariasis
    Brug f.
    periodic f.
Filatov disease
Filatov-Dukes disease
filling defect
film
    scout f.
Filmtab
    E.E.S. 400 F.
filter
    Greenfield f.
    inferior vena cava f.
    leukocyte-depleting f.
filtration
    autoregulation f.
    glomerular f.
    f. rate
filtrum ventriculi
FIM
    functional independence measure
financial constraint
finasteride
finding
    dearth of f.'s
fine hand movement
fine-needle
    f.-n. aspiration (FNA)
    f.-n. aspiration cytology
    f.-n. biopsy
finger
    clubbed f.'s
    hippocratic f.
    f. oximeter
    f. percussion

fingerbreadth
finger-nose-finger
fingerstick blood sugar (FSBS)
finger-to-nose test
Finkelstein
    F. feeding
    F. test
Fioricet
Fiorinal
fire
    St. Anthony f.
first
    f. aid
    f. disease
    f. heart sound (S_1)
    f. messenger
    f. rank symptom (FRS)
    f. voiding sensation
first-degree
    f.-d. atrioventricular block
    f.-d. burn
first-line pharmacologic therapy
first-pass method
first-set phenomenon
first-trimester abortion
Fischer sign
fish
    f. oil
    f. tapeworm anemia
fish-mouth meatus
fissura in ano
fissure
    Sylvian f.
fistula, pl. **fistulae, fistulas**
    aortoenteric f.
    arteriovenous f. (AVF)
    atrioventricular f.
    AV f.
    biliary f.
    Brescio-Cimino arteriovenous f.
    bronchopleural f.
    lymphatic f.
    pancreatic f.
    pulmonary arteriovenous f.
fistulogram
fistulous
fitness
    clinical f.
    National Association for Health
      & F. (NAHF)
    physical f.

NOTES

F

Fitz
> F. law
> F. syndrome

Fitz-Hugh-Curtis syndrome
five-day fever
five-year survival rate
fixate and follow
fixation device
fixative
> Zenker f.

fixed
> f. drug eruptions
> f. splitting

flaccidity
flag
> red f.

flagellate diarrhea
flagellosis
Flagyl
Flajani disease
flank pain
flap
> liver f.
> mucoperichondrial f.

flapping tremor
flare
> hormone f.

flash
> f. burn
> hot f.

flat affect
flattening of diaphragm
flatulence
flatulent dyspepsia
flatus enema
flavivirus
flavonoid
flavum
> ligamentum f.

flavus
> *Aspergillus f.*

flax-dresser's disease
flaxseed
flea-borne typhus
flecainide
flecks of calcium
Fleet Phospho-Soda
Fleischer ring
Fleischer-Strümpell ring
Flesch formula
flesh
> goose f.

Flex-all
Flexeril
flexibility
> waxy f.

flexible
> f. fiberoptic sigmoidoscopy (FFS)

> f. sigmoidoscopy (flex sig)
> f. torticollis

flexion
> Williams f.

Flexner bacillus
flexneri
> *Shigella f.*

Flexner-Strong bacillus
flexor
> f. carpi radialis
> f. tenosynovitis

flex sig
> flexible sigmoidoscopy

flexure
> hepatic f.
> splenic f.

flint disease
flip test
floating-beta proteinemia
Flonase nasal spray
flood fever
flopping
Florical
florid adenosis
Florinef
Florone cream 0.05%
Flovent inhaler
flow
> antegrade f.
> blood f.
> cerebral blood f.
> color f.
> forced expiratory f. (FEF)
> mesenteric blood f.
> f. obstruction
> peak expiratory f. (PEF)
> renal blood f.
> f. tract
> Wright peak f.

flow-by
flower
> purple cone f.

flowmetry
> urine f.

Floxin
flu
> influenza

fluconazole
fluctuance
fluctuant
fluctuating mental status
fluctuation
fludarabine
fludrocortisol
fludrocortisone
fluency
> verbal f.

fluffy pulmonary infiltrate

fluid
>
> ascitic f.
> body f.
> cerebrospinal f. (CSF)
> intravenous f.'s
> f. loss
> f. management
> f. overload
> f. restriction
> f. retention
> f. shift
> f. wave

fluke
>
> Chinese liver f.
> human blood f.
> intestinal f.
> liver f.
> lung f.

Flumadine
flumazenil
flunarizine
flunisolide
fluocinonide
fluorescein staining
fluorescence
fluorescent bronchoscopy
fluoric cachexia
fluorohydrocortisone therapy
fluoroquinolone
>
> f. antibiotic
> f. therapy

fluoroscopic monitoring
fluoroscopy
5-fluorouracil (5-FU)
>
> 5-f. cream
> 5-f. pulsed regimen

fluorourodynamic study (FUDS)
Fluothane
fluoxetine
fluphenazine
flurazepam
flush
>
> carcinoid f.
> hectic f.
> histamine f.
> malar f.

flushing
fluticasone propionate
fluticasone/salmeterol
flutter
>
> atrial f.

fluttering

fluvastatin sodium
fluvoxamine
flux
>
> blood f.

fly
>
> tsetse f.

FNA
>
> fine-needle aspiration

FNIC
>
> Food and Nutrition Information Center

foam
>
> f. cell
> f. mattress

FOBT
>
> fecal occult blood test

focal
>
> f. appendicitis
> f. granuloma
> f. metastatic disease
> f. necrosis
> f. neurologic sign
> f. neuropathy
> f. nodular hyperplasia
> f. nodular myositis
> f. peritonitis
> f. segmental glomerulosclerosis
> f. stenotic lesion

focus, pl. **foci**
Fogarty catheter
folate
fold
>
> aryepiglottic f.
> crural f.
> epicanthal f.

Foley catheter
foliaceus
>
> pemphigus f.

folic
>
> f. acid deficiency
> f. acid deficiency anemia

folk medicine
follicle
follicle-stimulating
>
> f.-s. hormone (FSH)
> f.-s. principle

follicular
>
> f. cancer
> f. goiter
> f. hormone
> f. hyperkeratosis
> f. hyperplasia
> f. thyroid carcinoma

F

NOTES

folliculitis
>f. barbae traumatica
>"hot-tub" f.

folliculosis

Fölling
>F. disease
>F. phenylketonuria

follitropin

follow
>fixate and f.

followup
>routine f.
>short-term f.

Folstein
>F. Mini-Mental State Examination
>Mini-Mental State Examination of F.
>F. MMSE

fomentation

fomite

fomivirsen

fontanelle
>posterior f.

Fontan operation

food
>f. asthma
>caffeine, alcohol, pepper, spicy f.'s (CAPS)
>F. and Drug Administration (FDA)
>f. fever
>F. Guide Pyramid
>f. insufficiency
>F. and Nutrition Information Center (FNIC)
>f. poisoning
>thermic effect of f. (TEF)

FOOSH
>fall on outstretched hand

foot, pl. **feet**
>f. problem
>runner's f.
>sandal f.
>f. ulcer

footstrike hemolysis

Foradil

foramen, pl. **foramina**
>foramen encroachment
>neural foramina
>vertebral foramina

foraminal stenosis

foraminotomy

Forbes-Albright syndrome

Forbes disease

force
>gravitational f.
>shearing f.
>f. of stream

forced
>f. alimentation

f. alkaline diuresis
f. end-expiratory wheeze
f. enteral nutrition
f. expiratory flow (FEF)
f. expiratory volume (FEV)
f. expiratory volume in one second (FEV$_1$)
f. feeding
f. vital capacity (FVC)

force-velocity curve

Forchheimer sign

Fordyce granule

forebrain
>basal f.

forehead
>olympian f.

foreign-body appendicitis

foreign object ingestion

forensic medicine

Forestier disease

forgetfulness
>benign f.
>benign senescent f.
>senescent f.

form
>pentavalent f.

formation
>intravascular thrombus f.
>thrombus f.
>vasoconstriction thrombus f.

forme
>f. fruste
>f. tardive

formoterol

formula, pl. **formulae, formulas**
>Berkow f.
>DuBois f.
>Flesch f.
>Momentum Muscular Backache F.

formulation
>controlled-release f.

fornix, pl. **fornices**

Fortaz

Fort Bragg fever

Forte
>Norgesic F.
>Solaquin F.

fortification spectrum

fortified milk

Fortis
>Mepergan F.

Fosamax

foscarnet

fosfomycin

Fosfree

fosinopril

fosphenytoin

fossa, pl. **fossae**
>cubital f.

Fothergill disease
foundation
American Health F. (AHF)
American Health Assistance F.
(AHAF)
American Menopause F. (AMF)
Arthritis F. (AF)
Beverly F.
F. for Biomedical Research (FBR)
Epilepsy F.
Glaucoma Research F. (GRF)
Hysterectomy Educational Resources
and Services F. (HERS)
International Tremor F. (ITF)
John Douglas French
Alzheimer's F.
MedicAlert F.
National Hospital F. (NHF)
National Kidney F. (NKF)
National Osteoporosis F. (NOF)
National Psoriasis F. (NPF)
National Sleep F. (NSF)
Parkinson's Disease F. (PDF)
Pulmonary Fibrosis F. (PFF)
Restless Legs Syndrome F.
Robert Wood Johnson F. (RWJF)
Setting Priorities for Retirement
Years F.
SPRY F.
The Skin Cancer F.
Well Spouse F. (WSF)
foundryman's fever
four
F. IADL Score
F. Instrumental Activities of Daily
Living Score
f. times a day (q.i.d.)
fourchette
Fournier gangrene
fourth
f. disease
f. heart sound (S_4)
fourth-degree burn
four-vessel angiography
foxglove
FR
functional reach
FR test
fraction
ejection f. (EF)
growth f.
shunt f.

fractional dose
fracture (FX)
basilar skull f.
Colles f.
comminuted f.
cough f.
femoral neck f.
Frykman-8 f.
hip f.
intertrochanteric hip f.
Jones f.
march f.
metatarsal stress f.
Monteggia f.
osteoporotic compression f.
pelvic f.
stress f.
subcapital hip f.
subtrochanteric f.
supracondylar femoral f.
teardrop f.
tibial plateau f.
vertebral f.
vertebral compression f.
fragile X syndrome
fragilis
Bacteroides f.
fragility
skin f.
fragmentation hemolytic anemia
frail elderly
frailty
frambesia tropica
frambesioma
framboesioides
mycosis f.
Framingham Heart Study
Franceschetti-Valerio syndrome
Francis disease
fraud
National Council Against Health F.
(NCAHE)
FRCP
Fellow of the Royal College of
Physicians (England)
FRCP(C)
Fellow of the Royal College of
Physicians (Canada)
FRCP(E)
Fellow of the Royal College of
Physicians (Edinburgh)

F

NOTES

FRCP(I)
    Fellow of the Royal College of
      Physicians (Ireland)
freckling
    periorbital f.
free
    f. PSA
    f. radical
    f. radical production
    f. radical scavenger
    f. radical-scavenging vitamin
    f. radical theory
    f. T_4
    f. T_3
    f. thyroid
    f. thyroxine index (FTI)
    f. T_4 test
Freiberg infarction
fremitus
    bronchial f.
    hydatid f.
    pleural f.
    rhonchal f.
    subjective f.
    tactile f.
    tussive f.
    vocal f.
Frenzel lens
frequency, pl. **frequencies**
    Hertz f.
    nocturnal urinary f.
frequenting
frequent premature ventricular
    contraction
Frerichs theory
Fresenius machine
fresh frozen plasma (FFP)
Frey-Baillarger syndrome
Frey syndrome
friable
friction
    f. murmur
    f. rub
    f. sound
Friderichsen-Waterhouse syndrome
Friedländer
    F. bacillus
    F. bacillus pneumonia
    F. disease
Friedreich
    F. ataxia
    F. phenomenon
frog breathing
Fröhlich
    F. dwarfism
    F. syndrome
Frohse
    arcade of F.

froissement
    bruit de f.
frôlement
    bruit de f.
frontal
    f. abulic syndrome
    f. disinhibition syndrome
    f. hemisphere
    f. opercular syndrome
    f. plane vector
    f. release sign
frontotemporal dementia
frost
    urea f.
frostbite
    deep f.
    superficial f.
frostnip
frottement
    bruit de f.
frovatriptan
frozen
    f. shoulder
    f. with liquid nitrogen
FRS
    first rank symptom
FRSC
    Fellow of the Royal Society (Canada)
fructosamine test
fructose intolerance
fructosemia
fructosuria
    essential f.
fruste
    forme f.
Frykman-8 fracture
FSBS
    fingerstick blood sugar
FSH
    follicle-stimulating hormone
FTC
    Federal Trade Commission
FTI
    free thyroxine index
5-FU
    5-fluorouracil
        5-FU, Adriamycin, Cytoxan (FAC)
        5-FU, Adriamycin, Cytoxan
            chemotherapy
        5-FU pulsed regimen
Fuchs dystrophy
fucosidosis
FUDS
    fluorourodynamic study
fugax
    amaurosis f.
    proctalgia f.
fugitive
Fugl-Meyer Sensory-Motor Assessment

Fukuyama syndrome
fulgurant
fulgurating migraine
fulguration
full
    f. and equal without bruits
    f. florid diabetic retinopathy
      (FFDR)
    f. liquid diet
full-blown proteinuria
full-thickness burn
fulminans
    acne f.
    pestis f.
fulminant
    f. colitis
    f. hepatic failure
    f. hepatitis
    f. hyperpyrexia
    f. sepsis
fulminating
    f. dysentery
    f. meningococcal septicemia
    f. smallpox
Fulvicin
fumarate
    clemastine f.
fumigate
fumigation
functio laesa
function
    anal f.
    biological f.
    cardiac pump f.
    cell f.
    cellular humoral immunological f.
    cerebellar f.
    compromised renal f.
    executive f.
    gain of f.
    humoral immune f.
    immune f.
    immunological f.
    impaired psychomotor f.
    f. independence
    liver f.
    loss of f.
    memory f.
    myocardial contractile f.
    neurocognitive f.
    parietal lobe f.
    psychomotor f.

    psychosocial f.
    renal f.
    small intestine f.
    thyroid f.
functional
    f. abdominal pain
    f. activity
    f. alteration
    f. asplenia
    f. autonomy
    f. bowel disease
    f. capacity
    f. castration
    f. characteristic
    f. decline
    f. deterioration
    f. disability
    f. dyspepsia
    f. dyspnea
    f. gain
    f. gastrointestinal disorder
    f. hyperinsulinism
    f. illness
    f. impairment
    f. incontinence
    f. independence measure (FIM)
    f. outcome
    f. performance
    f. prepubertal castration syndrome
    f. proteinuria
    f. reach (FR)
    f. reach test
    f. reactive hypoglycemia
    f. reserve
    f. status
functionality
    decreased f.
functioning
    high f.
    logical f.
    visuospatial f.
fundoplication
    laparoscopic f.
    Nissen f.
fundus, pl. **fundi**
funduscopic examination
fungal
    f. arthritis
    f. infection
    f. keratitis
    f. skin infection
fungating tumor

F

NOTES

fungemia
fungi (*pl. of* fungus)
Fungizone
fungoides
    mycosis f.
funguria
fungus, pl. **fungi**
funicular myelosis
FUO
    fever of undetermined origin
    fever of unknown origin
Furadantin
furfur
    Malassezia f.
furosemide
furred tongue

furuncle
furunculosis
fusiform
fusion protein
Fusobacterium
fusospirochetal stomatitis
futile intervention
Futura wrist splint
FVC
    forced vital capacity
FVD
    fibrovascular tissue on disk
F-wave measurement
FX
    fracture

g
   gram
GABA
   gamma-aminobutyric acid
GABAergic transmission
gabapentin
GAD
   generalized anxiety disorder
gadolinium
Gaffky
   G. scale
   G. table
gain
   g. of function
   functional g.
   solute g.
Gaisböck
   G. disease
   G. syndrome
gait
   antalgic g.
   g. ataxia
   choreoathetotic g.
   g. disorder
   g. disturbance
   helicopod g.
   rapid g.
   g. speed
   stiffer g.
   g. training
gaited
galactacrasia
galactokinase deficiency
galactophagous
galactophlebitis
galactopoietic hormone
galactorrhea
   hyperprolactinemic g.
   normoprolactinemia g.
galactose diabetes
galactosemia
galactosylceramide lipoidosis
galactotherapy
galantamine HBr
galanthamine
gall
gallbladder
   g. cancer
   Courvoisier g.
   g. disease
   empyema of g.
   g. ultrasound
gallinarum
   Enterococcus g.
   polyneuritis g.

gallium scan
gallop
gallstone
   asymptomatic g.
   black pigment g.
   brown pigment g.
   cholesterol g.
   g. colic
   g. disease
   g. ileus
galop
   bruit de g.
galvanotherapy
Gambian
   G. fever
   G. trypanosomiasis
gametokinetic hormone
gamma
   g. glutamyl transferase (GGT)
   g. GT
gamma-aminobutyric acid (GABA)
gamma-hydroxybutyrate toxicity
gamma-seminoprotein
gammopathy
   benign monoclonal g. (BMG)
   monoclonal g.
Gamna
   G. disease
   G. nodule
Gamstorp disease
ganciclovir
Gandy-Gamna
   G.-G. disease
   G.-G. nodule
   G.-G. spleen
Gandy-Nanta disease
ganglion, pl. **ganglia**
   basal g.
   Bock g.
   g. cyst
   dorsal root g. (DRG)
   sympathetic g.
   Troisier g.
ganglioside lipidosis
gangliosidosis
   G_{M1} g.
   generalized g.
gangrene
   Fournier g.
   gas g.
   Meleney g.
   Pott g.
   Raynaud g.
   spontaneous gas g.
   venous limb g.

G

gangrenosa
    vaccinia g.
gangrenosum
    pyoderma g.
gangrenous
    g. abscess
    g. cellulitis
    g. pneumonia
    g. stomatitis
Gantrisin
    Azo G.
gap
    anion g.
    fecal osmotic g.
    g. junction protein
    osmolal g.
    osmotic g.
Garamycin
garapata disease
Garcinia cambogia
Gardnerella
Gardner syndrome
Gard Violet
Garland triangle
garlic
garment
    antishock g.
    pneumatic antishock g.
garnet
    yttrium, argon, g. (YAG)
Garré disease
Gärtner bacillus
gas
    arterial blood g. (ABG)
    blood g.
    g. dilution
    g. gangrene
    g. inhalation
    RA blood g.
    room air blood g.
gaseous cellulitis
gaseousness
gasp
    agonal g.
gastralgia
gastric
    g. acid analysis
    g. algid malaria
    g. artery aneurysm
    g. atrophy
    g. cancer
    g. cardia
    g. colic
    g. crisis
    g. II diet
    g. emptying
    g. feeding
    g. hyperplasia
    g. hypersecretion

    g. indigestion
    g. inhibitory peptide (GIP)
    g. inhibitory polypeptide (GIP)
    g. lavage
    g. lymphoma
    g. motor dysfunction
    g. mucosa
    g. neurasthenia
    g. outlet obstruction
    g. reduction
    g. tetany
    g. varix
gastrica
    achylia g.
    adenasthenia g.
    myxorrhea g.
gastrin
    serum g.
gastrinoma
    duodenal g.
gastritis
    antral g.
    antrum-predominant g.
    catarrhal g.
    corpus-predominant g.
    eosinophilic g.
    erosive g.
    Helicobacter pylori g.
    hemorrhagic g.
    reflux g.
gastroalbumorrhea
gastroatonia
gastroblennorrhea
gastrochronorrhea
gastrocnemius
gastrocolic
gastrocolitis
gastroduodenal
    g. artery aneurysm
    g. manometry
gastrodynia
gastroenteric
gastroenteritis
    acute infectious nonbacterial g.
    endemic nonbacterial infantile g.
    eosinophilic g.
    epidemic nonbacterial g.
    infantile g.
    infectious nonbacterial g.
    nonbacterial infantile g.
    viral g.
gastroenterocolitis
gastroenterologist
gastroenterology
gastroenteropathy
    diabetic g.
gastroepiploic artery aneurysm
gastroesophageal
    g. junction

g. reflux
g. reflux disease (GERD)
gastroesophagitis
gastrogavage
gastrogenic
gastrogenous diarrhea
Gastrografin
gastrohydrorrhea
gastrointestinal (GI)
    g. anthrax
    g. biopsy
    g. bleeding
    g. bleeding from an unknown
      source
    g. cancer
    g. candidiasis
    g. cocktail
    g. disease
    g. disorder
    g. dysfunction
    g. hormone
    g. infection
    g. lavage
    g. manometry
    g. neuropathy
    g. toxicity
    upper g. (UGI)
    g. water loss
gastrointestinalis
    mycetism g.
gastrojejunal loop obstruction syndrome
gastrojejunostomy
    Billroth II g.
gastrolithiasis
gastrologist
gastrology
gastromegaly
gastromyxorrhea
gastroparalysis
gastroparesis
    g. diabeticorum
gastropathic
gastropathy
    hypertrophic g.
    portal hypertensive g.
gastroplasty
    Stamm g.
gastrorrhea
gastroscope
    fiberoptic g.
gastroscopy
gastrospasm

gastrostogavage
gastrostomy
    percutaneous endoscopic g. (PEG)
gastrotonometer
gastrotonometry
gastrotoxic
gastrotropic
gastroxia
gastroxynsis
Gas-X
Gatch bed
gated
    g. blood pool method
    g. single-proton emission computed
      tomography
gatekeeping
gatifloxacin
Gaucher
    G. disease
    G. splenomegaly
gauge
    Dacomed snap g.
gauze
    iodoform g.
gavage feeding
Gaviscon
gaze
gaze-evoked nystagmus
GBV-C
    GB virus C
GB virus C (GBV-C)
GCA
    giant cell arteritis
GCM
    geriatric care manager
G-CSF
    granulocyte colony-stimulating factor
g/dL
    grams per deciliter
GDS
    Geriatric Depression Scale
gegenhalten
gel
    g. cast
    Cleocin T g.
    diclofenac g.
    testosterone g.
    Topicort g.
    tretinoin g.
gelastic epilepsy
gelatinous ascites
Gel-Cam ointment

G

NOTES

Gelfoam
Gellhorn pessary
gemcitabine
gemfibrozil
gender specific
gene
> amyloid precursor protein g.
> ApoE4 g.
> apolipoprotein E epsilon 4 g.
> APP g.
> HER-2/neu g.
> presenilin-1 g.
> presenilin-2 g.
> g. therapy

general
> g. adaptation reaction
> g. duty nurse
> g. health
> g. hospital
> g. malaise
> g. physician
> g. practice
> g. sensorium

generalisatus
> herpes g.

generalist
generalization
generalized
> g. adenopathy
> g. anxiety disorder (GAD)
> g. distal nephron dysfunction
> g. gangliosidosis
> g. glycogenosis
> g. lymphadenopathy
> g. motor seizure
> g. musculoskeletal pain
> g. plane xanthoma
> g. tuberculosis

generation
> G.'s Online
> G.'s Together (GT)

generic drug
genetic
> g. disorder
> g. hypertension
> g. lethal
> g. testing

genital
> g. herpes
> g. mycoplasma infection
> g. tract cancer
> g. ulcer disease
> g. wart

genitalia
genitalis
> herpes g.

genitalium
> *Mycoplasma* g.

genitourinary (GU)

> g. cancer
> g. infection
> g. tuberculosis

genome
> g. encode
> negative-sense g.
> positive-sense g.
> g. replication strategy
> g. segmentation
> viral g.

Genora
genotype
genotypic tolerance
genotyping
gentamicin ototoxicity
genu
> g. valgus
> g. varum

Geocillin
geographic tongue
geomedicine
geopathology
geophagia
geotrichosis
geranylgeranylpyrophosphate (GGPP)
geratology
GERD
> gastroesophageal reflux disease

Gerhardt-Mitchell disease
Geriatric
geriatric
> g. acute care
> g. care manager (GCM)
> G. Depression Scale (GDS)
> g. medicine
> G. Pain Assessment
> g. therapy

geriatrician
geri chair
German measles
germ cell tumor
germinal aplasia
germinoma
geroderma
geromarasmus
gerontal
Gerontological Society of America (GSA)
gerontologist
gerontology
> The Center for Social G. (TCSG)

gerontotherapeutics
gerontotherapy
geropsychiatry
Gerstmann syndrome
Gesell
gestational
> g. diabetes

g. thrombocytopenia
g. trophoblastic neoplasm
gestationis
herpes g.
gesture
gesturing
get-up-and-go test
GFR
glomerular filtration rate
GG
Slo-phyllin GG
G$_{M1}$ gangliosidosis
GGPP
geranylgeranylpyrophosphate
GGT
gamma glutamyl transferase
GH
growth hormone
GHD
growth hormone deficiency
Ghon complex
Ghon-Sachs bacillus
GHRF, GH-RF
growth hormone-releasing factor
GHRH, GH-RH
growth hormone-releasing hormone
GI
gastrointestinal
GI antimuscarinic
GI cocktail
upper GI
giant
g. cell
g. cell arteritis (GCA)
g. cell hepatitis
g. cell pneumonia
g. follicular hyperplasia
g. follicular lymphadenopathy
g. follicular lymphoblastoma
g. follicular thyroiditis
g. hairy nevus
g. lymph node hyperplasia
giantism
Giardia lamblia
giardiasis
gibbus
Gibney boot
giddiness
Giemsa stain
Gierke disease
gigantism
acromegalic g.

cerebral g.
eunuchoid g.
exomphalos, macroglossia, and g.
(EMG)
hyperpituitary g.
pituitary g.
primordial g.
Gilbert
G. cholemia
G. disease
G. sign
G. syndrome
Gilchrist
G. disease
G. mycosis
Gilles de la Tourette syndrome
ginger
gingivitis
gingivostomatitis
acute herpetic g.
Ginkgo biloba
ginkgo supplement
ginseng
Panax g.
Siberian g.
Giordano-Giovannetti diet
Giovannetti diet
GIP
gastric inhibitory peptide
gastric inhibitory polypeptide
girdle
shoulder g.
Gitelman syndrome
githagism
GITS
gut-derived infectious toxic shock
GITT
glucose insulin tolerance test
giveaway
Gjessing syndrome
glabella
glabellar
glabrata
Torulopsis g.
glabrous skin
gland
adrenal g.
Bonnot g.
Brunner g.
endocrine g.
exocrine g.
master g.

NOTES

G

gland *(continued)*
    meibomian g.
    merocrine g.
    multinodular g.
    parathyroid g.
    parotid g.
    pineal g.
    pituitary g.
    Sigmund g.
    Skene g.
    suprahyoid accessory thyroid g.
    suprarenal g.
    thymus g.
    thyroid g.
glandular
    g. abscess
    g. epithelium
    g. plague
    g. tularemia
glandularity
    diffuse g.
    normal g.
glans area
Glanzmann thrombasthenia
glargine
    insulin g.
Glasgow Coma Scale
glatiramer acetate
glaucoma
    acute angle-closure g.
    aphakic g.
    g. filtration surgery
    narrow-angle g.
    pigmentary g.
    primary angle-closure g.
    primary open-angle g. (POAG)
    pseudoexfoliation g.
    G. Research Foundation (GRF)
    steroid-induced g.
Gleason score
Gleevec
Glénard disease
Glenn shunt
glenohumeral
gliamilide
glimepiride
glioblastoma multiforme
glioma
gliosis
GLIP
    glucagonlike insulinotropic peptide
glipizide
Glisson
    G. capsule
    G. cirrhosis
    G. disease
global
    g. anoxia
    g. aphasia

globe cell anemia
globulin
    antithymocyte g.
    cytomegalovirus immune g.
    hepatitis B immune g.
    immune g.
    serum g.
    sex hormone-binding g. (SHBG)
    thyroid-binding g. (TBG)
    unbound thyroxine-binding g. (UTBG)
globulinuria
globus
    g. hystericus
    g. pallidus
    g. pallidus receptor
    g. pharyngeus
    g. sensation
glomerular
    g. capillary pressure
    g. filtration
    g. filtration rate (GFR)
glomerulocapillary sclerosis
glomerulonephritis
    acute poststreptococcal g.
    Berger focal g.
    crescentic g.
    membranoproliferative g. type II
    mesangiopathic g.
    pauci-immune crescentic g.
    poststreptococcal g.
glomerulonephropathy
glomerulopathy
    immune-mediated g.
    membranous g.
glomerulosa
    zona g.
glomerulosclerosis
    diabetic g.
    focal segmental g.
    intercapillary g.
    primary focal segmental g.
    secondary focal segmental g.
glomerulus
glomus
    aural g.
glossal
glossitis
    atrophic g.
    Hunter g.
    migratory g.
    Moeller g.
glossodynia
glossopharyngeal breathing
GLP-1
    glucagonlike peptide
glucagon
    gut g.

glucagonlike
    g. insulinotropic peptide (GLIP)
    g. peptide (GLP-1)
glucagonoma
    nonsecretory g.
    g. syndrome
Glucerna
glucocorticoid
    g. deficiency
    g. injection
    g. reduction fibromyalgia
glucocorticoid-induced osteoporosis
glucocorticosteroid
    inhaled g.
    oral g.
glucocorticosteroid-induced osteoporosis
glucocorticotrophic
glucokinase
glucometer
    Accu-Chek II g.
    Advantage g.
    G. DEX blood glucose monitor
    G. DEX system
    G. Elite XL machine
    Glucostar II g.
    GlucoWatch g.
    Mill Glucometer II g.
    One Touch g.
    g. strip
gluconate
    quinidine g.
gluconeogenesis
glucopenia
Glucophage
GlucoProtein test
glucosamine sulfate
glucose
    blood g.
    fasting blood g.
    fasting plasma g.
    impaired fasting g.
    insulin-mediated g.
    g. insulin tolerance test (GITT)
    g. intolerance
    g. intolerance and pregnancy
    g. monitor
    g. monitoring device
    g. monitoring system
    plasma g.
    g. reading
    g. suppression test
    g. test strip

    g. tolerance (GT)
    g. tolerance test (GTT)
glucose-6-phosphatase hepatorenal glycogenosis
glucose-dependent insulinotropic polypeptide
glucose-galactose malabsorption
glucose-6-phosphate
    g.-6-p. dehydrogenase (G6PD)
    g.-6-p. dehydrogenase deficiency
    g.-6-p. dehydrogenase deficiency anemia
glucosidase inhibitor
glucosinolates
Glucostar II glucometer
glucosuria
Glucotrol XL
Glucovance
GlucoWatch
    G. glucometer
    G. glucose monitoring device
glucuronidation
glutamic aciduria
gluteal
gluten
    g. ataxia
    g. enteropathy
gluten-free diet
gluten-sensitive enteropathy (GSE)
glyburide
glycation
glycemic
    g. control
    g. index
glycerol
    iodinated g.
glycinuria
    familial g.
glycogen
    g. cardiomegaly
    g. storage disease
glycogenic cardiomegaly
glycogenolysis defect
glycogenosis
    brancher deficiency g.
    generalized g.
    glucose-6-phosphatase hepatorenal g.
    hepatophosphorylase deficiency g.
    myophosphorylase deficiency g.
    type 1–7 g.
glycoglycinuria

G

NOTES

glycol
> polyethylene g.
> propylene g.

glycolic aciduria
glycolipid lipidosis
glycolysis
glycopenia
glycopeptide antibiotic
glycopeptide-resistant enterococci
glycophilia
glycoprotein (GP)
> g. IIb-IIIa receptor antagonist
> g. IIIa
> spike-like g.
> two-envelope g.

glycostatic
glycosuria
> alimentary g.
> benign g.
> digestive g.
> nondiabetic g.
> nonhyperglycemic g.
> normoglycemic g.
> orthoglycemic g.
> pathologic g.
> renal g.

glycosylate
glycosylated
> g. hemoglobin
> g. hemoglobin test

glycotropic
glycuresis
Glynase Pres Tabs
Glyset
GM
> hepatitis GM

GnRH, Gn-RH
> gonadotropin-releasing hormone

go
> timed up and g. (TUG)

goal
GOAT
> Galveston Orientation and Amnesia Test

goat's milk anemia
Godélier law
Goggia sign
goiter
> adenomatous g.
> Basedow g.
> cabbage g.
> colloid g.
> cystic g.
> endemic g.
> euthyroid g.
> exophthalmic g.
> familial g.
> fibrous g.
> follicular g.
> intrathoracic g.

> multinodular g.
> myxedematous g.
> nodular g.
> nontoxic g. (NTG)
> nontoxic nodular g. (NTNG)
> papillomatous g.
> parenchymatous g.
> substernal g.
> thoracic g.
> toxic multinodular g.

goitrous
gold
> oral g.
> g. salt
> g. standard
> g. treatment

Goldblatt
> G. hypertension
> G. kidney

goldenseal
Goldman elevator
golfer's elbow
GoLYTELY
gonadal
> g. dysfunction
> g. dysgenesis

gonadocrin
gonadoliberin
gonadopathy
gonadotrophic hormone
gonadotropic hormone (GTH)
gonadotropin, gonadotrophin
> g. agonist
> anterior pituitary g.
> chorionic g.
> g. deficiency
> g. excess
> human chorionic g. (hCG)
> human menopausal g. (HMG)
> human pituitary g. (hPG)
> menopausal urinary g.
> pituitary g.
> total urinary g. (TUG)

gonadotropin-releasing
> g.-r. factor (GRF)
> g.-r. hormone (GnRH, Gn-RH)
> g.-r. hormone agonist
> g.-r. hormone test

gonococcal
> g. arthritis
> g. bacteremia
> g. endocarditis
> g. infection
> g. pharyngitis
> g. septicemia
> g. stomatitis
> g. urethritis

gonococcus, pl. **gonococci**
gonorrhea

gonorrheal
>   g. arthritis
>   g. rheumatism
>   g. stomatitis

gonorrhoeae
>   *Neisseria g.*

Goodpasture syndrome
Goody's powders
goose flesh
Gordon syndrome
Gore-Tex
Gorlin sign
Göthlin test
Gottron papule
gotu kola
gout
>   abarticular g.
>   articular g.
>   calcium g.
>   chalky g.
>   g. diet
>   idiopathic g.
>   intercritical g.
>   interval g.
>   latent g.
>   lead g.
>   masked g.
>   misplaced g.
>   oxalic g.
>   polyarticular g.
>   primary g.
>   renal g.
>   retrocedent g.
>   rheumatic g.
>   saturnine g.
>   secondary g.
>   tophaceous g.

gouty
>   g. arthritis
>   g. diathesis
>   g. iritis
>   g. nephropathy
>   g. proteinuria
>   g. tophi
>   g. urethritis

government hospital
GP
>   glycoprotein
>   GP IIIa

G6PD
>   glucose-6-phosphate dehydrogenase
grab bar

gracile habitus
gradatim
grade
Gradenigo syndrome
gradient
>   alveolar-arterial oxygen g.
>   transtubular potassium
>   concentration g.

grading
>   Karnofsky tumor g.

gradual withdrawal
graduate nurse
Graefe sign
graft
>   Bonfiglio g.
>   coronary artery bypass g. (CABG)
>   g. failure
>   onlay g.
>   saphenous vein g.
>   Thiersch g.

grafting
>   coronary artery bypass g. (CABG)
>   osteochondral g.
>   Papineau g.

graft-versus-host
>   g.-v.-h. disease (GVHD)
>   g.-v.-h. reaction (GVHR)

gram (g)
>   g.'s per deciliter (g/dL)
>   G. stain

gram-negative
>   g.-n. bacillary meningitis
>   g.-n. cocci
>   g.-n. sepsis

gram-positive cocci
grand mal seizure
granisetron hydrochloride
granular cast
granulation
granule
>   alpha g.
>   Fordyce g.

Granulex
granuloblastosis
granulocyte
>   g. colony-stimulating factor (G-CSF)
>   g. transfusion

granulocytic
>   g. hypoplasia
>   g. leukemia

granulocytopenia

G

NOTES

granuloma
> amebic g.
> g. annulare
> coccidioidal g.
> eosinophilic g.
> focal g.
> hepatic g.
> Hodgkin g.
> g. inguinale
> midline g.
> necrotic g.
> paracoccidioidal g.
> pulmonary eosinophilic g.
> pyogenic g.
> silicotic g.
> g. tropicum

granulomatosis
> allergic g.
> beryllium g.
> bronchocentric g.
> g. infantiseptica
> lymphomatoid g.
> necrotizing sarcoid g.
> g. siderotica
> Wegener g.

granulomatous
> g. amebic encephalitis
> g. change
> g. colitis
> g. enteritis
> g. hepatitis
> g. nocardiosis
> g. peritonitis
> g. prostatitis
> g. vasculitis

granulopoiesis
grapefruit juice interaction
graphesthesia
graphic picture scale
grave
> delirium g.

Graves
> G. disease
> G. ophthalmopathy
> G. speculum

gravida
gravidarum
> hyperemesis g.

gravis
> icterus castrensis g.
> myasthenia g.

gravitational force
gravity
> specific g.

Grawitz
> G. cachexia
> G. tumor

grayfish
gray matter

gray-out
green
> g. sickness
> g. sputum
> g. tobacco sickness

Greenfield
> G. disease
> G. filter
> G. syndrome

gregarinosis
grelot
> bruit de g.

Greville bath
Grey Turner sign
GRF
> Glaucoma Research Foundation
> gonadotropin-releasing factor

grid
> Wetzel g.

grief support group
Griesinger
> bilious typhoid of G.

Grifulvin V
grimacing
grip
> devil g.

grippe
Grisactin
griseofulvin
Gris-PEG
Gritti amputation
Gritti-Stokes amputation
Grocco
> G. sign
> G. triangle

groove sign
gross
> g. examination of tissue
> G. leukemia

groundhog bite
ground itch anemia
group
> g. A, B, C, D, G streptococcal
> infection
> g. A, B, G streptococcus
> Colton blood g.
> diagnosis-related g. (DRG)
> grief support g.
> g. I hormone
> g. hospital
> g. II polypeptide hormone
> g. practice
> self-help g.
> sociodemographic g.
> streptococcal g. A, B, G
> sulfhydryl g.
> support g.
> symptom g.
> g. therapy

growth
> cell g.
> g. curve
> g. cycle
> g. factor
> g. factor receptor
> g. fraction
> g. hormone (GH)
> g. hormone deficiency (GHD)
> g. hormone-releasing factor (GHRF, GH-RF)
> g. hormone-releasing factor test
> g. hormone-releasing hormone (GHRH, GH-RH)
> g. hormone secretagogue
> g. hormone-secreting pituitary tumor
> g. hormone therapy
> g. plate
> g. regulation
> g. retardation

growth-onset diabetes
growth-stimulating hormone (GSH)
grumose
gryposis penis
GSA
> Gerontological Society of America

GSE
> gluten-sensitive enteropathy

GSH
> growth-stimulating hormone

GT
> Generations Together
> glucose tolerance
> > gamma GT

GTH
> gonadotropic hormone

GTT
> glucose tolerance test

GU
> genitourinary

guaiac
> stool g.

Guaifed
guaifenesin
Guaitab
Guaituss
guanabenz
guarana
guard
> plate g.

guarding
> abdominal g.

Gubler
> G. icterus
> G. sign

Guéneau de Mussy point
guided needle biopsy
guideline
> Bethesda g.'s
> clinical practice g. (CPG)
> dietary g.

Guillain-Barré
> G.-B. polyneuritis
> G.-B. syndrome

Gulf War syndrome
Gull
> G. disease
> G. renal epistaxis

gum disease
gumma
> multiple g.

gummatous syphilis
Gunn sign
Günther syndrome
gurgling rale
gustatory
> g. hyperhidrosis
> g. loss

gut
> g. glucagon
> g. specific

gut-derived infectious toxic shock (GITS)
guttata
guttate
> psoriasis g.

guttural rale
Guyon
> G. amputation
> G. sign

GVHD
> graft-versus-host disease

GVHR
> graft-versus-host reaction

GYN
> gynecology

gynecological oncology
gynecologic disease
gynecologist
> American College of Obstetricians and G.'s (ACOG)

gynecology (GYN)
> obstetrics and g. (OB-GYN)

NOTES

G

gynecomastia
    refeeding g.
Gyne-Lotrimin
gyrata
    cutis vertices g.
gyrus, pl. **gyri**

cingulate g.

H₂
  H₂ blocker
  H₂ receptor
HAART
  highly active antiretroviral therapy
habit
  altered eating h.
  personal h.
  psychological h.
Habitrol
habituation
  h. exercise
habitus
  gracile h.
  marfanoid body h.
  sthenic h.
HACEK
  *Haemophilus aphrophilus, Actinobacillus
  actinomycetemcomitans,
  Cardiobacterium hominis, Eikenella
  corrodens, Kingella kingae*
Hadfield-Clarke syndrome
HAE
  hereditary angioedema
haematobium
  Schistosoma h.
Haemophilus
  *H. aphrophilus, Actinobacillus
  actinomycetemcomitans,
  Cardiobacterium hominis,
  Eikenella corrodens, Kingella
  kingae* (HACEK)
  H. hemolyticus
  H. infection
  H. influenzae
  H. influenzae meningitis
  H. influenzae type b (HIB)
  H. influenzae type b cellulitis
  H. influenzae vaccine
Haff disease
hafussi bath
Hagedorn
  neutral protamine H. (NPH)
hagiotherapy
Haglund
  H. deformity
  H. disorder
HAI
  hemagglutination-inhibition
  history activity index
hair
  beaded h.
  corkscrew h.
  moniliform h.

hairy
  h. cell leukemia
  h. leukoplakia
  h. tongue
halazepam
Halcion
Haldane effect
Haldol
half-life
  drug h.-l.
Halfprin
halfway house
haliphagia
halisteresis phenomenon
halitosis
Hallé point
Hallervorden-Spatz disease
Hallopeau acrodermatitis
Hallpike maneuver
hallucination
  hypnagogic h.
  hypnopompic h.
hallucinatory
hallucinogen
hallucinosis
  peduncular h.
hallucis
  adductor h.
hallux
  h. limitus
  h. rigidus
  h. valgus
Halog cream
halo nevus
haloperidol
Halotex lotion
halothane toxicity
Halstead-Reitan battery
Halsted inguinal herniorrhaphy
hamartoma
  chondromatous h.
  leiomyomatous h.
HAMD
  Hamilton Rating Scale for Depression
Hamilton
  H. Depression Scale
  H. Rating Scale for Depression
  (HAMD)
Hamman sign
hammertoe
Hancock amputation
hand
  h. arthrocentesis
  H. disease
  drop h.

H

173

hand *(continued)*
    fall on outstretched h. (FOOSH)
    outstretched h.
    h. pain
    H. syndrome
hand-and-foot syndrome
handbook
    Diabetes Self-Help H.
    Harriet Lane H.
handcuff palsy
hand-foot-mouth disease
handicap
    mental h.
    physical h.
handicapped
    National Library Service for the
    Blind and Physically H.
    (NLSBPH)
handrail
Hand-Schüller-Christian
    H.-S.-C. disease
    H.-S.-C. syndrome
Hanger-Rose skin test
Hanot
    H. cirrhosis
    H. disease
    H. syndrome
Hanot-Chauffard syndrome
Hansen bacillus
Hanta virus
haploinsufficiency
haplotype
    HLA h.
haptoglobin
Harada disease
hard cord
hardening
    work h.
hard-metal lung disease
harlequin reaction
harness
    Pavlik h.
Harriet Lane Handbook
Harrington rod
Harris-Benedict equation
Hartnup
    H. disease
    H. syndrome
hasamiyami
Hashimoto
    H. disease
    H. struma
    H. thyroid
    H. thyroiditis
hat-band headache
haustral marking
HAV
    hepatitis A virus
Haven syndrome

Haverhill fever
Havrix vaccine
Hawes-Pallister-Landor syndrome
hawkinsinuria
hay
    h. asthma
    h. fever
Hayem
    H. icterus
Hayem-Widal syndrome
Hayflick limit phenomenon
hazard
    environmental h.
    occupational h.
HB
    hepatitis B
    Recombivax HB
HbA$_{1c}$
    hemoglobin A$_{1c}$
HBH disease
HBr
    hydrobromic acid
    citalopram HBr
    galantamine HBr
HBV
    hepatitis B virus
HC
    Carmol HC
    thiamine HC
HCFA
    Health Care Finance Administration
hCG
    human chorionic gonadotropin
    quantitative beta hCG
HCl
    hydrochloride
    amantadine HCl
    buspirone HCl
    desipramine HCl
    doxepin HCl
    encainide HCl
    imipramine HCl
    nortriptyline HCl
    pioglitazone HCl
    quinapril HCl
    raloxifene HCl
    rimantadine HCl
    ticlopidine HCl
hCS
    human chorionic somatomammotropin
HCT
    hematocrit
    hydrochlorothiazide
    Atacand HCT
    Micardis HCT
HCTZ
    hydrochlorothiazide
HCV
    hepatitis C virus

HDL
> high-density lipoprotein
> > HDL cholesterol

HDL-C
> high-density lipoprotein cholesterol

HDSA
> Huntington's Disease Society of America

head
> h. banging
> h., ears, eyes, nose, throat (HEENT)
> femoral h.
> hourglass h.
> h. lice
> Medusa h.
> h. and neck cancer
> h. nurse
> H. & Shoulders
> h. trauma
> H. zone

headache
> cervicogenic h.
> chronic tension-type h.
> cluster h.
> coital h.
> cough h.
> exertional h.
> hat-band h.
> Horton h.
> hypnic h.
> jolt h.
> meningeal h.
> migraine h.
> muscle contraction h.
> neuralgic h.
> nitroglycerin h.
> paraplegic h.
> postconcussion h.
> postconcussional h.
> pressor h.
> h. prone
> spinal fluid loss h.
> tension h.
> tension-type h.
> thunderclap h.
> traction h.
> traumatic h.
> vascular h.

head-up
> h.-u. tilt-table test
> h.-u. tilt test

healed tuberculosis

healer
healing
health
> adolescent h.
> h. care
> h. care cost
> h. care employee precaution
> h. care facility
> H. Care Finance Administration (HCFA)
> h. center
> Department of Public H. (DPH)
> Diploma of Public H. (DPH)
> Doctor of Public H. (DPH, DrPH)
> h. evaluation
> general h.
> H. Insurance Association of America (HIAA)
> H. Insurance Portability and Accountability Act (HIPAA)
> h. maintenance
> h. maintenance organization (HMO)
> National Alliance for Hispanic H.
> National Institute of Mental H. (NIMH)
> National Institutes of H. (NIH)
> Office on Smoking and H. (OSH)
> h. promotion
> public h.
> h. risk assessment (HRA)
> h. status

health-related quality of life (HRQL, HRQOL)
healthy old age
hearing
> h. aid
> h. loss

Hearing-Handicap Inventory for the Elderly
heart
> athlete's h.
> h. block
> h. disease
> ejection fraction of h.
> h. failure
> h. hormone
> h. murmur
> h. rate (HR)
> soldier's h.
> h. sound
> h. tone
> h. transplant

NOTES

H

heart *(continued)*
    h. transplant rejection
    h. valve
    h. valve hemolysis
heartburn
heart-lung
    h.-l. transplant
    h.-l. transplantation
heat
    h. apoplexy
    h. cramp
    h. exhaustion
    h. hyperpyrexia
    h. prostration
    h. pyrexia
    h. stroke
    h. syncope
heated
    h. nasogastric lavage
    h. peritoneal lavage
heat-induced illness
heatstroke
heave
    dry h.'s
    parasternal h.
heaviness
heavy chain deposition disease
Heberden
    H. asthma
    H. disease
    H. node
    H. nodosity
    H. rheumatism
    H. sign
    H. syndrome
Heberden angina
hebetic
hebiatrics
Hecht
    H. phenomenon
    H. pneumonia
hectic flush
Hedinger syndrome
heel
    h. cord stretching exercise
    h. pain
    h. spur
    h. spur syndrome
heel-knee-shin
heel-to-shin
    h.-t.-s. test
HEENT
    head, ears, eyes, nose, throat
Heerfordt
    H. disease
    H. syndrome
Hegglin anomaly
height
    laryngeal h.

    maximum laryngeal h.
    minimum laryngeal h.
heightened filtration rate
Heimlich maneuver
Heinz body
helical
Helicobacter
    H. pylori
    H. pylori gastritis
helicoids
helicopod gait
helioaerotherapy
heliosis
heliotherapy
heliotrope rash
HELLP
    hemolysis, elevated liver enzymes, low
        platelets
helminthemesis
helminthiasis
helminthic
    h. dysentery
    h. infection
helminthism
heloma
    h. durum
    h. molle
hemagglutination-inhibition (HAI)
hemagglutinin neuraminidase (HN)
hemagglutinin neuraminidase protein
hemangioendothelioma
hemangioma
    cardiac h.
    h. of liver
hemangiomatosis
    systemic h.
hemangiopericytoma
hemarthrosis
hematemesis
hematherapy
hematinics
hematochezia
hematocrit (HCT)
    hemoglobin and h. (H&H)
hematogenous
    h. dissemination
    h. metastasis
    h. osteomyelitis
    h. spread
hematologic
    h. dysfunction
    h. tumor
hematology
hematology/oncology
hematoma
    chronic subdural h.
    epidural h.
    intracerebral h.
    subdural h.

hematopathologist
hematopathology
hematopoiesis
hematopoietic
    h. growth factor
    h. stem cell transplantation
hematoporphyria
hematosepsis
hematospermia
hematoxylin stain
hematuria
    Egyptian h.
    endemic h.
    isolated h.
    march h.
    painful h.
    painless h.
heme
    h. negative
    h. positive
hemianopia
    absolute h.
hemianopic
    h. field loss
    h. prism spectacles
hemianopsia
hemiatrophy
hemiballismus
hemiblock
    left anterior h. (LAHB)
hemic distomiasis
hemicolectomy
hemicrania
    chronic paroxysmal h.
hemidiaphragm
hemifacial
    h. spasm
hemimelia
hemiparesis
hemiparetic
hemiplegia
hemiplegic migraine
hemisensory
hemispatial
hemisphere
    frontal h.
hemithorax
hemoblastic leukemia
Hemoccult test
hemochromatosis
    primary h.
    secondary h.

hemocytoblastic leukemia
hemodialysis amyloidosis
hemodynamic
    h. effect
    h. pressure
hemofiltration
    continuous venovenous h.
hemoglobin (HGB)
    h. A_2
    h. A_{1c} (HbA_{1c})
    Bart h.
    glycosylated h.
    h. and hematocrit (H&H)
    h. hemolytic anemia
    hereditary persistence of fetal h.
    high-affinity h.
    low-affinity h.
    mean corpuscular h. (MCH)
hemoglobinemia
hemoglobinopathies
hemoglobinuria
    malarial h.
    paroxysmal nocturnal h.
hemoglobinuric
    h. acute tubular necrosis
    h. fever
    h. nephrosis
hemolysin
    acid h.
hemolysis
    chronic h.
    h., elevated liver enzymes, low
      platelets (HELLP)
    footstrike h.
    heart valve h.
    phenylhydrazine h.
hemolytic
    h. anemia
    h. disease
    h. icterus
    h. splenomegaly
    h. transfusion reaction
    h. uremic syndrome (HUS)
hemolyticus
    Haemophilus h.
    icterus h.
hemoperitoneum
hemophagocytic syndrome
hemophilia
    h. A, B, C
    Leyden h. B

NOTES

H

hemophilia *(continued)*
   h. neonatorum
   vascular h.
hemophiliac
hemophilic
   h. arthritis
   h. arthropathy
hemopoietic
hemoptysis
   cryptogenic h.
   endemic h.
   parasitic h.
hemorrhage
   cerebellar h.
   deep cerebral h.
   dot-and-blot h.
   exsanguinating h.
   hypertensive intracerebral h.
   intracerebral h.
   intracranial h.
   serous h.
   splinter h.
   subarachnoid h. (SAH)
   subconjunctival h.
   variceal h.
hemorrhagic
   h. bronchitis
   h. colitis
   h. dengue
   h. familial angiomatosis
   h. fever
   h. fever with renal syndrome
   h. gastritis
   h. infarction
   h. insult
   h. measles
   h. plague
   h. rickets
   h. scurvy
   h. shock
   h. smallpox
   h. stroke
hemorrhagica
   aleukia h.
   purpura h.
   scarlatina h.
   variola h.
hemorrhagicum
   corpus h.
hemorrhoid
   external h.
   internal h.
   thrombosed external h.
hemorrhoidectomy
hemosialemesis
hemosiderin
hemosiderosis
   idiopathic pulmonary h.

   nutritional h.
   transfusional h.
hemostasis
   primary h.
   secondary h.
hemostat
hemostatic
   h. disorder
   h. therapy
hemotherapy
hemotympanum
HEMPAS
   hereditary erythroblastic multinuclearity
   associated with positive acidified serum
Henle loop
Henoch purpura
Henoch-Schönlein
   H.-S. purpura
   H.-S. syndrome
henselae
   Rochalimaea h.
heparin
   low-molecular-weight h.
   h. therapy
   unfractionated h.
heparin-induced thrombocytopenia
heparinize
hepatalgia
hepatatrophia
hepatectomy
   recipient h.
hepatic
   h. abscess
   h. amebiasis
   h. amyloidosis
   h. artery aneurysm
   h. colic
   h. coma
   h. copper level
   h. 2,6-dimethyliminodiacetic acid
    (HIDA)
   h. 2,6-dimethyliminodiacetic acid
    scan
   h. distomiasis
   h. drug clearance
   h. encephalopathy
   h. failure
   h. fibrosis
   h. flexure
   h. granuloma
   h. infantilism
   h. infiltrative disorder
   h. insufficiency
   h. intermittent fever
   h. iron concentration
   h. lipase deficiency
   h. metabolism
   h. 3-methylglutaryl coenzyme A
    reductase inhibitor

h. necrosis
h. neoplasm
h. osteodystrophy
h. porphyria
h. schistosomiasis
h. structure
h. tumor
hepatica
adiposis h.
facies h.
porphyria h.
pseudohemophilia h.
hepaticojejunostomy
hepaticus
fetor h.
hepatis
lues h.
porta h.
hepatism
hepatitic
hepatitis
h. A
active h.
acute parenchymatous h.
acute viral h.
aggressive h.
alcoholic h.
anicteric virus h.
autoimmune h.
h. A vaccine
h. A virus (HAV)
h. B (HB)
h. B DNA
h. B immune globulin
h. B vaccine
h. B virus (HBV)
h. C
cholangiolitic h.
cholestatic h.
chronic active h. (CAH)
chronic persistent h.
chronic persisting h.
chronic viral h.
h. C RNA
cryptogenic chronic h.
h. C virus (HCV)
h. D
h. delta virus
drug-induced h.
h. E
epidemic h.
fulminant h.

h. G
giant cell h.
h. GM
granulomatous h.
infectious h. (IH)
ischemic h.
long incubation h.
lupoid h.
mild chronic h.
moderate chronic h.
MS-1 h.
NANB h.
NANBNC h.
neonatal h.
non-A h.
non-A, non-B h. (NANB)
non-A, non-B, non-C h.
non-B h.
non-C h.
nonviral chronic h.
parenchymatous h.
peliosis h.
persistent h.
persisting h.
plasma cell h.
radiation h.
serum h. (SH)
severe chronic h.
short incubation h.
subacute h.
syphilitic h.
transfusion h.
viral h. (VH)
viral h. type A, B, C, E
virus h.
virus A, B, C h.
hepatitis-associated arthritis
hepatization
hepatobiliary
h. dysfunction
h. infection
h. scintigraphy
hepatoblastoma
hepatocellular
h. carcinoma
h. disease
h. injury
h. necrosis
hepatocerebral
hepatocyte plasma membrane
hepatodynia
hepatodysentery

NOTES

H

hepatodystrophy
hepatoerythropoietic porphyria
hepatofugal
hepatogenic
hepatography
hepatohemia
hepatoiminodiacetic
  h. acid (HIDA)
  h. acid scan
hepatojugular reflux
hepatolenticular degeneration
hepatologist
hepatology
hepatomegaly
hepatopathic
hepatopathy
hepatopetal
hepatophosphorylase deficiency
  glycogenosis
hepatopulmonary syndrome
hepatorenal syndrome
hepatosplenic candidiasis
hepatosplenomegaly
hepatosplenopathy
hepatotherapy
hepatotoxemia
hepatotoxic effect
hepatotoxicity
  idiosyncratic h.
hepatotoxin
Hepatovirus
Heptavax
herald patch
herbal
  h. concoction
  h. therapy
herbal-induced rash
hereditaria
  adynamia episodica h.
  anemia hypochromica
    siderochestica h.
  porphyria cutanea tarda h.
  protocoproporphyria h.
  syphilis h.
hereditary
  h. angioedema (HAE)
  h. elliptocytosis
  h. erythroblastic multinuclearity
    associated with positive acidified
    serum (HEMPAS)
  h. fructose intolerance
  h. hemorrhagic telangiectasia
  h. medullary thyroid cancer
  h. methemoglobinemia
  h. methemoglobinemic cyanosis
  h. motor and sensory neuropathy
    type 1–4
  h. myokymia
  h. nephropathy

  h. neuropathy
  h. neuropathy with liability to
    pressure palsy
  h. nonhemolytic hyperbilirubinemia
  h. nonpolyposis colorectal cancer
    (HNPCC)
  h. osteodystrophy
  h. persistence of fetal hemoglobin
  h. renal abnormality
  h. sensory and autonomic
    neuropathy type 1
  h. spherocytosis
  h. sucrase-alpha-dextrinase
    deficiency
  h. vitamin D-resistant rickets
heredofamilial
heredogenerative disorder
Hering phenomenon
hermaphroditism
  adrenal h.
HER-2/neu gene
hernia
  Barth h.
  diaphragmatic h.
  esophageal h.
  external h.
  fat h.
  femoral h.
  hiatal h.
  hiatus h.
  incarcerated inguinal h.
  incisional h.
  indirect inguinal h.
  inguinal h.
  nontender incarcerated inguinal h.
  reducible femoral h.
  reducible inguinal h.
  Richter h.
  sliding hiatal h.
  small neck incisional h.
herniated
  h. disk
  h. nucleus pulposus (HNP)
herniation
  brain h.
  cerebral h.
  fascial h.
  transtentorial h.
herniorrhaphy
  Halsted inguinal h.
heroic snoring
heroin
  h. addiction
  h. overdose
  h. withdrawal
Herophili
  torcular H.
herpangina

herpes
h. catarrhalis
cutaneous h.
h. eye infection
h. generalisatus
genital h.
h. genitalis
h. gestationis
h. labialis
h. meningoencephalitis
h. pneumonia
recurrent genital h.
h. simplex
h. simplex meningitis
h. simplex virus (HSV)
h. simplex virus esophagitis
h. simplex virus infection
h. varicella-zoster virus
h. zoster (HZ)
h. zoster virus (HZV)
herpes-type virus (HTV)
herpesvirus
human h. 6 (HHV-6)
herpete
zoster sine h.
herpetic
h. esophagitis
h. fever
h. lesion
h. pharyngotonsillitis
h. stomatitis
h. urethritis
h. whitlow
Herrick anemia
herring-worm disease
HERS
Hysterectomy Educational Resources and Services Foundation
Hers disease
Herter disease
Hertz frequency
herz hormone
hesitancy
heterocrine
heterocrisis
heterocytotropic anaphylaxis
heterogeneity
heterogeneous
heterogenous
heterologous
heteropathy
heterophile test

heterophyiasis
heterophyidiasis
heterozygote
heterozygous familial hypercholesterolemia
hexachlorophene
hexamethonium
hexaxial reference system
Hey amputation
Hg
mercury
HGB
hemoglobin
HGE
human granulocytic ehrlichiosis
HGH, hGH
human growth hormone
H&H
hemoglobin and hematocrit
HHV-6
human herpesvirus 6
HIAA
Health Insurance Association of America
5-HIAA
5-hydroxyindoleacetic acid
urine for 5-HIAA
hiatal hernia
hiatus hernia
HIB
Haemophilus influenzae type b
hibernating
Hibiclens
hiccup, hiccough
Hickey-Hare test
HIDA
hepatic 2,6-dimethyliminodiacetic acid
hepatoiminodiacetic acid
HIDA scan
hidradenitis
suppurative h.
hidrosis
hiemalis
arthritis h.
hiemis
hyperemesis h.
hierotherapy
high
h. bone turnover disease
h. cervical lymphadenopathy
h. dose
h. enema
h. functioning

NOTES

high *(continued)*
    h. power field
    h. resolution
high-affinity hemoglobin
high-altitude
    h.-a. cerebral edema
    h.-a. sickness
high-calorie diet
high-density
    h.-d. lipoprotein (HDL)
    h.-d. lipoprotein cholesterol (HDL-
    C)
high-dose
    h.-d. dexamethasone suppression
    test
    h.-d. diuretic therapy
high-fat diet
high-fiber diet
high-frequency acuity
high-grade non-Hodgkin lymphoma
high-hepatic clearance drug
high-lateral myocardial infarction
**highly active antiretroviral therapy
(HAART)**
**high-molecular-weight kininogen
deficiency**
high-osmolarity solution
high-output failure
**high-resolution computed tomography
(HRCT)**
high-tension burn
hila (*pl. of* hilum)
hilar adenopathy
**Hill-Burton Free Medical Care
Program**
hilum, pl. **hila**
hip
    h. arthritis
    h. click
    h. fracture
    h. pain
    h. prosthesis
    h. replacement
HIPAA
    Health Insurance Portability and
    Accountability Act
hippocampal sclerosis
hippocampus
hippocratic
    h. face
    h. facies
    h. finger
    H. nail
    h. succussion
    h. succussion sound
hippocratici
    digiti h.
hippuran

hippuria
HipSaver protective underwear
hircismus
hircus
Hirschsprung disease
hirsute
hirsuties
hirsutism
    Apert h.
    constitutional h.
    idiopathic h.
hirudiniasis
Hirudo
His
    bundle of H.
Hismanal
His-Purkinje
    H.-P. pathway
    H.-P. system
Histalet
histamine
    h. fast
    h. flush
    h. receptor antagonist
histamine-2
    h.-2 blocker
    h.-2 receptor antagonist
histidinemia
histidinuria
histiocytic
    h. cytophagic panniculitis
    h. leukemia
    h. medullary reticulosis
histiocytosis
    pulmonary h.
    h. X
histocompatibility
histologic benign prostatic hyperplasia
histology
histolytic
histolytica
    Entamoeba h.
    Escherichia h.
histopathologic
histopathology
Histoplasma capsulatum **infection**
histoplasmoma
histoplasmosis
    chronic progressive pulmonary h.
    progressive pulmonary h.
history (HX)
    h. activity index (HAI)
    h. of (H/O)
    past h. (PH)
    patient h.
    h. and physical (H&P)
    sexual h.
histotoxic anoxia

histrionic
>	h. personality
>	h. personality disorder

HIV
>	human immunodeficiency virus
>	HIV serology
>	HIV test
>	HIV wasting syndrome

HIV-1-associated nephropathy

HIV/AIDS Treatment Information Service (ATIS)

HIV-associated
>	HIV-a. arthritis
>	HIV-a. diarrhea
>	HIV-a. lung disease
>	HIV-a. nephropathy
>	HIV-a. neurologic disease
>	HIV-a. thrombocytopenia

HLA
>	human leukocyte antigen
>	HLA-B27
>	HLA haplotype

HMG
>	human menopausal gonadotropin

HMG-CoA
>	HMG-CoA reductase
>	HMG-CoA reductase inhibitor

HMO
>	health maintenance organization

HN
>	hemagglutinin neuraminidase

HNP
>	herniated nucleus pulposus

HNPCC
>	hereditary nonpolyposis colorectal cancer

H/O
>	history of

hoarseness

Hodge pessary

Hodgkin
>	H. disease
>	H. granuloma
>	H. lymphoma

Hodgkinson Mental Test

Hoesch test

Hofmann bacillus

hole
>	macular h.

holistic medicine

holoendemic

holomorphosis

holosystolic murmur

Holter monitor

Holt-Oram syndrome

Homans sign

home
>	h. access system
>	h. discharge
>	h. environment
>	h. exercise program
>	h. glucose monitoring
>	h. health nurse
>	nursing h.
>	h. nutrition therapy
>	residential h.
>	h. safety assessment

homebound

homeless

homeopath

homeopathic remedy

homeopathist

homeopathy

homeostasis
>	potassium h.

homeostatic

homeotherapeutic

homeotherapy

homing value

hominis
>	*Blastocystis h.*
>	*Mycoplasma h.*
>	*Staphylococcus h.*
>	*Trichomonas h.*

hominivorax
>	*Cochliomyia h.*

homocitrullinuria

homocysteine reduction

homocystinuria

homocytotropic anaphylaxis

homogeneous

homogenous

homologous serum jaundice

homonymous

homophobia

homosexual proctitis

homozygous
>	h. C2 deficiency
>	h. familial hypercholesterolemia
>	h. hypobetalipoproteinemia

honeycombing

honey-thick liquid

honey urine

Hong Kong influenza

NOTES

H

hookworm
    h. anemia
    h. disease
    h. infection
Hoover
    H. sign
    H. test
hops
hora somni (h.s.)
  at bedtime
hordeolum
hormesis
hormonal
    h. ablation therapy
    h. agent
    h. manipulation
    h. migraine
hormone
    adipokinetic h.
    adrenocorticotropic h. (ACTH)
    adrenomedullary h.
    adrenotropic h.
    androgenic h.
    anterior pituitary h.
    antidiuretic h. (ADH)
    atrial natriuretic h. (ANH)
    cardiac h.
    h. change
    chorionic gonadotropic h.
    cortical h.
    corticotropic h.
    corticotropin-releasing h. (CRH)
    h. deficiency
    ectopic h.
    end terminal parathyroid h.
    estrogenic h.
    exogenous h.
    h. flare
    follicle-stimulating h. (FSH)
    follicular h.
    galactopoietic h.
    gametokinetic h.
    gastrointestinal h.
    gonadotrophic h.
    gonadotropic h. (GTH)
    gonadotropin-releasing h. (GnRH, Gn-RH)
    group I h.
    group II polypeptide h.
    growth h. (GH)
    growth hormone-releasing h. (GHRH, GH-RH)
    growth-stimulating h. (GSH)
    heart h.
    herz h.
    human chorionic somatomammotropic h.
    human growth h. (HGH, hGH)
    human pituitary follicle-stimulating h. (hPFSH)
    hypophysiotropic h.
    inappropriate h.
    inappropriate antidiuretic h. (IADH)
    interstitial cell-stimulating h. (ICSH)
    lactation h.
    lactogenic h.
    h. level
    lipid-mobilizing h.
    lipotropic h. (LPH)
    little adrenocorticotrophic h.
    local h.
    luteinizing h. (LH)
    luteinizing hormone-releasing h. (LH-RH, LHRH, LRH)
    mammotropic h.
    melanocyte-stimulating h. (MSH)
    h. metabolism
    parathyroid h. (PTH)
    pituitary gonadotropic h.
    pituitary growth h.
    placental growth h.
    posterior pituitary h.
    progestational h.
    h. receptor
    releasing h. (RH)
    h. replacement
    h. replacement therapy (HRT)
    salivary gland h.
    serum thyroid-stimulating h.
    sex h.
    somatotropic h. (STH)
    syndrome of inappropriate secretion of antidiuretic h. (SIADH)
    h. synthesis
    h. therapy
    thyroid h.
    thyroid-stimulating h. (TSH)
    thyrotropic h.
    thyrotropin-releasing h. (TRH)
hormone-prolactin
    chorionic growth h.-p.
hormonotherapy
horn
    cutaneous h.
    dorsal h.
    H. sign
    H. sign
Horner syndrome
Horton
    H. arteritis
    H. cephalalgia
    H. disease
    H. headache
    H. syndrome
hose
    support h.

TED h.
thromboembolic disease h.
hospice care
hospital
h. admission
base h.
camp h.
closed h.
day h.
h. discharge
h. epidemiology
h. fever
general h.
government h.
group h.
h. insurance
maternity h.
mental h.
municipal h.
night h.
h. nurse
open h.
philanthropic h.
private h.
proprietary h.
public h.
h. record
special h.
state h.
h. stay
teaching h.
Veterans Administration h.
voluntary h.
weekend h.
hospital-acquired bloodstream infection
hospitalist
hospitalization
hospitalize
do not h. (DNH)
host disease
hot
h. caudate lobe
h. flash
Icy H.
h. lesion
h. pack
h. thyroid nodule
hotline
National STD and AIDS H.'s
"hot-tub" folliculitis
hour
every h. [L. *quaque hora*] (q.h.)

24-hour
24-h. RAI uptake
24-h. urine cortisol
hourglass head
house
h. dust mite
halfway h.
h. officer
h. staff
household ambulator
housemaid knee
housing
congregate h.
Houssay-Biasotti syndrome
Houssay syndrome
hOx monitor
Hoyne sign
H&P
history and physical
HPA
hypothalamic-pituitary axis
HPAA
hypothalamic-pituitary-adrenal axis
hPFSH
human pituitary follicle-stimulating
hormone
hPG
human pituitary gonadotropin
HPT
hyperparathyroidism
HPV
human papillomavirus
HR
heart rate
HRA
health risk assessment
HRCT
high-resolution computed tomography
H$_2$ receptor antagonist
H-reflex measurement
HRQL
health-related quality of life
HRQOL
health-related quality of life
HRT
hormone replacement therapy
HS
Covera HS
H.S.
Estratest H.S.
h.s.
hora somni

NOTES

H

H-shaped vertebra
HSV
  herpes simplex virus
5-HT
  5-hydroxytryptamine
5-HT$_{2A}$
  5-hydroxytryptamine 2A
HTLV
  human T-cell lymphotropic virus
HTLV-III
  human T-cell lymphotropic virus III
HTV
  herpes-type virus
Hubbard tank
Huber opponensplasty
Huchard
  H. disease
  H. sign
  H. symptom
Huët-Pelger nuclear anomaly
Hughes syndrome
hum
  cervical venous h.
Humalog humectant
human
  h. babesiosis
  h. bite
  h. blood fluke
  h. botfly myiasis
  h. chorionic gonadotropin (hCG)
  h. chorionic gonadotropin level
  h. chorionic somatomammotropic
    hormone
  h. chorionic somatomammotropin
    (hCS)
  h. ecology
  h. granulocytic ehrlichiosis (HGE)
  h. growth hormone (HGH, hGH)
  h. herpesvirus 6 (HHV-6)
  h. immunodeficiency virus (HIV)
  h. leptin receptor
  h. leukocyte antigen (HLA)
  h. menopausal gonadotropin (HMG)
  h. monkeypox
  h. papillomavirus (HPV)
  h. pituitary follicle-stimulating
    hormone (hPFSH)
  h. pituitary gonadotropin (hPG)
  h. T-cell lymphotropic virus
    (HTLV)
  h. T-cell lymphotropic virus III
    (HTLV-III)
  h. ultralente insulin
humectant
  Humalog h.
humectation
humerus
Humibid

humidifier
  cool mist h.
humor
  peccant h.
humoral
  h. doctrine
  h. hypercalcemia of benignancy
  h. immune deficiency
  h. immune function
  h. rejection
hump
  buffalo h.
  dowager's h.
Humulin N
hunger
  air h.
  h. pain
  h. swelling
hungry bone syndrome
Hunter
  H. canal
  H. glossitis
  H. syndrome
Huntington
  H. chorea
  H. disease
  H. Disease Society of America
    (HDSA)
Huperzia serrata
huperzine A
Hurler
  H. disease
  H. syndrome
Hürthle
  H. cell adenoma
  H. cell carcinoma
  H. cell tumor
HUS
  hemolytic uremic syndrome
Hutchinson
  H. facies
  H. triad
Hutinel disease
HX
  history
hyaline
  h. cartilage
  h. cell
  h. degeneration
hyaline-like material
hyalinosis
hyaluronic acid
hybaroxia
hybridization
  Southern blot h.
Hycodan
Hycomine
hydatid
  h. cyst

h. disease
h. fremitus
h. resonance
h. thrill
hydatidiform mole
Hydergine
hydralazine
h. lupus
h. syndrome
hydrallostane
hydrargyria
hydrate
chloral h.
hydrazide
isonicotinic acid h. (INH)
Hydrea
hydremia
hydremic edema
hydriatric
hydrobromic acid (HBr)
hydrocarbon toxicity
hydrocele
Dupuytren h.
hydrocephaloid
hydrocephalus
normal-pressure h.
posthemorrhagic h. (PHH)
hydrochloride (HCl)
anagrelide h.
benazepril h.
colesevelam h.
diltiazem h.
dobutamine h.
donepezil h.
fexofenadine h.
granisetron h.
meperidine h.
minocycline h.
naltrexone h.
nefazodone h.
ondansetron h.
papaverine h.
phenazopyridine h.
propafenone h.
raloxifene h.
sibutramine h.
tacrine h.
tiagabine h.
tizanidine h.
hydrochlorothiazide (HCT, HCTZ)
hydrocholeresis
hydrocholeretic

hydrocodone
hydrocolloid dressing
hydrocortisone
hydrodiuresis
HydroDIURIL
hydroelectric bath
hydrogel dressing
hydrogen
h. cyanide inhalation
h. fluoride inhalation
h. ion concentration (pH)
h. peroxide
h. sulfide inhalation
hydrolyze
hydromorphone
hydronephrosis
hydropathic
hydropathy
hydropenia
hydropenic
hydrophila
Aeromonas h.
hydropic
Hydropres
hydrops
endolymphatic h.
h. fetalis
hydroquinine
hydrorrhea
hydrosalpinx
hydrostatic pulmonary edema
hydrosudopathy
hydrosudotherapy
hydrotherapeutic
hydrotherapeutics
hydrotherapy
hydrothorax
chylous h.
cirrhotic h.
hydroureter
hydroxide
magnesium h.
potassium h. (KOH)
hydroxyapatite deposition disease
hydroxychloroquine
hydroxykynureninuria
21-hydroxyprogesterone
hydroxyproline
hydroxyprolinemia
5-hydroxytryptamine (5-HT)
-h. 2A (5-HT_{2A})
hydroxyurea

NOTES

H

187

hydroxyzine
hyfrecated
hygieiology
hygieist
hygiene
    Doctor of H. (DHy)
    industrial h.
    sleep h.
hygienic
hygienist
hyglucosamine sulfate
hygroma
Hygroton
hymenolepiasis
    h. diminuta
    h. nana
Hymenoptera
hyoid
hyoscyamine
hypalgesia
hypanakinesia
hyperacidity
hyperactivity
    detrusor h.
    viral airway h.
hyperacusis
hyperacute organ rejection
hyperadenosis
hyperadiposis
hyperadrenalcorticalism,
    hyperadrenocorticalism
hyperadrenalism
hyperadrenergic state
hyperadrenocorticalism (*var. of*
    hyperadrenalcorticalism)
hyperadrenocorticism
hyperadrenocorticoidism
hyperalbuminemia
hyperalbuminosis
hyperaldosteronemia
hyperaldosteronism
    dexamethasone-suppressible h.
    hyperreninemic h.
    idiopathic h. (IHA)
    h. syndrome
hyperaldosteronuria
hyperalgesia
    esophageal h.
    zone of h.
hyperalimentation
    parenteral h.
    total parenteral h.
hyperalphalipoproteinemia
    primary h.
hyperaminoacidemia
hyperammonemia
hyperammonuria
hyperamylasemia
    salivary h.

hyperandrogenism
hyperazotemia
hyperazoturia
hyperbaric
    h. medicine
    h. oxygen
    h. oxygenation
    h. oxygen therapy
    h. oxygen treatment
hyperbarism
hyperbetalipoproteinemia
    familial h.
hyperbilirubinemia
    congenital h.
    conjugated h.
    constitutional h.
    hereditary nonhemolytic h.
    neonatal h.
    unconjugated h.
hyperbradykininemia
hyperbradykinism
hypercalcemia
    familial hypocalciuric h.
    idiopathic h.
    malignant h.
    non-parathyroid-related h.
    parathyroid-related h.
hypercalcinuria
hypercalciuria
    absorptive h.
    idiopathic h.
    renal h.
    resorptive h.
    secondary h.
hypercalcuria
hypercapnia
    post h.
hypercapnic
    h. acidosis
    h. respiratory failure
hypercarbic respiratory failure
hypercarotenemia
hypercatabolic
hypercatabolism
hypercatharsis
hypercellularity
hyperchloremic
    h. metabolic acidosis
hyperchlorhydria
hyperchloruria
hypercholesteremia
    familial heterozygous h.
hypercholesterolemia
    essential h. (EHC)
    familial h. (FH)
    heterozygous familial h.
    homozygous familial h.
    polygenic h.
hypercholesterolemic splenomegaly

hyperchromaffinism
hyperchromatism
    macrocytic h.
hyperchromic anemia
hyperchylia
hyperchylomicronemia
    familial h.
hypercoagulability
    acquired h.
hypercoagulable state
hypercontractility
hypercorticoidism
hypercortisolism
hypercreatinemia
hypercystinuria
hyperdipsia
hyperemesis
    h. gravidarum
    h. hiemis
hyperemetic
hyperemia
    Bier passive h.
    constriction h.
    venous h.
hyperemic
hypereosinophilic syndrome
hyperesthesia
hyperestrogenemia
hyperestrogenosis
hyperexcitability
hyperexcretory
hyperexplexia
hyperextension
    cervical h.
hyperforin
hyperfunction
    pituitary h.
hyperfunctioning thyroid nodule
hypergammaglobulinemia
hypergammaglobulinemic purpura
hypergastrinemia
hypergenitalism
hyperglandular
hyperglobulinemia
hyperglobulinemica
    purpura h.
hyperglobulinemic purpura
hyperglucagonemia
hyperglycemia
    isolated postchallenge h. (IPH)
    nonketotic h.
    posthypoglycemic h.

hyperglycemic nonketotic coma
hyperglyceridemia
    endogenous h.
    exogenous h.
hyperglyceridemic
hyperglycerolemia
hyperglycinemia
    ketotic h.
    nonketotic h.
hyperglycogenolysis
hyperglycorrhachia
hyperglycosemia
hyperglycosuria
hypergonadism
hypergonadotropic eunuchoidism
hyperhemoglobinemia
hyperhemolytic
hyperheparinemia
hyperhidrosis
    axillary h.
    gustatory h.
    h. lateralis
    unilateral h.
hyperhidrotic
hyperhomocysteinemia
hyperhomocystinemia
hyperhormonism
hyperhydration
hyperhydrochloridia, hyperhydrochloria
hyperhydroxyprolinemia
hypericin
hyper-IgE syndrome
hyperimmunoglobulin E syndrome
hyperinfection
hyperinflation
hyperingestion
hyperinsulinar obesity
hyperinsulinemia
hyperinsulinemic hypoglycemia
hyperinsulinism
    alimentary h.
    functional h.
    iatrogenic h.
    obesity of h.
hyperkalemia
    spurious h.
hyperkalemic periodic paralysis
hyperkeratosis
    epidermolytic h.
    follicular h.
hyperketosis
hyperkinesia

NOTES

H

189

hyperkinetic
  h. pulmonary hypertension
  h. tardus
hyperkoria
hyperkyphosis
hyperlactacidemia
hyperlactatemia
hyperlecithinemia
hyperleukocytosis
hyperlipasemia
hyperlipemia
  carbohydrate-induced h.
  combined fat- and carbohydrate-
    induced h.
  familial fat-induced h.
  familial hypercholesterolemia
    with h.
  fat-induced h.
  idiopathic h.
  mixed h.
hyperlipidemia
  endogenous h. (EHL)
  familial combined h.
  mixed hyperlipoproteinemia familial
    type 5 h.
hyperlipoproteinemia
  acquired h.
  familial h. (type I–IV)
  primary h.
hyperlithemia
hyperlithuria
hyperlordosis
hyperlucency
hyperlysinemia
hypermagnesemia
hypermedication
hypermenorrhea
hypermetabolic
hypermetabolism
  extrathyroidal h.
hypermetaplasia
hypermethioninemia
hypermineralization
hypernatremia
  essential h.
hypernatremic encephalopathy
hypernephroma
hypernitremia
hypernutrition
hyperopia
hyperorexia
hyperornithinemia
hyperosmia
hyperosmolality
hyperosmolar
  h. hyperglycemic nonketotic coma
  h. laxative
  h. nonketotic state
hyperosmolarity

hyperostosis
  ankylosing h.
  diffuse idiopathic skeletal h.
    (DISH)
hyperovarianism
hyperoxaluria
  primary h.
hyperoxemia
hyperoxia
hyperoxic
hyperoxidation
hyperpancreatism
hyperparathyroid
hyperparathyroidism (HPT)
  nutritional secondary h.
  primary h. (PHP)
  secondary h.
  tertiary h.
hyperparotidism
hyperpathia
hyperpepsia
hyperpepsinia
hyperperistalsis
hyperpexia
hyperphagia
hyperphagic
hyperphenylalaninemia
  malignant h.
  maternal h.
  persistent h.
  transient h.
hyperphonesis
hyperphosphatasemia tarda
hyperphosphatasia
hyperphosphatemia
hyperphosphaturia
hyperphosphoremia
hyperphosphorylation
hyperpigmentation
hyperpinealism
hyperpipecolatemia
hyperpituitarism
  basophilic h.
  eosinophilic h.
hyperpituitary gigantism
hyperplasia
  adrenal h.
  adrenocortical h.
  angiofollicular mediastinal lymph
    node h.
  benign mediastinal lymph node h.
  benign prostatic h. (BPH)
  C-cell h.
  congenital adrenal h.
  congenital adrenocortical h.
  congenital virilizing adrenal h.
  endometrial h.
  focal nodular h.
  follicular h.

gastric h.
giant follicular h.
giant lymph node h.
inflammatory h.
islet cell h.
late-onset congenital adrenal h.
Leydig cell h.
lipoid adrenal h.
lymphoid h.
mediastinal lymph node h.
microscopic benign prostatic h.
nodular adrenal h.
nodular adrenocortical h.
ovarian stromal h.
prostatic h.
pseudoepitheliomatous h.
Schwann h.
sebaceous h.
squamous cell h.
stromal h.
thymic medullary h.
virilizing h.
hyperplasmic obesity
hyperplastic
    h. dystrophy
    h. osteoarthritis
hyperplastic-hypertrophic obesity
hyperpnea
hyperpolarization
hyperpolypeptidemia
hyperpotassemia
hyperprebetalipoproteinemia
    familial hyperbetalipoproteinemia
      and h.
    familial hyperchylomicronemia
      with h.
hyperprochoresis
hyperprogesteronemia
hyperproinsulinemia
hyperprolactinemia
hyperprolactinemic galactorrhea
hyperproliferative anemia
hyperprolinemia
    familial h.
    h. type I, II
hyperproteinemia
hyperproteosis
hyperpyretic
hyperpyrexia
    fulminant h.
    heat h.
    malignant h.

hyperpyrexial
hyperreactive malarious splenomegaly
hyperreflexia
    detrusor h.
hyperreninemia
hyperreninemic hyperaldosteronism
hyperresonance
hypersalemia
hypersaline
hypersarcosinemia
hypersecretion
    gastric h.
hypersensitive conjunctivitis
hypersensitivity
    carotid sinus h.
    delayed h. (DH)
    delayed-type h. (DTH)
    h. pneumonia
    h. pneumonitis
    visceral h.
hyperserotonemia
    vasculocardiac syndrome of h.
hyperserotonergic state
hypersexuality
hypersomatotropism
hypersomnia
    continuous h.
    paroxysmal h.
    periodic h.
hypersomnolence
    primary central nervous system h.
hypersplenic neutropenia
hypersplenism
hypersusceptibility
hypertension
    accelerated h.
    acute h.
    alcohol-induced h.
    arterial h.
    benign h.
    chronic thromboembolic
     pulmonary h.
    diastolic h.
    Dietary Approaches to Stop H.
     (DASH)
    episodic h.
    epoprostenol pulmonary h.
    essential primary h.
    estrogen-induced h.
    familial h.
    genetic h.
    Goldblatt h.

NOTES

H

hypertension *(continued)*
    hyperkinetic pulmonary h.
    idiopathic h.
    intracranial h.
    isolated systolic h. (ISH)
    malignant h.
    ocular h.
    oral contraceptive-induced h.
    paroxysmal h.
    passive pulmonary h.
    portal h.
    postcapillary pulmonary h.
    postoperative h.
    precapillary pulmonary h.
    h. and pregnancy
    pregnancy-induced h. (PIH)
    primary pulmonary h.
    pseudorefractory h.
    pulmonary arterial h.
    pulmonary artery h. (PAHA)
    pulmonary venous h.
    reactive pulmonary h.
    rebound h.
    refractory h.
    renal vascular h.
    renovascular h.
    secondary h.
    stable h.
    systemic arterial h.
    systolic h.
    systolic-diastolic h. (SDH)
    thromboembolic pulmonary h.
    vascular h.
    venous h.
    white-coat h.
hypertensive
    h. crisis
    h. emergency
    h. encephalopathy
    h. hypertrophic cardiomyopathy
    h. intracerebral hemorrhage
    h. lower esophageal sphincter
    h. urgency
hypertestoidism
hypertestosteronism
hyperthecosis
    ovarian h.
    testoid h.
hyperthermia
    malignant h.
hyperthrombinemia
hyperthymic
hyperthymism
hyperthymization
hyperthyrea
hyperthyroidism
    apathetic h.
    factitious h.
    iatrogenic h.

    iodine-induced h.
    masked h.
    ophthalmic h.
    h. in pregnancy
    primary h.
    secondary h.
    subclinical h.
    thyroid-stimulating hormone-
        mediated h.
    transient h.
hyperthyroid ophthalmoplegia
hyperthyroxinemia
hypertonia
hypertonic
    h. condition
    h. hyponatremia
hypertonica
    polycythemia h.
hypertonicity
hypertonus
hypertoxic
hypertoxicity
hypertransfusion
hypertrichosis lanuginosa
hypertriglyceridemia
    familial h.
hypertrophic
    h. arthritis
    h. dystrophy
    h. gastropathy
    h. obesity
    h. obstructive cardiomyopathy
    h. osteoarthritis
    h. osteoarthropathy
    h. polyneuritis
    h. spurring
    h. stenosis
hypertrophy
    asymmetric septal h. (ASH)
    atrial h.
    benign prostatic h. (BPH)
    concentric left ventricular h.
    facet h.
    left ventricular h. (LVH)
    Marie h.
    myocardial h.
    prostatic h.
    right ventricular h. (RVH)
    ventricular h.
hypertyrosinemia
hyperuresis
hyperuricemia
    asymptomatic h.
hyperuricosuria
hyperuricuria
hypervalinemia
hypervascular tumor
hyperventilate

hyperventilation
    h. syndrome
    h. tetany
hyperviscosity
hypervitaminosis D
hypervolemia
hypervolemic hyponatremia
hypesthesia
hypha, pl. **hyphae**
hyphal
hyphemia
    intertropical h.
hypnagogic hallucination
hypnic headache
hypnopompic hallucination
hypnotherapy
hypnotic medication
hypnotoxin
hypoacidity
hypoactive sexual desire disorder
hypoadrenalism
hypoadrenergic state
hypoadrenocorticism
    pituitary h.
    secondary h.
hypoalbuminemia
hypoalbuminosis
hypoaldosteronemia
hypoaldosteronism
    hyporeninemic h.
    isolated h.
    selective h.
hypoalert
hypoalimentation
hypoalphalipoproteinemia
    primary h.
hypoandrogenism
hypoattenuation
hypoazoturia
hypobaria
hypobarism
hypobaropathy
hypobetalipoproteinemia
    homozygous h.
hypobilirubinemia
hypocalcemia
    familial benign h.
hypocalcipectic
hypocalciuria
hypocapnia
hypocapnic
hypochloremia

hypochloremic alkalosis
hypochlorhydria
hypochloridation
hypochlorization
hypochloruria
hypocholesterolemia agent
hypocholesterolemic
hypocholia
hypocholuria
hypochondriasis
hypochromia
    idiopathic h.
hypochromic microcytic anemia
hypochylia
hypocitraturia
hypocitremia
hypocitruria
hypocorticalism
hypocorticism
hypocorticoidism
hypocupremia
hypocycloidal
hypodermatoclysis
hypodermic
    h. injection
    h. syringe
hypodermoclysis
hypodipsia
    primary h.
hypoeccrisis
hypoechoic
hypoelectrolytemia
hypoepinephrinemia
hypoesthesia
hypoestrogenic
hypoestrogenism
hypoferremia
hypoferric anemia
hypofibrinogenemia
hypofunction
    adrenal h.
    pituitary h.
hypogammaglobulinemia
    common variable h.
hypogastrium
hypogeusia
hypoglandular
hypoglossal nerve
hypoglucagonemia
hypoglycemia
    alimentary h.
    endogenous hyperinsulinemic h.

NOTES

H

hypoglycemia *(continued)*
  fasting h.
  functional reactive h.
  hyperinsulinemic h.
  insulin autoimmune h.
  leucine h.
  leucine-induced h.
  mixed h.
  neonatal h.
  postprandial h.
  reactive h.
  spontaneous h.
  true reactive h.
hypoglycemic
  h. coma
  h. convulsion
  h. reaction
  h. shock
hypoglycemosis
hypoglycin
hypoglycogenolysis
hypoglycorrhachia
hypogonadal
hypogonadism
  familial hypogonadotropic h.
  hypogonadotrophic h.
  hypogonadotropic h.
  male h.
  pituitary h.
  primary h.
  secondary h.
  h. with anosmia
hypogonadotrophic hypogonadism
hypogonadotropic
  h. eunuchoidism
  h. hypogonadism
hypohepatia
hypohidrosis
hypohormonal
hypohydration
hypohydrochloria
hypoinsulinemia
hypoinsulinism
hypoiodidism
hypokalemia
hypokalemic
  h. metabolic alkalosis
  h. nephropathy
  h. periodic paralysis
hypokinesia
hypokinesis
hypokinetic
hypolactasia
hypoleydigism
hypolipemia
hypolipidemia
  primary h.
hypolipidemic
hypoliposis

hypolymphemia
hypomagnesemia
hypomania
hypomelanosis
hypomenorrhea
hypometabolic
  h. state
  h. syndrome
hypometabolism
  euthyroid h.
hypomorphic
hypomotility
  esophageal h.
hypomyxia
hyponatremia
  depletional h.
  dilutional h.
  diuretic-induced h.
  euvolemic h.
  hypertonic h.
  hypervolemic h.
  hypotonic h.
  hypovolemic h.
hyponatremic
hyponatruria
hypoosmolality
hypoovarianism
hypopancreatism
hypopancreorrhea
hypoparathyroidism
  familial h.
  immunodeficiency with h.
  h. syndrome
hypoparathyroid tetany
hypopepsia
hypoperfusion
  organ h.
  peripheral h.
hypophagia
hypopharyngeal tumor
hypophonesis
hypophosphatasia
hypophosphatemia
hypophosphatemic
  h. vitamin D-deficient rickets
  h. vitamin D-resistant rickets
hypophosphaturia
hypophyseal cachexia
hypophysectomy
hypophyseogenea
  asthenia gravis h.
hypophyseopriva
  cachexia h.
hypophyseotropic *(var. of* hypophysiotropic)
hypophysial
  h. amenorrhea
  h. cachexia

h. dwarf
h. infantilism
hypophysioprivic, hypophyseoprivic
hypophysiotropic, hypophyseotropic
h. hormone
hypophysitis
autoimmune h.
hypopiesia
hypopietic
hypopigmentation
hypopituitarism
postpartum hemorrhagic h.
hypopituitary dwarf
hypoplasia
adrenal h.
granulocytic h.
Krabbe h.
thymic h.
hypoplastic
h. anemia
h. neutropenia
hypopnea
hypoposia
hypopotassemia
hypopotassemic
hypoproliferative anemia
hypoproteinemia
prehepatic h.
hypoproteinemic
hypoproteinia
hypoproteinosis
hypoprothrombinemia
hypopyon
recurrent h.
h. uveitis
hyporeactive
hyporeflexia
detrusor h.
hyporeninemia
hyporeninemic hypoaldosteronism
hyporiboflavinosis
hyposecretion
hyposensitivity
hyposmolarity
hyposomatotropism
hypospadia
hypospadiac urethra
hyposplenism
hypostasis
hypostatic pneumonia
hyposthenuria

hyposupradrenalism (*See also*
hypoadrenalism)
hypotension
chronic idiopathic orthostatic h.
hypovolemic h.
idiopathic orthostatic h.
intracranial h.
intradialytic h.
orthostatic h.
postexercise h. (PEH)
postprandial h.
postural h.
sympathetic orthostatic h. (SOH)
sympathicotonic orthostatic h.
vascular h.
hypotensive
hypothalamic
h. amenorrhea
h. diabetes insipidus
h. dysfunction
h. hypothyroidism
h. obesity
h. pituitary cachexia
h. secretory neuron
h. tumor
hypothalamic-pituitary
h.-p. axis (HPA)
h.-p. dysfunction
**hypothalamic-pituitary-adrenal axis
(HPAA)**
hypothalamus
hypothenar
hypothermal
hypothermia
accidental h.
endogenous h.
induced h.
moderate h.
profound h.
regional h.
hypothermic blanket
hypothesis, pl. **hypotheses**
insular h.
J-curve h.
h. testing
trade-off h.
hypothesize
hypothrepsia
hypothrombinemia
hypothymism
hypothyroid
h. dwarf

NOTES

H

hypothyroid *(continued)*
    h. dwarfism
    h. infantilism
    h. obesity
hypothyroidism
    amenorrhea, galactorrhea, h. (AGH)
    central h.
    familial goitrous h.
    hypothalamic h.
    iatrogenic h.
    infantile h.
    postoperative h.
    primary h.
    radiation-induced h.
    secondary h.
    subclinical h.
    tertiary h.
hypotonia
hypotonic hyponatremia
hypotonicity
    asymptomatic h.
    chronic asymptomatic h.
    symptomatic h.
hypotrophic cardiomyopathy
hypotryptophanic
hypouricemia
hypovarianism
hypoventilation
    alveolar h.
    central alveolar h.
    idiopathic alveolar h.
hypovitaminosis
hypovolemia
hypovolemic
    h. hyponatremia
    h. hypotension
    h. shock

hypoxanthine guanine
    phosphoribosyltransferase deficiency
hypoxemia
hypoxemic respiratory failure
hypoxia
    mixed venous h.
hypoxic
    h. nephrosis
    h. pulmonary vasoconstriction
    h. respiratory failure
    h. syncope
hypurgia
hysterectomy
    H. Educational Resources and
        Services Foundation (HERS)
    total abdominal h. (TAH)
hysteria
    Briquet h.
hysterical
    h. fainting
    h. pseudocoma
    h. seizure
    h. vomiting
hystericus
    globus h.
hysterography
hysterosalpingogram
hysterosalpingography
hysteroscopy
Hytone
Hytrin
Hyzaar
HZ
    herpes zoster
HZV
    herpes zoster virus

I2
    prostaglandin I2
I&A
    irrigation and aspiration
IABC
    intraaortic balloon catheter
IADH
    inappropriate antidiuretic hormone
IADL
    instrumental activities of daily living
IAP
    intermittent acute porphyria
IAPAAS
    Center for the Study of
      Aging/International Association of
      Physical Activity, Aging, and Sports
iatraliptics
iatric
iatrogenesis
iatrogenic
    i. complication
    i. diarrhea
    i. drug reaction
    i. hyperinsulinism
    i. hyperthyroidism
    i. hypothyroidism
    i. transmission
    i. volume overload
iatrology
iatrophysics
iatrotechnique
IBC
    iron-binding capacity
IBD
    inflammatory bowel disease
Iberet-500
IBM
    inclusion body myositis
IBS
    irritable bowel syndrome
ibuprofen
ibutilide
IC
    intermittent claudication
ICD
    implantable cardioverter-defibrillator
    International Classification of Diseases
    ischemic coronary disease
ICD-9
    International Classification of Diseases,
      Ninth Revision
      ICD-9 coding
ICDA
    International Classification of Diseases,
      Adapted for Use in the United States

ICD-9-CM
    International Classification of Diseases,
      Ninth Revision, Clinical Modification
Iceland disease
I-cell disease
ice-pick-like pain
ichor
ichoremia
ichoroid
ichorous
ichorrhea
ichorrhemia
ichthyosis
ICON
    tandem ICON
    urine tandem ICON
icon
iconic memory
ICSH
    interstitial cell-stimulating hormone
ICT
    insulin coma therapy
ictal
icteric
    i. leptospirosis
    i. phase
icteroanemia
icterogenic
icterohematuric
icterohemoglobinuria
icterohemolytic anemia
icterohemorrhagica
    leptospirosis i.
icterohemorrhagic fever
icteroid
icterus
    acholuric hemolytic i.
    acquired hemolytic i.
    benign familial i.
    bilirubin i.
    i. castrensis gravis
    i. castrensis levis
    i. catarrhalis
    choluric hemolytic i.
    chronic familial i.
    congenital hemolytic i.
    cythemolytic i.
    familial i.
    Gubler i.
    Hayem i.
    hemolytic i.
    i. hemolyticus
    i. infectiosus
    infectious i.
    Liouvilles i.

icterus *(continued)*
    i. melas
    i. neonatorum
    physiologic i.
    i. praecox
    scleral i.
    i. simplex
    spirochetal i.
    i. typhoides
    urobilin i.
    i. viridans
ictus solis
ICU
    intensive care unit
Icy Hot
ID
    identification
I&D
    incision and drainage
idarubicin
IDD
    insulin-dependent diabetes
IDDM
    insulin-dependent diabetes mellitus
ideation
    suicidal i.
Idebenone
identification (ID)
ideomotor
idiogenesis
idiopathetic
idiopathic
    i. adrenal atrophy
    i. adrenocortical insufficiency
    i. aldosteronism
    i. alveolar hypoventilation
    i. anaphylaxis
    i. avascular necrosis
    i. benign proteinuria
    i. blennorrheal arthritis
    i. constipation
    i. deep vein thrombosis
    i. dilated cardiomyopathy
    i. disease
    i. gout
    i. hirsutism
    i. hyperaldosteronism (IHA)
    i. hypercalcemia
    i. hypercalciuria
    i. hyperlipemia
    i. hypertension
    i. hypertrophic osteoarthropathy (IHO)
    i. hypertrophic subaortic stenosis (IHSS)
    i. hypochromia
    i. infantilism
    i. inflammatory myopathy
    i. interstitial pneumonia

    i. leg edema
    i. myocarditis
    i. neutropenia
    i. oligospermia
    i. orthostatic hypotension
    i. paroxysmal rhabdomyolysis
    i. polyneuritis
    i. proctitis
    i. pulmonary fibrosis (IPF)
    i. pulmonary hemosiderosis
    i. purpura
    i. thrombocytopenia
    i. thrombocytopenic purpura (ITP)
    i. ventricular tachycardia
idiopathy
idiosyncrasy
idiosyncratic hepatotoxicity
idioventricular rhythm
IDL
    intermediate-density lipoprotein
id reaction
IF
    initiation factor
    intrinsic factor
ifosfamide
Ig
    immunoglobulin
IgA
    immunoglobulin A
    IgA nephropathy
    secretory IgA
IgE
    immunoglobulin E
IgE-mediated
    IgE-m. food allergy
    IgE-m. rhinitis
IGF
    insulinlike growth factor
IgG
    immunoglobulin G
IgM
    immunoglobulin M
IGT
    impaired glucose tolerance
IH
    infectious hepatitis
IHA
    idiopathic hyperaldosteronism
IHO
    idiopathic hypertrophic osteoarthropathy
IHS
    Indian Health Service
IHSS
    idiopathic hypertrophic subaortic stenosis
IIIa
    glycoprotein IIIa
    GP IIIa
IL-2
    interleukin-2

ILD
  interstitial lung disease
ileac
ileal
  i. loop
  i. pouch-anal anastomosis
  i. varix
ileitis
  backwash i.
  Crohn i.
  distal i.
  regional i.
ileocecal
ileocolitis
  Crohn i.
  ischemic i.
  regional i.
ileojejunal bypass
ileojejunitis
  ulcerative i.
ileoproctostomy
ileorectal
ileostomy
ileum
ileus
  adynamic i.
  dynamic i.
  gallstone i.
  mechanical i.
  occlusive i.
  paralytic i.
  spastic i.
  terminal i.
  verminous i.
Ilhéus fever
iliac crest
iliofemoral
  i. bypass
  i. thrombophlebitis
ilioinguinal
iliopsoas bursitis
iliotibial band (ITB)
ill
  National Alliance for the
    Mentally I. (NAMI)
illicit
illness
  acute febrile respiratory i. (AFRI)
  altitude i.
  building-related i.
  chronic altitude i.
  cold-induced i.

  depressive i.
  environmental i.
  febrile i.
  functional i.
  heat-induced i.
  influenza-like i.
  opportunistic i.
  organ-specific i.
  refractory i.
illumination
Ilotycin ointment
IM
  infectious mononucleosis
  internal medicine
  intramuscular
  Bicillin IM
  Wycillin IM
image
  body i.
imaging
  cervical magnetic resonance i.
  color duplex i.
  diffusion i.
  liver i.
  magnetic resonance i. (MRI)
  oncologic i.
  pancreatic i.
  pituitary i.
  radionuclide i.
  real-time B-mode i.
  serial i.
  single-photon planar i.
  stress myocardial perfusion i.
imatinib mesylate
imbalance
  electrolyte i.
IMCU
  intermediate medical care unit
Imdur
Imerslund syndrome
Imferon
iminoglycinuria
iminopeptiduria
imipenem
imipenem-cilastatin
imipramine HCl
Imitrex
immediate
  i. auscultation
  i. percussion
immersion
  i. bath

NOTES

immersion *(continued)*
    i. burn
    i. injury
immitis
    Coccidioides i.
immobility
immobilization
immotile cilia syndrome
immune
    i. complex disease
    i. complex disorder
    i. complex-like syndrome
    i. function
    i. globulin
    i. system
    i. theory
    i. thrombocytopenia
    i. thrombocytopenic purpura
immune-mediated glomerulopathy
immunity
    cell-mediated i.
immunization
    adult i.
    National Coalition for Adult I.
    (NCAI)
immunoassay
    enzyme-linked i. (ELISA)
immunobiologic
immunoblastic lymphadenopathy
immunocompetent
immunocompromise
immunodeficiency
    cellular i.
    congenital i.
    i. and malabsorption
    i. with hypoparathyroidism
immunodeficient
immunodepressed
immunoelectrophoresis
immunofluorescence
immunofluorescent microscopy
immunogenicity
immunoglobulin (Ig)
    i. A (IgA)
    i. A deficiency
    i. A nephropathy
    i. E (IgE)
    i. G (IgG)
    i. M (IgM)
    thyroid-binding inhibitory i. (TBII)
    thyroid-stimulating i. (TSI)
immunohemolytic anemia
immunologic
immunological function
immunologist
immunology
immunomodulatory drug
immunoprophylaxis
immunosenescence

immunosuppressant
immunosuppressed
immunosuppression
immunosuppressive
immunotherapy
immunotoxin
Imodium
impaction
    delirium, infection, atrophic
      urethritis and vaginitis,
      pharmaceuticals, psychological
      disorders, excessive urine output,
      restricted mobility, stool i.
      (DIAPPERS)
    fecal i.
    mucus i.
impaired
    i. abstraction
    i. drug clearance
    i. fasting glucose
    i. glucose tolerance (IGT)
    i. mentation
    i. psychomotor function
    significantly i.
    i. tissue perfusion
    i. vision
impairment
    age-associated memory i. (AAMI)
    cognitive i.
    diffusion i.
    functional i.
    intellectual i.
    memory i.
impedance plethysmography
impediment
    language i.
imperfecta
    erythrogenesis i.
    osteogenesis i.
impetiginization
impetigo
implant
    cochlear i.
    Silastic i.
implantable
    i. cardioverter-defibrillator (ICD)
    i. defibrillator
implantation
    autogenous cartilage i.
    intraocular lens i.
    pellet i.
implicated
implicit memory
impotence
improvement
    continuous quality i.
    symptomatic i.
impulse
    point of maximal i. (PMI)

I

IMT
    intimal-medial thickness
Imuran
in
    In Charge diabetes control system
    in extremis
    in situ
    in situ thrombosis
    in vitro
    in vivo
inactive tuberculosis
inactivity atrophy
inadequate sleep
inanition fever
inapparent
inappropriate
    i. antidiuretic hormone (IADH)
    i. antidiuretic hormone secretion
      syndrome
    i. hormone
    i. polycythemia
Inapsine
inborn
    i. error
    i. error of metabolism
    i. lysosomal disease
incapacitated
incapacitating
incarcerated inguinal hernia
incarceration
    i. symptom
    tender i.
incarnatio unguis
incentive spirometry
incidence
incipient
incision
    curvilinear i.
    i. and drainage (I&D)
    fasciotomy i.
    Pfannenstiel i.
incisional hernia
incisura
inclusion
    i. body myositis (IBM)
    i. cell disease
    Dawson i.
incoherent
incompatible blood transfusion reaction
incompetence
    cervical i.

    congenital valvular i.
    pyloric i.
incomplete
    i. bundle-branch block
    i. emptying
incontinence
    acute i.
    chronic i.
    cough test for stress i.
    fecal i.
    i. of feces
    functional i.
    micturition urinary i.
    mixed type of i.
    nocturnal urinary i.
    overflow i.
    paradoxical i.
    postsurgical i.
    reflex i.
    stress i.
    total i.
    transient i.
    urge i.
    urinary i.
    i. of urine
incontinent
increased
    i. colorectal diameter
    markedly i.
incretin
incretion
incubation
incubative stage
incurability
incurable
incus necrosis
indapamide
independence
    function i.
independently
Inderal
Inderide
index, pl. **indices, indexes**
    ankle-brachial i. (ABI)
    apnea i.
    apnea-hypopnea i. (AHI)
    Barthel I.
    body mass i. (BMI)
    cardiac i. (CI)
    Charlson comorbidity i.
    diet quality i.
    end-diastolic volume i. (EDVI)

NOTES

index *(continued)*
    end-systolic volume i. (ESVI)
    free thyroxine i. (FTI)
    glycemic i.
    history activity i. (HAI)
    Life Satisfaction I. A (LSIA)
    Life Satisfaction I. B (LSIB)
    low body mass i.
    maturation i.
    Miller i.
    National Institutes of Health
      Chronic Prostatitis Symptom I.
      (NIH-CPSI)
    obesity i.
    Pirquet i.
    respiratory disturbance i. (RDI)
    shock i.
    Spitzer Quality of Life I.
    splenic localization i. (SLI)
    stroke volume i. (SVI)
    therapeutic i.
    thyroid-binding i. (TBI)
    thyroid hormone-binding i.
    vital i.
Indian
    I. Health Service (IHS)
    I. sickness
    I. tick typhus
Indiana-type amyloidosis
indicant
indication
indicator
    Andrade i.
    i. dilution
indices (*pl. of* index)
indigent
indigestion
    acid i.
    fat i.
    gastric i.
    nervous i.
indinavir sulfate
indirect
    i. diuretic
    i. hemagglutination test
    i. inguinal hernia
indiscriminate lesion
indispensable
indisposition
Indium scan
individual
    i. characteristic
    i. tolerance
indobufen
Indochron
Indocin SR
indoleamine

indolent
    i. bubo
    i. multiple myeloma
indomethacin
induce
induced
    i. fever
    i. hypothermia
    i. malaria
    pill i.
    radiation i.
    i. sensitivity
    i. symptom
induction chemotherapy
inductotherm
inductothermy
InDuo system
induration
    brawny i.
industrial
    i. bronchitis
    i. disease
    i. hygiene
indwelling urinary catheter
inebriation
ineffective cough
inequality
    ventilation/perfusion i.
inertance
infancy
Infanrix
    I. diphtheria and tetanus toxoid
    I. diphtheria, tetanus toxoid, and
      acellular pertussis
    I. DTaP
infant
    i. pneumonia
    postmature i.
infantile
    i. beriberi
    i. celiac disease
    i. colic
    i. dwarfism
    i. gastroenteritis
    i. hypothyroidism
    i. leishmaniasis
    i. myofibromatosis
    i. myxedema
    i. osteomalacia
    i. pellagra
    i. scurvy
    i. tetany
infantilis
    roseola i.
infantilism
    Brissaud i.
    dysthyroidal i.
    hepatic i.
    hypophysial i.

hypothyroid i.
idiopathic i.
Lorain-Lévi i.
myxedematous i.
pancreatic i.
pituitary i.
proportionate i.
renal i.
sexual i.
thyroid i.
universal i.

infantiseptica
granulomatosis i.

infantum
cholera i.
osteopathia hemorrhagica i.

infarct
cerebral autosomal dominant
  arteriopathy with subcortical i.
  (CADASIL)
lacunar brain i.
pontine i.
subcortical i.

infarction
acute myocardial i. (AMI)
adrenal i.
anterior i.
anterior wall i. (AWI)
anterior wall myocardial i.
  (AWMI)
anteroinferior myocardial i.
anterolateral myocardial i.
anteroseptal myocardial i.
apical myocardial i.
atrial i.
cardiac i.
diaphragmatic i.
Freiberg i.
hemorrhagic i.
high-lateral myocardial i.
inferior i.
inferolateral myocardial i.
lacunar i.
lateral myocardial i.
myocardial i. (MI)
non-Q-wave myocardial i.
  (NQWMI)
non-ST-elevation myocardial i.
nontransmural i.
posterior myocardial i.
posterolateral myocardial i.
postoperative myocardial i.

pulmonary i.
Q-wave myocardial i.
recurrent myocardial i.
right ventricle myocardial i.
right ventricular i.
Roesler-Dressler i.
septal myocardial i.
silent myocardial i.
ST-elevation myocardial i.
subendocardial i.
through-and-through myocardial i.
transmural myocardial i.

infected
i. pilonidal cyst
i. pilonidal sinus
i. pressure ulcer

infection
abdominal i.
Acanthamoeba i.
adenovirus i.
Aeromonas i.
agonal i.
anaerobic i.
antecedent streptococcal i.
antibiotic-resistant bacterial i.
arbovirus i.
atypical mycobacterial i.
Bacillus cereus i.
bacterial i.
Bartonella i.
beta-hemolytic streptococcal i.
bladder i.
Blastomyces dermatitidis i.
blood i.
bloodstream i. (BSI)
Bordetella i.
Brugia malayi i.
Brugia timori i.
burn i.
Campylobacter i.
Campylobacter fetus i.
catheter-associated i.
catheter-related i.
central nervous system i.
clostridial i.
Clostridium difficile i.
Clostridium perfringens i.
community-acquired bladder i.
corynebacterial i.
Coxiella i.
Cryptosporidium i.
cytomegalovirus i.

NOTES

infection (*continued*)
    deep neck i.
    dimorphic fungal i.
    disseminated fungal i.
    disseminated gonococcal i.
    disseminated herpes simplex
     virus i.
    Ehrlichia i.
    emebic i.
    enteric i.
    Escherichia coli i.
    eye i.
    fungal i.
    fungal skin i.
    gastrointestinal i.
    genital mycoplasma i.
    genitourinary i.
    gonococcal i.
    group A, B, C, D, G
     streptococcal i.
    Haemophilus i.
    helminthic i.
    hepatobiliary i.
    herpes eye i.
    herpes simplex virus i.
    Histoplasma capsulatum i.
    hookworm i.
    hospital-acquired bloodstream i.
    intracerebral i.
    intravenous catheter-associated i.
    invasive burn i.
    invasive group A streptococcal i.
    latent i.
    latent tuberculosis i.
    leptomyxid amebic i.
    lower respiratory tract i.
    lower urinary tract i.
    lymphogranuloma venereum i.
    MAC i.
    Mansonella ozzardi i.
    Mansonella perstans i.
    Mansonella streptocerca i.
    microsporidia i.
    Multiceps i.
    musculoskeletal i.
    mycobacterial i.
    Mycobacterium abscessus i.
    Mycobacterium avium complex i.
    Mycobacterium chelonei i.
    Mycobacterium fortuitum i.
    Mycobacterium haemophilum i.
    Mycobacterium kansasii i.
    Mycobacterium marinum i.
    Mycobacterium xenopi i.
    Mycoplasma i.
    Naegleria i.
    natural focus of i.
    neck i.
    necrotizing soft tissue i.

    nonclostridial i.
    nosocomial i.
    oculogenital i.
    opportunistic i.
    oral i.
    organ transplant i.
    oropharyngeal i.
    Paramyxovirus i.
    parvovirus B19 i.
    periodontal i.
    perirectal i.
    pharyngeal gonococcal i.
    Plesiomonas shigelloides i.
    Pneumocystis i.
    postoperative wound i.
    posttransfusion i.
    posttransplant i.
    protozoal i.
    protozoan i.
    puerperal i.
    pulmonary i.
    pyogenic i.
    rectal gonococcal i.
    recurrent i.
    recurrent upper respiratory tract i.
     (RURTI)
    respiratory tract i.
    Salinem i.
    Salmonella i.
    Shigella i.
    sinus i.
    skin i.
    soft tissue i.
    streptococcal soft tissue i.
    Streptococcus viridans i.
    surgical i.
    systemic fungal i.
    terminal i.
    toxin-mediated i.
    trematode i.
    tuberculosis i.
    upper respiratory i. (URI)
    upper respiratory tract i.
    urinary tract i. (UTI)
    Vibrio parahaemolyticus i.
    Vibrio vulnificus i.
    viral i.
    whipworm i.
    wound i.
    Wuchereria bancrofti i.
    Yersinia enterocolitica i.
infectiosity
infectiosus
    icterus i.
infectious
    i. agent
    i. anemia
    i. arthritis
    i. disease

i. esophagitis
i. flexor tenosynovitis
i. hepatitis (IH)
i. icterus
i. mononucleosis (IM)
i. myxomatosis
i. neuropathy
i. nonbacterial gastroenteritis
i. polyneuritis
i. stomatitis
infectiousness
infective
i. endocarditis
i. polyneuritis
infectivity
inferior
i. infarction
i. olive receptor
i. petrosal venous sampling
i. vena cava (IVC)
i. vena cava filter
inferius
tuberculum thyroideum i.
inferobasal
inferolateral myocardial infarction
infertility
female i.
male i.
infestation
tapeworm i.
infiltrate
basilar interstitial i.
bilateral i.'s
fluffy pulmonary i.
infiltrating carcinoma
infiltration
marrow i.
infiltrative ductal carcinoma
infirm
infirmary
infirmity
inflammation
acute i.
adhesive i.
cardinal sign of i.
chronic i.
intestinal i.
nociceptor-induced i.
ocular i.
parietal peritoneal i.
pleura i.

skin i.
subacute i.
inflammatory
i. airway disease
i. bowel disease (IBD)
i. bowel disease arthritis
i. bowel disease and the elderly
i. bowel disease and pregnancy
i. breast cancer
i. diarrhea
i. hyperplasia
i. mediator
i. musculoskeletal condition
i. osteoarthritis
i. rheumatism
infliximab
influence
psychosocial i.
seasonal i.
influenza (flu)
i. A, B, C
Asian i.
endemic i.
Hong Kong i.
i. nostras
i. pneumonia
Russian i.
Spanish i.
i. vaccine
influenzae
Haemophilus i.
Haemophilus i. type b (HIB)
influenzal
i. neuritis
i. virus pneumonia
influenza-like illness
Influenzavirus
informatics
medical i.
information
demographic i.
insufficient i.
informed consent
infraareolar
infraclavicular
infracorporeal pressure
infrapatellar
bursitis i.
infrared treatment
infraspinatus
infrastructure
infraumbilical area

NOTES

infundibular stenosis
infundibulum
infusion
    continuous extravascular i. (CEI)
    continuous subcutaneous insulin i.
      (CSII)
    isoproterenol i.
    multivitamin i. (MVI)
ingesta
ingestion
    foreign object i.
ingestive
ingravescent
ingrown toenail
inguinal
    i. adenopathy
    i. hernia
inguinale
    granuloma i.
    lymphogranuloma i.
inguinodynia
INH
    isonicotinic acid hydrazide
inhalant
    toxic i.
inhalation
    ammonia i.
    i. anthrax
    carbon monoxide i.
    chlorine gas i.
    gas i.
    hydrogen cyanide i.
    hydrogen fluoride i.
    hydrogen sulfide i.
    irritant gas i.
    isocyanate i.
    metallic compound i.
    phosgene gas i.
    i. pneumonia
    potassium cyanide i.
    i. powder
    smoke i.
    i. therapy apparatus
inhaled
    i. corticosteroid
    i. glucocorticosteroid
inhaler
    Alupent i.
    Atrovent i.
    Azmacort i.
    beclomethasone nasal i.
    Beclovent oral i.
    Brethaire i.
    Flovent i.
    Intal i.
    isoproterenol i.
    Maxair i.
    Metaprel i.
    metered-dose i. (MDI)

    Nasarel i.
    nicotine i.
    Proventil i.
    salbutamol i.
    Serevent i.
    terbutaline i.
    Vanceril i.
inherited
    i. bleeding disorder
    i. cardiac tumor
    i. complement deficiency
    i. connective tissue disorder
    i. immunoglobulin deficiency
    i. thromboembolic disorder
    i. thrombophilia
inhibin
inhibit
inhibition
    uncompetitive i.
inhibitor
    ACE i.
    acetylcholinesterase i. (AChEI)
    alpha-glucosidase i.
    5-alpha-reductase i.
    angiotensin-converting enzyme i.
      (ACEI)
    aromatase i.
    beta-lactamase i.
    calcineurin i.
    carbonic anhydrase i.
    catechol methyltransferase i.
    cholinesterase i.
    COMT i.
    COX-2 i.
    cyclooxygenase-2 i.
    glucosidase i.
    hepatic 3-methylglutaryl coenzyme
      A reductase i.
    HMG-CoA reductase i.
    MAO i.
    mitotic spindle i.
    monoamine oxidase i. (MAOI)
    monoamine oxidase B i.
    neuraminidase i.
    NMDA i.
    N-methyl-D-aspartate i.
    nonnucleoside reverse
      transcriptase i.
    nucleoside analog reverse
      transcriptase i.
    phosphodiesterase i.
    platelet aggregation i.
    protease i.
    proton pump i. (PPI)
    selective serotonin reuptake i.
      (SSRI)
    serotonin-norepinephrine reuptake i.
      (SNRI)
    serotonin reuptake i. (SRI)

substance P i.
topoisomerase i.
tumor necrosis factor i.
vasopeptidase i.
in-home caregiver
inhomogeneous
initial
    i. dose
    i. evaluation
initiation factor (IF)
initiative
    The Dana Alliance for Brain I.
initiator
injectable
injection
    adrenal cortex i.
    botulinum toxin i.
    collagen i.
    Deca-Durabolin i.
    depot i.
    epidural steroid i.
    facet joint i.
    glucocorticoid i.
    hypodermic i.
    intralesional i.
    intrathecal i.
    intraventricular i.
    jet i.
    joint i.
    lactated Ringer i.
    ligamentous i.
    steroid i.
    i. system
    Theelin i.
    Toradol i.
    trigger point i. (TPI)
    Z-tract i.
injector
    jet i.
injury
    acute lung i.
    acute respiratory i.
    brain i.
    clenched-fist i.
    corrosive i.
    cumulative i.
    distraction i.
    egg-white i.
    hepatocellular i.
    immersion i.
    ischemic liver i.
    liver i.

    lung i.
    nerve i.
    pigment-induced renal i.
    radial nerve i.
    renal i.
    respiratory i.
    rotator cuff i.
    spinal cord i.
    steering wheel i.
    transfusion-related acute lung i.
    traumatic brain i.
    traumatic spinal cord i.
    ventilator-associated lung i.
innate
innatus
    calor i.
innervated
innervation
    parasympathetic i.
innocens
    diabetes i.
innocent
    i. heart murmur
    i. murmur of elderly
innocuous
innominate
Innovo Dial-a-Dose insulin delivery
    device
Inocor
inoculate
inoculation
inoculum effect
inoscopic
inosine 5′-triphosphate (ITP)
inotrope
inotropic
inquest
INR
    international normalized ratio
insalubrious
insanitary
insect bite
insenescence
insensible thirst
insert
    Plastizote i.
insertion
insidious
insipidus
    central diabetes i.
    diabetes i.
    hypothalamic diabetes i.

NOTES

insipidus (*continued*)
  nephrogenic diabetes i.
  transient diabetes i.
  triphasic diabetes i.
insolation
insomnia
  acute i.
  chronic i.
  i. and the elderly
  psychophysiologic i.
  rebound i.
  short-term i.
  transient i.
insomniac
inspersion
inspiratory
  i. flow rate
  medium i.
  i. phase
  i. pressure
  i. stridor
  i. wheeze
inspire
InspirEase
inspissated syndrome
inspissation
instability
  detrusor motor i.
  microsatellite i.
  postural i.
instillation
instillator
institute
  Better Hearing I.
  Better Vision I. (BVI)
  National Cancer I. (NCI)
  National Heart, Lungs, and
    Blood I. (NHLBI)
  National Human Genome
    Research I. (NHGRI)
institutional dysentery
institutionalization
institutionalized
instrumental activities of daily living
  (IADL)
insudate
insufficiency
  acute adrenal i. (AAI)
  acute adrenocortical i.
  acute respiratory i.
  adrenal i.
  adrenocortical i.
  anterior pituitary i.
  aortic i. (AI)
  arterial i.
  autonomic i.
  chronic adrenal i.
  chronic adrenocortical i.
  chronic renal i.

chronic venous i.
exocrine pancreatic i. (EPI)
food i.
hepatic i.
idiopathic adrenocortical i.
latent adrenocortical i.
mesenteric i.
mitral valve i.
pancreatic i.
parathyroid i.
partial adrenocortical i.
pituitary i.
postural i.
primary adrenocortical i.
pyloric i.
renal i.
respiratory i.
rheumatic mitral i.
secondary adrenocortical i.
thyroid i.
valvular i.
venous i.
vertebrobasilar i.
insufficient information
insufflation
insular hypothesis
insulin
  i. allergy
  i. antibody
  i. aspart
  i. autoimmune hypoglycemia
  basal i.
  i. cartridge
  i. coma therapy (ICT)
  i. delivery
  i. delivery device
  i. delivery system
  i. doser
  i. glargine
  human ultralente i.
  i. injection system
  intermediate-acting i.
  i. lipoatrophy
  i. lipodystrophy
  i. lispro
  long-acting i.
  neutral protamine Hagedorn i.
  NPH i.
  pork i.
  prandial i.
  i. production
  i. pump
  rapid-acting i.
  i. reaction
  i. receptor substrate-1 (IRS-1)
  i. resistance
  i. secretagogue
  i. sensitizer
  i. shock

i. syringe
i. therapy
insulin-dependent
    i.-d. diabetes (IDD)
    i.-d. diabetes mellitus (IDDM)
insulinlike growth factor (IGF)
insulin-mediated glucose
insulinoma
insulinopenic diabetes
insulitis
insult
    hemorrhagic i.
insurance
    hospital i.
    long-term care i.
    supplementary medical i.
intact
    extraocular muscles i. (EOMI)
intake
    caloric i.
    potassium i.
    recommended nutrient i. (RNI)
    sodium i.
    water i.
Intal inhaler
Integrilin
integrin alpha$_2$beta$_1$ deficiency
integrity
    skin i.
intellectual
    i. impairment
    i. level
    i. performance
intense
intensification
    i. chemotherapy
    dose i.
intensity
    point of maximal i. (PMI)
intensive
    i. care medicine
    i. care unit (ICU)
    i. therapeutic care
intent
    suicidal i.
intentionem
    per primam i.
intention tremor
interaction
    drug i.
    drug-drug i.

grapefruit juice i.
pharmokinetic i.
interactive
interarticular
interarticularis
    pars i.
interbronchial
intercadent
intercalary
intercalatum
    Schistosoma i.
intercapillary glomerulosclerosis
intercarpal joint
intercellular adhesion
intercostal space
intercourse
    sexual i.
intercritical gout
intercurrent disease
interdigestive migratory motor complex
interdisciplinary
interest
    conflicts of i.
interferon
    i. alfa-2a
    i. alfa-2b
    i. alfacon-1
    alpha i.
    i. alpha
    i. alpha therapy
    i. beta
interfollicular
intergluteal
interhemispheric
interictal
interior vena cava interruption
interleukin
    recombinant i. 11
interleukin-2 (IL-2)
intermediate-acting insulin
intermediate-density lipoprotein (IDL)
intermediate-grade non-Hodgkin lymphoma
intermediate medical care unit (IMCU)
intermedin
intermenstrual
intermittence
intermittency
intermittens
    diabetes i.
intermittent
    i. abdominal pain

NOTES

intermittent *(continued)*
    i. acute porphyria (IAP)
    i. asthma
    i. claudication (IC)
    i. cramp
    i. malaria
    i. malarial fever
    i. porphyria
    i. positive-pressure breathing (IPPB)
    i. positive-pressure ventilation
      (IPPV)
intern, interne
internal
    i. fluid shift
    i. hemorrhoid
    i. medicine (IM)
    i. medicine physician
international
    I. Classification of Diseases (ICD)
    I. Classification of Diseases,
      Adapted for Use in the United
      States (ICDA)
    I. Classification of Diseases, Ninth
      Revision (ICD-9)
    I. Classification of Diseases, Ninth
      Revision, Clinical Modification
      (ICD-9-CM)
    I. Committee of the Red Cross
    I. Hearing Society
    i. normalized ratio (INR)
    I. Tremor Foundation (ITF)
    I. Unit (IU)
interne *(var. of* intern)
internist
internus
    calor i.
interosseous
interparoxysmal
interpersonal relations
interphalangeal
    i. osteoarthritis
    proximal i. (PIP)
    terminal i. (TIP)
interrelationship
interrupted respiration
interruption
    interior vena cava i.
interruptus
    coitus i.
interscapular
interseptal
intersexual
intersexuality
interstitial
    i. cell-stimulating hormone (ICSH)
    i. cystitis
    i. disease
    i. fibrosis
    i. lung disease (ILD)

    i. nephritis
    i. plasma cell pneumonia
    i. pneumonitis
interstitialis
    calcinosis i.
intertriginous
intertrigo
intertrochanteric
    i. hip fracture
intertropica
    stomatitis i.
intertropical hyphemia
interval
    i. gout
    PQRST i.
    PR i.
    RR i.
intervascular
intervention
    futile i.
    life-sustaining i.
    machine-based i.
    nutritional i.
    percutaneous coronary i.
interventional cardiology
intervertebral iliotibial band
intestinal
    i. absorption
    i. allergy
    i. angina
    i. anthrax
    i. capillariasis
    i. fluke
    i. inflammation
    i. intoxication
    i. ischemia
    i. lumen
    i. luminal amebicide
    i. lymphangiectasia
    i. myiasis
    i. myopathic disorder
    i. myxoneurosis
    i. obstruction
    i. parasite
    i. pseudoobstruction
    i. schistosomiasis
    i. stasis
    i. steatorrhea
    i. tumor
intestinalis
    mycosis i.
    pneumatosis i.
intestine
    acute obstruction of small i.
    large i.
    small i.
intimal-medial thickness (IMT)
intolerance
    cold i.

fructose i.
glucose i.
hereditary fructose i.
lactose i.
milk i.
intoxication
acid i.
cyanide i.
digitalis i.
intestinal i.
legal i.
septic i.
water i.
intraabdominal abscess
intraaortic
i. balloon catheter (IABC)
i. balloon pump
intraarterial
i. catheter
i. chemotherapy
intracalcaneal bursitis
intracapillary
intracellulare
    Mycobacterium avium-i.
intracellular water
intracerebral
i. hematoma
i. hemorrhage
i. infection
intracerebroventricular
intracranial
i. bruit
i. hemorrhage
i. hypertension
i. hypotension
i. suppuration
i. thrombophlebitis
intractable
intradermal
intradialytic hypotension
intraductal
intraepithelial lymphocyte
intrafebrile
intrahepatic
i. bile duct
i. cholestasis
intralesional
i. injection
i. therapy
intraluminal
i. conjugated bile acid
    concentration

i. maldigestion
i. obstruction
intramural practice
intramuscular (IM)
intramuscularly
intranasal
i. calcitonin
i. steroid
intraocular
i. lens implantation
i. pressure (IOP)
intraoperative cholangiogram
intraosseous
intraperitoneal (IP)
intrapyretic
intrarenal
i. acute renal failure
i. renin angiotensin system
intraretinal microvascular abnormality
  (IRMA)
intrasellar
intraspinal
intrastromal corneal ring segment
intrathecal
i. analgesia
i. chemotherapy
i. injection
intrathoracic
i. goiter
i. thyroid
intrauterine
i. device (IUD)
i. pneumonia
intravascular thrombus formation
intravenous (IV)
i. bolus
i. catheter-associated infection
i. drug abuser
i. fluids
i. narcosis
i. nitroglycerin
i. pyelogram (IVP)
intravenously
intraventricular (I-V)
i. conduction disturbance
i. injection
i. neurocysticercosis
i. septum
intravesical
intra vitam
intrinsic
i. asthma

NOTES

intrinsic *(continued)*
   i. deficit
   i. factor (IF)
   i. factor deficiency
   i. muscle
   i. pathway defect
   i. renal failure
   i. sphincter deficiency
introital
introitus
   vaginal i.
intromission
intubation
intussusception
inunction
inundation fever
inure
invalid
invalidism
invasion
   stage of i.
   tumor i.
invasive
   i. burn infection
   i. group A streptococcal infection
   i. testing
invasiveness
inventory
   alcohol use disorders i.
   Beck Depression I. (BDI)
invermination
inverse
   i. ratio ventilation
   i. syntropy
inversion
inveterate
involuntary weight loss
involution
   thymic i.
involutional melancholia
involutive process
Inwave Prism Hemianopic Lens
Iodamoeba butschlii
iodide
   supersaturated potassium i.
   i. transport defect
iodinated glycerol
iodine
   butanol-extractable i. (BEI)
   i. contrast angiography
   i.-I-131 uptake test
   protein-bound i. (PBI)
   i. thyroid product
iodine-131
   radioactive iodine-131
iodine-fast
iodine-fixed crystal violet stain
iodine-induced hyperthyroidism
iodism

iodize
iodoform gauze
iodoglobulin
iodoquinol
iodotherapy
iodotyrosine deiodinase defect
Ionamin
ionic medication
Ionil-T Plus
ionization
ionized PTH calcium
ionizing radiation
iontophoresis
iontophoretic
iontotherapy
IOP
   intraocular pressure
Iopidine
Iowa-type amyloidosis
IP
   intraperitoneal
ipecac syrup
IPF
   idiopathic pulmonary fibrosis
IPH
   isolated postchallenge hyperglycemia
IPPB
   intermittent positive-pressure breathing
IPPV
   intermittent positive-pressure ventilation
ipratropium bromide
ipsilateral pleural effusion
irbesartan
iridectomy
irides (*pl. of* iris)
iridis
   rubeosis i.
iridium wire
iridocyclitis septica
iridodiagnosis
iridology
irinotecan
iris, pl. **irides**
   neovascularization of i.
iritis
   diabetic i.
   gouty i.
IRMA
   intraretinal microvascular abnormality
iron (Fe)
   i. absorption
   i. chelation therapy
   i. deficiency
   i. lung
   oral i.
   i. overload
   stainable i.
   i. storage disease
iron-binding capacity (IBC)

iron-deficiency anemia
irradiation
    laser i.
    i. therapy
irregular pulse
irreversible
    i. dementia
    i. shock
irrigation
    bowel i.
    whole bowel i.
irritability
    ventricular i.
irritable
    i. bowel
    i. bowel syndrome (IBS)
    i. colon
irritant gas inhalation
irritation
    peritoneal i.
    vulvar i.
irritative lesion
IRS-1
    insulin receptor substrate-1
ischemia
    acute mesenteric i.
    asymptomatic cardiac i. (ACI)
    cardiac i.
    chronic intestinal i.
    chronic mesenteric i.
    intestinal i.
    mesenteric i.
    myocardial i.
    nonocclusive mesenteric i.
    splanchnic i.
ischemic
    i. attack
    i. bone necrosis
    i. colitis
    i. coronary disease (ICD)
    i. heart disease
    i. heart failure
    i. hepatitis
    i. ileocolitis
    i. liver injury
    i. lumbago
    i. optic neuropathy
    i. stroke
    i. ulcer
ischemic-anoxic brain damage
ischial
ischiocavernosus muscle

ischiogluteal bursitis
ischiorectal
ischium
ischochymia
ischuretic
ischuria
ISH
    isolated systolic hypertension
island
    bone i.
    I. of Calleja receptor
    i. disease
    i. fever
islet
    i. cell
    i. cell hyperplasia
    i. cell tumor
    i. of Langerhans
    pancreatic i.
    Walthard i.
Ismo
isoandrosterone
isochromic anemia
Isoclor
isocyanate inhalation
isodense
isoenzyme
    CK i.
    creatine kinase i.
isoflavone
isoform
    CYP1A2 enzyme i.
    CYP3A enzyme i.
    CYP2C enzyme i.
    CYP2D6 enzyme i.
isolated
    i. calf vein thrombosis
    i. hematuria
    i. hypoaldosteronism
    i. myocarditis
    i. postchallenge hyperglycemia
    (IPH)
    i. proteinuria
    i. systolic hypertension (ISH)
isolation
    pulmonary i.
isoleucine acid
isometheptene
isoniazid
isonicotinic acid hydrazide (INH)
isopathy
Isophane insulin suspension

NOTES

isopropyl alcohol toxicity
isoproterenol
    i. infusion
    i. inhaler
Isoptin
Isordil Tembid
isoserum treatment
isosexual precocious puberty
isosorbide
    i. dinitrate
    i. mononitrate
    i. nitrate
isosporiasis
isosthenuria
isotonic lipid
isotretinoin drug study
isovaleric acidemia
isradipine
Israels-Wilkinson anemia
issue
    ethical i.
    legal i.
isthmus, pl. **isthmi**
    Krönig i.
Itai-Itai disease
ITB
    iliotibial band
itch
    barber's i.
    Cuban i.

    kabure i.
    Saint Ignatius i.
    warehousemen's i.
    winter i.
itching
    psychogenic i.
ITF
    International Tremor Foundation
ITP
    idiopathic thrombocytopenic purpura
    inosine 5′-triphosphate
itraconazole
Itsenko disease
IU
    International Unit
IUD
    intrauterine device
IV
    intravenous
        Aredia IV
        IV cocktail
        IV drug abuser
        IV push
I-V
    intraventricular
IVC
    inferior vena cava
Ivemark syndrome
IVP
    intravenous pyelogram

jabbing
Jaboulay
    J. amputation
    J. button
Jaccoud
    J. arthritis
    J. arthropathy
    J. fever
    J. sign
    J. syndrome
jackknife position
jackscrew
Jackson-Pratt drain
JACL
    Japanese American Citizens League
jactation capitis nocturna
jactitation
jail fever
Jakob-Creutzfeldt
    J.-C. disease
    J.-C. syndrome
Jaksch anemia
Jamaica ginger polyneuritis
Jamaican vomiting sickness
Jamar dynamometer
jambes
    maladie des j.
Janeway
    J. lesion
    J. spot
Jansky-Bielschowsky
    J.-B. disease
    J.-B. syndrome
Japanese
    J. American Citizens League
    (JACL)
    J. encephalitis
    J. encephalitis vaccine
    J. river fever
japonica
    cutaneous *Schistosoma j.*
japonicum
    Schistosoma j.
jargonaphasia
jaundice
    acholuric j.
    anhepatic j.
    anhepatogenous j.
    benign postoperative intrahepatic j.
    cholestatic j.
    chronic acholuric j.
    chronic familial nonhemolytic j.
    chronic idiopathic j.
    congenital hemolytic j.
    constitutional j.

    familial nonhemolytic j.
    Hayem j.
    hematogenous j.
    hemolytic j.
    hemorrhagic j.
    hepatocellular j.
    hepatogenous j.
    homologous serum j.
    human serum j.
    idiopathic j.
    infectious j.
    intrahepatic j.
    leptospiral j.
    malignant j.
    mechanical j.
    nonhemolytic j.
    nonobstructive j.
    nuclear j.
    obstructive j.
    painless j.
    physiologic j.
    postarsphenamine j.
    postoperative j.
    progressive j.
    pump j.
    regurgitation j.
    retention j.
    Schmorl j.
    spherocytic j.
    spirochetal j.
    toxemic j.
    transfusion j.
jaw
    j. osteomyelitis
    j. wiring
Jaworski body
J-curve hypothesis
jejunal artery aneurysm
jejuni
    Campylobacter j.
jejunoileal
jejunoileitis
jejunostomy
jejunotomy
jejunum
Jellinek
    J. sign
    J. symptom
jelling
jelly
    K-Y j.
Jendrassik
    J. maneuver
    J. sign

J

jerk
    clonic j.
    j. nystagmus
jerking
    ballistic exercise j.
jerky respiration
Jervell and Lange-Nielsen syndrome
Jeryl-Lynn virus
jet
    j. injection
    j. injector
    j. lag
    j. lag syndrome
    regurgitant j.
Jevity
Jew
    Ashkenazi J.
Jobst stocking
Job syndrome
jocular
JOD
    juvenile-onset diabetes
Jod-Basedow
    J.-B. disease
    J.-B. phenomenon
JODM
    juvenile-onset diabetes mellitus
Joffroy sign
John Douglas French Alzheimer's
    Foundation
Johne bacillus
joint
    astragaloscaphoid j.
    carpometacarpal j.
    Charcot j.
    coccygeal j.
    J. Commission on Accreditation of
      Healthcare Organizations
    cubital j.
    DIP j.
    distal interphalangeal j.
    j. effusion
    facet j.
    j. injection
    intercarpal j.
    j. line
    Lisfranc j.
    mandibular j.
    MCP j.
    metacarpophalangeal j.
    metatarsophalangeal j.
    mortise j.
    MTP j.
    j. pain
    proximal interphalangeal j.
    sacroiliac j.
    SI j.
    j. space narrowing
    talocrural j.

    temporomandibular j. (TMJ)
    ulnocarpal j.
    weight bearing j.
jolt headache
Jones fracture
Jordan anomaly
joule
Jr.
    Absorbine, Jr.
JRA
    juvenile rheumatoid arthritis
judgment, judgement
jugal bone
jugular
    j. sign
    j. venous distention (JVD)
    j. venous pressure (JVP)
    j. venous pressure elevation
    j. venous pulsation (JVP)
    j. venous pulse (JVP)
jugulation
jugulodigastric
junction
    dermoepidermal j.
    esophagogastric j.
    gastroesophageal j.
    squamocolumnar j.
    ureterovesical j. (UVJ)
junctional tachycardia
jungle fever
juniper
jurisprudence
    medical j.
justice
    Department of J. (DOJ)
justo major
juvenile
    j. aldosteronism
    j. chronic arthritis
    j. cirrhosis
    j. Crohn disease
    j. dermatomyositis
    j. diabetes
    j. inflammatory bowel disease
    j. lentigo
    j. myopathy
    j. nephronophthisis
    j. polyposis coli
    j. rheumatoid arthritis (JRA)
    j. ulcerative colitis
juvenile-onset
    j.-o. diabetes (JOD)
    j.-o. diabetes mellitus (JODM)
    j.-o. rheumatoid arthritis
juxt
juxtaarticular osteopenia
juxtallocortex
JVD
    jugular venous distention

JVP
   jugular venous pressure

jugular venous pulsation
jugular venous pulse

NOTES

J

K
   potassium
KA
   ketoacidosis
kabure itch
Kadian
Kaffir pox
kafindo
Kahler disease
kala azar
kaleidoscope
kalemia
Kaletra
kallikrein-kinin system
Kallmann syndrome
Kanavel
Kansas Geriatric Education Center (KS-GEC)
kansasii
   Mycobacterium k.
kanyemba
Kaon-Cl
Kaopectate
Kaposi
   K. disease
   K. sarcoma (KS)
   K. varicelliform eruption
   K. xeroderma
Karnofsky
   K. Rating Scale
   K. status
   K. tumor grading
Kartagener
   K. syndrome
   K. triad
karyotype
kasai
Katayama
   K. disease
   K. fever
   K. syndrome
kathexis
Katz Activities of Daily Living Scale
katzenjammer
kava kava
Kawasaki
   K. disease
   K. syndrome
Kay Ciel
Kaye dissecting scissors
Kayexalate
Kayser-Fleischer ring
KB
   ketone body

KCl
   potassium chloride
K-Dur
kedani fever
Keftab
Kefurox
Kefzol
Kegel exercise
Kehr sign
keloid
kelp
Kempner diet
Kenalog
Kenya fever
keratinocyte
keratinocytic dysplasia
keratinolytic agent
keratinous
keratin plug
keratitis
   fungal k.
   seborrheic k.
   ulcerative k.
keratoacanthoma
keratoconjunctivitis
   epidemic k. (EKC)
   k. sicca
keratoconus
keratoderma blennorrhagica
keratolysis
   pitted k.
keratomalacia
keratopathy
   pseudophakic bullous k.
keratosis, pl. **keratoses**
   actinic k. (AK)
   k. blennorrhagica
   plantar k.
   seborrheic k.
   solar k.
keratotic horny projection
keratotomy
   radial k.
kerion
Kerley A, B line
Kerlix
Kerlone
kernicterus
Kernig sign
Keshan disease
Ketamine
ketoacidosis (KA)
   alcoholic k.
   diabetic k. (DKA)

K

ketoaciduria
    branched chain k.
ketoconazole
ketogenic diet
ketohydroxyestrin
ketone
    k. body (KB)
    urine k.
ketonuria
    branched chain k.
ketoprofen
ketorolac
    k. tromethamine
ketosis
ketosis-prone diabetes
ketosis-resistant diabetes
17-ketosteroids
ketotic
    k. hyperglycinemia
Kew Gardens fever
kg
    kilogram
kidney
    k. amyloidosis
    Armanni-Ebstein k.
    crush k.
    dysplastic k.
    Goldblatt k.
    malignant neoplasm of k.
    multicystic dysplastic k.
    ptotic k.
    upper pole of k.
    k.'s, ureters, bladder (KUB)
Kiesselbach
    K. area
    K. plexus
    K. triangle
Kikuchi disease
killing
    bystander k.
kilogram (kg)
Kiloh-Nevin syndrome
Kimmelstiel-Wilson
    K.-W. disease
    K.-W. retinopathy
    K.-W. syndrome
kinase
    creatine k. (CK)
    protein k. C
    thymidine k. (TK)
    viral thymidine k.
kinesia
kinetic
    urea k.'s
kingae
    Haemophilus aphrophilus,
    Actinobacillus
    actinomycetemcomitans,
    Cardiobacterium hominis,

Eikenella corrodens, Kingella k.
(HACEK)
kinin
kininase
Kinkiang fever
kinky-hair disease
Kirk amputation
Kirkland disease
kit ligand
Klaron
K-Lease
Klebsiella
    K. pneumonia
    K. pneumoniae
    K. rhinoscleromatis
Klebs-Löffler bacillus
Klein bacillus
Kleine-Levin syndrome
Klemperer disease
Klinefelter syndrome
Klippel disease
Klippel-Trenaunay syndrome
Klonopin
Klor-Con
Klorvess
Klüver-Bucy syndrome
K-Lyte
knee
    k. arthrocentesis
    housemaid k.
    k. pain
    k. replacement
    k. sprain
Knies sign
Kniest syndrome
knifelike pain
Kocher-Debré-Sémélaigne syndrome
Kocher sign
Koch-Weeks bacillus
Koenig syndrome
KOH
    potassium hydroxide
koilocytosis
koilonychia
kola
    gotu k.
Kondremul
König syndrome
Konsyl
Koplik
    K. lesion
    K. spot
Korean hemorrhagic fever
Korotkoff
    K. phase
    K. sound
Korsakoff psychosis
Kostmann neutropenia
K-Phos Neutral

Krabbe
  K. disease
  K. hypoplasia
  K. leukodystrophy
  K. syndrome
kraurosis vulva
Krebs-Henseleit urea cycle
Krishaber disease
Krönig isthmus
KS
  Kaposi sarcoma
KS-GEC
  Kansas Geriatric Education Center
K-Tab
KUB
  kidneys, ureters, bladder
Kufs disease
Kundrat lymphosarcoma
Kunkel syndrome
kuru
Kussmaul
  K. breathing

  K. coma
  K. disease
  K. respiration
  K. sign
Kussmaul-Kien respiration
Kussmaul-Maier disease
Kutapressin
Ku-Zyme
Kveim-Siltzbach test
kwashiorkor
  marasmic k.
Kwell
Kyasanur Forest disease
K-Y jelly
kyphos
kyphoscoliosis
kyphosis
kyphotic
Kyrle disease
Kytril
kyushin

K

NOTES

L
> liter

LA
> Comhist LA
> Entex LA
> Nolex LA

L.A.
> Atrohist L.A.

Labbé syndrome

labetalol

labia
> lingual l.
> l. majora
> l. minora

labial
> l. abscess
> l. herpes simplex

labialis
> herpes l.
> myxadenitis l.

labile

lability
> emotional l.

labor
> Department of L. (DOL)

laboratory
> l. diagnosis
> Venereal Disease Research L.
> (VDRL)

labored
> l. breathing
> l. respiration

laborious

labrum

labyrinth
> dead l.

labyrinthine

labyrinthitis
> acute l.

labyrinthopathy

lacerate

laceration
> stellate l.

Lacey LeBeau tea

Lachman examination

Lac-Hydrin

Lacri-Lube

lacrimal disorder

lacrimation

lactacidemia

lactacidosis

Lactaid

lactase deficiency

lactate
> l. dehydrogenase (LDH)
> Ringer l.

lactated
> l. Ringer
> l. Ringer injection

lactation
> l. amenorrhea
> l. hormone

lactic
> l. acid
> l. acidosis
> l. dehydrogenase (LDH)

lacticacidemia

LactiCare ointment

lactimorbus

Lactobacillus

lactogenic hormone

lacto-ovo-vegetarian

lactose intolerance

lactosuria

lactotherapy

lactotropin

lactovegetarian diet

Lactrase

lactulose

lacunar
> l. brain infarct
> l. infarction

LAD
> left anterior descending

Lady Windemere's syndrome

Laënnec
> L. cirrhosis
> L. disease

laesa
> functio l.

Lafora disease

lag
> jet l.
> lid l.

lagophthalmos

LAHB
> left anterior hemiblock

Lahore sore

lake
> venous l.

Lambert-Eaton myasthenic syndrome

lamblia
> *Giardia l.*

lambliasis

lambo lambo

Lamictal

lamina, pl. **laminae**
> l. propria

laminectomy
lumbar l.
Lamisil
lamivudine
lamotrigine seizure
Lamprene
Lanacaine
Lanacort
Lancereaux diabetes
Lancereaux-Mathieu disease
lancet
lancinating pain
land
no-man's l.
l. scurvy
Landouzy
L. disease
L. dystrophy
L. purpura
L. type
Landouzy-Déjèrine dystrophy
Langenbeck amputation
Langerhans
islet of L.
language impediment
Lanoxicaps
Lanoxin
lansoprazole
lanthanic
Lantus
lanuginosa
hypertrichosis l.
laparoscopic
l. cholecystectomy (LC)
l. fundoplication
l. retropubic urethropexy
laparoscopy
laparotomy
lardaceous
l. liver
l. spleen
large
l. bowel obstruction
l. intestine
l. joint mechanoreceptor
l. loop excision
l. loop excision of transition zone (LLETZ)
Lariam
Laron
L. dwarf
L. dwarfism
L. syndrome
Laron-type dwarfism
Larrey-Weil disease
larvaceous
larval plague
larvate

laryngeal
l. carcinoma
l. descent
l. diphtheria
l. edema
l. height
larynges (*pl. of* larynx)
laryngitis
acute l.
laryngopharyngitis
laryngotracheal diphtheria
laryngotracheobronchitis
larynx, pl. **larynges**
amyloidosis of l.
malignant neoplasm of l.
Larzel anemia
Lasègue
laser
l. irradiation
l. prostatectomy
l. resurfacing
l. therapy
tunable dye l.
Lasix
L-asparaginase
Lassa
L. hemorrhagic fever
L. virus
last menstrual period (LMP)
Latanoprost
late
l. asthmatic response
l. benign syphilis
l. latent syphilis
l. lupus syndrome
l. luteal phase dysphoric disorder (LLPDD)
l. potential
l. rickets
late-life
l.-l. depression
l.-l. migraine
l.-l. onset
latency
sleep l.
latens
scarlatina l.
latent
l. adrenocortical insufficiency
l. diabetes
l. gout
l. infection
l. stage
l. syphilis
l. tetany
l. tuberculosis infection
l. typhoid

late-onset
  l.-o. congenital adrenal hyperplasia
  l.-o. familial Alzheimer disease
lateral
  anteroposterior and l.
  bilateral l.
  l. collateral ligament
  l. diffusion
  l. lead
  l. myocardial infarction
lateralis
  hyperhidrosis l.
latex agglutination test
lathyrism
Latino
latissimus
LATS
  long-acting thyroid stimulator
laudable pus
Launois-Cléret syndrome
Launois syndrome
Laurence-Biedl syndrome
Laurence-Moon-Biedl
  L.-M.-B. law
  L.-M.-B. syndrome
Laurence-Moon syndrome
LAV
  lymphadenopathy-associated virus
lavage
  bronchoalveolar l. (BAL)
  gastric l.
  gastrointestinal l.
  heated nasogastric l.
  heated peritoneal l.
  nasogastric l.
  peritoneal l.
law
  Allen paradoxical l.
  Baruch l.
  Bernoulli l.
  Cannon l.
  Courvoisier l.
  Eldercare Initiative in Consumer L.
    (EICL)
  Fitz l.
  Godélier l.
  Laurence-Moon-Biedl l.
  Louis l.
  Marfan l.
  National Center on Poverty L.,
    Inc. (NCPL)
  paradoxical l.

  l. of parsimony
  Poiseuille l.
  l. of similars
Lawrence-Seip syndrome
Lawton instrumental activities of daily living
laxative
  l. abuse
  bulk l.
  hyperosmolar l.
  saline l.
  stimulant l.
laxity
  pelvic muscle l.
layer
  cortical l.
lazaret
LBBB
  left bundle-branch block
LC
  laparoscopic cholecystectomy
L-carnitine
LCAT
  lecithin-cholesterol acyltransferase
  LCAT deficiency
LCE
  Legal Counsel for the Elderly
LD
  lethal dose
LDH
  lactate dehydrogenase
  lactic dehydrogenase
LDL
  low-density lipoprotein
  LDL cholesterol
  LDL receptor disorder
LDL-C
  low-density lipoprotein cholesterol
L-DOPA
  Early versus Later L-DOPA
    (ELLDOPA)
lead
  l. anemia
  augmented voltage unipolar left
    arm l. (aVL)
  augmented voltage unipolar left
    foot l. (aVF)
  augmented voltage unipolar right
    arm l. (aVR)
  aVF l.
  aVL l.
  aVR l.

L

NOTES

lead *(continued)*
    l. colic
    esophageal l.
    l. gout
    l. I, II, III
    lateral l.
    l. paralysis
    l. poisoning
    l. stomatitis
    l. time
    l. V
lead-time bias
leaflet
    aortic l.
league
    Japanese American Citizens L. (JACL)
    National Consumer's L. (NCL)
    National Urban L.
    Older Women's L. (OWL)
    L. of Red Cross Societies
leak
    biliary l.
    l. point pressure
leaky cell membrane
lean body mass
lean-mass catabolism
learning ability
lecithin
    polyunsaturated l.
lecithin-cholesterol
    l.-c. acyltransferase (LCAT)
    l.-c. acyltransferase deficiency
LED
    lupus erythematosus disseminatus
Ledercillin
Lederer anemia
leech
Leede-Rumpel phenomenon
LEEP
    loop electrosurgical excision procedure
leflunomide
left
    l. anterior descending (LAD)
    l. anterior divisional block
    l. anterior hemiblock (LAHB)
    l. bundle-branch block (LBBB)
    l. eye (OS)
    l. gastric artery (LGA)
    l. lower lobe (LLL)
    l. lower quadrant (LLQ)
    l. lower quadrant (of abdomen)
    l. middle lobe (LML)
    l. parasternal lift
    l. posterior divisional block
    l. salpingo-oophorectomy (LSO)
    l. septal ventricular tachycardia
    l. upper lobe (LUL)
    l. upper quadrant (LUQ)

    l. upper quadrant (of abdomen)
    l. ventricle (LV)
    l. ventricular (LV)
    l. ventricular failure
    l. ventricular free wall rupture
    l. ventricular hypertrophy (LVH)
    l. ventricular mass
    l. ventricular obstruction
    l. ventricular systolic dysfunction (LVSD)
    l. ventriculography
left-hand dominant
left-sided
    l.-s. heart failure
left-sided appendicitis
leg
    creepy-craze crawly syndrome of l.'s
    l. edema
    l. mobility
    l. ulcer
legal
    L. Counsel for the Elderly (LCE)
    L. disease
    l. intoxication
    l. issue
    l. medicine
    L. Services for the Elderly (LSE)
Legg-Calvé-Perthes disease
Legionella
    L. birminghamensis
    nosocomial *L.*
    L. pneumoniae
legionellosis
Legionnaires
    L. disease
    L. pneumonia
Leiden
    factor V L.
leiomyoma
leiomyomatous hamartoma
leiomyosarcoma
    cardiac l.
Leishman anemia
leishmania
leishmaniasis
    infantile l.
    mucosal l.
    visceral l.
leishmanin test
leishmaniosis
leisure time
Lejeune syndrome
Lemierre syndrome
length
    l. bias
    l. of stay
lenitive
Lennhoff sign

Lennox-Gastaut-Dravet syndrome
lens
> Frenzel l.
> Inwave Prism Hemianopic L.
> l. opacification
> l. opacity
> Varilux l.

lenta
> cholangitis l.
> sepsis l.

Lente
> pork L.

lentigo, pl. **lentigines**
> juvenile l.
> lentigines, electrocardiographic abnormalities, ocular hypertelorism, pulmonary stenosis, abnormalities of genitalia, retardation of growth, deafness (LEOPARD)
> lentigines, electrocardiographic abnormalities, ocular hypertelorism, pulmonary stenosis, abnormalities of genitalia, retardation of growth, deafness syndrome
> l. maligna melanoma
> solar l.

LEOPARD
> lentigines, electrocardiographic abnormalities, ocular hypertelorism, pulmonary stenosis, abnormalities of genitalia, retardation of growth, deafness
> LEOPARD syndrome

Lépine-Froin syndrome
lepirudin
leptin
leptodactylous
leptodermic
leptomeningeal
leptomyxid amebic infection
leptospirosis
> anicteric l.
> icteric l.
> l. icterohemorrhagica

leptothricosis
Leptotrombidium akamushi
Leriche
> L. disease
> L. syndrome

LES
> lower esophageal sphincter

Lesch-Nyhan syndrome

Lescol XL
lesion
> adynamic bone l.
> angiocentric immunoproliferative l. (AIL)
> Armanni-Ebstein l.
> Blumenthal l.
> bone l.
> Cameron l.
> cavitary lung l.
> cold l.
> Councilman l.
> Dieulafoy l.
> Ebstein l.
> enhancing ring l.
> focal stenotic l.
> herpetic l.
> hot l.
> indiscriminate l.
> irritative l.
> Janeway l.
> Koplik l.
> lung l.
> mass l.
> optic nerve l.
> pancreatic l.
> polypoid l.
> primary skin l.
> ring-wall l.
> secondary skin l.
> skin l.
> space-occupying l.
> spinal l.
> squamous intraepithelial l. (SIL)
> subtentorial l.
> supratentorial l.
> vaginal l.
> vascular l.
> vulvar l.

lesser pancreas
let-down reflex
lethal
> clinical l.
> l. dose (LD)
> genetic l.

lethality rate
lethargic
lethargy
Letterer-Siwe disease
leucine
> l. hypoglycemia

leucine-induced hypoglycemia

L

NOTES

leucovorin
Leudet
- L. bruit
- bruit de L.
- L. tinnitus

leuenkephalin
leukemia
- acute lymphoblastic l. (ALL)
- acute monocytic l. (AML)
- acute myeloblastic l. (AML)
- acute myelocytic l. (AML)
- acute myelogenous l. (AML)
- acute myeloid l.
- acute myelomonoblastic l. (AMMOL)
- acute myelomonocytic l. (AMML)
- acute nonlymphocytic l. (ANLL)
- acute nonlymphoid l. (ANLL)
- acute promyelocytic l. (APL)
- adult T-cell l.
- aleukemic l.
- aleukocythemic l.
- aplastic l.
- basophilic l.
- Bennett l.
- blast cell l.
- blastic l.
- Burkitt-type acute lymphoblastic l.
- chronic granulocytic l.
- chronic lymphocytic l. (CLL)
- chronic myelocytic l.
- chronic myelogenous l. (CML)
- chronic myeloid l.
- chronic myelomonocytic l. (CML, CMMoL)
- l. cutis
- embryonal l.
- end-stage acute l.
- eosinophilic l.
- granulocytic l.
- Gross l.
- hairy cell l.
- hemoblastic l.
- hemocytoblastic l.
- histiocytic l.
- leukopenic l.
- lymphatic l.
- lymphoblastic l.
- lymphocytic l.
- lymphogenous l.
- lymphoid l.
- lymphoidocytic l.
- L. and Lymphoma Society, Inc. (LLS)
- lymphosarcoma cell l.
- mast cell l.
- megakaryocytic l.
- micromyeloblastic l.
- monoblastic l.
- monocytic l.
- myeloblastic l.
- myelocytic l.
- myelogenous l.
- myeloid granulocytic l.
- myelomonocytic l.
- Naegeli l.
- nonlymphocytic l.
- nonlymphoid l.
- plasma cell l.
- plasmacytic l.
- prolymphocytic l.
- promyelocytic l.
- reticuloendothelial cell l.
- Rieder cell l.
- Schilling l.
- secondary acute l.
- smoldering myeloid l.
- splenomedullary l.
- splenomyelogenous l.
- stem cell l.
- subacute myeloid l.
- subleukemic l.
- undifferentiated cell l.

leukemic
- l. adenia
- l. erythrocytosis
- l. reticuloendotheliosis
- l. synovitis

leukemogenic
leukemoid reaction
Leukeran
leukobilin
leukocyte-depleting filter
leukocytic pyrogen
leukocytoclastic vasculitis
leukocytosis
- relative l.

leukodystrophy
- Krabbe l.
- metachromatic l.

leukoencephalopathy
- progressive multifocal l.

leukoerythroblastic anemia
leukolymphosarcoma
leukomalacia
- periventricular l.

leukopenia
leukopenic leukemia
leukoplakia
- hairy l.
- oral l.

leukorrhea
leukotriene
- l. modifier
- l. receptor antagonist

leuprolide
- depot l.

levamisole

Levaquin
Levatol
LeVeen shunt
level
    acetylcholine receptor antibody l.
    adrenocorticotropic hormone l.
    aldolase l.
    aminotransferase l.
    antibody l.
    blood acetylcholine receptor
      antibody l.
    blood ethanol l.
    cholesterol l.
    CKMB l.
    l. of consciousness
    cortisol l.
    C peptide l.
    creatine kinase myocardial band l.
    elevated prostate-specific antigen l.
    ethanol l.
    hepatic copper l.
    hormone l.
    human chorionic gonadotropin l.
    intellectual l.
    lipid l.
    parathyroid hormone l.
    plasma adrenocorticotropic
      hormone l.
    PTH l.
    serum aminotransferase l.
    serum cholesterol l.
    serum ferritin l.
    serum iron l.
    T_4-binding globulin l.
    testosterone l.
Lévi disease
levis
    icterus castrensis l.
Levlen 28
levodopa test
levofloxacin
levonorgestrel
levorphanol
levoscoliosis
Levothroid
levothyroxine sodium
Levoxine
Levoxyl
Levsin
Levsinex Timecaps
levulosemia
levulosuria

Lewis
    substance P of L.
Lewy
    L. body
    L. body dementia
    L. body disease
Leyden hemophilia B
Leydig
    L. cell
    L. cell hyperplasia
LFA
    Lupus Foundation of America
LFS
    liver function series
LFT
    liver function test
LGA
    left gastric artery
***l*-glyceric aciduria**
LH
    luteinizing hormone
Lhermitte
    L. sign
    L. syndrome
LH/FSH-RF
    luteinizing hormone/follicle-stimulating
      hormone-releasing factor
LH-RF
    luteinizing hormone-releasing factor
LH-RH, LHRH
    luteinizing hormone-releasing hormone
      (*See also* LRH)
L-hyoscyamine sulfate
lib
    a.d. l.
      as desired
libido
Libman-Sacks
    L.-S. endocarditis
    L.-S. syndrome
Librax
Librium
licensed
    l. practical nurse (LPN)
    l. vocational nurse (LVN)
licentiate
    L. of the Royal College of
      Physicians (Edinburgh) (LRCP(E))
    L. of the Royal College of
      Physicians (Ireland) (LRCP(I))
    L. of the Royal College of
      Physicians (of England) (LRCP)

L

NOTES

lichen
    l. chronicus simplex
    l. planus
    l. sclerosis
    l. sclerosus et atrophicus
lichenification
lichenoid dermatitis
licorice
Liddle syndrome
Lidex-E
lid lag
lidocaine
lienteric diarrhea
lientery
life, pl. **lives**
    l. cycle
    l. expectancy
    health-related quality of l. (HRQL, HRQOL)
    postnatal l.
    quality of l.
    relational l.
    L. Satisfaction Index A (LSIA)
    L. Satisfaction Index B (LSIB)
    L. Satisfaction Rating (LSR)
    l. span
    L. Stream
    l. table
LifeGuard enteral feeding set
lifelong obesity
life-prolonging measures
LifeScan Ultra machine
lifespan
lifestyle
    l. adjustment
    sedentary l.
life-sustaining
    l.-s. intervention
    l.-s. treatment
life-table analysis
life-threatening event
Li-Fraumeni syndrome
lift
    left parasternal l.
lift-off test
ligament
    anterior cruciate l.
    Cooper l.
    lateral collateral l.
    medial collateral l.
    posterior cruciate l.
ligamentous
    l. injection
    l. tear
ligamentum, pl. **ligamenta**
    l. flavum
ligand
    kit l.

ligation
    bilateral tubal l. (BTL)
    endoscopic band l.
    variceal l.
light
    l. bath
    l. chain
    l. chain deposition disease
    l. chain-related amyloidosis
    l. microscopy
    pupils equal and reactive to l. (PERL)
    Questran L.
    l. therapy
    l. touch
    l. touch testing
    l. treatment
    Woods l.
light-dark cycle
light-headedness
    psychogenic l.-h.
Lighthouse National Center for Vision and Aging (LNCVA)
light-touch palpation
Lignac
    L. disease
    L. syndrome
Lignac-Fanconi
    L.-F. disease
    L.-F. syndrome
ligneous thyroiditis
likelihood ratio
Likert scale
lily of the valley
limb-girdle dystrophy
limbic
Limbitrol
lime
    bruit de l.
limit
    within normal l.'s (WNL)
limited
    organ l.
    l. scleroderma
limitus
    hallux l.
limnemia
limnemic
limophthisis
Lincocin
lincosamide antibiotic
lindane 1% cream
line
    Aldrich-Mees l.
    bismuth l.
    joint l.
    Kerley A, B l.
    PA l.
    peripherally inserted catheter l.

PIC l.
posteroanterior l.
Shenton l.
spigelian l.
Sydney l.
linea semilunaris
linezolid
lingua
lingual
    l. labia
    l. thyroid
linguatuliasis
liniment cream
linkage
    medical record l.
Lioresal
Liouvilles icterus
lip
    cleft l.
lipasemia
lipedema
lipemia
    alimentary l.
    diabetic l.
    postprandial l.
lipid
    isotonic l.
    l. level
    l. peroxidation
    l. profile
    l. reduction
    l. storage disease
lipid-lowering
    l.-l. agent
    l.-l. drug
    l.-l. medication
    l.-l. therapy
lipid-mobilizing hormone
lipidolytic
lipidosis
    cerebral l.
    cerebroside l.
    ganglioside l.
    glycolipid l.
    sulfatide l.
lipiduria
Lipisorb
Lipitor
lipoatrophia
lipoatrophic diabetes
lipoatrophy
    insulin l.

lipochondrodystrophy
lipodystrophia progressiva
lipodystrophy
    congenital total l.
    insulin l.
    membranous l.
lipoflavonoid
lipofuscinosis
    ceroid l.
lipogenic enzyme propensity
lipogenous diabetes
lipogranuloma
lipogranulomatosis
    disseminated l.
lipoid
    l. adrenal hyperplasia
    l. proteinosis
lipoides
    arcus l.
lipoidica
    necrobiosis l.
lipoidosis
    cerebroside l.
    l. cutis et mucosae
    galactosylceramide l.
lipolysis
lipoma
    cardiac l.
    Madelung l.
lipomatosis
    epidural l.
    l. neurotica
lipomucopolysaccharidosis
liponephrosis
lipophilic
lipopolysaccharide porins
lipoprotein
    elevated l.
    high-density l. (HDL)
    intermediate-density l. (IDL)
    l. lipase deficiency
    low-density l. (LDL)
    very high density l. (VHDL)
    very low density l. (VLDL)
lipoprotein-triglyceride
    very low density l.-t. (VLDL-TG)
liposis
liposomal
    l. amphotericin B
    l. doxorubicin
lipoteichoic acid
lipotrophic

NOTES

L

lipotrophy
lipotropic hormone (LPH)
lipotropin
lipotropy
liquefaction
Liquibid
liquid
honey-thick l.
l. nitrogen (LN$_2$)
Titralac Plus L.
Liquifilm
Betagen L.
Lisfranc joint
lisinopril
lispro
insulin l.
listerial
Listeria monocytogenes
listeriosis
liter (L)
millimoles per l. (mmol/L)
lithium
l. carbonate
l. toxicity
Lithobid
lithotomy
lithotripsy
extracorporeal shock-wave l.
shock-wave l.
little adrenocorticotrophic hormone
livedoid dermatitis
livedo reticularis
liver
acute yellow atrophy of l.
amyloid l.
l. biopsy
l. breath
brimstone l.
capsular cirrhosis of l.
cirrhotic l.
l. disease
l. dysfunction
l. enzyme elevation
l. failure
l. flap
l. fluke
l. function
l. function series (LFS)
l. function test (LFT)
hemangioma of l.
l. imaging
l. injury
l. kidney syndrome
lardaceous l.
l. metastasis
omental tuberosity of l.
pigmented l.
l. scan
l. smear

l. toxicity
l. transplant
l. transplant rejection
venoocclusive disease of l.
yellow atrophy of l.
lives (*pl. of* life)
livid
Livierato sign
living
activities of daily l. (ADL)
l. donor
l. donor bilobar transplant
instrumental activities of daily l.
(IADL)
Lawton instrumental activities of
daily l.
l. will
Livingston insomnia scale
lizard bite
LLETZ
large loop excision of transition zone
LLL
left lower lobe
Lloyd syndrome
LLPDD
late luteal phase dysphoric disorder
LLQ
left lower quadrant
LLS
Leukemia and Lymphoma Society, Inc.
LML
left middle lobe
LMP
last menstrual period
LN$_2$
liquid nitrogen
LNCVA
Lighthouse National Center for Vision
and Aging
load
viral l.
loading
l. dose
excessive l.
repetitive l.
salt l.
lobar
l. atrophy
l. pneumonia
lobe
caudal l.
caudate l.
hot caudate l.
left lower l. (LLL)
left middle l. (LML)
left upper l. (LUL)
Riedel l.
right lower l. (RLL)

right middle l. (RML)
right upper l. (RUL)
lobectomy
thyroid l.
lobular
l. carcinoma
l. carcinoma in situ
lobulation
portal l.
lobule
local
l. death
l. disease
l. hormone
l. sign
l. symptom
localization-related seizure
localized
l. adenopathy
l. myositis
localizing
l. electrode
l. symptom
location
ostium primum l.
locator
Eldercare L.
lockjaw
Locoid cream
locomotion
loculated
l. pleural effusion
l. pus
loculus, pl. **loculi**
locum
l. tenant
l. tenens
Lodine
Lodosyn
Loestrin Fe
Löffler
L. eosinophilia
L. syndrome
Löfgren syndrome
logical functioning
Logistic Organ Dysfunction Score
loliism
lomefloxacin
Lomotil
lone
l. atrial fibrillation
l. episode

long
l. incubation hepatitis
l. QT syndrome
l. R-P tachycardia
l. thoracic nerve entrapment
long-acting
l.-a. beta agonist
l.-a. inhaled beta-agonist
l.-a. insulin
l.-a. oxycodone
l.-a. testosterone ester
l.-a. thyroid stimulator (LATS)
longevity
long-handled sock donner
longissimus dorsi
longitudinal study
long-leg cast
long-term
l.-t. care
l.-t. care facility
l.-t. care insurance
l.-t. memory
l.-t. RBC transfusion therapy
long-tract sign
longus
adductor l.
extensor digitorum l.
extensor hallucis l.
Loniten
loop
l. diuretic
car l.
l. electrosurgical excision procedure (LEEP)
Henle l.
ileal l.
l. recorder
loopogram
loose body
Looser zone
Lo-Ovral
loperamide
Lopid
lopidine
lopinavir
Lopressor
Loprox cream
Lorabid
loracarbef
Lorain disease
Lorain-Lévi
L.-L. dwarfism

L

NOTES

233

Lorain-Lévi *(continued)*
    L.-L. infantilism
    L.-L. syndrome
loratadine
lorazepam
Lorcet Plus
lordosis
    lumbar l.
Lorenz sign
Lortab
losartan potassium
Losec
loss
    acute blood l.
    bilateral vestibular l.
    blood l.
    conductive hearing l.
    fluid l.
    l. of function
    gastrointestinal water l.
    gustatory l.
    hearing l.
    hemianopic field l.
    involuntary weight l.
    nonrenal potassium l.
    nonrenal water l.
    potassium l.
    renal potassium l.
    renal water l.
    sensory l.
    water l.
    weight l.
loss-of-function disorder
Lotensin
lotion
    Caladryl l.
    calamine l.
    Halotex l.
    Sea and Ski l.
    Tinver l.
Lotrel 5/10
Lotrimin solution
Lotrisone
loud snoring
Lou Gehrig disease
Louis law
louse
    head l.'s
louse-borne typhus
lovastatin
Lovenox
Lovibond
    L. angle
    L. profile sign
low
    l. air-loss bed
    l. back pain
    l. body mass index

    l. bone turnover disease
    l. delirium
low-affinity hemoglobin
low-calorie diet
low-density
    l.-d. lipoprotein (LDL)
    l.-d. lipoprotein apheresis
    l.-d. lipoprotein cholesterol (LDL-C)
    l.-d. lipoprotein receptor
    l.-d. lipoprotein receptor disorder
low-dose
    l.-d. CT scan
    l.-d. dexamethasone suppression test
LowDye
lower
    l. abdominal pain
    l. esophageal ring
    l. esophageal sphincter (LES)
    l. eyelid
    l. gastrointestinal bleeding
    l. motor neuron
    l. respiratory tract
    l. respiratory tract infection
    l. urinary tract cancer
    l. urinary tract infection
    l. urinary tract obstruction
Lowe syndrome
Lowe-Terrey-MacLachlan syndrome
low-fat diet
low-grade non-Hodgkin lymphoma
low-hepatic clearance drug
low-molecular-weight heparin
low-purine diet
low-residue diet
low-salt
    l.-s. diet
    l.-s. syndrome
low-sodium diet
low-vision rehabilitation therapist
Loxitane
loxoscelism
Lozol
LP
    lumbar puncture
LPH
    lipotropic hormone
LPN
    licensed practical nurse
LRCP
    Licentiate of the Royal College of
    Physicians (of England)
LRCP(E)
    Licentiate of the Royal College of
    Physicians (Edinburgh)
LRCP(I)
    Licentiate of the Royal College of
    Physicians (Ireland)
LRF
    luteinizing hormone-releasing factor

LRH
    luteinizing hormone-releasing hormone
LSE
    Legal Services for the Elderly
LSIA
    Life Satisfaction Index A
LSIB
    Life Satisfaction Index B
LSO
    left salpingo-oophorectomy
LSR
    Life Satisfaction Rating
lubricant
    vaginal l.
Lucas sign
lucency, pl. **lucencies**
    punctate l.
Lucio phenomenon
Ludiomil
Ludwig angina
lues
    l. hepatis
    l. venerea
luetic
Luft
    L. disease
    L. syndrome
Lufyllin
LUL
    left upper lobe
luliberin
lumbago
    ischemic l.
lumbar
    l. disk syndrome
    l. laminectomy
    l. lordosis
    l. puncture (LP)
    l. root disease
    l. sympathetic blockade
    l. syringomyelia
lumborum
    quadratus l.
lumbosacral
lumbricoides
    Ascaris l.
lumen, pl. **lumina, lumens**
    intestinal l.
    vessel l.
lumpectomy
lunata
    Curvularia l.

lunate bone
Lund-Browder burn scale
lung
    l. abscess
    air-conditioner l.
    alveolar proteinosis of l.
    l. biopsy
    bird-breeder's l.
    bird-fancier's l.
    black l.
    l. blast
    brown l.
    l. cancer
    cheese-worker's l.
    coal miner's l.
    collier l.
    l. donor
    farmer's l.
    l. field
    l. fluke
    l. fluke disease
    l. injury
    iron l.
    l. lesion
    malt-worker's l.
    mason's l.
    miner's l.
    mushroom-worker's l.
    pump l.
    l. scan
    shock l.
    silo-filler's l.
    thresher's l.
    l. transplant
    l. transplant rejection
    vanishing l.
    l. volume
    l. volume reduction
    l. volume reduction surgery
        (LVRS)
    welder's l.
    wet l.
**lung-protective pressure-targeted
    ventilation**
lunula, pl. **lunulae**
lupinosis
lupoid hepatitis
Lupron Depot
lupus
    chilblain l.
    discoid l.
    drug-induced l.

NOTES

L

lupus *(continued)*
    l. erythematosus
    l. erythematosus disseminatus
      (LED)
    L. Foundation of America (LFA)
    hydralazine l.
    neonatal l.
    l. nephritis
    l. pernio
    l. profundus
lupuslike syndrome
LUQ
    left upper quadrant
lurch
    adductor l.
luteal
    l. phase defect
    l. phase deficiency
    l. phase therapy
luteinize
luteinizing
    l. hormone (LH)
    l. hormone/follicle-stimulating
      hormone-releasing factor (LH/FSH-
      RF)
    l. hormone-releasing factor (LH-RF,
      LRF)
    l. hormone-releasing hormone (LH-
      RH, LHRH, LRH)
    l. principle
luteohormone
luteolysin
luteum
lutropin
Lutz-Splendore-Almeida disease
Luvox
luxans
    coxa vara l.
luxus
LV
    left ventricle
    left ventricular
      LV mass
LVH
    left ventricular hypertrophy
LVN
    licensed vocational nurse
LVRS
    lung volume reduction surgery
LVSD
    left ventricular systolic dysfunction
lycoperdonosis
Lyme
    L. arthritis
    L. disease
    L. disease vaccine
    L. titer
lymph
    l. node

    l. node biopsy
    l. node dissection
    l. sinus
lymphadenectomy
lymphadenitic
lymphadenitis
    caseous l.
    paratuberculous l.
    regional granulomatous l.
lymphadenocyst
lymphadenoid thyroiditis
lymphadenopathy
    angioimmunoblastic l.
    cervical l.
    dermatopathic l.
    generalized l.
    giant follicular l.
    high cervical l.
    immunoblastic l.
    persistent generalized l.
    subcarinal l.
    tuberculous l.
lymphadenopathy-associated virus (LAV)
lymphangiectasia
    intestinal l.
lymphangiogram
lymphangioleiomyomatosis
lymphangitis
lymphatic
    l. abscess
    l. disease
    l. dyscrasia
    l. fistula
    l. leukemia
lymphatica
    pseudoleukemia l.
lymphaticus
    status l.
lymphedema
    l. praecox
    l. pump
lymphoblastic leukemia
lymphoblastoma
    giant follicular l.
lymphocyte
    atypical l.
    l. cell
    intraepithelial l.
    tumor-infiltrating l. (TILS)
lymphocyte-mediated response
lymphocytic
    l. choriomeningitis
    dermal l.
    l. interstitial pneumonia
    l. interstitial pneumonitis
    l. leukemia
    l. lymphoma
    l. lymphosarcoma

l. thyroiditis
l. thyroiditis neoplasia
lymphogenous
l. leukemia
l. metastasis
lymphogranuloma
l. inguinale
venereal l.
l. venereum
l. venereum infection
lymphoid
l. hyperplasia
l. leukemia
l. precursor B-cell
l. prccursor T-cell
l. tissue lymphoma
lymphoidocytic leukemia
lymphokine
lymphoma
African Burkitt l.
AIDS-related non-Hodgkin l.
B-cell l.
Burkitt l.
central nervous system l.
centrocytic l.
cutaneous T-cell l. (CTCL)
gastric l.
high-grade non-Hodgkin l.
Hodgkin l.
intermediate-grade non-Hodgkin l.
low-grade non-Hodgkin l.
lymphocytic l.
lymphoid tissue l.
mucosa-associated lymphoid
   tissue l.
non-Hodgkin l.

primary central nervous system l.
small-intestinal l.
T-cell l.
thyroid l.
well-differentiated lymphocytic l.
   (WDLL)
lymphomatoid granulomatosis
lymphomatosa
struma l.
lymphomatosum
papillary adenocystoma l.
lymphomatous
lymphonodus
lymphopathia
lymphopathy
lymphoproliferative syndrome
lymphoreticulosis
benign inoculation l.
lymphosarcoma
l. cell leukemia
fascicular l.
Kundrat l.
lymphocytic l.
sclerosing l.
lymphoscintigraphy
lymphotropic virus
lypressin
lyse
lysed horse blood
lysis
lysly hydroxylase deficiency
lysogenic conversion
lysolecithin hemolytic anemia
lysosomal disease
lytes, electrolytes
lytic

NOTES

M
monoclonal
M spike
m
meter
m²
meters squared
MA
mental age
Maalox
MAC
membrane attack complex
mitral annulus calcification
Mycobacterium avium complex
disseminated MAC
MAC infection
MacCallum patch
macerate
Machida scope
machine
Fresenius m.
Glucometer Elite XL m.
LifeScan Ultra m.
machine-based intervention
Mackenzie
M. amputation
M. disease
Maclagan thymol turbidity test
Macleod
M. capsular rheumatism
M. syndrome
macroadenoma
prolactin-secreting m.
macroamylasemia
Macrobid
macrobiosis
macrobiota
macrobiote
macrobiotic diet
macrobiotics
macrocrystal
nitrofurantoin m.
macrocytic
m. achylic anemia
m. anemia of pregnancy
m. anemia tropical
m. hyperchromatism
macrocytosis
Macrodantin
macrogenitosomia
m. praecox
m. praecox suprarenalis
macroglobulinemia
Waldenström m.
macroglossia

macrolide
m. antibiotic
m. therapy
macronodular cirrhosis
macronutrient
m. deficiency syndrome
m. supplementation
macrophage
macropodia
macroscopic BPH
macrosomatia adiposa congenita
macrovascular disease
macrovesicular
macula, pl. **maculae**
macular
m. degeneration
m. disease
m. hole
maculation
pernicious m.
macule
maculopapular
m. eruption
m. rash
maculopathy
cellophane m.
mad cow disease
Madelung
M. collar
M. disease
M. lipoma
M. neck
M. syndrome
Mad Hatter syndrome
madre
buba m.
magenta tongue
magna
coxa m.
magnesia
milk of m. (MOM)
magnesium
m. balance
esomeprazole m.
m. hydroxide
magnetic
m. resonance angiography (MRA)
m. resonance
cholangiopancreatography
m. resonance imaging (MRI)
m. resonance venography (MRV)
magnetotherapy
magnet therapy
magnification
symptom m.

M

Magnus sign
Mag-Ox 400
ma huang
maidica
    psychoneurosis m.
maidism
maintain
maintenance
    m. chemotherapy
    m. dose
    m. drug therapy
    health m.
Maisonneuve amputation
maitake mushroom
Maixner cirrhosis
major
    justo m.
    pestis m.
    thalassemia m.
    variola m.
majora
    labia m.
majority
making
    end-of-life decision m.
mal
    m. de la rosa
    m. de mer
    m. rouge
malabsorption
    fat m.
    glucose-galactose m.
    immunodeficiency and m.
    selective cobalamin m.
    m. symptom
    m. syndrome
    vitamin D m.
malacoplakia
maladie (*See also* malady)
    m. de plongeurs
    m. des jambes
malady
malaise
    general m.
malar flush
malaria
    acute m.
    algid m.
    autochthonous m.
    benign tertian m.
    bilious remittent m.
    cerebral m.
    chronic m.
    m. comatosa
    double tertian m.
    dysenteric algid m.
    falciparum m.
    gastric algid m.
    induced m.

    intermittent m.
    malariae m.
    malignant tertian m.
    nonan m.
    ovale m.
    pernicious m.
    quartan m.
    quotidian m.
    relapsing m.
    remittent m.
    tertian m.
    vivax m.
malariae
    m. malaria
    Plasmodium m.
malarial
    m. cachexia
    m. fever
    m. hemoglobinuria
malariology
malarious
Malarone
Malassezia furfur
malassimilation
malathion
malayi
    Brugia m.
maldigestion
    intraluminal m.
maldistribution
    fat m.
male
    m. breast cancer
    m. hypogonadism
    m. infertility
    m. sterility
maleate
    enalapril m.
male-pattern baldness
malformation
    Arnold-Chiari m.
    arteriovenous m. (AVM)
maligna
    polyadenitis m.
    scarlatina m.
    variola m.
malignancy
    cervical m.
    transplant m.
    uterine corpus m.
    vulvar m.
malignant
    m. acanthosis nigricans
    m. anemia
    m. ascites
    m. bubo
    m. carcinoid syndrome
    m. dysentery
    m. hepatic neoplasm

m. hypercalcemia
m. hyperphenylalaninemia
m. hyperpyrexia
m. hypertension
m. hyperthermia
m. hyperthermia syndrome
m. malnutrition
m. melanoma
m. mesothelioma
m. neoplasm of bladder
m. neoplasm of bone
m. neoplasm of bronchus
m. neoplasm of kidney
m. neoplasm of larynx
m. neoplasm of scrotum
m. neutropenia
m. otitis externa
m. pericardial effusion
m. pleural effusion
m. smallpox
m. spinal disease
m. tertian fever
m. tertian malaria
m. thyroid nodule
malignum
chorioepithelioma m.
malingering
malleolus stasis ulcer
malleosa
pneumonia m.
mallet
m. deformity
m. toe
Mallinckrodt
Mallory body
Mallory-Weiss
M.-W. syndrome
M.-W. tear
malnourishment
malnutrition
malignant m.
protein m.
protein-energy m. (PEM)
malpighian stigma
malposition
cardia m.
malpractice
Malta fever
Maltese cross
maltreatment
malt-worker's lung

malum
m. articulorum senilis
m. perforans pedis
m. venereum
mamillary nuclei receptor
mammary souffle
mammillate
mammillation
mammogram
mammography
screening m.
mammoplasty
mammotropic
m. factor
m. hormone
man
well-nourished m. (WNM)
managed
m. care
m. care organization
management
airway m.
fluid m.
medication m.
pain m.
pharmacologic m.
routine health m. (RHM)
stress m.
ventilator m.
manager
geriatric care m. (GCM)
National Association of
Progressional Geriatric Care M.'s
(NAPGCM)
Manchurian
M. hemorrhagic fever
M. typhus
Mandelamine
Mandel Social Adjustment Scale (MSAS)
mandible
angle of m.
mandibular joint
maneuver
Adson m.
Apley compression m.
Bárány m.
Cawthorne m.
Dix-Hallpike m.
doll's head m.
Hallpike m.
Heimlich m.

M

NOTES

maneuver *(continued)*
    Jendrassik m.
    Nylen-Bárány m.
    piano key m.
    Valsalva m.
    Wright m.
manganese
    m. dioxide aerosol
    m. poisoning
mania
manifestation
manipulation
    hormonal m.
    spinal m.
Manning criteria
mannitol
mannosidosis
Mann sign
manometer
    calibrated aneroid m.
manometry
    anorectal m.
    esophageal m.
    gastroduodenal m.
    gastrointestinal m.
Manson
    M. disease
    M. schistosomiasis
Mansonella
    M. ozzardi infection
    M. perstans infection
    M. streptocerca infection
mansonelliasis
mansonellosis
mansoni
    Schistosoma m.
mantle
Mantoux
    M. reaction
    M. testing
manual
    m. counting
    m. dexterity
manubrium
manus
    tinea m.
manuum
    tinea m.
MAO
    monoamine oxidase
    MAO inhibitor
MAOI
    monoamine oxidase inhibitor
MAP
    mean arterial pressure
maple
    m. bark disease
    m. syrup urine
    m. syrup urine disease

mapping
maprotiline
Marañón sign
marantic
    m. atrophy
    m. edema
    m. thrombosis
    m. thrombus
marasmic kwashiorkor
marasmoid
marasmus
    nutritional m.
Marburg
    M. disease
    M. hemorrhagic fever
    M. virus disease
Marcaine
    plain M.
march
    m. fracture
    m. hematuria
Marchand adrenals
Marchiafava-Bignami syndrome
Marchiafava-Micheli
    M.-M. anemia
    M.-M. disease
    M.-M. syndrome
marcid
marcor
Marcus Gunn pupil
Marek disease
Marfan
    M. law
    M. sign
    M. syndrome
marfanoid body habitus
marginal sinus
marginatum
    erythema m.
margin of safety
Marie
    M. disease
    M. hypertrophy
    M. sign
    M. syndrome
Marie-Robinson syndrome
Marie-Strümpell
    M.-S. arthritis
    M.-S. disease
    M.-S. spondylitis
    M.-S. syndrome
marijuana, marihuana
marination
marine envenomation
marinum
    Mycobacterium m.
marinus
    vomitus m.
marital status

markedly
   m. increased
   m. tender
marker
   molecular m.
   risk m.
   tumor m.
   m. X syndrome
marking
   haustral m.
Marlex mesh
marmorata
   cutis m.
Maroteaux-Lamy
   M.-L. disease
   M.-L. syndrome
marrow infiltration
Marshall-Marchetti
Marshall syndrome
Marsh disease
marsh fever
marshmallow
Martin-Bell syndrome
Martin-Gruber
   M.-G. anastomosis
   M.-G. phenomenon
masculinity
masculinization
masculinize
masculinizing
mask
   m. face
   Parkinson m.
   sleep m.
   Venturi m.
masked
   m. facies
   m. gout
   m. hyperthyroidism
mason's lung
masquerade
mass
   abdominal m.
   adnexal m.
   adrenal m.
   body m.
   breast m.
   epigastric m.
   fat-free m. (FFM)
   lean body m.
   left ventricular m.
   m. lesion

   LV m.
   m. media
   mediastinal m.
   neck m.
   pelvic m.
   perihilar m.
   pulsatile epigastric m.
   retroperitoneal m.
   m. screening
   scrotum m.
   soft tissue m.
massage therapy
masseter
massive
   m. bowel resection syndrome
   m. pneumonia
   m. transfusion
MAST
   medical antishock trousers
mast
   m. cell disease
   m. cell leukemia
mastalgia
mastectomy
   modified radical m.
   radical m.
   simple m.
   total m.
master
   m. gland
   M. of Surgery (MC)
mastication
mastocytosis
   cutaneous m.
   diffuse m.
   diffuse cutaneous m.
   systemic m.
mastodynia
mastoiditis
MAT
   multifocal atrial tachycardia
matching
material
   hyaline-like m.
materies morbi
maternal
   m. death
   m. fetal medicine
   m. hyperphenylalaninemia
maternity hospital
Mathieu disease
matricectomy

M

NOTES

matrix
matter
    gray m.
    white m.
mattress
    air m.
    egg crate foam m.
    foam m.
    static air m.
maturation index
maturity
maturity-onset
    m.-o. diabetes
    m.-o. diabetes of the young
      (MODY)
matutinus
    vomitus m.
Mauriac syndrome
Mavik
Maxair inhaler
Maxaquin
maxillary sinusitis
maximal
    m. permissible dose
    m. urinary flow rate (MUFR)
maximum
    m. inspiratory pressure
    m. laryngeal height
    m. urinary concentration (MUC)
    m. voluntary ventilation (MVV)
Maxipime
Maxivate
Maxzide
May-Hegglin anomaly
mayidism
Mayo-Robson point
MC
    Master of Surgery
    Medical Corps
McArdle
    M. disease
    M. syndrome
McArdle-Schmid-Pearson disease
MCBR
    minimum concentration of bilirubin
McBurney
    M. point
    M. sign
McCune-Albright syndrome
mcg
    microgram
MCH
    mean corpuscular hemoglobin
MCHC
    mean corpuscular hemoglobin
      concentration
McMurray test

MCP
    metacarpophalangeal
      MCP joint
MCS
    Mental Component Summary
MCT
    motor coordination test
MCTD
    mixed connective tissue disease
MCV
    mean corpuscular volume
MD
    muscular dystrophy
MD
    Doctor of Medicine
MDF
    myocardial depressant factor
MDI
    metered-dose inhaler
MDS
    myelodysplastic syndrome
M/E
    myeloid/erythroid
      M/E ratio
MEA
    multiple endocrine adenomatosis
meal
    after a m. [L. *post cibum*] (p.c.)
      post cibum
    before m.'s [L. *ante cibum*] (a.c.)
    Boyden m.
    M.'s on Wheels Association of
      America (MOWAA)
    m. planning
    test m.
meal-related
    m.-r. buffering
    m.-r. treatment
mean
    m. arterial pressure (MAP)
    behavioral m.'s
    m. corpuscular hemoglobin (MCH)
    m. corpuscular hemoglobin
      concentration (MCHC)
    m. corpuscular volume (MCV)
Means sign
measles
    atypical m.
    black m.
    German m.
    hemorrhagic m.
    m., mumps, rubella (MMR)
    m. and rubella (MR)
    m. and rubella vaccine
    three-day m.
    tropical m.
measure
    ancillary m.'s
    comfort m.'s

functional independence m. (FIM)
life-prolonging m.'s
prolonging m.'s
measurement
anthropometric m.
bone mass m.
m. of exposure
F-wave m.
H-reflex m.
meatus
fish-mouth m.
Mebaral
mebendazole
mechanica
acne m.
mechanical
m. esophageal obstruction
m. heart valve
m. ileus
m. pressure
m. ventilation
mechanism
biomolecular m.
mechanoreceptor
large joint m.
ventricular m.
mechanotherapy
mechlorcthamine
Meckel diverticulum
meclizine
Meclomen
MEDCO Sonicator
media (*pl. of* medium)
medial
m. collateral ligament
m. component
medialis
median survival time
mediastinal
m. disease
m. lymph node hyperplasia
m. mass
m. pleurisy
mediastinitis
chronic m.
mediastinoabdominal
mediastinoscopy
cervical m.
mediastinotomy
mediastinum

mediate
m. auscultation
m. percussion
mediated
vagally m.
mediator
inflammatory m.
polypeptide m.
medicable
Medicaid
medical
m. anatomy
m. care
m. castration
m. condition
M. Corps (MC)
m. decision-maker
m. diathermy
m. emergency
m. ethics
m. evaluation
m. examiner
m. informatics
m. intensive care unit (MICU)
m. jurisprudence
M. Literature Analysis and
Retrieval System (MEDLARS)
M. Officer (MO)
M. Outcomes Study (MOS)
M. Outcomes Study SF-36
m. record
m. record linkage
m. technology
m. thyroidectomy
m. transcriptionist
m. treatment
MedicAlert Foundation
medically restricted diet
medicament
medicamentosa
stomatitis m.
struma m.
thyrotoxicosis m.
medicamentosus
Cushing syndrome m.
Medicare
National Committee to Preserve
Social Security and M.
(NCPSSM)
M. part A
M. part B
M. Rights Center (MRC)

M

NOTES

medicate
medicated
> m. urethral system
> m. urethral system for erection (MUSE)
> m. urethral system for erection therapy

medication
> antidepressant m.
> antihypertensive m.
> m. compliance
> hypnotic m.
> ionic m.
> lipid-lowering m.
> m. management
> OTC m.
> outpatient m.
> over-the-counter m.
> prophylactic m.
> m. rebound syndrome
> sequestration of m.

medicator
medicinal
medicine
> adolescent m.
> aerospace m.
> alternative m.
> American Board of Internal M. (ABIM)
> American College of Physicians-American Society of Internal M. (ACP-ASIM)
> American College of Sports M. (ACSM)
> American Society of Internal M. (ASIM)
> aviation m.
> behavioral m.
> clinical m.
> comparative m.
> complementary m.
> defensive m.
> Doctor of M. (MD)
> evidence-based m.
> experimental m.
> family m.
> folk m.
> forensic m.
> geriatric m.
> holistic m.
> hyperbaric m.
> intensive care m.
> internal m. (IM)
> legal m.
> maternal fetal m.
> military m.
> National Library of M. (NLM)
> osteopathic m.
> preventive m.

> proprietary m.
> psychosomatic m.
> reproductive m.
> social m.
> socialized m.
> space m.
> sports m.
> theory of m.
> transplant m.
> tropical m.
> vascular m.
> women's m.

medicobiologic
medicochirurgical
medicolegal
medicomechanical
medicophysical
medicus
> Cumulative Index M.

MediSense
> M. Pen 2 blood glucose meter
> M. Precision meter
> M. Precision Q-I-D blood glucose monitoring system
> M. Precision Sure Dose insulin syringe
> M. Sof-Tact monitor

Mediterranean
> M. anemia
> M. erythematous fever
> M. exanthematous fever
> M. spotted fever

medium, pl. **media**
> acute otitis media
> barotitis media
> chronic otitis media
> external otitis media (EOM)
> m. inspiratory
> mass media
> otitis media
> pneumococcal acute otitis media
> radiocontrast media

MEDLARS
> Medical Literature Analysis and Retrieval System

MEDLARS-on-line (MEDLINE)
MEDLINE
> MEDLARS-on-line

Medrol Dosepak
medroxyprogesterone
> depot m. (DMPA)

Medtronic Pulsor Intrasound pain reliever
medulla, pl. **medullae**
> adrenal m.

medullary
> m. cystic disease
> m. sinus

m. thyroid cancer
m. thyroid carcinoma
medullated
medullation
medusae
caput m.
Medusa head
mefloquine
Mefoxin
Megace
megacolon
acquired m.
megakaryocyte
megakaryocytic leukemia
megaloblastic anemia
megaloblastoid
megalocytic anemia
megalopodia
megalosplenica
erythrocytosis m.
megarectum
meglitinide
meibomian gland
meibomianitis
meibomitis
Meige disease
Meigs syndrome
meiosis
mekongi
Schistosoma m.
melagra
melalgia
melancholia
involutional m.
melancholic
melancholic-endogenous
melanin
melanocyte-stimulating hormone (MSH)
melanoma
acral lentiginous m.
lentigo maligna m.
malignant m.
metastatic m.
nodular m.
superficial spreading m.
melanophore-expanding principle
melanorrhagia
melanorrhea
melanosis coli
melanotic
melanotransferrin
melanotropin

melas
icterus m.
melasma
m. addisonii
m. suprarenale
melatonin
Meleda disease
melena
m. neonatorum
m. spuria
m. vera
melenemesis
Meleney
M. chronic undermining ulcer
M. gangrene
melenic
melioidosis
melitensis
Brucella m.
febris m.
Mellaril
mellitus
adult-onset diabetes m.
diabetes m. (DM)
insulin-dependent diabetes m.
(IDDM)
juvenile-onset diabetes m. (JODM)
non–insulin-dependent diabetes m.
(NIDDM)
secondary diabetes m.
type 1, 2 diabetes m.
melon
bitter m.
meloplasty
melorheostosis
Meltzer-Lyon test
memantine
member
M. of the Royal College of
Physicians (Edinburgh) (MRCP(E))
M. of the Royal College of
Physicians (Ireland) (MRCP(I))
M. of the Royal College of
Physicians (of England) (MRCP)
membrane
m. attack complex (MAC)
bilayered m.
Bowman m.
canalicular m.
Descemet m.
epiretinal m.
hepatocyte plasma m.

M

NOTES

247

membrane *(continued)*
    leaky cell m.
    mucous m.
    m. permeability
    schneiderian m.
    synovial m.
    m. transport defect
    tympanic m. (TM)
    tympanitic m.
membranoproliferative glomerulonephritis type II
membranous
    m. glomerulopathy
    m. lipodystrophy
    m. stomatitis
memorial
memory
    echoic m.
    episodic m.
    m. function
    iconic m.
    m. impairment
    implicit m.
    long-term m.
    prospective m.
    recent m.
    retrospective m.
    rote m.
    semantic m.
    short-term m. (STM)
    wrote m.
MEN
    multiple endocrine neoplasia
    multiple endocrine neoplasm
menarche
mendelian disorder
Mendelson syndrome
Menest
Menetrier disease
Ménière
    M. disease
    M. syndrome
menieriformis
    polyneuritis cerebralis m.
meningeal headache
meninges *(pl. of* meninx)
meningioma
    clival m.
meningismus
meningitidis
    Neisseria m.
meningitis, pl. **meningitides**
    acute aseptic m.
    acute bacterial m.
    aseptic m.
    bacillary m.
    bacterial m.
    carcinomatous m.
    cryptococcal m.

    gram-negative bacillary m.
    Haemophilus influenzae m.
    herpes simplex m.
    Mollaret m.
    tuberculous m.
    viral m.
meningococcal
    m. carrier state
    m. conjugate vaccine
    m. disease
    m. polysaccharide vaccine
    m. septicemia
meningococcemia
    acute fulminating m.
meningoencephalitis
    arboviral m.
    herpes m.
meningomyelocele
meningotyphoid fever
meningovascular syphilis
meninx, pl. **meninges**
meniscal
    m. tear
    m. tearing
meniscectomy
menisci (*pl. of* meniscus)
meniscocytic anemia
meniscocytosis
meniscus, pl. **menisci**
Menkes
    M. disease
    M. syndrome
menometrorrhagia
menopausal urinary gonadotropin
menopause
    secondary m.
    surgical m.
menorrhagia
Menrium
menses
menstrual
    m. migraine
    m. pain
menstruation
    vicarious m.
mentagrophytes
    Trichophyton m.
mental
    m. age (MA)
    M. Component Summary (MCS)
    m. coprolalia
    m. degradation
    m. handicap
    m. health specialist
    m. hospital
    m. status
    m. status change
    m. status examination

mentation
    impaired m.
menthol
mentis
    compos m.
Mepergan Fortis
meperidine hydrochloride
Mephyton
mepivacaine
meprobamate
mEq
    milliequivalent
mer
    mal de m.
meralgia paresthetica
mercaptopurine (MP)
6-mercaptopurine (6-MP)
mercurial
    m. necrosis
    m. stomatitis
mercurialism
Mercurochrome
mercury (Hg)
    millimeters of m. (mmHg)
    m. poisoning
    m. sphygmomanometer
merocrine gland
meromicrosomia
meropenem
merosmia
Merrem
Merseburg triad
merthiolate
mesalamine
mesangial proliferation
mesangiocapillary
mesangiopathic glomerulonephritis
mesangioproliferative
mesenchymal cell
mesenteric
    m. adenitis
    m. artery aneurysm
    m. artery syndrome
    m. blood flow
    m. insufficiency
    m. ischemia
    m. microcirculation
    m. vascular occlusive disease
    m. venous thrombosis
mesenterica
    tabes m.
mesenteritis

mesentery
mesh
    Marlex m.
mesna
mesocardia
mesolimbic dopamine system
mesomelic
mesothelial cell
mesothelioma
    malignant m.
mesothelium
messenger
    first m.
Mestinon
mesylate
    bromocriptine m.
    delavirdine m.
    dihydroergotamine m.
    ergoloid m.
    imatinib m.
    nelfinavir m.
metabasis
metabolic
    m. acidosis
    m. alkalosis
    m. antagonist
    m. bone disease
    m. calculus
    m. condition
    m. craniopathy
    m. dementia
    m. disorder
    m. encephalopathy
    m. liver disease
    m. organ transplant complication
    m. rate
    m. syndrome
metabolism
    basal m.
    m. disorder
    drug m.
    hepatic m.
    hormone m.
    inborn error of m.
    renal sodium m.
metabolization
metabolized
metacarpal
metacarpophalangeal (MCP)
    m. joint
metachromatic leukodystrophy
metachronous

M

NOTES

metadysentery
metahypophysial diabetes
metaicteric
metainfective
metal fume fever
metallic
    m. compound inhalation
    m. rale
metalloproteinase
metaluetic
metamorphosis
    fatty m.
Metamucil
metamyelocyte
metanephrine
metaphysics
metaphysis, pl. metaphyses
metaplasia
    myeloid m.
    pseudopyloric m.
    squamous m.
metaplastic anemia
Metaprel inhaler
metaproterenol
metapyretic
metastasis, pl. metastases
    bone marrow m.
    brain m.
    hematogenous m.
    liver m.
    lymphogenous m.
    osseous m.
    tumor, necrosis, m. (TNM)
metastasize
metastasizing septicemia
metastatic
    m. arthritis
    m. brain tumor
    m. breast cancer
    m. carcinoid syndrome
    m. cardiac tumor
    m. colon cancer
    m. epidural spinal cord
      compression
    m. lung cancer
    m. melanoma
    m. mumps
    m. myonecrosis
    m. pneumonia
    m. prostate cancer
    m. tumor of unknown origin
metasyphilis
metasyphilitic
metatabus primus varus
metatarsalgia
metatarsal stress fracture
metatarsophalangeal (MTP)
    m. joint
metathesis

metenkephalin
meteorism
meteoropathy
meteorotropic
meter (m)
    blood glucose m.
    Exaclesh blood glucose m.
    MediSense Pen 2 blood
      glucose m.
    MediSense Precision m.
    One Touch Ultra m.
    m.'s squared (m^2)
metered-dose inhaler (MDI)
metformin
methacholine
methadone
methamphetamine addiction
methanol toxicity
methemalbuminemia
methemoglobinemia
    acquired m.
    congenital m.
    hereditary m.
    primary m.
    toxic m.
methemoglobinuria
methicillin-resistant *Staphylococcus*
  aureus (MRSA)
methimazole (MMI)
methocarbamol
method
    Brehmer m.
    Confusion Assessment M. (CAM)
    first-pass m.
    gated blood pool m.
    Ochsner m.
    paracelsian m.
    Rehfuss m.
    Schweninger m.
    single-photon emission computed
      tomography m.
    Thezac-Porsmeur m.
    Westergren m.
methodology
methotrexate, vinblastine, Adriamycin,
  cisplatin (M-VAC)
methylation
    MLH1 promoter m.
methylcellulose
methyldopa
methylene blue
methylmalonic
    m. acid
    m. acidemia
    m. aciduria
methylphenidate
methyl-phenyl-tetrahydropyridine (MPTP)
    m.-p.-t. parkinsonism
    m.-p.-t. poisoning

methylprednisolone
4-methylpyrazole
methylsalicylate
methyl tert-butyl ether
methyltransferase
    catechol m. (COMT)
methylxanthine
methysergide
Metimyd
metoclopramide
metoprolol succinate
MET 1 program
metrifonate
MetroGel Topical
metronidazole
metrorrhagia
metyrapone test
Meulengracht diet
Mevacor
Mexican
    M. spotted fever
    M. typhus
mexiletine
Mexitil
Meyer-Betz
    M.-B. disease
    M.-B. syndrome
Meynert
    nucleus basalis of M.
mezlocillin
MF heel cup
mg
    milligram
mg/dL
    milligram per deciliter
MI
    myocardial infarction
Miacalcin nasal spray
mianserin
mibefradil
Mibelli
    M. disease
    M. syndrome
Micardis HCT
Micatin
micatosis
micelle
    bilayered m.
Micheli
    microelliptopoikilocytic anemia of
      Rietti, Greppi, and M.
Michigan alcohol screening test

miconazole
Micral urine test strip
microabscess
microadenoma
    nonsecretory m.
microadenopathy
microalbuminuria
microaneurysm
microangiopathic hemolytic anemia
microangiopathy
    thrombohemolytic m.
microaspiration
Microbacterium
microbial antigenic phase shift
microbiology
microcalcification
microcardia
microcephaly
microcirculation
    mesenteric m.
microcolitis
microcolony
microcrystalline disease
microcytic
    m. anemia
    m. red cell
microcytosis
microdialysis
microdilution
    broth m.
microdose
microdrepanocytic anemia
microdroplet
    aerosolized m.
microelliptopoikilocytic
    m. anemia
    m. anemia of Rietti, Greppi, and
      Micheli
microflora
microglia
micrognathia
microgram (mcg)
micrographia
microhematuria
Micro-K
micrometastasis
micromyelia
micromyeloblastic leukemia
Micronase
micronodular cirrhosis
Micronor

M

NOTES

micronutrient
    m. supplementation
microobstructive uropathy
microorganism
microsatellite
    m. instability
    m. instability screening
microscope
    scanning electron m. (SEM)
microscopic
    m. benign prostatic hyperplasia
    m. BPH
    m. colitis
    m. polyangiitis
    m. polyarteritis nodosa
microscopy
    electron m.
    immunofluorescent m.
    light m.
MicroSpacer unit
microsplenia
microsplenic
microsporidia infection
microsporidiosis
microstethoscope, microstethophone
microsyringe
microtubule
microunits per milliliter
microvascular
    m. disease
    m. thrombosis
microvasculature
microvesicular
microwave
    m. diathermy treatment
    m. therapy
micturate
micturition
    m. syncope
    m. urinary incontinence
MICU
    medical intensive care unit
MID
    multiinfarct dementia
Midamor
MIDAS
    Migraine Disability Assessment Scale
midbulb
middiastolic
    apical m.
    basal m.
    m. murmur
middle lobe syndrome
midline granuloma
mid lumbar region
Midrin
midsystolic murmur
Mifeprex
mifepristone

mifepristone/misoprostol
miglitol
migraine
    abdominal m.
    acute confusional m.
    basilar artery m.
    Bickerstaff m.
    classic m.
    common m.
    complicated m.
    confusional m.
    M. Disability Assessment Scale
      (MIDAS)
    epileptic m.
    familial hemiplegic m.
    fulgurating m.
    m. headache
    hemiplegic m.
    hormonal m.
    late-life m.
    menstrual m.
    neurologic m.
    ocular m.
    ophthalmic m.
    ophthalmoplegic m.
    retinal m.
    vertebrobasilar m.
    vestibular m.
    m. with aura
    m. without aura
migrans
    erythema chronicum m.
    visceral larva m.
migration
migratory
    m. glossitis
    m. necrolytic erythema
    m. pneumonia
Mikulicz disease
Mikulicz-Radecki syndrome
Mikulicz-Sjögren syndrome
mild
    m. chronic hepatitis
    m. intermittent asthma
milestone
milia
miliaria rubra
miliaris
    variola m.
miliary
    m. fever
    m. pulmonary aspergillosis
    m. tuberculosis
milieu
military medicine
milium
milk
    acidophilus m.
    m. anemia

m. of bismuth
m. fever
fortified m.
m. intolerance
m. let-down reflex
m. of magnesia (MOM)
m. protein allergy
m. sickness
m. thistle
milk-alkali syndrome
milkpox
mill
m. fever
M. Glucometer II glucometer
Miller-Fisher test
milleri
Streptococcus m.
Miller index
miller's asthma
milliequivalent (mEq)
milligram (mg)
m. per deciliter (mg/dL)
milliliter (mL)
microunits per m.
nanograms per m. (ng/mL)
m.'s per minute (mL/min)
m.'s per second (mL/sec)
millimeter (mm)
m.'s of mercury (mmHg)
millimole (mmol)
m.'s per liter (mmol/L)
million international units (MIU)
Milroy
M. disease
M. edema
Milton
M. disease
M. edema
Milwaukee shoulder
mimesis
mimetic
mimic
mimicry
molecular m.
min
minute
mineral
m. deficiency
m. supplementation
mineralocoid
mineralocorticoid replacement

miner's
m. anemia
m. asthma
m. disease
m. lung
miniature scarlet fever
minilaparotomy
minimal-change nephrotic syndrome
minimal dose
Mini-Mental
M.-M. State Examination (MMSE)
M.-M. State Examination of
Folstein
minimum
m. concentration of bilirubin
(MCBR)
m. laryngeal height
Minipress
Minitran patch
Minkowski-Chauffard syndrome
Minocin
minocycline hydrochloride
minor
beta thalassemia m.
pestis m.
thalassemia m.
variola m.
minora
labia m.
Minot-Murphy diet
minoxidil
topical penile m.
Mintezol
minute (min)
milliliters per m. (mL/min)
m. ventilation
7-minute
7-minute neurocognitive battery
7-minute screen
miosis
miotic
mirabilis
Proteus m.
MiraLax
Mirapex
Mirchamp sign
Mirena
mirtazapine
misconduct
sexual m.
misdiagnosis

M

NOTES

mismatch
    ventilation/perfusion m.
misoprostol
misplaced gout
mist
    Bronkaid m.
    Primatene M.
mite
    house dust m.
    m. typhus
mite-born typhus
mithramycin
mitigate
mitior
    typhus m.
mitis
mitochondria
mitochondrial
    m. ataxia
    m. cardiomyopathy
    m. disorder
mitomycin C
mitotic spindle inhibitor
Mito-Velban
mitoxantrone
mitral
    m. annular calcification
    m. annuloplasty
    m. commissurotomy
    m. leaflet syndrome
    m. regurgitant murmur
    m. stenosis
    m. stenosis in pregnancy
    m. valve
    m. valve disease
    m. valve insufficiency
    m. valve prolapse (MVP)
    m. valve regurgitation
    m. valve surgery
    m. valvulotomy
Mitran
mittelschmerz
MIU
    million international units
mixed
    m. acid-base disorder
    m. aortic valve disease
    m. connective tissue disease
      (MCTD)
    m. hyperlipemia
    m. hyperlipoproteinemia familial
      type 5 hyperlipidemia
    m. hypoglycemia
    m. mitral disease
    m. respiratory failure
    m. type of incontinence
    m. uremic osteodystrophy
    m. venous hypoxia
    m. venous oxygen

mixed-tissue tumor
Miyoshi myopathy
mL
    milliliter
MLH1 promoter methylation
mL/min
    milliliters per minute
MLNS
    mucocutaneous lymph node syndrome
mL/sec
    milliliters per second
MM
    multiple myeloma
mm
    millimeter
mmHg
    millimeters of mercury
MMI
    methimazole
mmol
    millimole
mmol/L
    millimoles per liter
MMR
    measles, mumps, rubella
MMSE
    Mini-Mental State Examination
    Folstein MMSE
MO
    Medical Officer
Moban
mobility
    m. aid
    leg m.
    prefracture m.
Mobitz
    M. type I, II block
Möbius
    M. disease
    M. sign
    M. syndrome
moccasin
modality
    atypical sensory m.
Modane
model
    role m.
moderate
    m. category
    m. chronic hepatitis
    m. hypothermia
    m. persistent asthma
moderately disabled
Modicon
modicum
modification
    International Classification of
    Diseases, Ninth Revision,
    Clinical M. (ICD-9-CM)

National Resource Center on
Supportive Housing &
Home M.'s
structural m.
modified
m. acid
m. Blalock-Taussig
M. Mini-Mental State Examination
(3MSE)
m. radical mastectomy
m. smallpox
modifier
leukotriene m.
modulation
modulator
selective estrogen receptor m.
(SERM)
Moduretic
MODY
maturity-onset diabetes of the young
Moeller glossitis
moexipril
mofetil
mycophenolate m.
Mohs
M. micrographic surgery
M. scale
moist rale
molar pregnancy
mold
nondermatophytic m.
mole
hydatidiform m.
molecular
m. disease
m. marker
m. mimicry
molecule
extracellular matrix m.
molimen, pl. molimina
molimina of puffiness
molindone
Moll
apocrine gland of M.
Mollaret meningitis
molle
heloma m.
mollicute
molluscicidal
molluscum
m. contagiosum
m. contagiosum virus

molybdenum
MOM
milk of magnesia
Momentum Muscular Backache Formula
monarticular
Mönckeberg arrhythmia
Mondor
M. disease
M. syndrome
Monge
M. disease
M. syndrome
monilethrix
Monilia
moniliasis
chronic m.
moniliform hair
Monistat Dual-Pak
monitor
ambulatory blood pressure m.
(ABPM)
ambulatory Holter m. (AHM)
blood glucose m.
blood pressure m.
BpTRU blood pressure m.
CardioBeeper CB-12L cardiac m.
Co2smo Plus! respiratory m.
Glucometer DEX blood glucose m.
glucose m.
Holter m.
hOx m.
MediSense Sof-Tact m.
Precision m.
respiratory m.
Rigiscan m.
Sof-Tact glucose m.
monitoring
AECG m.
ambulatory electrocardiography m.
ambulatory Holter m. (AHM)
fluoroscopic m.
home glucose m.
pH m.
therapeutic drug m.
monkeypox
human m.
mono
mononucleosis
monoamine
m. oxidase (MAO)
m. oxidase B inhibitor
m. oxidase inhibitor (MAOI)

M

NOTES

255

monoarticular arthritis
monoblastic leukemia
Monocid
monoclonal (M)
    m. anti-IgE antibody
    m. gammopathy
    m. spike
monocyte
monocytic
    m. angina
    m. leukemia
monocytogenes
    Listeria m.
monofilament
    Semmes-Weinstein m.
monograph
monoleptic fever
monomer
monomicrobial
monomorphic ventricular tachycardia
mononeuritis
mononeuropathy
    diabetic m.
mononitrate
    isosorbide m.
mononuclear
    m. cell pleocytosis
    m. phagocyte
mononucleosis (mono)
    infectious m. (IM)
monoparesis
monopathic
monopathy
monophagism
monoplegia
monopolar
Monopril
monorchia
monorchidic
monorchidism
monorchism
monosomy x
Monospot test
monosymptomatic
monotherapy
    beta-lactam m.
    perindopril m.
monothermia
monounsaturated fatty acid
monoxide
    diffusing capacity of carbon m.
    diffusing capacity of lung for
      carbon m. (DLCO)
monozygotic twin
mons pubis
Monteggia fracture
montelukast
Montenegro test

mood
    m. disorder
    m. stabilizer
moon
    m. face
    m. facies
moon-shaped face
Moore syndrome
Morax-Axenfeld bacillus
Moraxella phenylpyruvica
morbi
    materies m.
morbid
    m. obesity
    m. thirst
morbidity
    cardiovascular m.
    premature m.
    puerperal m.
    m. rate
morbific
morbigenous
morbility
morbilli
morbilliform
Morbillivirus
morbilous
morbus
    cholera m.
Morel
    M. disease
    M. syndrome
Morel-Wildi syndrome
Morgagni syndrome
Morgan bacillus
Morganella morganii
morganii
    Morganella m.
morgue
moribund
moricizine
Morley peritoneocutaneous reflex
morning
    m. diarrhea
    every m. [L. *quaque mane*]
      (q.a.m., q.m.)
Moro reflex
morpheaform basal cell
morphine
    m. injector's septicemia
    m. sulfate
    m. sulfate immediate release
      (MSIR)
    sustained-release m.
morphogenetic
morphologically
morphology
    P-QRS m.
    QRS m.

Morquio
  M. disease
  M. sign
  M. syndrome
Morquio-Brailsford syndrome
Morquio-Ullrich
  M.-U. disease
  M.-U. syndrome
Morris syndrome
mors thymica
mortal
mortality
  all-cause m.
  CAD m.
  cardiovascular m.
  coronary artery disease m.
  m. rate
  m. rate doubling time
mortise
  ankle m.
  m. joint
Morton neuroma
mortuary
Morvan chorea
MOS
  Medical Outcomes Study
  MOS SF-36
mosaic
  Turner m.
mosaicism
  XO/XY m.
Moschcowitz
  M. disease
  M. sign
  M. test
Mosler
  M. diabetes
  M. sign
Mosse syndrome
Mossman fever
mother yaw
motilide
motilin
motility disorder
motion
  range of m. (ROM)
  m. sickness
  systemic anterior m. (SAM)
motivation
motor
  m. aphasia transcortical
  m. coordination

  m. coordination test (MCT)
  corticospinal m.
  m. neuron
  m. neuron disease
  m. pattern
  m. radiculopathy
  m. response
  m. strength 5+/5+
  m. tic
  m. unit
  m. vehicle accident (MVA)
Motrin
mottling
moulin
  bruit de la roue de m.
mount
mountain
  m. anemia
  m. disease
  m. sickness
mouth
  dry m.
  by m. [L. *per os*] (p.o.)
movement
  bowel m. (BM)
  constraint-induced m.
  m. disorder
  eye m.
  fine hand m.
  periodic limb m. (PLM)
  rapid eye m. (REM)
  repetitive leg-jerking m.
  m. therapy
moving toes, painful leg syndrome
MOWAA
  Meals on Wheels Association of America
moxa
moxalactam
moxibustion
moxifloxacin
MP
  mercaptopurine
6-MP
  6-mercaptopurine
MPD
  myofascial pain-dysfunction
MPTP
  methyl-phenyl-tetrahydropyridine
  N-methyl-4-phenyl-1,2,3,6-
    tetrahydropyridine
  MPTP parkinsonism
  MPTP poisoning

M

NOTES

MPTP-induced parkinsonism
MR
    measles and rubella
      MR vaccine
MRA
    magnetic resonance angiography
MRC
    Medicare Rights Center
MRCP
    Member of the Royal College of
      Physicians (of England)
MRCP(E)
    Member of the Royal College of
      Physicians (Edinburgh)
MRCP(I)
    Member of the Royal College of
      Physicians (Ireland)
MRI
    magnetic resonance imaging
      cervical MRI
MRSA
    methicillin-resistant *Staphylococcus*
    aureus
MRV
    magnetic resonance venography
MS
    multiple sclerosis
      MS Contin
MS-1 hepatitis
MSA
    multiple system atrophy
MSAS
    Mandel Social Adjustment Scale
3MSE
    Modified Mini-Mental State Examination
MSEL
    myasthenic syndrome of Eaton-Lambert
MSH
    melanocyte-stimulating hormone
MSIR
    morphine sulfate immediate release
MSK
    musculoskeletal
MTB
    Mycobacterium tuberculosis
MTP
    metatarsophalangeal
      MTP joint
MUC
    maximum urinary concentration
mucinosis
mucinous
    m. ascites
    m. tumor
Muckle-Wells syndrome
mucocele
mucocolitis
mucocutaneous
    m. candidiasis

    m. lymph node syndrome (MLNS)
    m. ocular syndrome
mucoenteritis
mucoepidermoid
mucoid impaction of bronchus
mucolipid
mucolipidosis, pl. **mucolipidoses**
    m. I–IV
mucolytic
mucomembranous enteritis
mucoperichondrial flap
mucoperiosteal
mucopolysaccharidosis
    type IH m.
    type IS m.
    type II m.
    type III m.
    type IVA m.
    type IVB m.
    type V m.
    type VI m.
    type VII m.
mucopolysacchariduria
mucopurulent cervicitis
Mucor
mucormycosis
    rhinocerebral m.
    m. sinusitis
mucosa
    atrophic gastric m.
    buccal m.
    gastric m.
mucosa-associated lymphoid tissue
  lymphoma
mucosae
    lipoidosis cutis et m.
mucosal
    m. erythema
    m. leishmaniasis
mucositis necroticans agranulocytica
mucous
    m. colitis
    m. diarrhea
    m. membrane
    m. rale
mucoviscidosis
mucus impaction
mucus-secreting cell
mud bed
Muenster cast
MUFR
    maximal urinary flow rate
MUGA
    multigated angiogram
    multiple gaited acquisition
      exercise MUGA
mulberry spot
Mulder click

müllerian
    m. duct
    m. mixed tumor
    m. regression factor
Müller sign
multiagent chemotherapy
multibacillary
Multiceps **infection**
multichannel
    m. cystometrogram
    m. cystometry
multicystic dysplastic kidney
multidisciplinary pain management center
multidrug resistant
multidrug-resistant tuberculosis
multifactorial
    m. disease
    m. disorder
MULTIFIT trial
multifocal atrial tachycardia (MAT)
multiforme
    erythema m.
    glioblastoma m.
multigated angiogram (MUGA)
multiinfarct
    m. dementia (MID)
    m. dementia with delirium
    m. disease
multinodular
    m. gland
    m. goiter
multiparous
multiphasic
multiple
    m. chemical sensitivity
    m. cholesterol emboli syndrome
    m. endocrine adenomatosis (MEA)
    m. endocrine deficiency syndrome
    m. endocrine neoplasia (MEN)
    m. endocrine neoplasia type I, II
    m. endocrine neoplasm (MEN)
    m. gaited acquisition (MUGA)
    m. glandular deficiency syndrome
    m. gumma
    m. lentigines syndrome
    m. myeloma (MM)
    m. organ dysfunction syndrome
    m. sclerosis (MS)
    m. sensory defect dizziness
    m. sensory deficit
    m. system atrophy (MSA)

multiplex
    dysostosis m.
multiresistant
    m. bacteria
multisystem
    m. atrophy
    m. disease
multivariate
multivessel disease
multivitamin infusion (MVI)
multocida
    Pasteurella m.
mumps
    metastatic m.
    m. orchitis
    m. vaccine
mumu fever
Münchausen by proxy syndrome
municipal hospital
Munro point
Mupirocin
mural thrombus
mu receptor
murine typhus
murmur
    aortic systolic ejection m.
    apical m.
    Austin-Flint m.
    blowing diastolic m.
    blowing systolic ejection m.
    crescendo-decrescendo m.
    diastolic m.
    false-negative m.
    false-positive m.
    friction m.
    heart m.
    holosystolic m.
    innocent heart m.
    middiastolic m.
    midsystolic m.
    mitral regurgitant m.
    physiologic m.
    protodiastolic m.
    regurgitation m.
    respiratory m.
    Steell m.
    systolic ejection m. (SEM)
    systolic heart m.
    vesicular m.
Murphy
    M. percussion
    M. sign

M

NOTES

Murray Valley rash
muscarine
muscarinic agonist
muscarinism
muscle
    m. asthenia
    bulbocavernosus m.
    m. contraction headache
    m. cramp
    cricopharyngeus m.
    m. disease
    extraocular m.
    intrinsic m.
    ischiocavernosus m.
    paraspinous m.
    m. phosphorylase deficiency
    m. relaxant
    smooth m.
    soleus m.
    m. sound
    sternocleidomastoid m.
    m. tonicity
    m. wasting
    m. weakness
muscle-strengthening exercise
muscular
    m. dystrophy (MD)
    m. pain-fasciculation syndrome
    pseudohypertrophic m.
    m. rheumatism
muscularis
musculoligamentous
musculoskeletal (MSK)
    m. adaptation
    m. infection
    m. pain
MUSE
    medicated urethral system for erection
    MUSE therapy
mushroom
    maitake m.
    m. poisoning
mushroom-worker's lung
musical bruit
mussitans
    delirium m.
mustard
    M. atrial baffle repair
    nitrogen m.
Mustargen
mutagen
mutagenic
mutant
mutation
mutilans
    arthritis m.
mutism
    akinetic m.
mutual resistance

MVA
    motor vehicle accident
M-VAC
    methotrexate, vinblastine, Adriamycin,
    cisplatin
MVI
    multivitamin infusion
MVP
    mitral valve prolapse
MVV
    maximum voluntary ventilation
Myadec
Myà disease
myalgia
    epidemic m.
    m. thermica
Myambutol
myasthenia
    m. gravis
    m. gravis pseudoparalytica
myasthenic
    m. crisis
    m. syndrome
    m. syndrome of Eaton-Lambert
    (MSEL)
myatonia congenita
Mycelex troche
mycetes
mycetism
    m. choliformis
    m. gastrointestinalis
    m. nervosa
    m. sanguinareus
mycetoma
Mycitracin
mycobacteria
    nontuberculous m.
mycobacterial infection
mycobacteriosis
Mycobacterium
    M. abscessus infection
    M. avium
    M. avium complex (MAC)
    M. avium complex infection
    M. chelonei infection
    M. fortuitum infection
    M. haemophilum infection
    M. kansasii
    M. kansasii infection
    M. marinum
    M. marinum infection
    M. tuberculosis (MTB)
    M. xenopi infection
Mycocide NS
mycogastritis
Mycolog
Mycolog-II
mycology
mycophenolate mofetil

Mycoplasma
  M. *fermentans*
  M. *genitalium*
  M. *hominis*
  M. **infection**
  M. *pneumoniae*
  M. *urealyticum*
mycoplasma, pl. **mycoplasmata**
  m. pneumonia
mycoplasmal pneumonia
mycosis, pl. **mycoses**
  m. framboesioides
  m. fungoides
  Gilchrist m.
  m. intestinalis
  splenic m.
  systemic m.
mycostasis
mycostat
Mycostatin elixir
mycotic stomatitis
mycotoxicosis
mydriasis
myelin
  abnormal tubular m. (ATM)
myelination, myelinization
myeloblastic leukemia
myelocytic leukemia
myelodysplasia
myelodysplastic syndrome (MDS)
myelofibrosis
myelofibrotic
myelogenous leukemia
myelogram
myeloid
  m. basic protein
  m. granulocytic leukemia
  m. metaplasia
myeloid/erythroid (M/E)
  myeloid/erythroid ratio
myelokathexis
myeloma
  amyloidosis of multiple m.
  Bence Jones m.
  indolent multiple m.
  multiple m. (MM)
  smoldering multiple m.
myelomatosis
myelomonocytic leukemia
myelopathic polycythemia

myelopathy
  diabetic m.
  transverse m.
myelophthisic
  m. anemia
  m. splenomegaly
myeloproliferative
  m. disease
  m. disorder
myeloradiculopathy
myelosarcoma
myelosarcomatosis
myelosclerosis
myelosclerotic anemia
myelosis
  aleukemic m.
  aplastic m.
  chronic nonleukemic m.
  erythremic m.
  funicular m.
  nonleukemic m.
myelosuppression
Myerson sign
myiasis
  human botfly m.
  intestinal m.
Mykrox
Myleran
Mylicon
myoadenylate deaminase deficiency
myocardial
  m. anoxia
  m. contractile function
  m. contraction
  creatine kinase m.
  m. damage
  m. depressant factor (MDF)
  m. disease
  m. hypertrophy
  m. infarction (MI)
  m. ischemia
  m. necrosis
  m. perfusion scan
  m. resection
  m. revascularization
myocarditis
  acute bacterial m.
  acute isolated m.
  bacterial m.
  chronic m.
  diphtheritic m.
  fibrous m.

M

NOTES

myocarditis *(continued)*
   idiopathic m.
   isolated m.
   rheumatic m.
   tuberculoid m.
   tuberculous m.
myocardium
   contractile state of m.
   inotropic state of m.
myocelialgia
myoclonic
myoclonus
   sleep m.
myocrismus
myocyte necrosis
myodemia
myofascial
   m. pain
   m. pain-dysfunction (MPD)
   m. pain syndrome
myofibrillar
myofibroblast
myofibromatosis
   infantile m.
Myoflex
myoglobinemia
myoglobinuria
myoglobinuric rhabdomyolytic acute renal failure
myoglobulinuria
myokymia
   hereditary m.
myolysis cardiotoxica
myoma
myomectomy
myometrial
myonecrosis
   anaerobic m.
   clostridial m.
   metastatic m.
   uterine m.
myopalmus
myopathic
myopathy
   centronuclear m.
   Cushing disease m.
   dysthyroid m.
   idiopathic inflammatory m.
   juvenile m.
   Miyoshi m.
myophone
myophosphorylase deficiency glycogenosis

myopia
myorelaxant property
myositis
   epidemic m.
   focal nodular m.
   inclusion body m. (IBM)
   localized m.
   nodular m.
   m. ossificans
   m. purulenta tropica
   tropical m.
myotomal
myotonic dystrophy
myriad
myringa
myringitis
myringomycosis
Mysoline
Mytrex cream
myurous
myxadenitis labialis
myxedema
   m. coma
   congenital m.
   infantile m.
   operative m.
   pituitary m.
   pretibial m.
myxedematoid
myxedematous
   m. arthropathy
   m. dementia
   m. facies
   m. goiter
   m. infantilism
   m. neuropathy
myxocystoma
myxoid cyst
myxoma
   atrial m.
   cardiac m.
   cystic m.
   m. fibrosum
   m. nabothian
   m. sarcomatosum
myxomatosis
   infectious m.
myxomatous degeneration
myxomembranous colitis
myxoneurosis
   intestinal m.
myxorrhea gastrica

N4A
    National Association of Area Agencies
    on Aging
NAAP
    National Association of Activity
    Professionals
nabothian
    n. cyst
    myxoma n.
nabumetone
NACHC
    National Association of Community
    Health Centers
NaCl
    sodium chloride
    sterile NaCl
NAD
    National Association of the Deaf
    no appreciable disease
nadir
nadolol
Naegeli
    N. leukemia
    N. syndrome
Naegleria **infection**
NAELA
    National Academy of Elder Law
    Attorneys, Inc.
nafarelin
NAFC
    National Association for Continence
nafcillin
NAHC
    National Association for Home Care
NAHD
    National Association for Human
    Development
NAHF
    National Association for Health &
    Fitness
NAHOE
    National Association on HIV Over Fifty
nail
    Hippocratic n.
    n. patella syndrome
    n. plate
    Schneider n.
    Terry n.
Naldecon Senior
Nalfon
naloxone
naltrexone hydrochloride
NAMI
    National Alliance for the Mentally Ill

NAMS
    North American Menopause Society
nana
    hymenolepiasis n.
NANASP
    National Association of Nutrition and
    Aging Service Programs
NANB
    non-A, non-B hepatitis
    NANB hepatitis
NANBNC
    non-A, non-B, non-C
    NANBNC hepatitis
nanism
nanogram (ng)
nanograms per milliliter (ng/mL)
nanukayami fever
NAPCA
    National Asian Pacific Center on Aging
NAPGCM
    National Association of Progressional
    Geriatric Care Managers
Naphcon-A
NAPNES
    National Association for Practical Nurse
    Education and Services
Naprelan
Naprosyn
naproxen
Naqua
naratriptan
Narcan
narcissistic personality
narcolepsy
narcosis
    intravenous n.
    nitrogen n.
    n. paralysis
    prolonged n.
narcotic analgesic
Nardil
NARIC
    National Rehabilitation Information
    Center
naris, pl. **nares**
narrow-angle glaucoma
narrow-complex tachycardia
narrowing
    joint space n.
NAS
    no added salt
    NAS diet
Nasacort AQ
nasal
    n. cavity

N

nasal *(continued)*
>   n. congestion
>   n. feeding
>   n. papillomatosis
>   n. pillow
>   n. regurgitation
>   n. secretion
>   n. septoplasty
>   n. turbinate

Nasalcrom
Nasalide
Nasarel inhaler
nasi
>   ala n.

nasogastric (NG)
>   n. lavage
>   n. tube

nasojejunal (NJ)
>   n. feeding
>   n. tube

nasopharyngeal
>   n. cancer

Nasostat hemostatic nasal balloon
NASUA
>   National Association of State Units on Aging

NASW
>   National Association of Social Workers

natal sore
nateglinide
natiform skull
national
>   N. Academy of Elder Law Attorneys Inc.
>   N. Alliance for Hispanic Health
>   N. Alliance for the Mentally Ill (NAMI)
>   N. Arthritis and Musculoskeletal and Skin Diseases Information Clearinghouse
>   N. Asian Pacific Center on Aging (NAPCA)
>   N. Association of Activity Professionals (NAAP)
>   N. Association of Area Agencies on Aging (N4A)
>   N. Association of Community Health Centers (NACHC)
>   N. Association for Continence (NAFC)
>   N. Association of the Deaf (NAD)
>   N. Association for Health & Fitness (NAHF)
>   N. Association for Hispanic Elderly
>   N. Association for Home Care (NAHC)
>   N. Association for Human Development (NAHD)

>   N. Association of Nutrition and Aging Service Programs (NANASP)
>   N. Association on HIV Over Fifty (NAHOE)
>   N. Association for Practical Nurse Education and Services (NAPNES)
>   N. Association of Progressional Geriatric Care Managers (NAPGCM)
>   N. Association of Social Workers (NASW)
>   N. Association of State Units on Aging (NASUA)
>   N. Bar Association (NBA)
>   N. Cancer Institute (NCI)
>   N. Caucus and Center on Black Aged, Inc. (NCBA)
>   N. Center for Complementary and Alternative Medicine Clearinghouse (NCCAM)
>   N. Center for Health Statistics (NCHS)
>   N. Center on Elder Abuse (NCEA)
>   N. Center on Minority Health and Health Disparities (NCMHD)
>   N. Center on Poverty Law, Inc. (NCPL)
>   N. Cholesterol Education Program (NCEP)
>   N. Citizen's Coalition for Nursing Home Reform (NCCNHR)
>   N. Coalition for Adult Immunization (NCAI)
>   N. Committee to Preserve Social Security and Medicare (NCPSSM)
>   N. Consumer's League (NCL)
>   N. Council Against Health Fraud (NCAHE)
>   N. Council of La Raza (NCLR)
>   N. Council on Aging, Inc. (NCOA)
>   N. Council on Alcoholism and Drug Dependence (NCADD)
>   N. Council on Patient Information and Education (NCPIE)
>   N. Diabetes Information Clearinghouse (NDIC)
>   N. Digestive Diseases Information Clearinghouse (NDDIC)
>   N. Eye Health Education Program (NEHEP)
>   N. Family Caregivers Association (NFCA)
>   N. Gerontological Nursing Association (NGNA)

N. Health Information Center (NHIC)

N. Health and Nutrition Examination Follow-Up Study

N. Health and Nutrition Examination Survey (NHANES)

N. Health Service (England) (NHS)

N. Heart, Lungs, and Blood Institute (NHLBI)

N. Heart, Lungs, and Blood Institute Information Center

N. Hispanic Council on Aging (NHCoA)

N. Hospice and Palliative Care Organization (NHPCO)

N. Hospital Foundation (NHF)

N. Human Genome Research Institute (NHGRI)

N. Indian Council on Aging (NICOA)

N. Information and Referral Support Center (NIRSC)

N. Institute of Allergy and Infectious Disease (NIAID)

N. Institute of Child Health and Human Development (NICHD)

N. Institute of Child Health and Human Development Information Clearinghouse

N. Institute of Dental and Craniofacial Research (NIDCR)

N. Institute of Environmental Health Sciences (NIEHS)

N. Institute of General Medical Sciences (NIGMS)

N. Institute of Mental Health (NIMH)

N. Institute of Neurological Disorders and Stroke (NINDS)

N. Institute of Nursing Research (NINR)

N. Institute on Aging (NIA)

N. Institute on Alcohol Abuse and Alcoholism (NIAAA)

N. Institute on Deafness and Other Communication Disorders (NIDCD)

N. Institute on Drug Abuse (NIDA)

N. Institutes of Health (NIH)

N. Institutes of Health Chronic Prostatitis Symptom Index (NIH-CPSI)

N. Institutes of Health Stroke Scale

N. Interfaith Coalition on Aging (NICA)

N. Kidney Foundation (NKF)

N. Kidney and Urological Diseases Information Clearinghouse (NKUDIC)

N. Legal Support for Elderly People with Mental Disabilities Project

N. Library of Medicine (NLM)

N. Library Service for the Blind and Physically Handicapped (NLSBPH)

N. Long-Term Care Ombudsman Research Center (NLTCORC)

N. Long-Term Care Research Center (NLTCRC)

N. Medical Association (NMA)

N. Mental Health Association (NMHA)

N. Multiple Sclerosis Society (NMSS)

N. Organization of Rare Disorders (NORD)

N. Organization of Victim Assistance (NOVA)

N. Osteoporosis Foundation (NOF)

N. Policy and Resource Center on Nutrition and Aging

N. Policy and Resource Center on Women and Aging (NPRCWA)

N. Prevention Information Network (NPIN)

N. Psoriasis Foundation (NPF)

N. Rehabilitation Information Center (NARIC)

N. Resource Center Diversity and Long-Term Care (NRCDLTC)

N. Resource Center on Native American Aging (NRCNAA)

N. Resource Center on Supportive Housing & Home Modifications

N. Resource and Information Center (NRIC)

N. Rural Health Association (NRHA)

N. Self-Help Clearinghouse (NSHC)

N

NOTES

national *(continued)*
    N. Senior Citizens' Education and Research Center (NSCERC)
    N. Senior Citizens' Law Center (NSCLC)
    N. Senior Games Association (NSGA)
    N. Sleep Foundation (NSF)
    N. STD and AIDS Hotlines
    N. Stroke Association (NSA)
    N. Urban League
    N. Women's Health Information Center (NWHIC)
    N. Women's Health Network (NWHN)
native
    N. Elder Health Care Resource Center (NEHCRC)
    n. valve endocarditis
natriuretic peptide
natural
    n. focus of infection
    n. killer cell
naturopath
naturopathic
naturopathy
Nauheim
    N. bath
    N. treatment
naupathia
nausea
    epidemic n.
    n. and vomiting (N&V)
    n., vomiting, diarrhea (NVD)
nauseant
nauseate
nauseating
nauseous
Navane
Navelbine
navicula
navicular
    carpal n.
    talar n.
NBA
    National Bar Association
NBTE
    nonbacterial thrombotic endocarditis
NCADD
    National Council on Alcoholism and Drug Dependence
NCAHE
    National Council Against Health Fraud
NCAI
    National Coalition for Adult Immunization
NCBA
    National Caucus and Center on Black Aged, Inc.

NCCAM
    National Center for Complementary and Alternative Medicine Clearinghouse
NCCNHR
    National Citizen's Coalition for Nursing Home Reform
NCEA
    National Center on Elder Abuse
NCEP
    National Cholesterol Education Program
NCHS
    National Center for Health Statistics
NCI
    National Cancer Institute
NCL
    National Consumer's League
NCLR
    National Council of La Raza
NCMHD
    National Center on Minority Health and Health Disparities
NCOA
    National Council on Aging, Inc.
NCPIE
    National Council on Patient Information and Education
NCPL
    National Center on Poverty Law, Inc.
NCPSSM
    National Committee to Preserve Social Security and Medicare
NCT
    number connection test
NDC
    nondifferentiated cell
NDDIC
    National Digestive Diseases Information Clearinghouse
NDIC
    National Diabetes Information Clearinghouse
near-drowning
near-syncope
necatoriasis
neck
    bull n.
    femoral n.
    n. infection
    Madelung n.
    n. mass
    n. pain
    n. strain
    turkey gobbler n.
    webbed n.
    wry n.
necklace
    Casal n.
necrobiosis lipoidica
necrocytosis

necrologist
necrology
necrolysis
    toxic epidermal n.
necrosis
    avascular n.
    bland n.
    bone n.
    cold-induced n.
    decubital n.
    focal n.
    hemoglobinuric acute tubular n.
    hepatic n.
    hepatocellular n.
    idiopathic avascular n.
    incus n.
    ischemic bone n.
    mercurial n.
    myocardial n.
    myocyte n.
    pancreatic n.
    phosphorus n.
    piecemeal n.
    pituitary n.
    postpartum pituitary n.
    pressure n.
    quiet n.
    radiation n.
    simple n.
    spontaneous n.
    submassive hepatic n.
    tubular n.
necrotic
    n. cell death
    n. cirrhosis
    n. granuloma
necroticans
    enteritis n.
necrotizing
    n. cellulitis
    n. enterocolitis
    n. fasciitis
    n. pancreatitis
    n. pneumonia
    n. sarcoid granulomatosis
    n. soft tissue infection
    n. ulcerative stomatitis
    n. vasculitis
NED
  no evidence of disease
nedocromil sodium

needed
    as n. (p.r.n.)
    as much as n. (q.l.)
needle
    n. aspiration
    n. aspiration lung biopsy
    n. bath
    Chiba n.
    n. management system
    NovoFine n.
    scalp vein n.
    transtracheal n.
    Tuohy n.
needle-free injection system
Neer test
nefazodone hydrochloride
neg
  negative
negative (neg)
    n. correlation
    predictive value n.
    n. predictive value
    n. symptom
negative-sense genome
NegGram
neglect
NEHCRC
  Native Elder Health Care Resource
  Center
NEHEP
  National Eye Health Education Program
Neisseria
    N. gonorrhoeae
    N. meningitidis
Nélaton catheter
nelfinavir mesylate
Nelson syndrome
nematode
Nembutal
neoadjuvant chemotherapy
Neo-Calglucon
neocortex
NeoDecadron
neoformans
    Cryptococcus n.
neomorphic
neomycin
neonatal
    n. hepatitis
    n. hyperbilirubinemia
    n. hypoglycemia
    n. lupus

NOTES

N

neonatal *(continued)*
    n. placing
    n. tetanus
neonatology
neonatorum
    hemophilia n.
    icterus n.
    melena n.
    pemphigus n.
    tetanus n.
neoplasia
    cervical intraepithelial n., grade 2
      (CIN II)
    lymphocytic thyroiditis n.
    multiple endocrine n. (MEN)
    multiple endocrine n. type I, II
    silent n.
    synchronous colonic n.
    thyroid malignant n.
    vulvar intraepithelial n. (VIN)
neoplasm
    adrenal n.
    benign hepatic n.
    colorectal n.
    gestational trophoblastic n.
    hepatic n.
    malignant hepatic n.
    multiple endocrine n. (MEN)
    poorly differentiated n.
    prostatic n.
    trophoblastic n.
neoplastic
    n. disease
    n. pathology
    n. pericardial effusion
    n. process
neoprene brace
Neosporin
Neo-Synephrine
neovascularization
    n. of disk (NVD)
    n. elsewhere on retina (NVE)
    n. of iris
NEPD
    no evidence of pulmonary disease
nephralgia
nephralgic
nephrectomy
nephredema
nephritic syndrome
nephritis
    chronic interstitial n.
    dropsical n.
    interstitial n.
    lupus n.
    salt-losing n.
nephritogenic
nephrocalcinosis

nephrogenic
    n. ascites
    n. diabetes insipidus
nephrogenous
nephrolithiasis
nephrology
nephronophthisis
    juvenile n.
nephropathia epidemica
nephropathy
    acute bone marrow transplant-
      associated n.
    allograft n.
    Balkan n.
    bone marrow transplant-
      associated n.
    cast n.
    chronic bone marrow transplant-
      associated n.
    Danubian endemic familial n.
    diabetic n.
    dropsical n.
    familial n.
    gouty n.
    hereditary n.
    HIV-associated n.
    HIV-1-associated n.
    hypokalemic n.
    IgA n.
    immunoglobulin A n.
    obstructive n.
    radiocontrast n.
    sickle cell n.
    transplant-associated n.
    urate n.
nephropexy
nephroptosis
nephropyelitis
nephrosclerosis
nephrosclerotic
nephrosis
    acute n.
    amyloid n.
    familial n.
    hemoglobinuric n.
    hypoxic n.
    osmotic n.
    toxic n.
    vacuolar n.
nephrostolithotomy
nephrotic syndrome
nephrotomogram
nephrotoxicity
    aminoglycoside n.
nephrotuberculosis
nephroureterectomy
Neptazane
NER
    no evidence of recurrence

NERD
no evidence of recurrent disease
nerve
n. block
Bock n.
n. compression
n. conduction
n. conduction study
cranial n.
n. entrapment
hypoglossal n.
n. injury
n. palsy
peripheral n.
phrenic n.
n. root compression
n. root stimulation
n. root syndrome
somatic pudendal n.
nervosa
angina n.
anorexia n.
bulimia n.
mycetism n.
nervous
n. asthma
n. breakdown
n. dyspepsia
n. indigestion
n. tinnitus
nettle
Nettleship syndrome
network
artificial neural n. (ANN)
National Prevention Information N.
(NPIN)
National Women's Health N.
(NWHN)
neuf
bruit de cuir n.
neural
n. foramina
n. foraminal canal
neuralgia
cranial n.
postherpetic n.
pudendal n.
Sluder n.
trigeminal n.
Wartenberg n.
neuralgic headache
neuraminidase inhibitor

neurapraxia
neurasthenia
gastric n.
neurasthenic
neurectomy
neurinoma
neuritic plaque
neuritis
brachial plexus n.
dietetic n.
endemic n.
influenzal n.
optic n.
retrobulbar n.
rheumatic n.
neuroablation
neuroacanthocytosis
neuroanatomic change
neurobehavioral deficit
neuroblastoma
neurocardiogenic syncope
neurocognitive function
NeuroCom EquiTest
neurocutaneous
neurocysticercosis
intraventricular n.
parenchymal n.
subarachnoid n.
neurocyte
neurodegeneration
neurodegenerative disease
neurodermatitis
neuroectodermal
neuroeffector
neuroendocrine
n. theory
n. tumor
neuroendocrinology
neurofibrillary tangle
neurofibroma
neurofibromatosis, pl. **neurofibromatoses**
n. 2
von Recklinghausen n.
neurogenic
n. bladder
n. cachexia
neuroglycopenia
neurohormonal abnormality
neurohormone
neuroimaging study
neurokinin A
neurokinin-1 receptor antagonist

NOTES

N

neurolabyrinthitis
neurolathyrism
neuroleptic
    n. toxicity
neurologic
    n. disease
    n. migraine
    n. specialist
neurology
    American Academy of N. (AAN)
neuroma
    acoustic n.
    Morton n.
neuromuscular
    n. blockade
    n. disease
    n. weakness
neuromyasthenia
    epidemic n.
neuromyelitis optica
neuromyopathic
neuromyositis
neuromyotonia
neuron
    corticobulbar n.
    hypothalamic secretory n.
    lower motor n.
    motor n.
    pain-transmission n.
    raphe n.
    sympathetic postganglionic n.
    upper motor n.
neuronal
    n. cell
    n. migration disorder
    n. somata
neuronitis
    vestibular n.
neuronopathy
Neurontin
neuroophthalmologic examination
neuropathic
    n. arthropathy
    n. pain
neuropathy
    amyloid n.
    autonomic n.
    carcinomatous n.
    cardiovascular autonomic n.
    diabetic n.
    diabetic autonomic n. (DAN)
    femoral n.
    focal n.
    gastrointestinal n.
    hereditary n.
    hereditary motor and sensory n.
     type 1–4
    hereditary sensory and
     autonomic n. type 1

infectious n.
ischemic optic n.
myxedematous n.
optic n.
peripheral n.
toxic n.
neuropeptide
neurophysiologic change
neuroprotective
    n. drug
    n. therapy
neuropsychiatric
    n. disease
    n. systemic lupus erythematosus
neuropsychological test battery
neurorehabilitation
neuroroentgenologic
neuroroentgenology
neurosarcoidosis
neuroscience
    Society for N.
neurostimulation
    dorsal column n.
    thalamic column n.
neurosurgery
neurosyphilis
neurotensinoma
neurotica
    lipomatosis n.
neurotoxin
neurotransmitter change
neurotrophin
    recombinant brain-derived n.
neurourologic
neurovascular sheath
neutraceutical
neutral
    K-Phos N.
    n. lipid storage disease
    n. protamine Hagedorn (NPH)
    n. protamine Hagedorn insulin
Neutra-Phos
Neutrogena
neutropenia
    chronic hypoplastic n.
    chronic idiopathic n.
    congenital n.
    cyclic n.
    drug-induced n.
    familial benign chronic n.
    hypersplenic n.
    hypoplastic n.
    idiopathic n.
    Kostmann n.
    malignant n.
    periodic n.
    peripheral n.
    primary splenic n.

splenic n.
transient n.
neutropenic
neutrophil
n. defect
polymorphonuclear segmented n.'s
(polys)
polynuclear n.'s
segmented n.'s (segs)
neutrophilia
acquired n.
chronic n.
neutrophilic dermatosis
neutropic drug
nevertheless
nevirapine
nevus, pl. **nevi**
blue n.
choroidal n.
compound n.
congenital melanocytic n.
dermal n.
dysplastic n.
giant hairy n.
halo n.
Newcastle disease
Newcastle-Manchester bacillus
New World hemorrhagic fever
Nexium
NFCA
National Family Caregivers Association
NG
nasogastric
NG tube
ng
nanogram
ng/mL
nanograms per milliliter
NGNA
National Gerontological Nursing
Association
NHANES
National Health and Nutrition
Examination Survey
NHANES Battery
NHCoA
National Hispanic Council on Aging
NHF
National Hospital Foundation
NHGRI
National Human Genome Research
Institute

NHIC
National Health Information Center
NHLBI
National Heart, Lungs, and Blood
Institute
NHP
Nottingham Health Profile
NHPCO
National Hospice and Palliative Care
Organization
NHS
National Health Service (England)
NIA
National Institute on Aging
NIAAA
National Institute on Alcohol Abuse and
Alcoholism
niacin
NIAID
National Institute of Allergy and
Infectious Disease
NICA
National Interfaith Coalition on Aging
nicardipine
NICHD
National Institute of Child Health and
Human Development
nicking
NICOA
National Indian Council on Aging
Nicobid
Nicoderm patch
Nicolas-Favre disease
nicotina
stomatitis n.
nicotine
n. inhaler
n. nasal spray
n. replacement therapy (NRT)
transdermal n.
Nicotinex
NIDA
National Institute on Drug Abuse
NIDCD
National Institute on Deafness and Other
Communication Disorders
NIDCR
National Institute of Dental and
Craniofacial Research
NIDD
non–insulin-dependent diabetes

NOTES

N

NIDDM
non–insulin-dependent diabetes mellitus
nidus, pl. **nidi**
NIEHS
National Institute of Environmental
Health Sciences
Niemann
N. disease
N. splenomegaly
Niemann-Pick
N.-P. C (NPC)
N.-P. C disease
N.-P. C1 disease
nifedipine
Niferex
nifurtimox
niger
Aspergillus n.
vomitus n.
night
n. blindness
n. eating syndrome
every n. [L. *quaque nocte*] (q.n.)
every other n. [L. *quaque altera nocte*] (q.o.n.)
n. hospital
n. sweats
nightmare
NIGMS
National Institute of General Medical
Sciences
nigricans
acanthosis n.
malignant acanthosis n.
pseudoacanthosis n.
NIH
National Institutes of Health
NIH Osteoporosis and Related
Bone Diseases National Resource
Center (NIH-ORBD-NRC)
NIH-CPSI
National Institutes of Health Chronic
Prostatitis Symptom Index
nihilism
therapeutic n.
NIH-ORBD-NRC
NIH Osteoporosis and Related Bone
Diseases National Resource Center
Nike shoe
Nikolsky sign
NIMH
National Institute of Mental Health
nimodipine
NINDS
National Institute of Neurological
Disorders and Stroke
NINR
National Institute of Nursing Research

nipple
n. discharge
n. resection
NIRSC
National Information and Referral
Support Center
nisoldipine
Nissen fundoplication
niter paper
nitrate
econazole n.
isosorbide n.
nitrendipine
nitrite
nitritoid reaction
Nitro-Bid
Nitrodisc
Nitro-Dur
nitrofurantoin macrocrystal
nitrogen
blood urea n. (BUN)
frozen with liquid n.
liquid n. (LN_2)
n. mustard
n. narcosis
urea n.
nitroglycerin
n. headache
intravenous n.
sublingual n.
nitroid shock
Nitrol ointment
nitroprusside sodium
Nitrostat
Nizoral 1%, 2%
NJ
nasojejunal
NJ feeding
NJ tube
njovera
NKA
no known allergies
NKDA
no known drug allergies
NKF
National Kidney Foundation
NKUDIC
National Kidney and Urological Diseases
Information Clearinghouse
NLM
National Library of Medicine
NLSBPH
National Library Service for the Blind
and Physically Handicapped
NLTCORC
National Long-Term Care Ombudsman
Research Center

NLTCRC
National Long-Term Care Research
Center
NMA
National Medical Association
NMDA
N-methyl-D-aspartate
NMDA inhibitor
N-methyl-D-aspartate (NMDA)
N-methyl-D-aspartate inhibitor
**N-methyl-4-phenyl-1,2,3,6-
tetrahydropyridine (MPTP)**
NMHA
National Mental Health Association
NMSS
National Multiple Sclerosis Society
no
no added salt (NAS)
no added salt diet
no appreciable disease (NAD)
no evidence of disease (NED)
no evidence of pulmonary disease
(NEPD)
no evidence of recurrence (NER)
no evidence of recurrent disease
(NERD)
Nocard bacillus
nocardiasis
nocardiosis
granulomatous n.
nociceptive pain
nociceptor
afferent n.
silent n.
nociceptor-induced inflammation
nocte
quaque n.
quaque altera n.
nocturia
nocturna
jactation capitis n.
nocturnal
n. caffeine
n. diarrhea
n. dyspnea
n. enuresis
n. erection
n. paroxysmal dystonia
n. penile tumescence (NPT)
n. polysomnography (NPSG)
n. symptom

n. urinary frequency
n. urinary incontinence
nod
bishop's n.
nodal
n. fever
n. tachycardia
node
anterior cervical lymph n.
Bouchard n.
Delphian n.
Heberden n.
lymph n.
Osler n.
Parrot n.
Schmorl n.
sentinel n.
shotty n.
sinoatrial n.
sinus n.
submental n.
Troisier n.
nodosa
arthritis n.
microscopic polyarteritis n.
periarteritis n. (PAN)
polyarteritis n.
trichorrhexis n.
nodosity
Heberden n.
nodosum
erythema n.
nodular
n. adrenal hyperplasia
n. adrenocortical hyperplasia
n. bronchiectasis
n. goiter
n. melanoma
n. myositis
n. panniculitis
nodularis
prurigo n.
nodule
adrenal n.
Albini n.
apple jelly n.
Aschoff n.
Bohn n.
Bouchard n.
Caplan n.
cold n.
colloid n.

N

NOTES

nodule *(continued)*
    Gamna n.
    Gandy-Gamna n.
    hot thyroid n.
    hyperfunctioning thyroid n.
    malignant thyroid n.
    prostate n.
    pulmonary n.
    rheumatoid n.
    Schmorl n.
    single thyroid n.
    single toxic n.
    solitary pulmonary n. (SPN)
    thyroid n.
    toxic n.
    Wilson n.
nodulous
NOF
    National Osteoporosis Foundation
noise
    background n.
    n. induced
Nolex LA
Nolvadex
noma
no-man's land
nomenclature
non-A
    non-A hepatitis
    non-A, non-B
    non-A, non-B hepatitis (NANB)
    non-A, non-B, non-C (NANBNC)
    non-A, non-B, non-C hepatitis
    non-A syndrome
nonadherence
    regimen n.
nonalcoholic steatohepatitis
nonallergic rhinitis
nonambulator
nonanion gap acidosis
nonan malaria
nonarticular rheumatism
non-B
    non-B hepatitis
    non-A, non-B
nonbacteremic
nonbacterial
    n. infantile gastroenteritis
    n. infectious arthritis
    n. prostatitis
    n. thrombotic endocarditis (NBTE)
non-C
    non-C hepatitis
    non-A, non-B, non-C (NANBNC)
noncardiac chest pain
nonclostridial infection
noncolicky epigastric pain
noncompliance
noncoronary cause

nondeforming arthritis
nondermatophytic mold
nondiabetic glycosuria
nondifferentiated cell (NDC)
nondihydropyridine calcium channel blocker
nondipper
nondipping
nondisclosure
nondisease
nonenveloped virus
nongonococcal septic arthritis
nonhemolytic
    n. febrile transfusion reaction
non-Hodgkin lymphoma
nonhospitalized
nonhydrostatic pulmonary edema
nonhyperglycemic glycosuria
nonimmunity
noninfectious diarrheal disease
noninflammatory
noninherited factor
non–insulin-dependent
    n.–i.-d. diabetes (NIDD)
    n.–i.-d. diabetes mellitus (NIDDM)
noninvasive
    n. cardiac testing
    n. positive pressure ventilation
nonionizing radiation
nonischemic chest pain
nonislet cell tumor
nonisolated proteinuria
nonketotic
    n. hyperglycemia
    n. hyperglycinemia
    n. hyperosmolar syndrome
    n. state
nonleukemic myelosis
nonlymphocytic leukemia
nonlymphoid leukemia
nonmegaloblastic
    n. macrocytic anemia
nonmelancholic
nonmelanoma
nonnarcotic analgesic
Nonne-Milroy disease
Nonne-Milroy-Meige syndrome
nonnephrotic proteinuria
nonnucleoside reverse transcriptase inhibitor
nonocclusive mesenteric ischemia
nonorganic
nonpalpable purpura
nonparalytic
non-parathyroid-related hypercalcemia
nonparoxysmal atrioventricular junctional tachycardia
nonpharmacologic therapy
nonpitting edema

nonplague yersiniosis
nonpolyposis colorectal cancer
non-potassium-sparing diuretic
nonproductive cough
non-Q
non-Q-wave myocardial infarction
   (NQWMI)
nonrandomized study
nonrenal
   n. potassium loss
   n. water loss
nonreplicative
nonrespiratory acidosis
nonresponsive tumor
nonrestorative sleep
nonroutine
nonsecretory
   n. glucagonoma
   n. microadenoma
non-small-cell lung cancer (NSCLC)
nonspecific
   n. arthralgia
   n. effector cell
   n. interstitial pneumonia
   n. ST change
   n. stomatitis
   n. tachycardia
non-ST-elevation myocardial infarction
nonsteroidal antiinflammatory drug
   (NSAID)
nonstochastic
nonsulfonylurea
nonsuppurative panniculitis
nonsurgical therapeutic abortion
nonsurvival
nonsustained ventricular tachycardia
   (NSVT)
nontender incarcerated inguinal hernia
nonthrombocytopenic purpura
nonthyroidal illness syndrome
nontoxic
   n. goiter (NTG)
   n. nodular goiter (NTNG)
nontransmural infarction
nontreponemal test
nontropical sprue
nontuberculin mycobacterial disease
nontuberculous mycobacteria
nonulcer dyspepsia
nonunion gap metabolic acidosis
nonurgent problem
nonvariceal bleeding

nonvenereal
   n. syphilis
   n. treponematosis
nonviral chronic hepatitis
nonweightbearing exercise
Noonan syndrome
Nootropil
noradrenaline
NORD
   National Organization of Rare Disorders
Nordette-28
Norel
norepinephrine
Norethin
Norflex
norfloxacin
Norgesic Forte
Norinyl
Norlestrin
normal
   n. extracellular fluid volume
   n. glandularity
   n. pressure
   n. sinus rhythm (NSR)
normal-pressure hydrocephalus
Norman-Wood syndrome
normeperidine
normetanephrine
normochromic
   n. normocytic anemia
normocyte
normocytic anemia
Normodyne
normoglycemia
normoglycemic glycosuria
normokalemic periodic paralysis
normoprolactinemia galactorrhea
normospermatogenic sterility
normotension
   white-coat n.
normotensive
normotopia
normotopic
Noroxin
Norpace
Norplant
Norpramin
north
   N. American blastomycosis
   N. American Menopause Society
   (NAMS)

NOTES

N

north *(continued)*
    N. Queensland tick fever
    N. Queensland tick typhus
nortriptyline HCl
Norvasc
Norvir
Norwalk-like agent virus
nosetiology
nosochthonography
nosocomial
    n. aspergillosis
    n. infection
    n. *Legionella*
    n. pneumonia
    n. septicemia
nosogenesis
nosogenic
nosogeography
nosographic
nosography
nosologic
nosology
nosometry
nosonomy
nosopoietic
nosotaxy
nosotoxic
nosotoxicosis
nosotrophy
nosotropic
nostras
    cholera n.
    influenza n.
nostrum
notariorum
    paralysis n.
notch
    suprasternal n.
Nothnagel
    N. sign
    N. syndrome
Nothnagel-type acroparesthesia
notifiable disease
Nottingham Health Profile (NHP)
not yet diagnosed (NYD)
nourishment
NOVA
    National Organization of Victim
      Assistance
Novafed
Novartis
novel diet
novo
    de n.
Novocain
NovoFine needle
Novolin
    N. L
    N. PenFill cartridge

NovoLog
Novoste Beta-Cath System
noxa
noxious stimulus
NPC
    Niemann-Pick C
NPF
    National Psoriasis Foundation
NPH
    neutral protamine Hagedorn
      NPH insulin
NPIN
    National Prevention Information Network
NPRCWA
    National Policy and Resource Center on
      Women and Aging
NPSG
    nocturnal polysomnography
NPT
    nocturnal penile tumescence
NQWMI
    non-Q-wave myocardial infarction
NRCDLTC
    National Resource Center Diversity and
      Long-Term Care
NRCNAA
    National Resource Center on Native
      American Aging
NRHA
    National Rural Health Association
NRIC
    National Resource and Information
      Center
NRT
    nicotine replacement therapy
NS
      Mycocide NS
NSA
    National Stroke Association
NSAID
    nonsteroidal antiinflammatory drug
NSCERC
    National Senior Citizens' Education and
      Research Center
NSCLC
    National Senior Citizens' Law Center
    non-small-cell lung cancer
NSF
    National Sleep Foundation
NSGA
    National Senior Games Association
NSHC
    National Self-Help Clearinghouse
NSR
    normal sinus rhythm
NSVT
    nonsustained ventricular tachycardia
n-telopeptide

NTG
    nontoxic goiter
NTNG
    nontoxic nodular goiter
Nubain
nucha
nuchal rigidity
nuclear
    n. multiple gaited acquisition
    n. sclerosis
nuclei (*pl. of* nucleus)
nucleocapsid
nucleoid
nucleolar pattern
nucleoprotein
nucleoside analog reverse transcriptase inhibitor
nucleotide
    antidiphosphopyridine n.
    n. sequence
nucleus, pl. nuclei
    n. basalis
    n. basalis of Meynert
    n. pulposus
    reticular n.
nudge
    sternum n.
null
nulligravid
nulligravida
nulliparous
nullisomic
number connection test (NCT)
numbness
numerous
nummiform
nummular eczema
nummulation
Nuprin
nurse
    American Association of Critical-Care N.'s (AACN)
    charge n.
    community health n.
    dry n.
    general duty n.
    graduate n.
    head n.
    home health n.
    hospital n.
    licensed practical n. (LPN)
    licensed vocational n. (LVN)

    practical n.
    n. practitioner
    private duty n.
    public health n.
    registered n. (RN)
    school n.
    scrub n.
    special n.
    student n.
    visiting n.
    wet n.
nurse-midwife
    certified n.-m. (CNM)
nursing
    n. care
    Fellow of the American Academy of N. (FAAN)
    n. home
nutans
    spasmus n.
nutation
nutatory
nutcracker esophagus
Nutraderm
nutrient
    n. enema
    essential n.'s
nutrition
    central parenteral n.
    delirium, dementia, depression, drugs; eyes and ears; physical performance and "phalls" (falls); incontinence; n. (DEEP-IN)
    enteral n.
    forced enteral n.
    parenteral n.
    partial parenteral n.
    peripheral parenteral n.
    n. status
    total parenteral n. (TPN)
    total peripheral parenteral n. (TPPN)
nutritional
    n. characteristic
    n. cirrhosis
    n. dropsy
    n. edema
    n. hemosiderosis
    n. intervention
    n. macrocytic anemia
    n. marasmus
    n. polyneuropathy

N

NOTES

nutritional *(continued)*
    n. secondary hyperparathyroidism
    n. state
    n. status
    n. support
    n. therapy
nutritive
nutriture
N&V
    nausea and vomiting
NVD
    nausea, vomiting, diarrhea
    neovascularization of disk
NVE
    neovascularization elsewhere on retina
NWHIC
    National Women's Health Information
    Center

NWHN
    National Women's Health Network
nycturia
NYD
    not yet diagnosed
Nylen-Bárány maneuver
Nyquil
nystagmus
    Baer n.
    downbeat n.
    gaze-evoked n.
    jerk n.
nystatin
Nytol

OA
  osteoarthritis
OAA
  Opticians Association of America
OAD
  obstructive airway disease
    spirometry-defined OAD
oasthouse urine disease
oat cell carcinoma
obelion
Ober test
obese
obesity
    adrenocortical o.
    adult-onset o.
    alimentary o.
    endogenous o.
    exogenous o.
    hyperinsulinar o.
    o. of hyperinsulinism
    hyperplasmic o.
    hyperplastic-hypertrophic o.
    hypertrophic o.
    hypothalamic o.
    hypothyroid o.
    o. hypoventilation syndrome
    o. index
    lifelong o.
    morbid o.
    simple o.
obesity-associated diabetes
OB-GYN
  obstetrics and gynecology
objective
    o. sign
    o. swelling
    o. symptom
    o. tinnitus
obliterans
    arteriosclerosis o. (ASO)
    bronchiolitis fibrosa o.
    thromboangiitis o. (TAO)
obliterative
    o. bronchiolitis
    o. bronchitis
OBS
  organic brain syndrome
observation
observational study
obsessive-compulsive
    o.-c. disorder (OCD)
    o.-c. personality disorder
obstetrics and gynecology (OB-GYN)
obstinate
obstipation

obstruction
    acute o.
    airway o.
    bile duct o.
    bladder outlet o.
    blood flow o.
    bowel o.
    bronchial o.
    common duct o.
    cystic duct o.
    extrahepatic o.
    flow o.
    gastric outlet o.
    intestinal o.
    intraluminal o.
    large bowel o.
    left ventricular o.
    lower urinary tract o.
    mechanical esophageal o.
    partial small bowel o. (PSBO)
    prostatic o.
    renal artery o.
    small bowel o.
    unilateral nasal o.
    upper airway o.
    upper urinary tract o.
    ureteric vesical junction o.
    ureterovesical junction o.
    urinary tract o.
    UVJ o.
obstruction/incompetence
    urethral o./i.
obstructive
    o. airflow disease
    o. airway disease (OAD)
    o. cardiomyopathy
    o. cirrhosis
    o. lung disease
    o. nephropathy
    o. pneumonia
    o. shock
    o. sleep apnea (OSA)
    o. sleep apnea syndrome (OSAS)
obtund
obtundation
obtunded
    somnolent and o.
obturation
obturator sign
OC
  oral contraceptive
OCA
  Organization of Chinese Americans
occipital
occipitonuchal

O

occipitotemporal
occiput
Occlusal
occlusion
    acute arterial o.
    branch retinal artery o. (BRAO)
    branch retinal vein o. (BRVO)
    central retinal artery o. (CRAO)
    central retinal vein o. (CRVO)
    cerebral artery o.
    embolic mesenteric vascular o.
occlusive
    o. disease
    o. ileus
occult
    o. blood
    o. blood test
    o. gastrointestinal bleeding
occulta
    spina bifida o.
occupational
    o. airway disease
    o. asthma
    o. hazard
    o. lung disease
    o. paralysis
    o. parenchymal disease
    o. radiation
    O. Safety and Health
      Administration (OSHA)
    o. therapist (OT)
    o. therapy (OT)
occurrence
OCD
    obsessive-compulsive disorder
ochronosis
ochronotic arthritis
Ochsner method
OCP
    oral contraceptive pill
octan
octogenarian
octreotide
OcuCaps
Ocufen
OcuHist antihistamine decongestant eye drops
ocular
    o. bobbing
    o. chemical burn
    o. convergence
    o. cysticercosis
    o. dipping
    o. hypertension
    o. inflammation
    o. migraine
    o. toxoplasmosis
    o. trauma
oculobuccogenital syndrome

oculocephalic test
oculocerebrorenal syndrome
oculocutaneous albinism
oculogenital infection
oculoglandular tularemia
oculographic
oculogyria
oculomotor
    o. palsy
oculopharyngeal dystrophy
oculopneumoplethysmography (OPG, OPPG)
oculosympathetic syndrome
oculovestibular
oculus
    o. sinister (OS)
    o. uterque (OU)
Ocuvite
ocytocin
OD
    overdose
    right eye
odd
    posttest o.'s
    o.'s ratio
Oddi
    sphincter of O.
O-desmethylvenlafaxine
odontoid
odontoprisis
odor
odorant
odynophagia
of
    complains of (C/O)
    history of (H/O)
Office on Smoking and Health (OSH)
officer
    house o.
    Medical O. (MO)
offset
    sleep o.
ofloxacin
Ogen
Ogilvie syndrome
ogival point
OGTT
    oral glucose tolerance test
Ohara disease
oil
    fish o.
    o. pneumonia
    progesterone in o.
    o. retention enema
ointment
    clobetasol o.
    Gel-Cam o.
    Ilotycin o.
    LactiCare o.

Nitrol o.
   tacrolimus o.
olanzapine toxicity
Older Women's League (OWL)
Oldfield syndrome
oleandrism
olecranon
oleotherapy
olestra
olfaction
olfactogenital dysplasia
olfactorial ability
olfactory
oligemia
oligoarthritis
oligocholia
oligochylia
oligochymia
oligodendrocyte
oligodendroglioma
oligodipsia
oligohydramnios
oligohydruria
oligomenorrhea
oligopepsia
oligophrenia
   phenylpyruvic o.
oligophrenic
oligopnea
oligoptyalism
oligospermia
   idiopathic o.
oligosymptomatic
oligotrophia
oliguria
olivopontocerebellar atrophy
Ollier disease
olympian forehead
Olympus videoscope
ombudsman
omega-3 polyunsaturated fatty acid
Omenn syndrome
omental
   o. tuberosity
   o. tuberosity of liver
   o. tuberosity of pancreas
omentitis
omentum
   Cushing disease of o.
omeprazole
omithosis
Omniflox tablets

omphalic
omphalitis
omphalophlebitis
omphalorrhagia
omphalorrhea
omphalospinous
Omsk hemorrhagic fever
once
   at o. (stat., STAT)
onchocerciasis
onchocercoma
oncogene
oncogenic
oncologic
   o. emergency
   o. imaging
oncology
   gynecological o.
oncolysis
oncotherapy
oncotic pressure
Oncovin
ondansetron hydrochloride
Ondine curse
one
   O. Touch glucometer
   O. Touch Ultra meter
oneiric delirium
onlay graft
online
   Generations O.
onset
   dim light melatonin o. (DMLO)
   late-life o.
   sleep o.
ontologist
ontology
onyalai
onychocryptosis
onychogryphosis
onycholysis
onychomadesis
onychomycosis
onychoschizia
o'nyong-nyong fever
oophorectomy
   prophylactic o.
oophoritis parotidea
O&P
   ova and parasites
opacification
   lens o.

O

NOTES

opacity
  lens o.
open
  o. hospital
  o. lung biopsy
  o. tuberculosis
opening snap
open-loop pump therapy
operation
  arterial switch o.
  Fontan o.
  Wertheim o.
  Whipple o.
  Whitman o.
operative
  o. myxedema
  o. procedure
operculum, pl. **opercula**
operon promoter sequence
OPG
  oculopneumoplethysmography
ophiasis
ophthalmic
  o. Graves disease
  o. hyperthyroidism
  o. migraine
ophthalmodynamometry
ophthalmologic
ophthalmology
  American Academy of O. (AAO)
ophthalmopathy
  Graves o.
ophthalmoplegia
  diabetic o.
  exophthalmic o.
  hyperthyroid o.
  thyrotoxic o.
ophthalmoplegic migraine
ophthalmoscope
ophthalmovascular
opiate
opioid
  o. addiction
  o. analgesic
  o. cell membrane receptor
  continuous-infusion o.
  o. toxicity
  o. withdrawal
opisthion
opisthorchiasis
opisthotic
opisthotonos
Opitz
  O. disease
  O. syndrome
OPPG
  oculopneumoplethysmography
opponensplasty
  Huber o.

opponens weakness
opportunistic
  o. illness
  o. infection
  o. pneumonia
opsoclonus
optic
  o. ataxia
  o. nerve disease
  o. nerve lesion
  o. neuritis
  o. neuropathy
  o. tectum
optica
  neuromyelitis o.
Opticrom
OPTIMA
  Oxford Project to Investigate Memory
  and Aging
Optimine
optimism
  therapeutic o.
optimize
optimum dose
OptiPranolol
Optised
Orabase
Orajel
oral
  o. administration
  o. antibiotic
  o. antidiabetic agent
  o. antihistamine
  o. cancer
  o. candidiasis
  o. conjugated estrogen
  o. contraceptive (OC)
  o. contraceptive-induced
  hypertension
  o. contraceptive pill (OCP)
  o. corticosteroid
  o. disease
  o. glucocorticosteroid
  o. glucose tolerance
  o. glucose tolerance test (OGTT)
  o. gold
  o. health care
  o. health status
  o. infection
  o. iron
  o. leukoplakia
  o. phosphate
  o. phosphodiesterase
  o. rehydration
  o. rehydration therapy (ORT)
  o. vasodilator
oral-cervicofacial
Oramorph
Orap

Orasone
OraSure test
orbicular
orbital osteomyelitis
orbitopathy
Orbivirus
orchialgia
orchica
    adiposis o.
orchichorea
orchiectomy
orchiodynia
orchioneuralgia
orchiopathy
orchiotherapy
orchitis
    mumps o.
    o. parotidea
    o. variolosa
order
    DNH o.
    DNR o.
    do-not-hospitalize o.
    do-not-resuscitate o.
orderly
orectic
Oretic
orexia
organ
    o. confined
    end o.
    o. hypoperfusion
    o. limited
    o. rejection
    target o.
    o. transplant
    o. transplant infection
organic
    o. brain syndrome (OBS)
    o. delirium
    o. disease
    o. solvent poisoning
organicism
organicist
Organidin elixir
organification defect
organism carriage
organization
    O. of Chinese Americans (OCA)
    health maintenance o. (HMO)
    Joint Commission on Accreditation
      of Healthcare O.'s

managed care o.
National Hospice and Palliative
    Care O. (NHPCO)
social health maintenance o.
    (SHMO)
World Health O. (WHO)
organomegaly
organomercurials
organopathy
organophosphate toxicity
organophosphorous compound poisoning
organotherapy
organ-specific illness
orgasmic dysfunction
Oriental schistosomiasis
orientation
    spatial o.
orifice
origin
    fever of undetermined o. (FUO)
    fever of unknown o. (FUO)
    metastatic tumor of unknown o.
    pyrexia of unknown o. (PUO)
Orinase
oris
    cancrum o.
orlistat
Ormond disease
Ornade Spansules
ornithine transcarbamylase deficiency
ornithinuria
ornithosis
oromandibular
oropharyngeal
    o. aspiration
    o. candidiasis
    o. dysphagia
    o. infection
    o. tumor
oropharynx
Oropouche virus
orotic aciduria
Oroya fever
Orpington Prognostic scale
ORT
    oral rehydration therapy
Ortho
    O. All-Flex
    O. Tri-Cyclen
Ortho-Cept
orthocrasia
Ortho-Cyclen

O

NOTES

orthodromic reciprocating tachycardia
Ortho-Ex
orthogenics
orthoglycemic glycosuria
orthomolecular therapy
orthonasal perception
Ortho-Novum
orthopedic rehabilitation
orthopedics
orthophoria
    asthenic o.
orthopnea position
orthopneic position
orthosis, pl. orthoses
    ankle-foot o. (AFO)
orthostasis
orthostatic
    o. hypotension
    o. proteinuria
    o. purpura
    o. stress
orthothanasia
orthotic
    Spenco Polysorb O.'s
orthotist
Ortolani sign
Orudis
Oruvail
OS
    left eye
    oculus sinister
os
    os calcis
    os cervix
    per os (p.o.)
    os perineum
    os trigonum
OSA
    obstructive sleep apnea
OSAS
    obstructive sleep apnea syndrome
Os-Cal 250/500
oscillation
    to-and-fro o.
oscillometry
oseltamivir
Osgood-Schlatter disease
OSH
    Office on Smoking and Health
OSHA
    Occupational Safety and Health
    Administration
Osler
    O. disease
    O. node
    O. sign
    O. syndrome II
    O. triad
Osler-Vaquez disease

Osler-Weber-Rendu
    O.-W.-R. disease
    O.-W.-R. syndrome
osmolal gap
osmolality
    plasma o.
    serum o.
    urine o.
osmolarity
osmoregulation
osmotherapy
osmotic
    o. diarrhea
    o. diuresis
    o. gap
    o. nephrosis
    o. regulation
    o. stimulus
osseous
    o. metastasis
    o. pain
ossificans
    myositis o.
ossifying fibroma
osteitis
    o. condensans
    o. deformans
    o. fibrosa
    o. fibrosa cystica
    o. symphysis pubis
    synovitis, acne, pustulosis,
      hyperostosis, o. (SAPHO)
osteoarthritic change
osteoarthritis (OA)
    o. deformans
    o. deformans endemica
    endemic o.
    erosive inflammatory o.
    hyperplastic o.
    hypertrophic o.
    inflammatory o.
    interphalangeal o.
    primary generalized hypertrophic o.
osteoarthropathy
    diabetic neuropathic o. (DNOA)
    hypertrophic o.
    idiopathic hypertrophic o. (IHO)
osteoarthrosis
osteoblast
osteoblastoma
osteocalcin
osteocartilaginous
osteochondral grafting
osteochondritis dissecans
osteochondrodysplasia
osteochondrodystrophia deformans
osteochondrodystrophy
    familial o.
osteoclast

osteodystrophy
    Albright hereditary o.
    hepatic o.
    hereditary o.
    mixed uremic o.
    parathyroid o.
    renal o.
    uremic o.
osteogenesis
    endochondral o.
    o. imperfecta
    o. imperfecta congenita
    o. imperfecta cystica
    o. imperfecta tarda
    periosteal o.
osteoid osteoma
osteoma
    osteoid o.
osteomalacia
    infantile o.
    tumor-induced o.
osteomalacic
osteomyelitis
    acute hematogenous o.
    chronic o.
    hematogenous o.
    jaw o.
    orbital o.
    vertebral o.
osteomyelosclerosis
osteonecrosis
osteoonychial
osteoonychodysplasia
osteopath
osteopathia hemorrhagica infantum
osteopathic
    o. medicine
    o. physician
osteopathy
    alimentary o.
    Doctor of O. (DO)
osteopenia
    juxtaarticular o.
osteopetrosis
osteophagia
osteophyte
osteopoikilosis
osteopontin
osteoporosis
    glucocorticoid-induced o.
    glucocorticosteroid-induced o.

    postmenopausal o. (PMO)
    steroid-induced o.
osteoporotic compression fracture
osteosarcoma
osteosis
    renal fibrocystic o.
osteotomy
    Chiari o.
    derotative o.
    distal chevron o.
ostial
ostium, pl. **ostia**
    o. primum
    o. primum location
    o. secundum
ostreotoxism
OT
    occupational therapist
    occupational therapy
OTC
    over the counter
    OTC medication
other
    significant o. (SO)
otic
    Coly-Mycin O.
otitis
    o. externa
    o. media
    serous o.
otoacoustic
otolaryngology
otomycosis
otorhinolaryngology
otorrhea
otosclerosis
    cochlear o.
otoscope
otospongiosis
ototoxicity
    gentamicin o.
ototoxin
Otto
    O. disease
    O. pelvis
OU
    oculus uterque
ounce (oz)
out
    rule o. (R/O)
outcome
    functional o.

O

NOTES

outlook
  Bayesian o.
out-of-pocket expense
outpatient medication
output
  cardiac o. (CO)
outrigger splint
outstretched hand
outweigh
ovale
  o. malaria
  patent foramen o. (PFO)
  Pityrosporum o.
  Plasmodium o.
ovalocytary anemia
ovalocyte
ovalocytosis
  southeast Asian o.
ova and parasites (O&P)
ovarian
  o. amenorrhea
  o. cancer
  o. dysfunction
  o. failure
  o. hyperthecosis
  o. stromal hyperplasia
  o. vein thrombosis
ovarii
  struma o.
ovary
  sclerocystic disease of o.
Ovcon-35
over
  o. the counter (OTC)
  o. diagnose
  o.-the-counter medication
overactive bladder
overactivity
  detrusor o.
overdialysis
overdiuresis
overdose (OD)
  alcohol o.
  heroin o.
  o. toxicity
overflow incontinence
overgrowth
  small intestinal bacterial o.
overhydration
overlap syndrome
overlay
overload
  fluid o.
  iatrogenic volume o.
  iron o.
  volume o.
overnight
  o. dexamethasone suppression test

  o. oximeter
  o. oximetry
overproduction
  thyroid-stimulating hormone o.
overt diabetes
overuse syndrome
overweight
Ovral
ovulatory bleeding
ovulocyclic porphyria
OWL
  Older Women's League
Owren
  O. deficiency
  O. disease
oxacillin
oxalate
  calcium o.
  urine o.
oxalic gout
oxalosis
  primary hyperoxaluria and o.
oxaluria
  enteric o.
oxazepam
oxazolidinone
Oxford Project to Investigate Memory
  and Aging (OPTIMA)
oxidase
  cytochrome o.
  monoamine o. (MAO)
oxidation
  protein o.
oxide
  vasodilating nitric o.
oximeter
  finger o.
  overnight o.
  pulse o.
oximetry
  overnight o.
  pulse o.
Oxipor VHC
Oxistat cream
Oxpam
OXT
  oxytocin
Oxy 10
oxybutynin chloride
oxycodone
  long-acting o.
  sustained-release o.
OxyContin
oxygen
  o. delivery
  o. demand
  hyperbaric o.
  mixed venous o.
  partial pressure of o. (PO_2)

partial pressure alveolar o. (PAO_2)
partial pressure arterial o. (PAO_2)
o. poisoning
o. tent
o. therapy
o. toxicity

oxygenation
apneic o.
arterial o.
hyperbaric o.

OxyIR
oxykrinin
oxylalia
oxyrygmia
oxytocin (OXT)
oz
ounce
ozonator

NOTES

O

P450

cytochrome P450

PA

physician assistant
posteroanterior
PA line

P&A

percussion and auscultation

PAB

prealbumin

Pabalate

pabular

pabulum

PAC

Platinol, Adriamycin, cyclophosphamide

pacchionian depression

PACE

Program of All-Inclusive Care for the
Elderly

pacemaker

Biotronik p.
Chardack p.
demand p.
permanent p.

pacemaker-mediated tachycardia

pachycholia

pachychymia

pachydermodactyly

pachydermoperiostitis

pachydermoperiostosis

pacing

dual p.

pack

cold p.
dry p.
hot p.
wet p.

packed red blood cells (PRBC)

packing

paclitaxel

PAD

peripheral arterial disease

pad

Carrington p.
Silipos p.
Spenco metatarsal p.

PA&E

present, active, equal

Paget

P. disease
P. disease of bone
P. Foundation for Paget's Disease
of Bone and Related Disorders

Paget-von Schroetter syndrome

pagophagia

PAHA

p-aminohippuric acid
pulmonary artery hypertension

Pahvant

P. Valley fever
P. Valley plague

PAHVC

pulmonary alveolar hypoxic
vasoconstriction

pain

abdominal p.
acid-induced p.
acute pelvic p.
back p.
bone p.
cancer p.
cardiac chest p.
chest wall p.
chronic functional abdominal p.
chronic intermittent abdominal p.
chronic low back p. (CLBP)
chronic pelvic p.
chronic persistent abdominal p.
colicky p.
duality of p.
elbow p.
epigastric p.
esophageal chest p.
exertional chest p.
eye p.
facial p.
flank p.
functional abdominal p.
generalized musculoskeletal p.
hand p.
heel p.
hip p.
hunger p.
ice-pick-like p.
intermittent abdominal p.
joint p.
knee p.
knifelike p.
lancinating p.
low back p.
lower abdominal p.
p. management
p. management center
menstrual p.
musculoskeletal p.
myofascial p.
neck p.
neuropathic p.
nociceptive p.
noncardiac chest p.

P

pain *(continued)*
    noncolicky epigastric p.
    nonischemic chest p.
    osseous p.
    parietal p.
    pediatric back p.
    pelvic p.
    periumbilical p.
    persistent abdominal p.
    pleuritic chest p.
    postprandial p.
    psychogenic pelvic p.
    radicular p.
    referred p.
    referred abdominal p.
    scrotum p.
    p. sensitive
    sexual p.
    shoulder p.
    somatic p.
    p. therapy
    thoracic p.
    visceral p.
pain-dysfunction
    myofascial p.-d. (MPD)
pain-free
painful hematuria
painkiller
painless
    p. hematuria
painter's colic
pain-transmission neuron
palatable
palatal petechiae
palate
    cleft p.
palatinus
    tori p.
    a torus p.
palindromia
palindromic rheumatism
palliate
palliation
palliative
    p. care
    p. shunt
    p. treatment
pallidum
    Treponema p.
pallidus
    globus p.
pallor
    cachectic p.
palmar
    p. and dorsal aspects
    p. erythema
    p. xanthoma
palmare
    xanthoma striatum p.

Palmer acid test for peptic ulcer
palmetto
    saw p.
palmin test
palmomental
palpable
    p. purpura
    p. rale
palpate
palpation
    bimanual p.
    deep p.
    light-touch p.
palpatopercussion
palpatory percussion
palpebra
palpitation
palsy
    Bell p.
    cerebral p.
    cranial nerve p.
    diver's p.
    extraocular p.
    facial nerve p.
    handcuff p.
    hereditary neuropathy with liability to pressure p.
    nerve p.
    oculomotor p.
    peroneal nerve p.
    pressure p.
    progressive supranuclear p.
    supranuclear p.
Paltauf dwarf
paludal fever
Pamelor
pamidronate
p-**aminobenzoate**
p-**aminohippuric acid (PAHA)**
PAN
    periarteritis nodosa
panacea
panacinar
Panafil
Panax ginseng
panbronchiolitis
pancarditis
Pancoast tumor
Pancof HC syrup
pancreas
    aberrant p.
    p. accessorium
    accessory p.
    annular p.
    cystic fibrosis of p. (CFP)
    divided p.
    p. divisum
    fibrocystic disease of p.
    lesser p.

omental tuberosity of p.
polycystic p.
unciform p.
Willis p.
Winslow p.
Pancrease
pancreatalgia
pancreatic
    p. abscess
    p. arteriole
    p. artery aneurysm
    p. cancer
    p. cholera
    p. colic
    p. diabetes
    p. diarrhea
    p. fistula
    p. function test
    p. imaging
    p. infantilism
    p. insufficiency
    p. islet
    p. islet adenomatosis
    p. lesion
    p. necrosis
    p. pseudocyst
    p. steatorrhea
    p. tumor
pancreatica
    achylia p.
    diarrhea p.
    phthisis p.
    sialorrhea p.
pancreaticobiliary disorder
pancreaticoduodenal artery aneurysm
pancreaticoduodenectomy
pancreatitis
    acute p.
    biliary p.
    calcareous p.
    calcific p.
    calcifying p.
    chronic calcifying p. (CCP)
    chronic relapsing p.
    necrotizing p.
    Ranson criteria for severity of
      acute p.
    relapsing p.
pancreatoduodenectomy
pancreatogenic

pancreatogenous
    p. diarrhea
    p. fatty diarrhea
pancreatography
pancreatopathy
pancreatorenal syndrome
pancreopathy
pancreozymin
pancreozymin-secretin test
pancytopenia
    congenital p.
    Fanconi p.
pandemic
panencephalitis
    progressive rubella p.
    rubella p.
    sclerosing p. (SSPE)
    sclerosis p.
    subacute sclerosing p.
panendoscopy
pang
pangastritis
panhypopituitarism (PHP)
panic disorder
panneuritis epidemica
panniculitis
    febrile p.
    histiocytic cytophagic p.
    nodular p.
    nonsuppurative p.
    relapsing febrile nodular
      nonsuppurative p.
pannus
panophthalmitis
Panoxyl
pansystolic
Pantene Blue
pantomime
Pantopaque
pantoprazole delayed-release tablet
PAO₂
    arterial oxygen pressure
    partial pressure alveolar oxygen
    partial pressure arterial oxygen
Pap
    Papanicolaou
      class III Pap
      Pap smear
      Pap test
Papanicolaou (Pap)
    P. smear (Pap smear)
    P. test

NOTES

P

papaverine hydrochloride
paper
    p. mill worker's disease
    niter p.
    potassium nitrate p.
    saltpeter p.
papilla, pl. papillae
    Vater p.
papillary
    p. adenocystoma lymphomatosum
    p. fibroelastoma
    p. muscle fibrosis
    p. muscle rupture
    p. response
    p. thyroid carcinoma
papilledema
papillitis
papilloma
    zymotic p.
papillomatosis
    nasal p.
    respiratory p.
papillomatous goiter
papillomavirus
    human p. (HPV)
Papineau grafting
pappataci fever
papule
    Gottron p.
papulonodular
papulosquamous
papulovesicular
para
paraactinomycosis
para-**aminosalicylic acid (PASA)**
paraaortic
paracelsian method
paracenesthesia
paracentesis
    diagnostic p.
paracholera
paracicatricial
paracmasis
paracmastic
paracme
paracoagulation
    plasma protamine p.
paracoccidioidal granuloma
paracoccidioidomycosis
paracolon
    Citrobacter p.
paradigm
paradipsia
paradox
    abdominal p.
paradoxical
    p. aciduria
    p. diaphragm phenomenon
    p. incontinence

    p. law
    p. pulse
paradoxically split S$_2$
paradoxic splitting
paradoxus
    pulsus p.
paraffin
    p. bath
    p. section
Paraflex
Parafon Forte DSC
paraganglioma
paraganglion
    adrenergic p.
    aortic p.
    cardiac p.
    cholinergic p.
paragnomen
paragonimiasis
paragonorrheal
parahaemolyticus
    Vibrio p.
parahormone
parainfluenza
    p. viral disease
    p. virus
parakeratosis
paralimbic region
parallax
paralumbar
paralysis, pl. paralyses
    p. agitans
    alcoholic p.
    arsenical p.
    ascending flaccid p.
    Bell p.
    diphtheritic p.
    diver's p.
    familial hyperkalemic periodic p.
    familial hypokalemic periodic p.
    hyperkalemic periodic p.
    hypokalemic periodic p.
    lead p.
    narcosis p.
    normokalemic periodic p.
    p. notariorum
    occupational p.
    periodic p.
    postdiphtheritic p.
    pressure p.
    serum p.
    tourniquet p.
    Vernet p.
    vocal cord p.
    Werdnig-Hoffman p.
paralytic ileus
paramedic
paramedical staff
parameningeal

parameter
paramnesia
paramphistomiasis
paramyloidosis
paramyotonia congenita
Paramyxovirus infection
paranasal sinus tumor
paraneoplastic
    p. acrokeratosis
    p. syndrome
paranesthesia
parangi
paranoia
paraosmia
paraparesis
paraparetic
parapedesis
parapestis
paraphasia
    phonemic p.
    semantic p.
paraphimosis
paraplegia
paraplegic headache
parapneumonic empyema
paraprotein
parapsoriasis en plaques
parasagittal
parascarlatina
parasite
    intestinal p.
    ova and p.'s (O&P)
    protozoan p.
parasitic
    p. disease
    p. hemoptysis
    p. thyroiditis
parasomnia
paraspinal
paraspinous muscle
parasternal
    p. chondrodynia
    p. heave
parasympathetic innervation
parasyphilis
parasyphilitic
parasyphilosis
parasystole
    ventricular p.
parathormone (PTH)
parathyrin

parathyroid
    p. adenoma
    p. gland
    p. hormone (PTH)
    p. hormone level
    p. hormone-related peptide (PTHrP)
    p. insufficiency
    p. osteodystrophy
    p. tetany
parathyroidectomy
    acute p. (APTX)
parathyroidoma
parathyroid-related hypercalcemia
parathyroprival tetany
parathyroprivous
    status p.
paratonia
paratripsis
paratuberculous lymphadenitis
paratyphoid fever
paraventricular
paravertebral triangle
parchemin
    bruit de p.
paregoric
parenchyma
    pulmonary p.
parenchymal
    p. disease
    p. neurocysticercosis
parenchymatous
    p. disease
    p. goiter
    p. hepatitis
parent
    Children of Aging P.'s (CAPS)
parental consent
parenteral
    p. alimentation
    p. anticonvulsant
    p. antihypertensive agent
    p. hyperalimentation
    p. nutrition
    p. therapy
    p. vasodilator
parenteral-controlled analgesia (PCA)
parenteric fever
paresis
    bibrachial p.
    canal p.
paresthesia
    circumoral p.

NOTES

P

paresthetica
    meralgia p.
paretic
parietal
    p. lobe function
    p. pain
    p. peritoneal inflammation
parietitis
parietofrontal
parietooccipital dysfunction
Parinaud syndrome
parity
Park aneurysm
Parkes-Weber syndrome
Parkinson
    P. complex
    P. crisis
    P. dementia complex
    P. disease
    P. facies
    P. mask
    P. rigidity
    P. sign
    P. syndrome
parkinsonian
    p. facies
    p. reaction
parkinsonism
    drug-induced p.
    methyl-phenyl-tetrahydropyridine p.
    MPTP p.
    MPTP-induced p.
    postencephalitic p. (PEP)
    postencephalitis p.
    primary p.
    secondary p.
    vascular p.
Parkinson-like facies
Parkinson's Disease Foundation (PDF)
Parlodel
Parnate
paromomycin
paronychia
parorexia
parosmia
parosteal
parosteitis
parotid
    p. bubo
    p. gland
    p. tenderness
parotidea
    oophoritis p.
    orchitis p.
parotiditis
    epidemic p.
parotitis phlegmonosa
parous
paroxetine

paroxysm
paroxysmal
    p. ataxia
    p. atrial tachycardia
    p. dyskinesia
    p. hypersomnia
    p. hypertension
    p. nocturnal dyspnea (PND)
    p. nocturnal hemoglobinuria
    p. nodal tachycardia (PNT)
    p. peritonitis
    p. positional vertigo
    p. rhabdomyolysis
    p. supraventricular tachycardia
      (PSVT)
    p. tachyarrhythmia
    p. ventricular tachycardia
parrot
    P. disease
    p. fever
    P. node
    p. tongue
    P. ulcer
Parry disease
pars, pl. **partes**
    p. interarticularis
    p. plana vitrectomy
    p. space
parsimony
    law of p.
Parsons disease
partes (*pl. of* pars)
parthenolide
partial
    p. adrenocortical insufficiency
    p. complex seizure
    p. liquid ventilation
    p. parenteral nutrition
    p. pressure alveolar oxygen (PAO_2)
    p. pressure arterial oxygen (PAO_2)
    p. pressure of carbon dioxide
      (PCO_2)
    p. pressure of oxygen (PO_2)
    p. prothrombin time (PPT)
    p. small bowel obstruction (PSBO)
    p. thromboplastin time (PTT)
partial-thickness burn
Partnership for Caring (PFC)
parulis
parvovirus-associated arthritis
parvovirus B19 infection
parvum
    Chrysosporium p.
parvus
PASA
    para-aminosalicylic acid
passive
    p. external rewarming
    p. pulmonary hypertension

past
>p. history (PH)
>p. pointing

Pasteurella
>*P. multocida*
>*P. tularensis*

pasteurellosis
Pastia sign
Patanol
patch
>clonidine p.
>Deponit P.
>herald p.
>MacCallum p.
>Minitran p.
>Nicoderm p.
>Peyer p.
>salon pain p.
>Testoderm p.
>testosterone p.

patchy atelectasis
patella, pl. **patellae**
>baja p.
>chondromalacia patellae

patellar
patellofemoral
patency
>shunt p.

patent
>p. ductus
>p. ductus arteriosus (PDA)
>p. foramen ovale (PFO)

Paterson-Brown-Kelly syndrome
Paterson-Kelly syndrome
Paterson syndrome
pathema
pathoamine
pathoanatomic
pathocrinia
pathoformic
pathogen
>respiratory p.

pathogenesis
pathogenic
pathogenicity
pathogeny
pathognomonic symptom
pathognomy
pathognostic
pathologic
>p. amenorrhea
>p. diagnosis

>p. glycosuria
>p. secondary erythrocytosis

pathological
>p. characteristic
>p. stealing

pathology
>neoplastic p.
>speech and language p.

pathometric
pathometry
pathomimesis
pathomimicry
pathomiosis
pathophysiological
pathophysiology
pathopoiesis
pathosis
pathway
>aldose reductase p.
>ascending p.
>central hypothalamic
> neurochemical p.
>descending p.
>descending motor p.
>His-Purkinje p.
>somatosensory p.

patient (pt)
>airway obstruction in conscious p.
>airway obstruction in
> unconscious p.
>p. autonomy
>p. bill of rights
>p. care technician (PCT)
>community-dwelling p.
>p. compliance
>conscious p.
>p. history
>p. profile
>unconscious p.

patient-controlled analgesia (PCA)
Patrick test
pattern
>cholestatic p.
>circadian p.
>dermatomal p.
>endogenous p.
>motor p.
>nucleolar p.

patulous
pauciarticular
paucibacillary

NOTES

P

pauci-immune crescentic
  glomerulonephritis
paucity
Paul treatment
Pautrier abscess
Pavabid caps
Pavlik harness
Pavy disease
Paxil
Paxipam
payer, payor
    private p.
    third party p.
Payr
    P. disease
    P. sign
PBA
    Prevent Blindness America
PBC
    primary biliary cirrhosis
PBI
    protein-bound iodine
PC
    Rubramin PC
p.c.
    after a meal [L. *post cibum*]
    post cibum
PCA
    parenteral-controlled analgesia
    patient-controlled analgesia
PCF
    pharyngoconjunctival fever
PCO$_2$
    partial pressure of carbon dioxide
PCOS
    polycystic ovary syndrome
PCP
    primary care physician
PCPFS
    President's Council on Physical Fitness
      and Sports
PCR
    percutaneous coronary revascularization
    polymerase chain reaction
    protein catabolic rate
PCS
    Physical Component Summary
PCT
    patient care technician
PD
    pediatric dose
PDA
    patent ductus arteriosus
    personal digital assistant
PDF
    Parkinson's Disease Foundation
PDGF
    platelet-derived growth factor

PDR
    proliferative diabetic retinopathy
PE
    pulmonary embolism
    pulmonary embolus
PEA
    Pulseless Electrical Study
peak
    p. airway pressure
    p. end-expiratory pressure
    p. exercise
    p. expiratory flow (PEF)
    p. oxygen uptake
peau d'orange
peccant humor
Pecquet
    P. cisterna
    P. duct
    P. reservoir
pectora (*pl. of* pectus)
pectoralis
pectoriloquy
    aphonic p.
    whispered p.
pectoris
    angina p.
    postinfarction angina p.
pectorophony
pectus, pl. pectora
    p. e. excavatum
pedal
    p. edema
    p. pulse
    p. spasm
pedatrophia
Pederson speculum
pedes (*pl. of* pes)
Pediamycin
pediatric
    p. back pain
    p. dose (PD)
pediatrician
pediatrics
pediatrist
pediatry
Pediazole
pedicle tip amputation
pediculosis pubis
pedis
    dorsalis p. (DP)
    malum perforans p.
    tinea p.
peduncle
peduncular hallucinosis
peel
    chemical p.
PEEP
    positive end-expiratory pressure

PEF
    peak expiratory flow
PEG
    percutaneous endoscopic gastrostomy
    pneumoencephalogram
        PEG tube
Pegasys
PEH
    postexercise hypotension
pejorative
Pel-Ebstein
        P.-E. disease
        P.-E. fever
        P.-E. pyrexia
        P.-E. symptom
Pelger-Huët nuclear anomaly
peliosis
        bacillary p. (BP)
        bacterial p.
        p. hepatitis
        p. rheumatica
Pelizaeus-Merzbacher disease
pellagra
        infantile p.
        pellagra sine p.
        secondary p.
        typhoid p.
pellagroid
pellagrous
Pellegrini-Stieda disease
pellet implantation
Pellizzi syndrome
pellucid
pellucidi
        septi cavum p.
pelopathy
pelotherapy
pelvic
        p. floor dyssynergia
        p. floor weakness
        p. fracture
        p. inflammatory disease (PID)
        p. mass
        p. muscle exercise
        p. muscle laxity
        p. organ prolapse
        p. pain
        p. ultrasound
        p. vein thrombosis
pelvis, pl. **pelves**
        Otto p.
        platypellic p.

pelvitherm
PEM
    protein-energy malnutrition
Pemberton sign
pemoline
pemphigoid
        bullous p.
pemphigosa
        variola p.
pemphigus
        cicatricial p.
        p. erythematosus
        p. foliaceus
        p. neonatorum
        p. vegetans
        p. vulgaris
penbutolol sulfate
penciclovir
pencil tenderness
Pendred
        P. disease
        P. syndrome
pendulous abdomen
pendulum exercise
penes (*pl. of* penis)
penetrans
        ulcera p.
PenFill insulin cartridge
penicillamine
penicillin
        benzathine p.
        p. benzathine
        phenoxymethyl p.
penicillus
penile prosthesis
penis, pl. **penes**
        gryposis p.
Penrose drain
pension
        P. Rights Center (PRC)
        P. and Welfare Benefits
            Administration (PWBA)
pentaerythritol tetranitrate
pentalogy
Pentam
pentamidine
        aerosolized p.
Pentasa
pentastomiasis
pentavalent form
Pentolair
pentostatin

NOTES

P

Pentothal
pentoxifylline
penumbra
Pen-Vee K
people
>Self Help for Hard of Hearing P., Inc. (SHHH)

PEP
>postencephalitic parkinsonism

Pepcid
Pepper
>P. syndrome
>P. type

pepsic
peptic
>p. stricture
>p. ulcer
>p. ulcer disease (PUD)

peptide
>C p.
>endogenous opioid p.
>gastric inhibitory p. (GIP)
>glucagonlike p. (GLP-1)
>glucagonlike insulinotropic p. (GLIP)
>natriuretic p.
>parathyroid hormone-related p. (PTHrP)
>procollagen p.

peptidoglycan rigid cell wall
Pepto-Bismol
Peptostreptococcus
per
>p. diem
>p. os (p.o.)
>p. primam intentionem
>p. rectum
>p. se
>p. tubam

peracute
peratodynia
perception
>orthonasal p.
>retronasal p.

perceptual-spatial deficit
Percocet
Percodan
Percogesic
percuss
percussible
percussion
>p. and auscultation (P&A)
>auscultatory p.
>bimanual p.
>clavicular p.
>deep p.
>direct p.
>finger p.
>immediate p.

>mediate p.
>Murphy p.
>palpatory p.
>piano p.
>p. sound
>threshold p.

percussor
percutaneous
>p. balloon aortic valvuloplasty
>p. cholangiography
>p. coronary intervention
>p. coronary revascularization (PCR)
>p. endoscopic gastrostomy (PEG)
>p. endoscopic gastrostomy tube
>p. femoral approach
>p. liver biopsy
>p. needle aspiration biopsy (PNAB)
>p. on-surface stimulation (POSS)
>p. transluminal coronary angioplasty (PTCA)
>p. transluminal coronary arteriography (PTCA)

Perdiem
perennial rhinitis
Perez sign
perforated
>p. peptic ulcer

perforating appendicitis
perforation
>colonic p.
>valvular p.

performance
>cognitive p.
>functional p.
>intellectual p.
>physician p.

perfringens
>*Clostridium p.*

perfusate
perfuse
perfusion
>p. defect
>impaired tissue p.
>p. lung scan
>regional p.
>tissue p.

pergolide
Periactin
perianal disease
periaortic
periapical
periappendicitis
periareolar
periarteritis nodosa (PAN)
periarticular
peribronchial
pericallosal
pericardial
>p. cyst

p. disease
p. effusion
p. friction rub
p. tuberculosis
pericardiocentesis
pericarditis
acute p.
postinfarction p.
pyogenic p.
viral p.
pericardium
congenital absence of p.
dropsy of p.
pericaval
pericholangiolitic cirrhosis
pericholangitis
perichondritis
peristernal p.
perichondrium
Peri-Colace
pericolic membrane syndrome
Peridex
Peridium
perihepatitis
perihilar
p. calcification
p. mass
perimembranous
perimenopausal
perimenopause
perinatal HIV transmission
perindopril
p. (Aceon) protection against
recurrent stroke study
(PROGRESS)
p. monotherapy
perineal candidiasis
perinephric abscess
perineum
os p.
period
absolute refractory p. (ARP)
last menstrual p. (LMP)
prodromal p.
quarantine p.
periodic
p. arthralgia
p. disease
p. fever
p. filariasis
p. hypersomnia
p. limb movement (PLM)

p. limb movement disorder
(PLMD)
p. neutropenia
p. paralysis
p. peritonitis
p. polyserositis
p. vomiting
periodicity
periodontal
p. disease
p. infection
perioperative
p. cardiac complication
perioral dermatitis
periorbital freckling
periosteal osteogenesis
periostosis
peripartum
peripatetic
peripheral
p. ageusia
p. agglutinin
p. arterial disease (PAD)
p. arthritis
p. blood pressure
p. blood smear
p. edema
p. hypoperfusion
p. nerve
p. nerve root syndrome
p. nervous system disorder
p. neuropathy
p. neutropenia
p. parenteral nutrition
p. polyneuropathy
p. root compression
p. vascular disease
p. vascular resistance (PVR)
p. venous disease
peripherally
p. inserted catheter (PIC)
p. inserted catheter line
p. inserted central catheter (PICC)
periportal cirrhosis
perirectal infection
peristalsis
reversed p.
peristasis
peristernal perichondritis
peritheliomatous
perithoracic

NOTES

P

peritoneal
    p. cavity
    p. irritation
    p. lavage
    p. tuberculosis
peritonealgia
peritoneopathy
peritoneoscopic
peritoneum
peritonitis
    acute p.
    benign paroxysmal p.
    chemical p.
    p. deformans
    focal p.
    granulomatous p.
    paroxysmal p.
    periodic p.
    primary p.
    secondary p.
    tuberculous p.
peritonsillar
peritovenous
peritracheal
Peritrate SA
perityphlitis actinomycotica
periumbilical pain
periungual
perivalvular abscess
periventricular leukomalacia
perkinism
PERL
    pupils equal and reactive to light
PERLA
    pupils equal and reactive to light and
      accommodation
perléche
Perles
    Tessalon P.
perlingual
permanent pacemaker
Permapen
Permax
PermCath
    Davol P.
permeability
    membrane p.
pernicieux
    accès p.
perniciosiform
pernicious
    p. anemia
    p. maculation
    p. malaria
    p. vomiting
pernio
    lupus p.
peroneal nerve palsy
peroneus brevis

peroral endoscopy
peroxidation
    lipid p.
peroxide
    benzoyl p.
    carbamide p.
    hydrogen p.
Perphenazine
PERRLA
    pupils equal, round and reactive to light
      and accommodation
PERS
    personal emergency response system
Persa-Gel
Persantine
Persantine-thallium stress test
persecutory delusion
perseverate
Persian
    P. Gulf syndrome
    P. relapsing fever
persistence
persistent
    p. abdominal pain
    p. asthma
    p. generalized lymphadenopathy
    p. hepatitis
    p. hyperphenylalaninemia
    p. proteinuria
persisting hepatitis
person
    American Association of
      Retired P.'s (AARP)
    community-residing p.
personal
    p. digital assistant (PDA)
    p. emergency response system
      (PERS)
    p. habit
personality
    p. disorder
    histrionic p.
    narcissistic p.
person-years
perspective
perspiration
Perthes
    P. disease
    P. test
pertinent
perturbation
pertussis
    Bordetella p.
    diphtheria, tetanus toxoids, and
      acellular p. (DTaP)
    Infanrix diphtheria, tetanus toxoid,
      and acellular p.
    p. syndrome
pertussis-like syndrome

peruana
    verruca p.
    verruga p.
perusal
Peruvian wart
perversion
    taste p.
pes, pl. **pedes**
    p. anserinus
    p. anserinus bursitis
    p. cavus
    p. planus
pessary
    cube p.
    doughnut p.
    Gellhorn p.
    Hodge p.
    ring p.
pessimism
    therapeutic p.
pest
pesticemia
pestiferous
pestilence
pestilential
pestis
    p. ambulans
    p. bubonica
    p. fulminans
    p. major
    p. minor
    p. siderans
PET
    positron emission tomography
petechia, pl. **petechiae**
    palatal petechiae
petechial purpura
petit mal seizure
pétrissage
petrositis
Peutz-Jeghers syndrome
Peyer patch
Peyronie
    P. disease
    P. plaque
Pfannenstiel incision
Pfaundler-Hurler syndrome
PFC
    Partnership for Caring
Pfeiffer
    P. bacillus

    P. disease
    P. test
PFF
    Pulmonary Fibrosis Foundation
Pfizerpen
PFO
    patent foramen ovale
PFT
    pulmonary function test
Pfuhl sign
pg
    picogram
PGA
    prostaglandin A
PGWB
    Psychological General Well-Being Scale
PH
    past history
pH
    hydrogen ion concentration
    pH monitoring
phacolysin
phacomatosis
phagocyte
    mononuclear p.
phagocytophilia
    Ehrlichia p.
phagocytosis
phakomatosis
phalangeal
phalanx, pl. **phalanges**
Phalen
    P. sign
    P. test
phalilalia
phallalgia
phallodynia
phanerogenic
pharmaceutical
pharmacodiagnosis
pharmacodynamic change
pharmacodynamics
    altered p.
pharmacokinetic change
pharmacologic
    p. management
    p. stress testing
    p. therapy
    p. treatment
pharmacology
pharmacotherapy
    symptomatic p.

NOTES

P

pharmokinetic interaction
pharyngeal
    p. candidiasis
    p. gonococcal infection
    p. pouch syndrome
pharynges (*pl. of* pharynx)
pharyngeus
    globus p.
pharyngitis
    candidal p.
    gonococcal p.
    p. sicca
pharyngoconjunctival
    acute p. (APC)
    p. fever (PCF)
    p. fever virus
pharyngoesophageal diverticulum
pharyngotonsillitis
    herpetic p.
pharynx, pl. **pharynges**
    erythematous p.
phase
    expiratory p.
    icteric p.
    inspiratory p.
    Korotkoff p.
    p. O potential
    preicteric p.
Phazyme
Phenaphen
phenazopyridine hydrochloride
Phenchlor
phencyclidine toxicity
Phenergan with codeine
phenobarbital
phenol
phenolphthalein
phenolsulfonphthalein (PSP)
phenomenology
phenomenon, pl. **phenomena**
    anaphylactoid p.
    Becker p.
    Cushing p.
    Danysz p.
    dawn p.
    fall-and-rise p.
    first-set p.
    Friedreich p.
    halisteresis p.
    Hayflick limit p.
    Hecht p.
    Hering p.
    Jod-Basedow p.
    Leede-Rumpel p.
    Lucio p.
    Martin-Gruber p.
    paradoxical diaphragm p.
    Raynaud p.
    Rumpel-Leede p.

    second-set p.
    Somogyi p.
    Staub-Traugott p.
    Trousseau p.
    vacuolization p.
    vacuum joint p.
phenothiazine
phenotype
    atherogenic low-density lipoprotein
        pattern B p.
phenoxybenzamine
phenoxymethyl penicillin
phentermine
    fenfluramine and p.
phentolamine test
phenylalanine
phenylalkylamine
phenylbutazone
phenylephrine
phenylhydrazine hemolysis
phenylketonuria (PKU)
    Fölling p.
phenylpropanolamine
phenylpyruvica
    Moraxella p.
phenylpyruvic oligophrenia
phenytoin
pheochrome
pheochromoblast
pheochromocytoma
PHH
    posthemorrhagic hydrocephalus
Philadelphia
    P. chromosome
    P. Geriatric Center Morale Scale
philanthropic hospital
philiater
Philippine hemorrhagic fever
philtrum, pl. **philtra**
phimosis
pHisoDerm
pHisoHex
phlebalgia
phlebitic
phlebitis
    superficial p.
phleboclysis
    drip p.
phlebolith
phlebology
phlebotomize
phlebotomus fever
phlebotomy
phlegm
phlegmasia
phlegmatic
phlegmon
phlegmonosa
    parotitis p.

phlegmonous
    p. adenitis
    p. enteritis
phlogistic
phlorizin diabetes
phobia
    social p.
Phoma
phonacoscope
phonacoscopy
phonating
phonemic paraphasia
phonendoscope
phonic tic
phonocardiogram
phonophobia
phonophore
phosgene gas inhalation
Phosphaljel
phosphatase
    acid p.
    alkaline p.
    prostatic acid p.
phosphate
    p. depletion
    p. diabetes
    oral p.
    p. supplementation
    p. tetany
    tubular reabsorption p. (TRP)
phosphatidosis
phosphatidylinositide
3′-phosphoadenosine-5′-phosphosulfate
phosphodiesterase
    p. inhibitor
    oral p.
phosphokinase
    creatine p. (CPK)
phospholipid
phosphopenia, phosphorpenia
phosphorus necrosis
phosphorylase
Phospho-Soda
    Fleet P.-S.
phosphuresis
phosphuria
photoallergy
photochemical radiation
photocoagulation
    argon laser p.
photodamage
photodermatitis

photodynamic therapy
photography
    stereoscopic fundus p.
photopathy
photophobia
photoplethysmography
photoprotection
photoreceptor
photosensitivity
phototherapy
PHP
    panhypopituitarism
    primary hyperparathyroidism
phrenic
    p. nerve
    p. pressure test
phrenospasm
phrygian cap
PHS
    Public Health Service
phthisiologist
phthisis, pl. **phthises**
    diabetic p.
    p. pancreatica
phylaxis
phyllode
    cystosarcoma p.
physalopteriasis
physiatrician
physiatrics
physiatrist
physic
physical
    p. activity
    p. age
    p. allergy
    P. Component Summary (PCS)
    p. diagnosis
    p. disimpaction
    p. examination
    p. fitness
    p. handicap
    history and p. (H&P)
    p. self-endangerment
    p. sign
    p. therapist (PT)
    p. therapy (PT)
physician
    American Academy of Family P.'s
    (AAFP)
    p. assistant (PA)
    attending p.

NOTES

P

physician *(continued)*
  family p.
  Fellow of the American College of P.'s (FACP)
  Fellow of the American College of Chest P.'s (FACCP)
  Fellow of the Royal College of P.'s (Canada) (FRCP(C))
  Fellow of the Royal College of P.'s (Edinburgh) (FRCP(E))
  Fellow of the Royal College of P.'s (England) (FRCP)
  Fellow of the Royal College of P.'s (Ireland) (FRCP(I))
  general p.
  internal medicine p.
  Licentiate of the Royal College of P.'s (Edinburgh) (LRCP(E))
  Licentiate of the Royal College of P.'s (Ireland) (LRCP(I))
  Licentiate of the Royal College of P.'s (of England) (LRCP)
  Member of the Royal College of P.'s (Edinburgh) (MRCP(E))
  Member of the Royal College of P.'s (Ireland) (MRCP(I))
  Member of the Royal College of P.'s (of England) (MRCP)
  osteopathic p.
  p. performance
  primary care p. (PCP)
  resident p.
  Royal College of P.'s (Edinburgh) (RCP(E))
  Royal College of P.'s (Ireland) (RCP(I))
  Royal College of P.'s (of England) (RCP)
physician-assisted suicide
Physick pouch
physiognomy
physiognosis
physiologic
  p. anemia
  p. dwarfism
  p. icterus
  p. murmur
  p. splitting
  p. vertigo
physiological condition
physiologist
physiology
  Eisenmenger p.
  pulmonary p.
physiopsychic
physiopyrexia
physiotherapeutic
physiotherapist
physiotherapy

phytobezoar
phytochemical
phytohemagglutinin
phytosis
phytotherapy
phytotrichobezoar
pial
  p. vein
pian
piano
  p. key maneuver
  p. percussion
piaulement
  bruit de p.
PIC
  peripherally inserted catheter
  PIC line
pica
PICC
  peripherally inserted central catheter
Pick
  P. adenoma
  P. atrophy
  P. body
  P. cell
  P. disease
  P. syndrome
pickwickian syndrome
picogram (pg)
picolinate
  chromium p.
Picornaviridae
PID
  pelvic inflammatory disease
PIE
  pulmonary interstitial emphysema
piecemeal necrosis
Pierini
  atrophoderma of Pasini and P.
Pierre Robin syndrome
piezogenic
pigbel
pig bronchus
pigeon chest
piggyback
pigmentary
  p. cirrhosis
  p. glaucoma
pigment cirrhosis
pigmented
  p. liver
  p. villonodular synovitis
pigment-induced renal injury
pigmentosa
  retinitis p. (RP)
pigmentosum
  xeroderma p.
pigmenturia
pigtail catheter

PIH
 pregnancy-induced hypertension
pilar
pilaris
 pityriasis rubra p.
pili (*pl. of* pilus)
pill
 birth control p.
 p. burden
 p. induced
 oral contraceptive p. (OCP)
 serenity-tranquility-peace p.
 sleeping p.
 STP p.
pill-induced esophagitis
pillow
 nasal p.
pill-rolling tremor
pilocarpine
pilocystic
piloerection
pilonidal
 p. cyst
 p. sinus
pilorum
 arrectores p.
pilos
pilosis
pilus, pl. **pili**
 pili incarnati barbae
pimclorrhea
pimelorthopnea
pimozide
pin
 Steinmann p.
pindolol
pineal
 p. calcification
 p. disease
 p. gland
 p. tumor
pinguecula
pink
 p. disease
 p. puffer
pinna, pl. **pinnae**
pinprick
 decreased p.
 p. test
pins-and-needles
pinta fever
pioglitazone HCl

piorthopnea
PIP
 proximal interphalangeal
piperacillin
 p. and tazobactam
piperonyl
pipe stem cirrhosis
piqûre diabetes
piracetam
pirbuterol
piriform
piriformis muscle spasm
Pirogoff
 P. amputation
 P. edema
piroxicam
Pirquet index
PIS
 primary immunodeficiency syndrome
pisotriquetral
pitted keratolysis
pitting edema
Pittsburgh pneumonia
pituitarism
pituitary
 p. adenoma
 p. basophilia
 p. basophilism
 p. cachexia
 p. disorder
 p. dwarf
 p. dwarfism
 p. enlargement
 p. eunuchism
 p. function test
 p. gigantism
 p. gland
 p. gonadotropic hormone
 p. gonadotropin
 p. growth hormone
 p. hyperfunction
 p. hypoadrenocorticism
 p. hypofunction
 p. hypogonadism
 p. imaging
 p. infantilism
 p. insufficiency
 p. myxedema
 p. necrosis
 p. tumor
pityriasis
 p. alba

NOTES

P

pityriasis *(continued)*
   p. lichenoides et varioliformis
   p. rosea
   p. rubra pilaris
   p. versicolor
Pityrosporon
Pityrosporum ovale
pizotifen
pizotyline
PKU
   phenylketonuria
placebo effect
placement
placental growth hormone
placenta protein
placentotherapy
placing
   neonatal p.
plafond
plagiocephaly
plague
   ambulant p.
   black p.
   bubonic p.
   glandular p.
   hemorrhagic p.
   larval p.
   Pahvant Valley p.
   p. pneumonia
   pneumonic p.
   pulmonic p.
   p. septicemia
   septicemic p.
plain
   p. Marcaine
   p. spine radiograph
plan
   aftercare p.
   capitated health p.
   subjective, objective, assessment,
      and p. (SOAP)
   treatment p.
plana *(pl. of* planum)
planar xanthoma
planimetry
planning
   care p.
   meal p.
planocellular
plant alkaloid
plantar
   p. fasciitis
   p. keratosis
   p. reflex
   p. wart
plantigrade
planum, pl. **plana**
   plana verruca
planuria

planus
   lichen p.
   pes p.
plaque
   amyloid p.
   atherosclerotic p.
   en p.'s
   fibroproliferative p.
   fibrous p.
   neuritic p.
   parapsoriasis en p.'s
   Peyronie p.
   senile p.
Plaquenil
plasma
   p. adrenocorticotropic hormone
      level
   p. cell
   p. cell hepatitis
   p. cell leukemia
   p. cortisol
   p. free T4
   fresh frozen p. (FFP)
   p. glucose
   p. iodoprotein disorder
   p. leptin concentration
   p. osmolality
   p. protamine paracoagulation
   p. somatomedin C
   p. testosterone
   p. therapy
   p. thyroid-stimulating hormone
      assay
plasmacytic leukemia
plasmacytoma
   solitary p.
plasmacytosis
plasmapheresis
plasminogen
   fibrin-bound p.
Plasmodium
   P. falciparum
   P. malariae
   P. ovale
   P. vivax
plaster
   Sal-Acid p.
plastic bronchitis
plasticity
Plastizote insert
plate
   growth p.
   p. guard
   nail p.
plateau
platelet
   p. activation defect
   p. adhesion
   p. aggregation

p. aggregation inhibitor
p. alloimmunization
p. count
p. destruction
p. disorder
p. function study
hemolysis, elevated liver enzymes, low p.'s (HELLP)
p. transfusion
platelet-derived growth factor (PDGF)
platelet-stimulating factor
Platinol, Adriamycin, cyclophosphamide (PAC)
platinum-containing agent
platypellic pelvis
platypelloid
platypnea
platypodia
Plaut angina
Plavix
playing
role p.
pleconaril
pledget
Erycette p.
soaked cotton p. 4%
Plendil
pleocytosis
mononuclear cell p.
pleomorphic
Plesiomonas shigelloides **infection**
plessesthesia
plessimeter
plessimetric
plessor
plethora
plethysmography
impedance p.
pleura, pl. **pleurae**
p. inflammation
pleuracentesis
pleural
p. biopsy
p. crackle
p. disease
p. effusion
p. fluid cytologic examination
p. fluid eosinophilia
p. fremitus
p. friction rub
p. rale
p. tuberculosis

pleuralgia
pleurisy
benign dry p.
bilateral p.
chronic p.
chyliform p.
diaphragmatic p.
double p.
epidemic benign dry p.
epidemic diaphragmatic p.
mediastinal p.
typhoid p.
pleuritic
p. chest pain
p. pneumonia
p. rub
pleuritis
pleurocentesis
pleurocholecystitis
pleurodynia
epidemic p.
pleurogenic
pleurogenous
pleurohepatitis
pleuropulmonary disease
pleurotyphoid
pleximeter
plexitis
plexometer
plexopathy
benign brachial p.
brachial p.
plexor
plexus
Auerbach p.
brachial p.
choroid p.
Kiesselbach p.
plicamycin
plication
PLM
periodic limb movement
PLMD
periodic limb movement disorder
plombage
plongeurs
maladie de p.
plug
keratin p.
punctal p.
plumbism
plumbotherapy

NOTES

P

Plummer
- P. disease
- P. sign

Plummer-Vinson syndrome
pluricausal
pluriresistant
plus
- Ionil-T P.
- Lorcet P.

PMC
- pseudomembranous colitis

PMDD
- premenstrual dysphoric disorder

PMDS
- premenstrual dysphoric syndrome

PMI
- point of maximal impulse
- point of maximal intensity

PMMA
- polymethylmethacrylate

PMN
- polymorphonuclear

PMO
- postmenopausal osteoporosis

PMR
- polymyalgia rheumatica

PNAB
- percutaneous needle aspiration biopsy

PND
- paroxysmal nocturnal dyspnea

pneopneic reflex
pneumatic
- p. dilation

pneumatoscope
pneumatosis
- p. cystoides intestinalis
  pneumococcus
- p. intestinalis

pneumobilia
pneumocholecystitis
pneumococcal
- p. acute otitis media
- p. empyema
- p. pneumonia
- p. polysaccharide vaccine

pneumococcal-CRM197 conjugate vaccine
pneumococci (*pl. of* pneumococcus)
pneumococcosis
Pneumococcus
pneumococcus, pl. **pneumococci**
- pneumatosis cystoides intestinalis p.

pneumocolon
pneumoconiosis, pneumokoniosis
- asbestosis p.
- bauxite p.
- coal worker's p. (CWP)
- collagenous p.
- rheumatoid p.

p. siderotica
silicate p.
Pneumocystis
- *P. carinii*
- *P. carinii* pneumonia
- *P. infection*

pneumocystosis
pneumoempyema
pneumoencephalogram (PEG)
pneumokoniosis (*var. of* pneumoconiosis)
pneumology
pneumolysin
- p. antibody
- p. antigen-antibody

pneumomediastinum
pneumomycosis
pneumonectomy
pneumonia
- acute eosinophilic p.
- acute interstitial p.
- adenoviral p.
- alcoholic p.
- amebic p.
- anthrax p.
- apex p.
- apical p.
- aspiration p.
- atypical p.
- bacillary p.
- bacterial p.
- bilious p.
- bronchial p.
- bronchiolitis obliterans organizing p.
- candidal p.
- caseous p.
- catarmal p.
- central p.
- cerebral p.
- chemical p.
- chlamydial p.
- chronic eosinophilic p.
- community-acquired p. (CAP)
- congenital p.
- core p.
- croupous p.
- cytomegalovirus p.
- deglutition p.
- desquamative p.
- desquamative interstitial p. (DIP)
- p. dissecans
- double p.
- eosinophilic p.
- fibrous p.
- Friedländer bacillus p.
- gangrenous p.
- giant cell p.
- Hecht p.
- herpes p.
- hypersensitivity p.

hypostatic p.
idiopathic interstitial p.
infant p.
influenza p.
influenzal virus p.
inhalation p.
p. interlobularis purulenta
interstitial plasma cell p.
intrauterine p.
Klebsiella p.
Legionnaires p.
lobar p.
lymphocytic interstitial p.
p. malleosa
massive p.
metastatic p.
migratory p.
Mycoplasma p.
mycoplasmal p.
necrotizing p.
nonspecific interstitial p.
nosocomial p.
obstructive p.
oil p.
opportunistic p.
Pittsburgh p.
plague p.
pleuritic p.
pneumococcal p.
Pneumocystis carinii p.
primary atypical p.
progressive p.
purulent p.
rheumatic p.
segmental p.
septic p.
simple eosinophilic p.
staphylococcal p.
Staphylococcus aureus p.
streptococcal p.
superficial p.
suppurative p.
terminal p.
toxemic p.
traumatic p.
tuberculous p.
tularemic p.
typhoid p.
unilateral p.
unresolved p.
uremic p.
usual interstitial p.

p. vaccine
ventilator-associated p. (VAP)
viral p.
walking p.
wandering p.
white p.
woolsorter's p.
pneumoniae
    Chlamydia p.
    Klebsiella p.
    Legionella p.
    Mycoplasma p.
    Streptococcus p.
pneumonic plague
pneumonitis
    acute interstitial p.
    aspiration p.
    chemical p.
    chronic aspiration p.
    cryptogenic organizing p.
    hypersensitivity p.
    interstitial p.
    lymphocytic interstitial p.
pneumonoconiosis, pneumonokoniosis
pneumonopathy
    eosinophilic p.
pneumonopleuritis
pneumoperitoneum
pneumophagia
pneumopleuritis
pneumoretroperitoneum
pneumoscope
pneumotachygraph
pneumothorax, pl. **pneumothoraces**
    pressure p.
Pneumovax
PNT
    paroxysmal nodal tachycardia
PO₂
    partial pressure of oxygen
p.o.
    by mouth [L. *per os*]
    per os
POAG
    primary open-angle glaucoma
pocket
    rheumatoid p.
podagra
podagral
poditis
    tourniquet p.
podocyte

NOTES

P

309

podophyllin
Podospora anserina
POEMS
    polyneuropathy, organomegaly,
    endocrinopathy, monoclonal
    gammopathy, skin change
      POEMS syndrome
pogoniasis
poietin
poikilocyte
poikilocytosis
poikiloderma
poikilothermia
poikilothermy
poikilothymia
point
    Clado p.
    de Mussy p.
    Desjardins p.
    p. epidemic
    Guéneau de Mussy p.
    Hallé p.
    p. of maximal impulse (PMI)
    p. of maximal intensity (PMI)
    Mayo-Robson p.
    McBurney p.
    Munro p.
    ogival p.
    Ramond p.
    trigger p. (TP)
pointes
    torsades de p.
pointing
    past p.
Poiseuille law
poison
    acrid p.
    puffer p.
    shellfish p.
poisoning
    acetaminophen p.
    ackee p.
    bacterial food p.
    blood p.
    carbon disulfide p.
    carbon monoxide p.
    central nervous system p.
    djenkol p.
    food p.
    lead p.
    manganese p.
    mercury p.
    methyl-phenyl-tetrahydropyridine p.
    MPTP p.
    mushroom p.
    organic solvent p.
    organophosphorous compound p.
    oxygen p.
    salicylate p.

    Salmonella food p.
    silver p.
    Staphylococcus food p.
    sulfur dioxide p.
    tetraethyl p.
    thallium p.
Poitou colic
Poland syndrome
Polaramine
polar anemia
pole
poliodystrophy
polioencephalitis
    superior hemorrhagic p.
poliomyelitis
    bulbar p.
    p. vaccine
poliovirus
polka fever
pollakidipsia
pollakiuria
pollicis longus brevis
pollinosis
polyadenitis maligna
polyangiitis
    microscopic p.
    p. overlap syndrome
polyarcuate
polyarteritis nodosa
polyarthralgia
polyarthritis
    p. chronica
    epidemic p.
    p. rheumatica acuta
    seronegative p.
polyarthropathy
polyarthrosis
polyarticular
    p. arthritis
    p. gout
polyavitaminosis
polycarbophil
    calcium p.
polychondritis
    relapsing p.
polychondropathia
polychondropathy
polychromasia
Polycillin
Polycitra-K crystal
polyclinic
polyclonal
polycystic
    p. kidney disease
    p. ovary disease
    p. ovary syndrome (PCOS)
    p. pancreas
polycythemia
    compensatory p.

p. hypertonica
inappropriate p.
myelopathic p.
primary p.
relative p.
p. rubra
p. rubra vera
secondary p.
splenomegalic p.
spurious p.
stress p.
polydipsia
primary p.
polydystrophy
pseudo-Hurler p.
polyendocrine
p. adenomatosis
p. deficiency syndrome
polyendocrinopathy
polyene antibiotic
polyethylene glycol
polygenic hypercholesterolemia
polyglandular endocrine syndrome
polyhedral
polyhydramnios
polyleptic fever
polymenorrhea
polymerase
p. chain reaction (PCR)
p. chain reaction test
polymer fume fever
polymethylmethacrylate (PMMA)
p. bone cement
polymicrobial
p. bacteriuria
p. etiology
polymorbidity
polymorphism
polymorphonuclear (PMN)
p. cell
p. segmented neutrophils (polys)
polymyalgia rheumatica (PMR)
polymyositis
trichinous p.
polymyositis/dermatomyositis
polymyxin B-neomycin-cortisone drop
polyneuritis
acute febrile p.
acute idiopathic p.
acute infective p.
acute postinfectious p.
alcoholic p.

anemic p.
ascending p.
p. cerebralis menieriformis
cranial p.
diabetic p.
endemic p.
febrile p.
p. gallinarum
Guillain-Barré p.
hypertrophic p.
idiopathic p.
infectious p.
infective p.
Jamaica ginger p.
postinfectious p.
p. potatorum
progressive hypertrophic p.
p. syndrome
triorthocresyl phosphate p.
polyneuropathy
erythredema p.
nutritional p.
p., organomegaly, endocrinopathy, monoclonal gammopathy, skin change (POEMS)
p., organomegaly, endocrinopathy, monoclonal gammopathy, skin change syndrome
peripheral p.
uremic p.
polynuclear neutrophils
polyopsia
polyostotic
polyp
cervical p.
colorectal p.
polypapilloma
polyparesis
polypathia
polypectomy
polypeptide
gastric inhibitory p. (GIP)
glucose-dependent insulinotropic p.
p. mediator
vasoactive intestinal p. (VIP)
polypeptide-secreting tumor
polyphagia
polypharmacy
polyplasmia
polypnea
polypoid lesion

NOTES

P

polyposa
> enteritis p.

polyposia

polyposis coil syndrome

polypragmasy

polypropylene brace

polyrrhea

polys
> polymorphonuclear segmented
> neutrophils

polysaccharide vaccine

polyserositis
> familial paroxysmal p.
> periodic p.
> recurrent p.

polysomnography
> nocturnal p. (NPSG)

Polytrim

polytrophic

polyunsaturated
> p. fatty acid (PUFA)
> p. lecithin

polyuria test

polyvalent

polyvinyl

Pompe disease

pompholyx

POMS
> Profile of Mood States
> POMS Questionnaire

Poncet
> P. disease
> P. rheumatism

Pondimin

ponos

Ponstel

pontine infarct

pontis
> cisterna p.

pool
> abdominal p.

poorly
> p. contractile bladder
> p. differentiated neoplasm

poor posture

poples

popliteal
> p. artery aneurysm
> p. artery entrapment syndrome
> p. cyst
> p. cystic degeneration

population
> baby boomer p.

POR
> problem-oriented record

porcine valve

porencephalia

porins
> lipopolysaccharide p.

pork
> p. insulin
> p. Lente

porokeratosis

porphobilinogen

porphyria
> acute intermittent p.
> congenital erythropoietic p.
> p. cutanea tarda
> p. cutanea tarda hereditaria
> p. cutanea tarda symptomatica
> erythropoietic p.
> hepatic p.
> p. hepatica
> hepatoerythropoietic p.
> intermittent p.
> intermittent acute p. (IAP)
> ovulocyclic p.
> South African-type p.
> symptomatic p.
> variegate p.

porphyrin

porphyrinopathy

porphyrism

portacaval shunt

porta hepatis

portal
> p. cirrhosis
> p. hypertension
> p. hypertensive gastropathy
> p. lobulation
> p. pressure
> p. vein
> p. vein thrombosis

portasystemic

Porter-Silber

portopulmonary syndrome

portosystemic shunt

Portuguese-type amyloidosis

port-wine
> p.-w. stain
> p.-w. stain birthmark

Posadas disease

Posadas-Wernicke disease

position
> jackknife p.
> orthopnea p.
> orthopneic p.
> prone p.
> supine p.
> Trendelenburg p.

positional vertigo

positive
> p. end-expiratory pressure (PEEP)
> predictive value p.
> p. predictive value
> trace p.

positive-sense genome

positron emission tomography (PET)

Posner-Schlossman syndrome
posologic
posology
POSS
    percutaneous on-surface stimulation
possible
    as soon as p. (ASAP)
post
    p. acute care
    p. cibum (after a meal [L. *post cibum*], p.c.)
    p. hypercapnia
    p. resuscitation
    p. resuscitation care
    p. resuscitative care
    status p. (S/P)
postadenectomy cellulitis
postadolescence
postadrenalectomy syndrome
postcapillary pulmonary hypertension
postcardiotomy delirium
postcibal metabolic rate
postconcussional headache
postconcussion headache
postconcussive syndrome
postdiphtheritic paralysis
postencephalitic parkinsonism (PEP)
postencephalitis parkinsonism
posterior
    anterior and p. (A&P)
    p. cortical atrophy
    p. cruciate ligament
    p. fontanelle
    p. interosseous syndrome
    p. myocardial infarction
    p. pituitary hormone
    p. tibial (PT)
    p. tibial pulse
    p. tibial tendinitis
    p. urethral valve
    p. vitreous detachment (PVD)
posteroanterior (PA)
    p. line
posteroinferior
posterolateral myocardial infarction
postexercise hypotension (PEH)
postexertional asthma
postexposure
postfall syndrome
postfebrile
postganglionic

postgastrectomy syndrome
posthemorrhagic hydrocephalus (PHH)
posthepatic
posthepatitic cirrhosis
postherpetic neuralgia
posthitis
posthypoglycemic hyperglycemia
postictal state
postinfarction
    p. cardiomyopathy
    p. pericarditis
postinfectious
    p. bradycardia
    p. polyneuritis
    p. psychosis
postinfluenzal encephalitis
postintervention
postmalarial
postmastectomy
postmature infant
postmenopausal
    p. bleeding
    p. hormonal replacement
    p. osteoporosis (PMO)
postmenopause
postmicturition syncope
postmortem examination
postnatal life
postnecrotic cirrhosis
postoperative
    p. adjuvant chemotherapy
    p. bronchopneumonia
    p. delirium
    p. heart failure
    p. hypertension
    p. hypothyroidism
    p. intraabdominal abscess
    p. myocardial infarction
    p. premature ventricular contraction
    p. pulmonary complication
    p. shock
    p. supraventricular tachycardia
    p. tetany
    p. wound infection
postpartum
    p. amenorrhea
    p. hemorrhagic hypopituitarism
    p. iliofemoral thrombophlebitis
    p. pituitary necrosis
    p. renal failure
    p. thyroiditis
postphlebitic syndrome

NOTES

P

postpneumonic
postpolio syndrome
postprandial
    p. blood sugar (PPBS)
    p. glycemic control
    p. hypoglycemia
    p. hypotension
    p. lipemia
    p. pain
postprimary tuberculosis
postprostate massage urine
postpuberal
postpuberty
postpubescent
postradiation complication
postreceptor
postremission
postrenal acute renal failure
postrotatory
postscarlatinal
poststatic dyskinesia
poststreptococcal glomerulonephritis
postsurgical incontinence
posttest odds
postthrombotic syndrome
posttransfusion
    p. infection
    p. purpura
posttransplantation
posttransplant infection
posttraumatic
    p. acute renal failure (PTARF)
    p. stress disorder
    p. vertigo
posttussis suction sound
posttussive
    p. rale
    p. suction
    p. syncope
posttyphoid
postulate
postural
    p. ability
    p. blood pressure
    p. collapse
    p. drainage therapy
    p. hypotension
    p. instability
    p. insufficiency
    p. reflex
    p. tremor
    p. vertigo
posture
    poor p.
posturography
    computerized dynamic p. (CDP)
postvaccinal
postvenectomy cellulitis
postviral syndrome

postvoid
    p. residual (PVR)
    p. residual determination
    p. residual volume
potassium (K)
    p. balance
    p. chloride (KCl)
    clavulanate p.
    p. cyanide inhalation
    p. deficit
    p. depletion
    diclofenac p.
    p. homeostasis
    p. hydroxide (KOH)
    p. intake
    losartan p.
    p. loss
    p. nitrate paper
    p. redistribution
    p. salt
potassium-sparing diuretic
potatorum
    polyneuritis p.
potency
    sexual p.
potent
potentia
potential
    p. bias
    compound muscle action p.
      (CMAP)
    p. drawback
    late p.
    phase O p.
potion
Pott
    P. aneurysm
    P. disease
    P. gangrene
    P. syndrome
Potter
    P. facies
    P. syndrome
Potts anastomosis
pouch
    Physick p.
    Rathke p.
poudrage
    talc p.
Poulet disease
poultry handler's disease
pounding
powder
    p. burn
    Goody's p.'s
    inhalation p.
power of attorney
pox
    Kaffir p.

Ppa
    pulmonary artery
PPBS
    postprandial blood sugar
PPD
    purified protein derivative
PPDR
    preproliferative diabetic retinopathy
PPI
    proton pump inhibitor
PPT
    partial prothrombin time
Ppv
    pulmonary vein
P-QRS morphology
PQRST interval
PR
    PR interval
    PR segment
practical nurse
practice
    extramural p.
    family p.
    general p.
    group p.
    intramural p.
practitioner
    alternative p.
    nurse p.
Prader-Willi-Angelman syndrome
Prader-Willi syndrome
praecox
    icterus p.
    lymphedema p.
    macrogenitosomia p.
praesens
    status p.
pralidoxime
pramipexole
Pramosone
Pramoxine
prandial insulin
Prandin
Pravachol
pravastatin
prazepam
praziquantel
prazosin
PRBC
    packed red blood cells
PRC
    Pension Rights Center

preagonal
prealbumin (PAB)
preauthorization
precapillary pulmonary hypertension
precaution
    airborne p.
    contact p.
    droplet p.
    health care employee p.
    universal p.'s
precipitate
precipitating
    p. cause
    p. factor
precipitous
precirrhotic
precision
    P. monitor
    P. Q-I-D blood glucose monitoring system
    P. Sure Dose insulin syringe
preclinical
precocious
    p. pseudopuberty
    p. puberty
precocity
    sexual p.
precordia
precordial catch syndrome
Precose
precritical
precursor
    dopamine p.
prediabetes
predictive
    p. value
    p. value negative
    p. value positive
predictor
predilection
    ethnic p.
predispose
predisposing cause
predisposition
prednisolone
prednisone
    p. burst
    cyclophosphamide, hydroxydaunomycin, Oncovin, p. (CHOP)
preeclampsia
preejaculatory

NOTES

P

preexcitation
 ventricular p.
prefracture mobility
preganglionic
pregnancy
 abdominal pain in p.
 acute abdomen in p.
 arrhythmia in p.
 asthma and p.
 bacterial endocarditis in p.
 breast cancer and p.
 chronic hypertension in p.
 diabetes of p.
 p. diabetes
 epilepsy and p.
 glucose intolerance and p.
 hypertension and p.
 hyperthyroidism in p.
 inflammatory bowel disease and p.
 macrocytic anemia of p.
 mitral stenosis in p.
 molar p.
 primary pulmonary hypertension
 in p.
 pulmonary tuberculosis and p.
 radiation exposure in p.
 renal disease and p.
 renal transplantation and p.
 sarcoidosis and p.
 p. in systemic lupus erythematosus
 p. test
 unplanned p.
 urinary tract infection and p.
 valvular heart disease in p.
pregnancy-induced hypertension (PIH)
pregnane
pregnanediol
pregnanedione
pregnanetriol
pregnenolone
prehepatic
 p. edema
 p. hypoproteinemia
prehormone
preicteric phase
preintervention
Preisz-Nocard bacillus
preleukemia
preleukemic
preload
premalignant
Premarin
premature
 p. aging
 p. atherosclerosis
 p. atrial complex
 p. atrioventricular junctional
 complex
 p. ejaculation

 p. morbidity
 p. ventricular complex
 p. ventricular contraction (PVC)
premenopausal
premenopause
premenstrual
 p. dysphoric disorder (PMDD)
 p. dysphoric syndrome (PMDS)
premonitory symptom
premorbid
Premphase
Prempro
preoperative
 p. anemia
 p. assessment
 p. cardiac evaluation
 p. medical evaluation
prep
 preparation
preparation (prep)
 thick and thin p.
 tissue p.
prepartum
prepatellar bursitis
preponderance
preproliferative diabetic retinopathy
 (PPDR)
prepuberal
prepubescent
prepuce
preputii
 smegma p.
prepyloric
prerenal
 p. acute renal failure
 p. azotemia
prerogative
presacral
Presalin
presbyastasis
presbyatrics
presbycusis
presbyopia
prescription (Rx)
 shotgun p.
presence
presenile dementia
presenilin-1
 p.-1 gene
 p.-1 gene on chromosome 1, 14
presenilin-2 gene
presenility
presenium
present, active, equal (PA&E)
presenting symptom
preseptal cellulitis
President's Council on Physical Fitness
 and Sports (PCPFS)

pressor
    p. headache
    p. stress
pressure
    arterial p.
    arterial blood p. (ABP)
    arterial oxygen p. (PAO$_2$)
    autopositive end-expiratory p.
    bilevel positive airway p. (BiPAP)
    blood p. (BP)
    carbon monoxide p.
    continuous positive airway p.
      (CPAP)
    diurnal blood p.
    p. effect
    end-expiratory p.
    glomerular capillary p.
    hemodynamic p.
    infracorporeal p.
    inspiratory p.
    intraocular p. (IOP)
    jugular venous p. (JVP)
    leak point p.
    maximum inspiratory p.
    mean arterial p. (MAP)
    mechanical p.
    p. necrosis
    normal p.
    oncotic p.
    p. palsy
    p. paralysis
    peak airway p.
    peak end-expiratory p.
    peripheral blood p.
    p. pneumothorax
    portal p.
    positive end-expiratory p. (PEEP)
    postural blood p.
    pulmonary artery occlusion p.
    pulmonary capillary wedge p.
    pulmonary venous p.
    p. sore
    systolic blood p. (SBP)
    p. ulcer
    urethral closure p.
    venous p.
pressure-flow study
pressure-graded stocking
pressure-support ventilation
PreSun Spray
presynaptic rundown
presyncopal episode

presyncope
pretibial
    p. fever
    p. myxedema
pretreatment evaluation
preulcer disease
preurethritis
Prevacid
prevalence
prevalent
prevention
    Centers for Disease Control and P.
      (CDC)
    secondary p.
    tertiary p.
preventive
    p. dose
    p. medicine
    p. treatment
priapism
pricking
Prilosec
primary
    p. adrenal failure
    p. adrenocortical insufficiency
    p. aging
    p. aldosteronism
    p. amenorrhea
    p. amyloidosis
    p. angle-closure glaucoma
    p. atypical pneumonia
    p. benign cardiac tumor
    p. biliary cirrhosis (PBC)
    p. bubo
    p. cardiac tumor
    p. caregiver
    p. care physician (PCP)
    p. care setting
    p. central nervous system
      hypersomnolence
    p. central nervous system
      lymphoma
    p. degenerative dementia
    p. degenerative dementia of
      Alzheimer type, presenile onset,
      with delirium
    p. degenerative dementia of
      Alzheimer type, presenile onset,
      with delusions
    p. degenerative dementia of
      Alzheimer type, senile onset, with
      delusions

NOTES

P

primary *(continued)*
    p. disease
    p. erythroblastic anemia
    p. extrapulmonary
      coccidioidomycosis
    p. focal segmental
      glomerulosclerosis
    p. generalized genetic epilepsy
    p. generalized hypertrophic
      osteoarthritis
    p. gout
    p. gouty arthritis
    p. graft failure
    p. headache syndrome
    p. hemochromatosis
    p. hemostasis
    p. hyperalphalipoproteinemia
    p. hyperlipoproteinemia
    p. hyperoxaluria
    p. hyperoxaluria and oxalosis
    p. hyperparathyroidism (PHP)
    p. hyperthyroidism
    p. hypoalphalipoproteinemia
    p. hypodipsia
    p. hypogonadism
    p. hypolipidemia
    p. hypothyroidism
    p. immunodeficiency syndrome
      (PIS)
    p. malignant cardiac tumor
    p. medical care
    p. methemoglobinemia
    p. open-angle glaucoma (POAG)
    p. parkinsonism
    p. peritonitis
    p. polycythemia
    p. polydipsia
    p. pulmonary hypertension
    p. pulmonary hypertension in
      pregnancy
    p. refractory anemia
    p. renal tubular acidosis
    p. reninism
    p. sensory afferent
    p. sex characteristics
    p. site
    p. skin lesion
    p. sleep disorder
    p. splenic neutropenia
    p. syphilis
    p. tuberculosis
    p. union
    p. writing tremor
Primatene Mist
Primaxin
primidone
primigravid

primordial
    p. dwarfism
    p. gigantism
primum
    ostium p.
Principen
principle
    follicle-stimulating p.
    luteinizing p.
    melanophore-expanding p.
PRIND
    prolonged reversible ischemic neurologic
    deficit
Prinivil
Prinzide
Prinzmetal angina
prison fever typhus
1974 Privacy Act
private
    p. duty nurse
    p. hospital
    p. payer
PRL
    prolactin
p.r.n.
    as needed
    pro re nata
Proampacin
proarrhythmia
Pro-Banthine
probe
    Doppler p.
probenecid
problem
    behavioral p.
    clotting factor p.
    concomitant medical p.
    p. drinking
    foot p.
    nonurgent p.
problematic behavior
problem-oriented record (POR)
procainamide
Procan SR
procarbazine
Procardia XL
procatarctic
procatarxis
procedure
    Blalock-Taussig p.
    Bristow p.
    Clagett p.
    loop electrosurgical excision p.
      (LEEP)
    operative p.
    seton p.
    sling p.
procelous

process
    aging p.
    coracoid p.
    degenerative p.
    disease p.
    involutive p.
    neoplastic p.
    sideroachrestic p.
    spinous p.
    styloid p.
    tissue-damaging p.
    xiphoid p.
procidentia
procollagen peptide
proctalgia fugax
proctitis
    chronic ulcerative p.
    epidemic gangrenous p.
    homosexual p.
    idiopathic p.
    radiation p.
proctocolectomy
proctocolitis
    ulcerative p.
Proctocort
ProctoCream
ProctoFoam
proctoscopic
proctoscopy
proctosigmoid
proctosigmoidoscopy
    fiberoptic p.
prodromal
    p. period
    p. stage
prodrome
prodromic sign
prodromus
prodrug
    acid-labile p.
product
    advanced glycosylation end p.'s
    end p.'s
    iodine thyroid p.
production
    congenital deficiency of
      testosterone p.
    free radical p.
    insulin p.
    sebum p.
    testosterone p.
proemial

proenkephalin
proestrogen
professional
    allied health p.
    National Association of
      Activity P.'s (NAAP)
profile
    basic metabolic p. (BMP)
    blood chemistry p.
    lipid p.
    P. of Mood States (POMS)
    P. of Mood States Questionnaire
    Nottingham Health P. (NHP)
    patient p.
    rapid p. 11
    Sickness Impact P. (SIP)
    transcriptional p.
profilometry
    urethral pressure p.
profound
    p. anemia
    p. hypothermia
profunda
    colitis cystica p.
profundoplasty
profundus
    lupus p.
progeria
Progestasert
progestational
    p. agent
    p. hormone
progesterone in oil
progestin
    subdermal p.
progestogen
prognathic
prognathism
prognose
prognosis, pl. **prognoses**
prognostic
prognosticate
prognostication
prognostician
Prograf
program
    P. of All-Inclusive Care for the
      Elderly (PACE)
    captioned media p. (CMP)
    Center for the Advancement of
      State Community Services P.'s
      (CASCSP)

NOTES

P

program *(continued)*
    Hill-Burton Free Medical Care P.
    home exercise p.
    MET 1 p.
    National Association of Nutrition
      and Aging Service P.'s
      (NANASP)
    National Cholesterol Education P.
      (NCEP)
    National Eye Health Education P.
      (NEHEP)
    rehabilitation p.
    12-step p.
    work stabilization p.
programmed ventricular stimulation
PROGRESS
    perindopril (Aceon) protection against
    recurrent stroke study
      PROGRESS trial
progress
progression
    dementia p.
    disease p.
    R-wave p.
progressiva
    lipodystrophia p.
progressive
    p. hypertrophic polyneuritis
    p. inflammatory arthritis
    p. massive fibrosis
    p. multifocal leukoencephalopathy
    p. myoclonus epilepsy
    p. pneumonia
    p. pulmonary histoplasmosis
    p. rubella panencephalitis
    p. supranuclear palsy
progressive-relapsing
proguanil
prohormone
proinflammatory
project
    P. Aliento
    Captopril Prevention P.
    Cooperative Cardiovascular P.
      (CCP)
    National Legal Support for Elderly
      People with Mental Disabilities P.
projectile vomiting
projection
    keratotic horny p.
prokinetic
    p. agent
    p. drug
prolactin (PRL)
    p. deficiency
    p. testosterone
prolactin-inhibiting factor
prolactinoma

prolactin-secreting
    p.-s. macroadenoma
    p.-s. pituitary tumor
prolapse
    mitral valve p. (MVP)
    pelvic organ p.
    rectal p.
    uterine p.
    valve p.
prolepsis
proleptic
proliferans
    angioendotheliomatosis p.
proliferation
    mesangial p.
proliferative
    p. arthritis
    p. bronchiolitis
    p. capacity
    p. diabetic retinopathy (PDR)
    p. vitreoretinopathy (PVR)
Prolixin
Proloid
prolongation
    cardiac conduction p.
prolonged
    p. activated partial thromboplastin
      time
    p. fast
    p. narcosis
    p. prothrombin time
    p. QT syndrome
    p. reversible ischemic neurologic
      deficit (PRIND)
prolonging measures
Proloprim
prolymphocytic leukemia
prometaphase
promethazine
ProMod
promoter
promotility agent
promotion
    health p.
promulgated
promyelocyte
promyelocytic leukemia
pronation
pronator drift
prone
    headache p.
    p. position
Pronestyl
Propacet
propafenone hydrochloride
Propagest
propanol
propantheline bromide
Propecia

propellant
    beclomethasone with CFC p.
    beclomethasone with HFA p.
propensity
    lipogenic enzyme p.
property
    anticonvulsant p.
    anxiolytic p.
    myorelaxant p.
prophylactic
    p. medication
    p. oophorectomy
    p. treatment
prophylaxis, pl. **prophylaxes**
    antibiotic p.
    anti-*Toxoplasma* p.
    tuberculosis p.
Propine
propionate
    fluticasone p.
propionibacterium acne
propionic acidemia
proportionate infantilism
propositus
propoxyphene
propranolol
propria
    lamina p.
proprietary
    p. hospital
    p. medicine
proprioception
proprioceptive
proprioceptive-oculocephalic reflex
proptosis
Propulsid
propylene glycol
propylthiouracil (PTU)
pro re nata (p.r.n.)
Proscar
ProSobee
prosody
ProSom
prosopagnosia
prosopopilary virilism
prospective memory
prostacyclin
prostaglandin
    p. A (PGA)
    p. E_1
    p. I2
prostatalgia

prostate
    p. cancer
    p. nodule
    transurethral electrovaporization
      of p. (TUEVP)
    transurethral incision of p. (TUIP)
    transurethral resection of p.
      (TURP)
prostatectomy
    laser p.
    radical p.
    transurethral ultrasound-guided laser-
      induced p. (TULIP)
prostate-specific
    p.-s. antigen (PSA)
    p.-s. antigen transition zone (PSA-
      TZ)
prostatic
    p. acid phosphatase
    p. hyperplasia
    p. hypertrophy
    p. neoplasm
    p. obstruction
prostatism
prostatitis
    acute bacterial p.
    asymptomatic inflammatory p.
    bacterial p.
    chronic bacterial p.
    granulomatous p.
    nonbacterial p.
prostatodynia
prostatomy
prostatorrhea
prostatotomy
ProStep
prosthesis, pl. **prostheses**
    Aufranc-Turner hip p.
    Austin Moore p.
    hip p.
    penile p.
    Small-Carrion penile p.
prosthetic
    p. heart valve
    p. valve endocarditis (PVE)
prosthetica
    stomatitis p.
prosthetist
prosthodontist
prostration
    heat p.
protease inhibitor

NOTES

P

protect
protected specimen brush (PSB)
protective
  p. extension resection
  p. underwear
protein
  amyloid precursor p. (APP)
  Bence Jones p.
  bone-specific p.
  p. C
  p. catabolic rate (PCR)
  Charcot-Leyden crystal p.
  C-reactive p. (CRP)
  p. C, S deficiency
  p. deficiency
  dietary p.
  E1A p.
  extracellular p.'s
  p. fever
  fibronectin-binding p.
  fusion p.
  gap junction p.
  hemagglutinin neuraminidase p.
  p. kinase C
  p. malnutrition
  myeloid basic p.
  p. oxidation
  placenta p.
  purified placental p.
  p. S
  p. synthesis
  urinalysis showed trace p.
protein-bound iodine (PBI)
proteinemia
  Bence Jones p.
  broad-beta p.
  floating-beta p.
protein-energy
  p.-e. malnutrition (PEM)
  p.-e. undernutrition
protein-losing enteropathy
proteinosis
  lipoid p.
  pulmonary alveolar p.
  tissue p.
proteinuria
  Bence Jones p.
  benign p.
  dipstick-positive p.
  full-blown p.
  functional p.
  gouty p.
  idiopathic benign p.
  isolated p.
  nonisolated p.
  nonnephrotic p.
  orthostatic p.
  persistent p.
  tubular p.

proteohormone
Proteus
  P. mirabilis
  P. rettgeri
  P. vulgaris
prothrombin
  p. time (pro time, PT)
pro time
  prothrombin time
protocol
  Bruce p.
  research p.
  treatment p.
protocoproporphyria hereditaria
protodiastolic murmur
Protonix
proton pump inhibitor (PPI)
protooncogene
protopianoma
Protopic
protoporphyria
  erythropoietic p.
protoporphyrin
  erythrocyte p. (EP)
protozoal infection
protozoan
  p. infection
  p. parasite
protriptyline
protrusio acetabuli
protuberant
Proventil
  P. inhaler
  P. Repetabs
Provera
Providencia stuartii
provocation typhoid
provocative
  p. stimulus
  p. technique
  p. test
prowazekii
  Rickettsia p.
proxetil
  cefpodoxime p.
proximal
  distal to p.
  p. interphalangeal (PIP)
  p. interphalangeal joint
  p. renal tubule dysfunction
proximate cause
Prozac Weekly
prudent heart diet
prune
  p. belly syndrome
prune-juice
  p.-j. expectoration
  p.-j. sputum
prurigo nodularis

pruritic rash
pruritus
    p. ani
    jaundice p.
    symptomatic p.
    p. vulva
    vulvar p.
Prussian blue treatment
PSA
    prostate-specific antigen
    free PSA
psammoma
PSA-TZ
    prostate-specific antigen transition zone
    PSA-TZ density
PSB
    protected specimen brush
PSBO
    partial small bowel obstruction
pseudacusis
pseudallescheriasis
pseudoacanthosis nigricans
pseudoactinomycosis
pseudoanemia
pseudoaneurysm
    ventricular p.
pseudoappendicitis
pseudobulbar
pseudocholinesterase deficiency
pseudoclaudication
pseudocoma
    hysterical p.
pseudocrisis
pseudo-Cushing syndrome
pseudocyesis
pseudocyst
    pancreatic p.
pseudodiabetes
pseudodiphtheria
pseudodipsia
pseudodysentery
pseudoephedrine
pseudoepileptic seizure
pseudoepitheliomatous hyperplasia
pseudoexfoliation glaucoma
pseudofolliculitis barbae
pseudofracture
pseudogout
pseudo-Graefe sign
pseudohemophilia hepatica

pseudo-Hurler
    p.-H. disease
    p.-H. polydystrophy
pseudohydronephrosis
pseudohyperparathyroidism
pseudohypertension
pseudohypertrophic muscular
pseudohypha, pl. pseudohyphae
pseudohypoaldosteronism
    p. type I, II
pseudohypoparathyroidism
pseudoileus
pseudoinfluenza
pseudoleukemia lymphatica
pseudolithiasis
pseudolymphocytic choriomeningitis
pseudomegacolon
pseudomembranous
    p. angina
    p. bronchitis
    p. colitis (PMC)
    p. enteritis
    p. enterocolitis
Pseudomonas
    P. aeruginosa
    P. cellulitis
pseudomucinous adenofibroma
pseudoobstruction
    intestinal p.
pseudoparalysis
pseudoparalytica
    myasthenia gravis p.
pseudoparaplegia
    Basedow p.
pseudophakic bullous keratopathy
pseudoplegia
pseudopolydystrophy
pseudopolyp
pseudoporphyria
pseudoprimary aldosteronism
pseudopterygium
pseudopuberty
    precocious p.
pseudopyloric metaplasia
pseudorefractory hypertension
pseudorheumatism
pseudorickets
pseudorubella
pseudoscarlatina
pseudosclerosis
    Westphal-Strümpell p.
pseudoseizure

NOTES

P

pseudosmallpox
pseudotubercular yersiniosis
pseudotuberculosis
    Yersinia p.
pseudotumor cerebri
pseudovariola
pseudo-vitamin D deficiency rickets
pseudoxanthoma elasticum
psilosis
psittaci
    Chlamydia p.
psittacosis
psoas sign
psomophagia
psoralen
    p. ultraviolet A-range therapy
    p. ultraviolet A-range treatment
      (PUVA)
    p. with radiation
Psorcon
psorenteritis
psoriasiform rash
psoriasis
    p. guttate
    pustular p.
psoriatic arthritis
PSP
    phenolsulfonphthalein
PSVT
    paroxysmal supraventricular tachycardia
psychiatric
    p. disorder
    p. disturbance
    p. specialist
psychiatry
    American Association for
      Geriatric P. (AAGP)
psychoactive drug
psychoendocrinology
psychogenic
    p. cough
    p. dizziness
    p. erection
    p. itching
    p. light-headedness
    p. pelvic pain
    p. vomiting
psychogeriatric
psychological
    p. distress
    P. General Well-Being Scale
      (PGWB)
    p. habit
psychometric scale
psychomotor
    p. agitation/retardation
    p. function
    p. retardation
psychoneurosis maidica

psychopharmacology
psychophysical health status
psychophysiologic insomnia
psychosis, pl. psychoses
    Korsakoff p.
    postinfectious p.
    Wernicke-Korsakoff p.
psychosocial
    p. care
    p. development
    p. function
    p. influence
psychosomatic medicine
psychotherapeutic agent
psychotherapy
psychotic
    p. depression
    p. symptom
psychotropic
psyllium
PT
    physical therapist
    physical therapy
    posterior tibial
    prothrombin time
pt
    patient
PTARF
    posttraumatic acute renal failure
PTCA
    percutaneous transluminal coronary
      angioplasty
    percutaneous transluminal coronary
      arteriography
pterion
pterygium
PTH
    parathormone
    parathyroid hormone
      PTH level
PTHrP
    parathyroid hormone-related peptide
ptosis, pl. ptoses
ptotic kidney
PTT
    partial thromboplastin time
PTU
    propylthiouracil
pubarche
puberal
puberty
    p. and anovulatory bleeding
    delayed p.
    isosexual precocious p.
    precocious p.
pubescence
pubescent
pubic ramus

pubis
    mons p.
    osteitis symphysis p.
    pediculosis p.
    symphysis p.
public
    p. health
    p. health nurse
    P. Health Service (PHS)
    p. hospital
puborectalis
PUD
    peptic ulcer disease
puddle sign
puddling
pudendal
    p. area
    p. neuralgia
pudendum, pl. **pudenda**
Pudenz button
puerperal
    p. infection
    p. morbidity
    p. sepsis
puerperium, pl. **puerperia**
PUFA
    polyunsaturated fatty acid
puff
    veiled p.
puffer
    pink p.
    p. poison
puffiness
    molimina of p.
pugilistic
pugilistica
    dementia p.
pull test
Pulmicort
Pulmo-Aide
pulmonale
    cor p.
pulmonary
    p. adenomatosis
    p. alveolar hypoxic vasoconstriction
      (PAHVC)
    p. alveolar proteinosis
    p. amebiasis
    p. angiography
    p. anthrax
    p. arterial hypertension
    p. arteriogram

    p. arteriolar resistance
    p. arteriovenous fistula
    p. aspergilloma
    p. aspergillosis
    p. aspiration syndrome
    p. atresia
    p. capillary wedge pressure
    p. circuit
    p. cirrhosis
    p. congestion
    p. disease
    p. distomiasis
    p. edema
    p. embolism (PE)
    p. embolus (PE)
    p. eosinophilic granuloma
    p. fibrosis
    P. Fibrosis Foundation (PFF)
    p. function test (PFT)
    p. gas exchange
    p. histiocytosis
    p. infarction
    p. infection
    p. interstitial emphysema (PIE)
    p. isolation
    p. nodule
    p. parenchyma
    p. physiology
    p. rehabilitation
    p. schistosomiasis
    p. siderosis
    p. talcosis
    p. toilet
    p. tuberculosis
    p. tuberculosis and pregnancy
    p. tularemia
    p. valve stenosis
    p. vascular resistance (PVR)
    p. vasculature
    p. vein (Ppv)
    p. venous hypertension
    p. venous pressure
pulmonary-renal syndrome
pulmonic
    p. plague
    p. regurgitation
    p. tularemia
    p. valve
    p. valvular stenosis
pulmonitis
pulmonology
Pulmozyme

NOTES

P

pulposus
    herniated nucleus p. (HNP)
    nucleus p.
pulsatile
    p. epigastric mass
pulsation
    jugular venous p. (JVP)
pulse
    abdominal p.
    collapsing p.
    distal p.
    irregular p.
    jugular venous p. (JVP)
    p. oximeter
    p. oximetry
    paradoxical p.
    pedal p.
    posterior tibial p.
    p. therapy
    waterhammer p.
pulsed Doppler
pulseless
    P. Electrical Study (PEA)
    p. ventricular tachycardia
pulsus
    p. abdominalis
    p. alternans
    p. paradoxus
pump
    p. bump
    D-TRON insulin p.
    insulin p.
    intraaortic balloon p.
    p. lung
    lymphedema p.
    sodium p.
    stomach p.
puna
punchdrunk syndrome
puncta (*pl. of* punctum)
punctal plug
punctate
    p. basophilia
    p. lucency
    p. rash
punctum, pl. puncta
puncture
    p. diabetes
    lumbar p. (LP)
    Quincke p.
pungent
punjatensis
    Ceratophyllus p.
PUO
    pyrexia of unknown origin
pupil
    Adie tonic p.
    Argyll Robertson p.

    p.'s equal and reactive to light (PERL)
    p.'s equal and reactive to light and accommodation (PERLA)
    p.'s equal, round and reactive to light and accommodation (PERRLA)
    Marcus Gunn p.
puréed diet
purgation
purge
purging
    bingeing and p.
purified
    p. placental protein
    p. protein derivative (PPD)
purine
purine-free diet
purine-restricted diet
Purkinje
    P. cell
    P. cell body
purple
    p. cone flower
    p. toe syndrome
purpura
    p. abdominalis
    allergic p.
    anaphylactoid p.
    p. cachectica
    cocktail p.
    dependent nonthrombocytopenic p.
    drug-induced vascular p.
    ecchymotic p.
    Echinacea p.
    p. hemorrhagica
    Henoch p.
    Henoch-Schönlein p.
    hypergammaglobulinemic p.
    hyperglobulinemic p.
    p. hyperglobulinemica
    idiopathic p.
    idiopathic thrombocytopenic p. (ITP)
    immune thrombocytopenic p.
    Landouzy p.
    nonpalpable p.
    nonthrombocytopenic p.
    orthostatic p.
    palpable p.
    petechial p.
    posttransfusion p.
    p. rheumatica
    Schamberg p.
    Schönlein p.
    Schönlein-Henoch p.
    secondary thrombocytopenic p.
    senile p.
    p. senilis

p. simplex
solar p.
symptomatic p.
p. symptomatica
thrombocytopenic p.
p. thrombolytica
thrombopenic p.
thrombotic thrombocytopenic p. (TTP)
thrombotic thrombohemolytic p.
p. variolosa
vascular p.
Waldenström hyperglobulinemic p.
purpuric
pursed-lip breathing
purulent
p. pneumonia
p. secretion
p. sputum
p. synovitis
p. thrombophlebitis
purulenta
pneumonia interlobularis p.
pus
p. basin
laudable p.
loculated p.
push
IV p.
pustular psoriasis
pustule
putrid bronchitis
PUVA
psoralen ultraviolet A-range treatment
PUVA therapy
PVC
premature ventricular contraction
PVD
posterior vitreous detachment
PVE
prosthetic valve endocarditis
PVR
peripheral vascular resistance
postvoid residual
proliferative vitreoretinopathy
pulmonary vascular resistance
PWBA
Pension and Welfare Benefits Administration
pyarthrosis
pyelitis
emphysematous p.

pyelocaliectasis
pyelogram
intravenous p. (IVP)
pyelonephritis
pyelonephrosis
pyemesis
pyemia
arterial p.
cryptogenic p.
pyemic
pygalgia
Pygeum africanum
pyknodysostosis
pylephlebitis
pyloralgia
pylori
Helicobacter p.
pyloric
p. channel ulcer
p. incompetence
p. insufficiency
p. stenosis
pyloroplasty
pylorospasm
pylorus
Pym fever
pyochezia
pyoderma
p. faciale
p. gangrenosum
pyogenic
p. fever
p. granuloma
p. infection
p. liver abscess
p. pericarditis
p. sterile arthritis
pyohemia
pyohemothorax
pyomyositis
tropical p.
pyopneumocholecystitis
pyopneumohepatitis
pyopneumoperitoneum
pyopneumoperitonitis
pyopneumothorax
subdiaphragmatic p.
pyorrhea
pyosalpinx
pyourachus
pyoureter

NOTES

pyramid
> Food Guide P.

pyramidal

pyrazinamide

pyrectic

pyrene

pyrenemia

pyrethrins

pyrethron

pyrethrum

pyretic

pyretogen

pyretogenesis

pyretogenetic

pyretogenous

pyretotherapy

pyrexia
> heat p.
> Pel-Ebstein p.
> p. of unknown origin (PUO)

pyrexial

pyribenzamine

Pyridiate

pyridinium

pyridinoline

Pyridium

pyridoxine

pyridoxine-responsive anemia

pyrogen
> endogenous p.
> exogenous p.
> leukocytic p.

pyrogenic cytokine

pyrophosphate crystal

pyropoikilocytosis

pyrosis

pyrotherapy

pyrotic

pyruvate
> p. kinase deficiency
> p. kinase deficiency anemia

pyuria
> abacterial p.

pyuric

Q

Q fever
Q 103 needle management system

q.
each
every

q.a.m.
every morning [L. *quaque mane*]
quaque ante meridiem

q.d.
every day [L. *quaque die*]

q.h.
every hour [L. *quaque hora*]

q.h.s.
quaque hora somni

q.i.d.
four times a day
quater in die

q.l.
as much as needed
quantum libet

q.m.
every morning [L. *quaque mane*]

q.n.
every night [L. *quaque nocte*]

q.o.d.
every other day [L. *quaque altera die*]

q.o.n.
every other night [L. *quaque altera nocte*]

QRS
QRS axis
QRS complex
QRS duration
QRS morphology
QRS voltage

QST
quantitative sensory testing

QT corrected

Q-tip

quack

quackery

quad cane

quadrant
left lower q. (LLQ)
left upper q. (LUQ)
right lower q. (RLQ)
right upper q. (RUQ)
upper left q. (ULQ)
upper right q. (URQ)

quadrantectomy

quadratum
caput q.

quadratus lumborum

quadriceps

quadriparesis

quadriplegia

qualitative
q. deficiency
q. platelet disorder
q. stool fat

quality
Agency for Healthcare Research & Q. (AHRQ)
q. assurance
q. of life
Q. of Well-Being Scale (QWB)

quantitative
q. analysis
q. beta-hCG
q. electroencephalographic activity
q. platelet defect
q. sensory testing (QST)
q. virology

quantity

Quant sign

quantum libet (q.l.)

quaque
q. altera die
q. altera nocte
q. ante meridiem (q.a.m.)
q. die
q. hora
q. hora somni (q.h.s.)
q. mane
q. nocte

quarantine period

quartan
double q.
q. fever
q. malaria
triple q.

quartile

quater in die (q.i.d.)

quaternary syphilis

quazepam

Queckenstedt sign

Queensland tick typhus

query fever

questionnaire
Cook-Medley q.
European Organization for Research and Treatment of Cancer Quality of Life Q. (EORTC QLQ)
POMS Q.
Profile of Mood States Q.
RAND Social Activities Q.
Short Portable Mental Status Q. (SPMSQ)

Questran Light

Queyrat erythroplasia
Quick test
quiescent migrainous syndrome
quiet necrosis
Quinaglute
quinapril
    q. HCl
Quincke
    Q. angioedema
    Q. disease
    Q. edema
    Q. I syndrome
    Q. puncture
    Q. sign
quinestradiol

Quinidex Extentabs
quinidine gluconate
quinine sulfate
quininism
quinolone
quinsy
quintan fever
quinupristin-dalfopristin
quotidian
    q. fever
    q. malaria
QVAR Inhalation Aerosol
Q-wave myocardial infarction
QWB
    Quality of Well-Being Scale

RA
> rheumatoid arthritis
> room air
>> RA blood gas

Raaf catheter
rabbit fever
rabeprazole sodium
rabid
raccoon sign
racemic epinephrine
rachiocampsis
rachiocentesis
rachitic diet
rachitism
rachitis tarda
rachitogenic
RAD
> reactive airway disease

radial
> r. keratotomy
> r. nerve injury

radialis
> flexor carpi r.

radiata
> corona r.

radiation
> r. anemia
> r. burn
> r. dermatosis
> r. enteritis
> r. exposure
> r. exposure in pregnancy
> r. hepatitis
> r. induced
> ionizing r.
> r. necrosis
> nonionizing r.
> occupational r.
> photochemical r.
> r. proctitis
> psoralen with r.
> r. sickness
> r. syndrome
> ultraviolet r.

radiation-induced hypothyroidism
radical
> r. external beam radiotherapy
> free r.
> r. mastectomy
> r. prostatectomy

radicle
> biliary r.

radicular pain
radiculitis
radiculoneuritis

radiculopathy
> cervical r.
> motor r.

radioactive
> r. iodine-131
> r. iodine therapy
> r. iodine uptake
> r. iodine uptake test

radioallergoabsorbent testing
radioallergosorbent
> r. assay test (RAST)
> r. screen
> r. test

radiocontrast
> r. media
> r. nephropathy
> r. sensitivity reaction

radiocurable tumor
radiofluorescent antibody (RFA)
radiofrequency catheter ablative therapy
radiograph
> plain spine r.

radiographic
radiography
> chest r.

radioimmunoassay (RIA)
radioiodinated
> r. serum albumin (RISA)
> r. serum albumin cisternogram

radioiodine uptake (RIU)
radioisotopic scan
radiologist
radiology
> diagnostic r.

radiolucency
radionuclide
> r. imaging
> r. scanning

radiopaque
radiopill
radioreceptor
radioresistant tumor
radiosensitive tumor
radiotelemetering capsule
radiotherapy
> external beam r.
> radical external beam r.

radiotoxemia
radius
radiffinosus
> *Enterococcus r.*

ragpicker's disease
ragsorter's disease
Raimondi spring catheter
raised toilet seat

R

raising
straight leg r. (SLR)

rale
amphoric r.
atelectatic r.
bibasilar r.
bubbling r.
cavernous r.
clicking r.
consonating r.
crackling r.
crepitant r.
dry r.
gurgling r.
guttural r.
metallic r.
moist r.
mucous r.
palpable r.
pleural r.
posttussive r.
sibilant r.
Skoda r.
sonorous r.
subcrepitant r.
Velcro r.
vesicular r.
whistling r.

raloxifene
r. HCl
r. hydrochloride

ramipril

Ramond
R. point
R. sign

Ramsay
R. Hunt syndrome
R. Hunt syndrome type 1

ramus
pubic r.

random blood sugar (RBS)
randomization
randomized trial
RAND Social Activities Questionnaire

range
r. of motion (ROM)
r. of motion test

ranitidine
Ransohoff sign
Ranson
R. criteria
R. criteria for severity of acute
pancreatitis

rape
bruit de scie ou de r.

raphania
raphe
dorsal r.
r. neuron

rapid
r. cycling
r. eye movement (REM)
r. eye movement sleep
r. gait
r. plasma reagent (RPR)
r. plasma reagin (RPR)
r. profile 11
r. strep-antigen test

rapid-acting insulin
rappel
bruit de r.

rarefaction
RAS
renin-angiotensin system

rash
butterfly r.
depigmented r.
heliotrope r.
herbal-induced r.
maculopapular r.
Murray Valley r.
pruritic r.
psoriasiform r.
punctate r.
shawl-sign r.
V-sign r.

Rasmussen
R. aneurysm
R. encephalitis

raspberry tongue
RAST
radioallergosorbent assay test
RAST screen

rat-bite
r.-b. disease
r.-b. fever

rate
accelerated r.
attack r.
basal metabolic r. (BMR)
case fatality r.
death r.
distal flow r.
erythrocyte sedimentation r. (ESR)
fatality r.
filtration r.
five-year survival r.
glomerular filtration r. (GFR)
heart r. (HR)
heightened filtration r.
inspiratory flow r.
lethality r.
maximal urinary flow r. (MUFR)
metabolic r.
morbidity r.
mortality r.
postcibal metabolic r.
protein catabolic r. (PCR)

renal excretion r.
respiratory r.
resting heart r.
resting metabolic r. (RMR)
Rourke-Ernstein sedimentation r.
sedimentation r.
survival r.
urine flow r.
ventricular r.
weak flow r.
Westergren sedimentation r.

Rathke pouch
rating
　Life Satisfaction R. (LSR)
ratio
　albumin-globulin r. (AG)
　A/V r.
　case fatality r.
　C/D r.
　cup-to-disk r.
　false-negative r.
　false-reassurance r.
　international normalized r. (INR)
　likelihood r.
　M/E r.
　myeloid/erythroid r.
　odds r.
　therapeutic-to-toxic r.
ration
　basal r.
rationale
rational symptom
Raudixin
RAV
　Rous-associated virus
raw
Rayer disease
Raymond apoplexy
Raynaud
　R. disease
　R. gangrene
　R. phenomenon
　R. sign
　R. syndrome
ray resection
Raza
　National Council of La R.
　　(NCLR)
razor bumps
RBBB
　right bundle-branch block

RBC
　red blood cell
r binder deficiency
RBS
　random blood sugar
RCA
　right coronary artery
RCP
　Royal College of Physicians (of England)
RCP(E)
　Royal College of Physicians (Edinburgh)
RCP(I)
　Royal College of Physicians (Ireland)
RD
　registered dietitian
RDA
　recommended dietary allowance
RDI
　respiratory disturbance index
RDS
　respiratory distress syndrome
reabsorption
　chlorine r.
　sodium r.
　tubular r.
reach
　functional r. (FR)
reactant
　acute-phase r.
reaction
　acute pharyngoconjunctival r.
　adverse drug r.
　allergic r.
　allergic drug r. (ADR)
　anaphylactoid r.
　APC r.
　Bittorf r.
　Cushing r.
　delayed hemolytic transfusion r.
　drug r.
　eosinopenic r.
　extrapyramidal r.
　febrile r.
　general adaptation r.
　graft-versus-host r. (GVHR)
　harlequin r.
　hemolytic transfusion r.
　hypoglycemic r.
　iatrogenic drug r.
　id r.
　incompatible blood transfusion r.
　insulin r.

NOTES

R

reaction *(continued)*
  leukemoid r.
  Mantoux r.
  nitritoid r.
  nonhemolytic febrile transfusion r.
  parkinsonian r.
  polymerase chain r. (PCR)
  radiocontrast sensitivity r.
  Roger r.
  Sahli r.
  serum r.
  r. time
  transfusion r.
  Weil-Felix r.
reactive
  r. airway disease (RAD)
  r. airways dysfunction syndrome
  r. erythrocytosis
  r. hypoglycemia
  r. pulmonary hypertension
  r. thrombocytosis
reading
  glucose r.
reagent
  rapid plasma r. (RPR)
reagin
  rapid plasma r. (RPR)
real-time B-mode imaging
rearrangement
  chromosomal r.
Rebetol
rebound
  r. hypertension
  r. insomnia
  tenderness and r. (T&R)
  r. tenderness
recalcification
recall test
recent memory
receptor
  adrenergic r.
  caudate putamen r.
  cerebral cortex r.
  claustrum r.
  globus pallidus r.
  growth factor r.
  H_2 r.
  hormone r.
  human leptin r.
  inferior olive r.
  Island of Calleja r.
  low-density lipoprotein r.
  mamillary nuclei r.
  mu r.
  opioid cell membrane r.
  ventral pallidum r.
  V1, V2 r.
recessive
recessus

recidivation
recipient hepatectomy
reciprocating tachycardia
Reclus disease
recognition domain
recombinant
  r. brain-derived neurotrophin
  r. human replacement therapy
  r. immunoblot assay (RIBA)
  r. interferon beta
  r. interleukin 11
  r. plasminogen activator (r-PA)
  r. tissue plasminogen activator
Recombivax HB
recommendation
recommended
  r. dietary allowance (RDA)
  r. nutrient intake (RNI)
reconstruction
  spiral r.
record
  computerized patient r.
  hospital r.
  medical r.
  problem-oriented r. (POR)
recorder
  loop r.
recording
  clinical r.
recovery
recrudescence
recrudescent
  r. typhus
  r. typhus fever
recruitment
recta (*pl. of* rectum)
rectal
  r. alimentation
  r. cancer
  r. dyschezia
  r. erythema
  r. evacuation
  r. gonococcal infection
  r. prolapse
  r. temperature
  r. ulcer
rectal-outlet delay
rectify
rectoabdominal
rectoanal angle
rectocele
rectorrhaphy
rectosigmoidectomy
rectosigmoidoscopy
rectosigmoid villous adenoma
rectum, pl. recta
  per r.
rectus sheath
recumbency

R

recumbent
    dorsal r.
recuperate
recuperation
recurrence
    no evidence of r. (NER)
    r. risk
recurrent
    r. anaphylaxis
    r. aphthous stomatitis
    r. appendicitis
    r. cystitis
    r. fever
    r. genital herpes
    r. hypopyon
    r. infection
    r. myocardial infarction
    r. polyserositis
    r. rhabdomyolysis
    r. sustained ventricular tachycardia
    r. upper respiratory tract infection
      (RURTI)
    r. vomiting
recurvation
red
    r. blood cell (RBC)
    r. blood cell scintigraphy
    r. blood cell transfusion
    r. cell aplasia
    R. Cross
    r. eye
    r. fever
    r. flag
    r. man syndrome
    r. rubber catheter
    r. strawberry tongue
    r., white, and blue sign
redintegration
redistribution
    potassium r.
redound
reduced
    r. capacity
    r. rectal sensation
reducible
    r. femoral hernia
    r. inguinal hernia
reducing diet
reductase
    CoA r.
    HMG-CoA r.

reduction
    closed r.
    gastric r.
    homocysteine r.
    lipid r.
    lung volume r.
    stride length r.
redundancy
reduplication
Redux
Reed-Hodgkin disease
Reed-Sternberg cell
reemergence of controlled disease
reentry
    r. pulmonary edema
    sinus nodal r.
reepithelialization
Reese syndrome
reexacerbartion
reexacerbate
refection
refeeding
    r. edema
    r. gynecomastia
    r. syndrome
referral
    Alzheimer's Disease Education
      and R. (ADEAR)
    r. filter bias
referred
    r. abdominal pain
    r. pain
Refetoff syndrome
refill
    brisk capillary r.
    capillary r.
reflex
    abdominocardiac r.
    r. asthma
    avoidance r.
    Babinski r.
    Barkman r.
    blink test r.
    bulbocavernosus r.
    Capps r.
    corneal r.
    deep tendon r. (DTR)
    r. dyspepsia
    r. incontinence
    let-down r.
    milk let-down r.
    Morley peritoneocutaneous r.

NOTES

reflex *(continued)*
    Moro r.
    plantar r.
    pneopneic r.
    postural r.
    proprioceptive-oculocephalic r.
    renal r.
    righting r.
    snout r.
    Somogyi r.
    r. sympathetic dystrophy (RSD)
    r. symptom
    r. therapy
    triceps r.
    viscerosensory r.
reflexogenic erection
reflexotherapy
reflux
    abdominojugular r.
    acid r.
    duodenogastric r.
    esophageal r.
    r. esophagitis
    r. gastritis
    gastroesophageal r.
    hepatojugular r.
    ureterorenal r.
    urine r.
    vesicoureteral r.
reform
    National Citizen's Coalition for
      Nursing Home R. (NCCNHR)
refraction
refractive
    r. error
    r. surgery
refractory
    r. anemia
    r. ascites
    r. emesis
    r. heart failure
    r. hypertension
    r. illness
    r. rickets
    r. sprue
refresh
refrigerant
refrigeration
Refsum
    R. disease
    R. syndrome
refusal
    treatment r.
regain
regimen
    antiretroviral r.
    dosing r.
    5-fluorouracil pulsed r.
    5-FU pulsed r.

    r. nonadherence
    stepped-care hypertensive r.
region
    mid lumbar r.
    paralimbic r.
regional
    r. cancer
    r. colitis
    r. enteritis
    r. enterocolitis
    r. granulomatous lymphadenitis
    r. hypothermia
    r. ileitis
    r. ileocolitis
    r. perfusion
registered
    r. dietitian (RD)
    r. nurse (RN)
registry
    cancer r.
    SEER cancer r.
    Surveillance, Epidemiology, and
      End Results cancer r.
    tumor r.
Regitine
Reglan
regression
regressive
regrinding
regular
    r. rate and rhythm (RRR)
    r. sleep schedule
regulation
    dietary r.
    growth r.
    osmotic r.
    renal r.
    volume r.
regurgitant jet
regurgitation
    acid r.
    acute mitral r.
    aortic r. (AR)
    chronic mitral r.
    mitral valve r.
    r. murmur
    nasal r.
    pulmonic r.
    rheumatic mitral r.
    tricuspid r.
    valvular r.
rehabilitation
    American Academy of Physical
      Medicine and R. (AAPMR)
    American Association of
      Cardiovascular and Pulmonary R.
      (AACVPR)
    amputation r.
    cardiac r.

cardiovascular r.
r. center
faith-based r.
orthopedic r.
r. program
pulmonary r.
stroke r.
subacute r.
therapeutic r.
r. therapist
visual r.
Rehfuss method
rehydration
oral r.
r. therapy
Reichmann
R. disease
R. syndrome
Reid sleeve
Reifenstein syndrome
reimbursement
reinfarction
early r.
reinfection tuberculosis
reinforcement
bovine pericardial strip r.
Reinke edema
Reiter
R. disease
R. syndrome
rejection
acute organ r.
chronic ductopenic r.
chronic organ r.
ductopenic r.
heart transplant r.
humoral r.
hyperacute organ r.
liver transplant r.
lung transplant r.
organ r.
steroid-resistant r.
transplant r.
Relafen
relapse
relapsing
r. appendicitis
r. febrile nodular nonsuppurative
   panniculitis
r. fever
r. malaria

r. pancreatitis
r. polychondritis
relapsing-remitting
relation
interpersonal r.'s
relational life
relationship
doctor-patient r.
relative
r. erythrocytosis
r. leukocytosis
r. polycythemia
relaxant
muscle r.
smooth-muscle r.
relaxation
cardioesophageal r.
deep muscle r.
r. technique
relaxin
relaxing activity
release
morphine sulfate immediate r.
   (MSIR)
sustained r.
releasing
r. factor
r. hormone (RH)
Relenza
relevant
reliability
reliever
Medtronic Pulsor Intrasound pain r.
REM
rapid eye movement
REM sleep
remediable
remedial
remedy
homeopathic r.
Remeron
remineralization
Reminyl Oral Solution
remission
remit
remittence
remittent
r. malaria
r. malarial fever
remodeling
bone r.
remotely

R

NOTES

removal
renal
    r. allograft dysfunction
    r. amyloidosis
    r. ballottement
    r. biopsy
    r. blood flow
    r. calculus
    r. carbuncle
    r. cell adenocarcinoma
    r. cell cancer
    r. colic
    r. crisis
    r. cyst
    r. diabetes
    r. disease and pregnancy
    r. drug clearance
    r. epistaxis
    r. excretion rate
    r. failure
    r. failure anemia
    r. fibrocystic osteosis
    r. function
    r. function test
    r. glycosuria
    r. gout
    r. hypercalciuria
    r. infantilism
    r. injury
    r. insufficiency
    r. osteitis fibrosa
    r. osteodystrophy
    r. potassium excretion
    r. potassium loss
    r. reflex
    r. regulation
    r. replacement therapy
    r. rickets
    r. sodium metabolism
    r. toxicity
    r. transplant
    r. transplantation
    r. transplantation and pregnancy
    r. tuberculosis
    r. tubular acidosis (RTA)
    r. tubular defect
    r. tubule dysfunction
    r. tubulointerstitial disease
    r. ultrasonography
    r. vascular hypertension
    r. vein thrombosis
    r. water loss
Rendu-Osler-Weber
    R.-O.-W. disease
    R.-O.-W. syndrome
renin-angiotensin-aldosterone system
renin-angiotensin system (RAS)
reninism
    primary r.

renin-secreting tumor
renogenic
renogram
renopathy
Renova
renovascular hypertension
reoperation
ReoPro
repaglinide
repair
    Fallot r.
    Mustard atrial baffle r.
    Senning atrial baffle r.
    surgical r.
repeat
    short tandem r.
repens
    Sernoa r.
reperfusion
    coronary r.
    r. therapy
Repetabs
    Proventil R.
repetition
repetitive
    r. leg-jerking movement
    r. loading
replacement
    alpha-1 protease inhibitor r.
    aortic valve r.
    estrogen r.
    hip r.
    hormone r.
    knee r.
    mineralocorticoid r.
    postmenopausal hormonal r.
    testosterone r.
    r. therapy
    total hip r. (THR)
    total knee r. (TKR)
    valve r.
    vitamin K r.
Replens
replication
    suppression of r.
repolarization
reportable disease
reproducibility
reproducible
reproductive medicine
reptilian stare
Rescon-GG
research
    Alliance for Aging R.
    American Federation of Aging R.
        (AFAR)
    Foundation for Biomedical R.
        (FBR)

National Institute of Dental and Craniofacial R. (NIDCR)
National Institute of Nursing R. (NINR)
  r. protocol

resection
  block r.
  bowel r.
  myocardial r.
  nipple r.
  protective extension r.
  ray r.
  small-intestine r.
  transurethral r. (TUR)
  wedge r.

reserpine

reservatus
  coitus r.

reserve
  functional r.

reservoir
  Pecquet r.

reset osmostat syndrome

residential
  r. care
  r. home

resident physician

residual
  postvoid r. (PVR)
  r. volume (RV)

residuum, pl. **residua**

resin
  bile acid sequestrant r.
  cation exchange r.
  r. sponge uptake
  r. sponge uptake of triiodothyronine
  r. triiodothyronine (RT_3)
  r. triiodothyronine uptake

resistance
  androgen r.
  arterial arteriolar r.
  insulin r.
  mutual r.
  peripheral vascular r. (PVR)
  pulmonary arteriolar r.
  pulmonary vascular r. (PVR)
  thyroid hormone r.
  viral r.

resistant
  multidrug r.

resisted hip extension

resonance
  amphoric r.
  bandbox r.
  bellmetal r.
  cavernous r.
  cracked-pot r.
  electron paramagnetic r. (EPR)
  hydatid r.
  skodaic r.
  tympanic r.
  tympanitic r.
  vesicular r.
  vesiculotympanic r.
  vesiculotympanitic r.
  vocal r. (VR)
  wooden r.

resorption
  bone r.

resorptive hypercalciuria

resource allocation

respectively

respiration
  agonal r.
  amphoric r.
  blowing r.
  bronchial r.
  bronchovesicular r.
  cavernous r.
  Cheyne-Stokes r.
  cogwheel r.
  diffusion r.
  interrupted r.
  jerky r.
  Kussmaul r.
  Kussmaul-Kien r.
  labored r.
  stertorous r.
  temperature, pulse, r. (TPR)
  tubular r.
  vesicular r.
  vesiculocavernous r.

respiratory
  r. acidosis
  r. alkalosis
  r. bronchiolitis-associated interstitial lung disease
  r. compliance
  r. distress syndrome (RDS)
  r. disturbance index (RDI)
  r. failure
  r. injury
  r. insufficiency

NOTES

respiratory *(continued)*
    r. monitor
    r. murmur
    r. muscle disease
    r. papillomatosis
    r. pathogen
    r. rate
    r. sound
    r. syncytial virus (RSV)
    Taiwan acute r. (TWAR)
    r. tract
    r. tract infection
respirophasic chest discomfort
respite care
response
    Arthus r.
    asthmatic r.
    auditory brainstem-evoked r.
    baroreflex r.
    brainstem auditory evoked r.
      (BAER)
    brainstem evoked r. (BSER)
    Cushing r.
    depletion r.
    early asthmatic r.
    late asthmatic r.
    lymphocyte-mediated r.
    motor r.
    papillary r.
responsibility
responsible
responsive
    cytotoxic T-cell r.
    r. tumor
rest
    r. attenuation
    bed r.
    r., ice, compression, elevation
      (RICE)
    r. tremor
resting
    r. electrocardiogram
    r. electrocardiography
    r. heart rate
    r. metabolic rate (RMR)
    r. tachycardia
    r. tremor
restless
    r. legs syndrome (RLS)
    R. Legs Syndrome Foundation
restlessness
restoration
restorative care
Restoril
restriction
    caloric r.
    fluid r.

restrictive
    r. cardiomyopathy
    r. obstructive lung disease
result
    false-positive r.
    Surveillance, Epidemiology, and
      End R.'s (SEER)
resurfacing
    laser r.
resuscitate
    do not r. (DNR)
resuscitation
    cardiopulmonary r. (CPR)
    post r.
retardation
    growth r.
    psychomotor r.
    X-linked mental r.
retarded ejaculation
Retavase
retch
retching
retention
    fluid r.
    urinary r.
    r. vomiting
reteplase
rete ridge
reticula (*pl. of* reticulum)
reticularis
    livedo r.
    zona r.
reticular nucleus
reticulocyte count
reticuloendothelial cell leukemia
reticuloendotheliosis
    leukemic r.
reticulonodular pulmonary density
reticulosis
    benign inoculation r.
    histiocytic medullary r.
reticulospinal
reticulum, pl. **reticula**
Retin-A
retina
    neovascularization elsewhere on r.
      (NVE)
retinaculum
retinae
    cyanosis r.
retinal
    r. abiotrophy
    r. detachment
    r. migraine
retinitis
    cytomegalovirus r.
    r. pigmentosa (RP)
Retinol

retinopathy
background diabetic r. (BDR)
diabetic r. (DR)
full florid diabetic r. (FFDR)
Kimmelstiel-Wilson r.
preproliferative diabetic r. (PPDR)
proliferative diabetic r. (PDR)
van Heuven anatomical
classification of diabetic r.
retinoschisis
retraction
retrobulbar neuritis
retrocalcaneal bursitis
retrocaval
retrocedent gout
retrocele
retrocession
retrogasserian
retrograde
retrolisthesis
retromolar trigone
retronasal perception
retroorbital
retroperitoneal
r. fibrosis
r. mass
retrospective memory
retrosternal thyroid
retroversion
Retrovir
retrovirus
AIDS-associated r. (ARV)
rettgeri
Proteus r.
Retzius space
Reusner sign
revascularization
myocardial r.
percutaneous coronary r. (PCR)
transmyocardial laser r.
reversal
reversed
r. peristalsis
r. splitting
reversible calcinosis
reviewer
utilization r.
revision
International Classification of
Diseases, Ninth R. (ICD-9)
revivescence
revivification

rewarming
active core r.
active external r.
core r.
external r.
passive external r.
Reye syndrome
Rezulin
RFA
radiofluorescent antibody
RH
releasing hormone
Rh
Rhesus
Rhabditis
rhabdomyolysis
acute recurrent r.
exertional r.
familial paroxysmal r.
idiopathic paroxysmal r.
paroxysmal r.
recurrent r.
rhabdomyoma
cardiac r.
rhabdomyosarcoma
cardiac r.
rhagades
rhaphania
rhegma
rhegmatogenous retinal detachment (RRD)
rheoencephalography
Rhesus (Rh)
R. factor
rheumatalgia
rheumatic
r. aortic valve disease
r. arthritis
r. fever
r. gout
r. heart disease
r. mitral insufficiency
r. mitral regurgitation
r. myocarditis
r. neuritis
r. pneumonia
r. tetany
rheumatica
peliosis r.
polymyalgia r. (PMR)
purpura r.
scarlatina r.

NOTES

R

341

rheumatism
> articular r.
> cerebral r.
> gonorrheal r.
> Heberden r.
> inflammatory r.
> Macleod capsular r.
> muscular r.
> nonarticular r.
> palindromic r.
> Poncet r.
> soft tissue r.
> subacute r.

rheumatismal

rheumatoid
> r. arthritis test
> r. disease
> r. factor
> r. factor test
> r. nodule
> r. pneumoconiosis
> r. pocket

rheumatologist

rheumatology

Rheumatrex

rhinitis
> allergic r.
> IgE-mediated r.
> nonallergic r.
> perennial r.
> seasonal allergic r.

rhinocerebral
> r. mucormycosis
> r. zygomycosis

Rhinocort

rhinolith

rhinophonia

rhinophyma

rhinoplasty

rhinorrhea

rhinoscleroma

rhinoscleromatis
> *Klebsiella r.*

rhinosinusitis

rhinovirus

Rhizopus

rhizotomy

RHM
> routine health management

Rhodesian trypanosomiasis

Rhodococcus equi

rhombencephalitis

rhomboidal

rhonchal fremitus

rhonchus, pl. **rhonchi**
> cavernous r.

rhus

rhusiopathiae
> *Erysipelothrix r.*

rhythm
> accelerated idioventricular r.
> agonal r.
> chronobiologic r.
> circadian r.
> idioventricular r.
> normal sinus r. (NSR)
> regular rate and r. (RRR)
> sinus r. (SR)

rhytidosis

RIA
> radioimmunoassay

RIBA
> recombinant immunoblot assay

Ribas-Torres disease

ribavirin

rib belt

riboflavin deficiency

ribonucleic acid (RNA)

ribonucleoprotein (RNP)
> r. antibody

Ricard amputation

RICE
> rest, ice, compression, elevation

rice disease

rice-field fever

rice-water stool

Richards-Rundle syndrome

Richet aneurysm

Richner-Hanhart syndrome

Richter hernia

ricinism

rickets
> acute r.
> adult r.
> celiac r.
> hemorrhagic r.
> hereditary vitamin D-resistant r.
> hypophosphatemic vitamin D-deficient r.
> hypophosphatemic vitamin D-resistant r.
> late r.
> pseudo-vitamin D deficiency r.
> refractory r.
> renal r.
> scurvy r.
> vitamin D-resistant r.

Rickettsia
> *R. akari*
> *R. australis*
> *R. conorii*
> *R. prowazekii*
> *R. rickettsii*
> *R. sibirica*
> *R. tsutsugamushi*
> *R. typhi*

rickettsialpox

rickettsii
>*Rickettsia r.*

rickettsiosis
>California flea r.
>vesicular r.

rickety

Ridaura

ridge
>rete r.

Riedel
>R. disease
>R. lobe
>R. struma
>R. thyroiditis

Rieder cell leukemia

Rieger syndrome

Riesman sign

rifabutin

Rifamate

rifampicin

rifampin

rifapentine

Rift Valley fever virus

right
>r. aortic arch
>r. bundle-branch block (RBBB)
>r. eye (OD)
>r. lower lobe (RLL)
>r. lower quadrant (RLQ)
>r. lower quadrant (of abdomen)
>r. middle lobe (RML)
>patient's bill of r.'s
>r. salpingo-oophorectomy (RSO)
>r. upper lobe (RUL)
>r. upper quadrant (RUQ)
>r. upper quadrant (of abdomen)
>r. ventricle (RV)
>r. ventricle myocardial infarction
>r. ventricular (RV)
>r. ventricular cardiomyopathy
>r. ventricular failure
>r. ventricular hypertrophy (RVH)
>r. ventricular infarction
>r. ventricular outflow tract
>r. ventriculography

right-hand dominant

righting reflex

right-left confusion

right-sided heart failure

right-side Ebstein anomaly

rigidity
>cogwheel r.

decerebrate r.
decorticate r.
extrapyramidal r.
nuchal r.
Parkinson r.

rigidus
>hallux r.

Rigiscan monitor

rigor

Riley-Day
>R.-D. dysautonomia
>R.-D. syndrome

Rilutek

rimae

rimantadine HCl

ring
>Fleischer r.
>Fleischer-Strümpell r.
>Kayser-Fleischer r.
>lower esophageal r.
>r. pessary
>Schatzki r.
>vaginal r.
>Waldeyer r.

Ringer
>R. lactate
>lactated R.

ring-wall lesion

Rinne test

Riopan

Ripault sign

RISA
>radioiodinated serum albumin
>RISA cisternogram

rise
>chair r.

risedronate sodium

risk
>r. behavior
>empiric r.
>r. factor
>r. marker
>recurrence r.
>r. stratification

risk-taking behavior

Risperdal

risperidone

ristocctin

Ritalin-SR

ritodrine

ritonavir

rituximab

R

NOTES

RIU
    radioiodine uptake
rivastigmine
rizatriptan
RLL
    right lower lobe
RLQ
    right lower quadrant
RLS
    restless legs syndrome
RML
    right middle lobe
RMR
    resting metabolic rate
RN
    registered nurse
RNA
    ribonucleic acid
      ectopic RNA
      hepatitis C RNA
RNI
    recommended nutrient intake
RNP
    ribonucleoprotein
      RNP antibody
R/O
    rule out
Robaxin
Robaxisal
robertsonian translocation
Robertson sign
Roberts syndrome
Robert Wood Johnson Foundation (RWJF)
Robinul
Robitussin A-C
Rocaltrol
Rocephin
Rochalimaea henselae
Rockwood exercise
Rocky Mountain spotted fever
rocuronium bromide
rod
    Harrington r.
rodent ulcer
Rodrigues aneurysm
roentgen
roentgenogram
roentgenographic
Roesler-Dressler infarction
roetheln
rofecoxib
Roger
    R. bruit
    bruit de R.
    R. disease
    R. reaction
    R. symptom
Roho bed

Rokitansky
    R. disease
    R. diverticulum
rolandic
role
    r. model
    r. playing
roll
    trochanter r.
ROM
    range of motion
Roman fever
Romberg
    R. sign
    R. test
Romberg-Paessler syndrome
Rome criteria
Rommelaere sign
rongeur
room
    r. air (RA)
    r. air blood gas
root
    aortic r.
    valerian r.
ropinirole
rosa
    mal de la r.
rosacea
    acne r.
rose
    r. gardener's disease
    r. spot
rosea
    pityriasis r.
Rosenbach
    R. sign
    R. syndrome
Rosenthal syndrome
roseola
    epidemic r.
    r. infantilis
roseoliform exanthem
roseolous
rosiglitazone
Ross River fever
rostrally
Rotacaps
rotation
rotator
    r. cuff
    r. cuff injury
rotavirus
Rot-Bielschowsky syndrome
rote
    r. fashion
    r. memory
röteln

Roth
 R. disease
 R. spot
Rothmann-Makai syndrome
Rotor syndrome
rouge
 mal r.
roughage
rouleau, pl. **rouleaux**
roundworm
 tissue r.
Rourke-Ernstein sedimentation rate
Rous-associated virus (RAV)
Roussy
 thalamic syndrome of Déjérine
  and R.
route
 transperineal r.
routine
 r. followup
 r. health management (RHM)
Roux-en-Y anastomosis
Rovsing sign
Rowasa
Roxanol
Roxicet
Roxicodone
Roxiprin
royal
 R. College of Physicians
  (Edinburgh) (RCP(E))
 R. College of Physicians (Ireland)
  (RCP(I))
 R. College of Physicians (of
  England) (RCP)
 r. touch
RP
 retinitis pigmentosa
r-PA
 recombinant plasminogen activator
RPR
 rapid plasma reagent
 rapid plasma reagin
RRD
 rhegmatogenous retinal detachment
RR interval
RRR
 regular rate and rhythm
RSD
 reflex sympathetic dystrophy
RSO
 right salpingo-oophorectomy

RSV
 respiratory syncytial virus
RT$_3$
 resin triiodothyronine
RTA
 renal tubular acidosis
RT$_3$ uptake
rub
 friction r.
 pericardial friction r.
 pleural friction r.
 pleuritic r.
rubella
 congenital r.
 measles and r. (MR)
 measles, mumps, r. (MMR)
 r. panencephalitis
 r. vaccine
rubella-associated arthritis
rubelliform
rubeola
rubeosis
 r. iridis
 r. iridis diabetica
Rubin test
Rubivirus
rubor
rubra
 miliaria r.
 polycythemia r.
 r. vera
Rubramin PC
rubrum
 Trichophyton r.
ructus
Rud syndrome
ruga, pl. **rugae**
rugitus
RUL
 right upper lobe
rule
 Clark weight r.
 Cowling r.
 r. out (R/O)
 Young r.
rumination
Rumpel-Leede
 R.-L. phenomenon
 R.-L. sign
 R.-L. test

R

NOTES

Rundles-Falls
    R.-F. anemia
    R.-F. syndrome
rundown
    presynaptic r.
Runeberg
    R. anemia
    R. disease
    R. type
runner's foot
rupia
rupture
    cardiac r.
    chordae r.
    left ventricular free wall r.
    papillary muscle r.
    pulmonary artery r.
    tendon r.
    ventricular free wall r.
    ventricular septal r.
RUQ
    right upper quadrant
RURTI
    recurrent upper respiratory tract infection
rush

Russell syndrome
Russian influenza
rust
    R. disease
    R. sign
    R. syndrome
rusty sputum
Rutherford syndrome
rutidosis
Ru-Tuss
RV
    residual volume
    right ventricle
    right ventricular
        RV dilatation
RVH
    right ventricular hypertrophy
R-wave progression
RWJF
    Robert Wood Johnson Foundation
Rx
    prescription
Rynatan
Rythmol

S_1
first heart sound
S_2
second heart sound
paradoxically split S_2
split S_2
S_3
third heart sound
S_4
fourth heart sound
SA
sinoatrial
SA exit block
Peritrate SA
SAA
severe aplastic anemia
sabeluzole
Sabin-Feldman dye test
sabre
coup de s.
saburra
saburral
sac
central thecal s.
saccade
Saccharomyces cerevisiae
saccular aneurysm
sacculated
saccule
sacculiform
sacculus, pl. **sacculi**
sacculi of Beale
Sach disease
sacra (*pl. of* sacrum)
sacral micturition center
sacroiliac (SI)
s. joint
sacroiliitis
sacrospinalis
sacrum, pl. **sacra**
SAD
seasonal affective disorder
saddle
s. anesthesia
s. bump deformity
saddleback fever
S-adenosylmethionine (SAM-e)
safety
contract for s.
margin of s.
saginata
taeniasis s.
sagittal
SAH
subarachnoid hemorrhage

Sahli reaction
saint
S. Ignatius itch
S. triad
sakushu fever
Sal-Acid plaster
salbutamol inhaler
Salflex
salicylate
s. poisoning
s. toxicity
salicylic acid
saline
s. diuresis
s. laxative
Salinem
S. fever
S. infection
Salinex
salivary
s. gland calculus
s. gland disease
s. gland hormone
s. gland swelling
s. gland tumor
s. hyperamylasemia
salivation
salmeterol xinafoate
Salmonella
S. enterica choleraesuis
S. enterica enteritidis
S. enterica subsp. typhimurium
S. food poisoning
S. infection
S. typhi
S. typhosa
salmonellosis
salon pain patch
salpingectomy
salpingitis
salpingo-oophorectomy
bilateral s.-o. (BSO)
left s.-o. (LSO)
right s.-o. (RSO)
unilateral s.-o. (USO)
salpingo-oophoritis
salsalate
salt
bile s.
calcium s.
cathartic s.
s. depletion syndrome
s. edema
s. fever
gold s.

salt *(continued)*
>   s. loading
>   no added s. (NAS)
>   potassium s.
>   s. wasting

saltans
>   thrombophlebitis s.

salt-depletion crisis

salt-losing
>   s.-l. defect
>   s.-l. nephritis
>   s.-l. syndrome

saltpeter paper

salubrious

salutarium

salutary

salutatory

Salutensin

salvage
>   s. chemotherapy
>   s. therapy

salvarsan

salvo

Salzmann

SAM
>   systemic anterior motion

SAM-e
>   S-adenosylmethionine

sampling
>   inferior petrosal venous s.

SAMSHA
>   Substance Abuse and Mental Health
>   Services Administration

Samter syndrome

San
>   S. Joaquin Valley disease
>   S. Joaquin Valley fever

sanative

sanatorium

sanatory

sandal foot

sandfly fever

Sandhoff disease

Sandwith bald tongue

Sanfilippo
>   S. disease
>   S. syndrome

sanguinareus
>   mycetism s.

sanguine

sanguineous

sanitarian

sanitarium

sanitary

sanitation

sanitization

Sansert

Santini booming sound

SaO₂
>   arterial oxygen saturation

São Paulo
>   S. P. fever
>   S. P. typhus

saphenous vein graft

SAPHO
>   synovitis, acne, pustulosis, hyperostosis,
>   osteitis
>   SAPHO syndrome

sapremia

saprophyte

saprophytic

saquinavir

sarcoid
>   s. arthritis
>   Boeck s.
>   Darier-Roussy s.
>   Schaumann s.
>   Spiegler-Fendt s.

sarcoidosis
>   beryllium s.
>   Boeck s.
>   s. and pregnancy
>   Schaumann s.

sarcoma
>   Ewing s.
>   Kaposi s. (KS)
>   soft tissue s.

sarcomatoid

sarcomatosum
>   myxoma s.

sarcomatous

sarcopenia

Sarcoptes scabiei

sarcosinemia

Sarna

sat
>   saturation

satiety

sativa
>   cannabis s.

saturation (sat)
>   arterial oxygen s. (SaO₂)

saturnine
>   arthralgia s.
>   s. colic
>   s. gout

saturnism

saucerize

Saunders disease

saw palmetto

SBE
>   subacute bacterial endocarditis

SBP
>   systolic blood pressure

scabiei
>   *Sarcoptes s.*

scabies

scalded skin syndrome
scalding
scale
  Activities-Specific Balance
    Confidence S. (ABC)
  adaptive s.
  alcohol dependence s.
  Alzheimer Disease Assessment S.
    (ADAS)
  Blessed Dementia Rating S.
  Bradburn Affect Balance S.
  Center for Epidemiologic Studies
    Depression S. (CES-D)
  Childhood Autism Rating S.
    (CARS)
  Children's Affective Rating S.
    (CARS)
  Clinical Global Impression-Severity
    of Illness S. (CGI-S)
  Falls Efficacy S. (FES)
  Gaffky s.
  Geriatric Depression S. (GDS)
  Glasgow Coma S.
  graphic picture s.
  Hamilton Depression S.
  Karnofsky Rating S.
  Katz Activities of Daily Living S.
  Likert s.
  Livingston insomnia s.
  Lund-Browder burn s.
  Mandel Social Adjustment S.
    (MSAS)
  Migraine Disability Assessment S.
    (MIDAS)
  Mohs s.
  National Institutes of Health
    Stroke S.
  Orpington Prognostic s.
  Philadelphia Geriatric Center
    Morale S.
  Psychological General Well-
    Being S. (PGWB)
  psychometric s.
  Quality of Well-Being S. (QWB)
  Short-Form Geriatric Depression S.
  sliding s.
  verbal s.
  visual analogue s.
  Wechsler Adult Intelligence S.-
    Revised
  Wechsler Memory S. (WMS)
  word descriptor s.

  Zubrod s.
  Zung Self-Rating Depression S.
scalene
scalenotomy
scalenus anticus syndrome
scaler treadmill
scalp vein needle
scaly
scan
  bone s.
  computed tomography s.
  CT s.
  DEXA s.
  diisopropyliminodiacetic acid s.
  DISIDA s.
  dual-energy x-ray absorptiometry s.
  gallium s.
  hepatic 2,6-dimethyliminodiacetic
    acid s.
  hepatoiminodiacetic acid s.
  HIDA s.
  Indium s.
  liver s.
  low-dose CT s.
  lung s.
  myocardial perfusion s.
  perfusion lung s.
  radioisotopic s.
  scintigraphic ventilation/perfusion s.
  single-photon emission computed
    tomography s.
  SPECT s.
  ventilation/perfusion lung s.
  V/Q s.
scanning
  s. electron microscope (SEM)
  radionuclide s.
  tagged red blood cell s.
scaphocephaly
scaphoid
scapholunate
scapula
  spine of s.
scarlatina
  anginose s.
  s. hemorrhagica
  s. latens
  s. maligna
  s. rheumatica
  s. simplex
  stomatitis s.
scarlatinal

S

NOTES

scarlatinella
scarlatiniform
scarlatinoid
scarlet fever
SCAT
    sickle cell anemia test
scatoma
scavenger
    free radical s.
SCC
    squamous cell carcinoma
SCCD
    subacute cortical cerebellar degeneration
scenario
Schafer syndrome
Schamberg
    S. disease
    S. purpura
Schatzki ring
Schaumann
    S. body
    S. disease
    S. sarcoid
    S. sarcoidosis
    S. syndrome
schedule
    dosing s.
    regular sleep s.
    sleep s.
scheduled toileting
Scheie syndrome
Schenck disease
schenckii
    Sporotrichum s.
Scheuermann disease
Scheuthauer-Marie-Sainton syndrome
Schilder disease
Schilling
    S. leukemia
    S. test
Schirmer test
schistocyte
Schistosoma
    S. haematobium
    S. intercalatum
    S. japonicum
    S. mansoni
    S. mekongi
schistosome
schistosomia
schistosomiasis
    Asiatic s.
    bladder s.
    cutaneous s.
    s. disorder
    ectopic s.
    hepatic s.
    intestinal s.

Manson s.
Oriental s.
pulmonary s.
urinary s.
schizoaffective disorder
schizophrenia
schizophrenic
schizophreniform disorder
schizotypal
schlammfieber
Schmidt
    S. diet
    S. syndrome
Schmidt-Strassburger diet
Schmitz bacillus
Schmorl
    S. bacillus
    S. node
    S. nodule
schneiderian membrane
Schneider nail
Schneidersitz
Scholl
    Dr. S.
Scholz disease
Schönlein-Henoch
    S.-H. purpura
    S.-H. syndrome
Schönlein purpura
school nurse
Schottmüller
    S. disease
    S. fever
Schott treatment
Schüffner dot
Schüller-Christian disease
Schüller disease
Schultz angina
Schultze acroparesthesia
Schultze-type acroparesthesia
Schwachman syndrome
Schwann hyperplasia
schwannoma
schwannosis
Schwartz
    S. leukemia virus
    S. test
Schwartz-Bartter syndrome
Schweninger method
sciatic
    s. nerve compression
    s. nerve syndrome
sciatica
SCIDS
    severe combined immunodeficiency
        syndrome
scie
    bruit de s.

science
    National Institute of Environmental
       Health S.'s (NIEHS)
    National Institute of General
       Medical S.'s (NIGMS)
scientific theory
scintigram
scintigraphic ventilation/perfusion scan
scintigraphy
    dipyridamole-thallium s.
    hepatobiliary s.
    red blood cell s.
    thallium s.
scintillating scotoma
scintillation
scintiphotography
scirrhous CA
scissoring
scissors
    Kaye dissecting s.
SCLC
    small-cell lung cancer
sclera
scleradenitis
sclerae anicteric
scleral
    s. icterus
    s. show
scleredema
scleritis
sclerocystic
    s. disease
    s. disease of ovary
sclerodactylia annularis ainhumoides
sclerodactyly
scleroderma
    diffuse s.
    limited s.
    systemic sclerosis sine s.
sclerodermatomyositis
sclerogenous
sclerosing
    s. cholangitis
    s. lymphosarcoma
    s. panencephalitis (SSPE)
sclerosis
    amyotrophic lateral s. (ALS)
    aortic s.
    glomerulocapillary s.
    hippocampal s.
    lichen s.
    multiple s. (MS)

    nuclear s.
    s. panencephalitis
    systemic s.
sclerotherapy
    endoscopic injection s.
SCM
    sternocleidomastoid
scoliosis
scope
    Machida s.
scopolamine
    Transderm S.
scorbutica
    stomatitis s.
scorbutic anemia
scorbutigenic
scorbutus
scordinema
score
    acute physiology and chronic
      health evaluation s.
    APACHE II s.
    Apgar s.
    Four IADL S.
    Four Instrumental Activities of
      Daily Living S.
    Gleason s.
    Logistic Organ Dysfunction S.
scorpion sting
Scotch short arm cast
scotoma, pl. **scotomata**
    absolute s.
    Bjerrum s.
    scintillating s.
Scott syndrome
Scot-Tussin
scout film
screen
    beta hCG s.
    7-minute s.
    radioallergosorbent s.
    RAST s.
    "up and go" s.
    vision s.
screening
    s. for Alzheimer disease
    carrier s.
    familial s.
    s. mammography
    mass s.
    microsatellite instability s.

S

NOTES

screening (*continued*)
    s. test
    s. urinalysis
screw
    AO s.
Scribner shunt
scrofula
scrotum, pl. **scrota, scrotums**
    malignant neoplasm of s.
    s. mass
    s. pain
    s. swelling
scrub
    s. nurse
    s. typhus
scurvy
    Alpine s.
    hemorrhagic s.
    infantile s.
    land s.
    s. rickets
    sea s.
scybala
scybalous feces
scybalum
SDAT
    senile dementia of Alzheimer type
SDH
    systolic-diastolic hypertension
se
    per se
sea
    s. scurvy
    s. sickness
    S. and Ski lotion
seagull bruit
seasickness
seasonal
    s. affective disorder (SAD)
    s. allergic rhinitis
    s. factor
    s. influence
    s. variation
seat
    raised toilet s.
sebaceous
    s. gland of Zeis
    s. hyperplasia
seborrhea
seborrheic
    s. blepharitis
    s. dermatitis
    s. keratitis
    s. keratosis
sebum production
Seconal
second
    forced expiratory volume in one s.
    (FEV$_1$)

    s. heart sound (S$_2$)
    milliliters per s. (mL/sec)
    s. sound
secondary
    s. acute leukemia
    s. adrenal failure
    s. adrenocortical insufficiency
    s. aging
    s. aldosteronism
    s. amenorrhea
    s. amyloidosis
    s. coccidioidomycosis
    s. diabetes
    s. diabetes mellitus
    s. drowning
    s. focal segmental
      glomerulosclerosis
    s. gout
    s. hemochromatosis
    s. hemostasis
    s. hypercalciuria
    s. hyperparathyroidism
    s. hypertension
    s. hyperthyroidism
    s. hypoadrenocorticism
    s. hypogonadism
    s. hypothyroidism
    s. liver disease
    s. medical care
    s. menopause
    s. parkinsonism
    s. pellagra
    s. peritonitis
    s. polycythemia
    s. prevention
    s. refractory anemia
    s. renal tubular acidosis
    s. sclerosis cholangitis
    s. sex characteristics
    s. skin lesion
    s. syphilis
    s. thrombocytopenic purpura
    s. tuberculosis
    s. union
    s. X zone
second-degree
    s.-d. atrioventricular block
    s.-d. burn
second-set phenomenon
second-trimester abortion
secreta
secretagogue
    growth hormone s.
    insulin s.
secrete
secretin test
secretion
    external s.
    nasal s.

purulent s.
syndrome of inappropriate
  antidiuretic hormone s.
secretomotor
secretory
  s. adenoma
  s. diarrhea
  s. IgA
  s. testing
section
  cesarean s.
  paraffin s.
  vaginal birth after cesarean s.
  (VBAC)
Sectral
secular
secundines
secundum
  s. artem
  ostium s.
security
  Social S.
sedating version tricyclic depressant
sedation
sedative
sedative-hypnotic
sedentary lifestyle
sedimentation rate
SEER
  Surveillance, Epidemiology, and End
    Results
    SEER cancer registry
segment
  intrastromal corneal ring s.
  PR s.
  ST s.
  TP s.
segmental
  s. atelectasis
  s. pneumonia
segmentation
  genome s.
segmented neutrophils (segs)
segmenter
segs
  segmented neutrophils (*See also* polys)
Seip-Lawrence syndrome
seizure
  s. activity
  breastfeeding and s.
  clonic s.
  febrile s.

generalized motor s.
grand mal s.
hysterical s.
lamotrigine s.
localization-related s.
partial complex s.
petit mal s.
pseudoepileptic s.
tonic s.
tonic-clonic s.
withdrawal s.
Seldane
Seldinger technique
selection
  s. bias
  donor s.
selective
  s. cobalamin malabsorption
  s. estrogen receptor modulator
    (SERM)
  s. hypoaldosteronism
  s. IgA deficiency
  s. neuronal death
  s. renal angiography
  s. serotonin reuptake inhibitor
    (SSRI)
  s. serotonin reuptake inhibitor
    toxicity
  s. transsphenoidal surgery
selegiline
selenious
selenium
  s. burdens
  s. toxicity syndrome
self-assessment
self-care
self-determination
self-efficacy
self-endangerment
  physical s.-e.
self-examination
  breast s.-e. (BSE)
self-help group
**Self Help for Hard of Hearing People,
  Inc. (SHHH)**
self-intermittent catheterization
self-limited
  s.-l. disease
  s.-l. inflammatory arthritis
self-limiting
self-perception
self-poisoning

S

NOTES

353

self-report of constipation
sella
sellar tumor
Selsun Blue
Selye adaptation syndrome
SEM
    scanning electron microscope
    systolic ejection murmur
semantic
    s. complaint
    s. memory
    s. paraphasia
semen analysis
semi
semilunaris
    linea s.
semimembranosus
seminiferous
    s. tubule
    s. tubule dysgenesis
seminoma
semiotic
semiotics
semitertian
Semmes-Weinstein monofilament
Semprex-D
Senear-Usher
    S.-U. disease
    S.-U. syndrome
senescence
    benign s.
    cell s.
senescent forgetfulness
senile
    s. atrophy
    s. cortical devastation
    s. delirium
    s. dementia
    s. dementia of Alzheimer type
    (SDAT)
    s. deterioration
    s. plaque
    s. purpura
    s. sinus node dysfunction
    s. skin
    s. systemic amyloidosis
    s. urethritis
senilis
    arcus s.
    malum articulorum s.
    purpura s.
senility
senior
    s. citizen
    S. Job Bank
    Naldecon S.
SeniorNet (SN)
senium

senna
    S. Tabs
Senning atrial baffle repair
Senokot
sensation
    chilling s.
    dissociated s.
    first voiding s.
    globus s.
    reduced rectal s.
sense
    vibration s.
sensitive
    pain s.
sensitivity
    acquired s.
    baroreceptor s.
    beta-lactam s.
    culture and s. (C&S)
    induced s.
    multiple chemical s.
sensitization
sensitize
sensitizer
    insulin s.
sensorimotor
sensorineural deafness
sensorium
    general s.
sensory
    s. deficit
    s. disorder
    s. loss
    S. Organization Test (SOT)
sentinel node
sepsis, pl. **sepses**
    community-acquired s.
    fulminant s.
    gram-negative s.
    s. lenta
    puerperal s.
    s. syndrome
septa (*pl. of* septum)
septal
    s. myocardial infarction
    s. ventricular tachycardia
septan
septemia
septic
    s. arthritis
    s. bursitis
    s. fever
    s. intoxication
    s. intracranial thrombophlebitis
    s. pneumonia
    s. shock
    s. shock syndrome
    s. wound

septica
    iridocyclitis s.
septi cavum pellucidi
septicemia
    acute fulminating meningococcal s.
    catheter-associated nosocomial s.
    fulminating meningococcal s.
    gonococcal s.
    meningococcal s.
    metastasizing s.
    morphine injector's s.
    nosocomial s.
    plague s.
septicemic plague
septicophlebitis
septicopyemia
septicum
    Clostridium s.
septooptic dysplasia
septoplasty
    nasal s.
septostomy
    atrial s.
Septra DS
septum, pl. **septa**
    intraventricular s.
sequela, pl. **sequelae**
sequence
    nucleotide s.
    operon promoter s.
sequential
    s. multiple analysis-20 (SMA-20)
    S. Multiple Analyzer Computer
        (SMAC)
sequestra (*pl. of* sequestrum)
sequestrant
    bile s.
    bile acid s.
sequestration
    s. of medication
    splenic s.
sequestrum, pl. **sequestra**
sequoiosis
sera (*pl. of* serum)
Serafem
Ser-Ap-Es
Serax
serenity-tranquility-peace (STP)
    s.-t.-p. pill
Serentil
Serevent inhaler

serial
    s. imaging
    s. testing
series
    liver function s. (LFS)
    upper gastrointestinal s. (UGIS)
SERM
    selective estrogen receptor modulator
Sernoa repens
serodiagnosis
seroepidemiology
serology
    HIV s.
    viral s.
seroma
seronegative
    s. arthritis
    s. polyarthritis
    s. spondyloarthropathy
Serophene
seropurulent
serosa
serosanguineous
serositis
    adhesive s.
serotherapy
serotonergic
serotonin
    s. receptor agonist
    s. receptor antagonist
    s. reuptake inhibitor (SRI)
    s. syndrome
**serotonin-norepinephrine reuptake
    inhibitor (SNRI)**
serotype
    adenovirus s.
serous
    s. adenofibroma
    s. diarrhea
    s. hemorrhage
    s. otitis
    s. tumor
Serpasil
serpiginous corneal ulcer
serrata
    Huperzia s.
Serratia
serrating
Sertoli cell
Sertoli-cell-only syndrome
sertraline
serum, pl. **sera**

S

NOTES

355

serum *(continued)*
- s. accident
- s. albumin
- s. aminotransferase
- s. aminotransferase level
- s. ammonia
- anticrotalus s.
- antirabies s.
- antitoxic s.
- s. carotene
- s. cholesterol level
- s. disease
- s. enzyme
- s. eruption
- s. ferritin level
- s. gastrin
- s. globulin
- s. glutamic oxaloacetic transaminase (SGOT)
- s. glutamic pyruvic transaminase (SGPT)
- s. hepatitis (SH)
- hereditary erythroblastic multinuclearity associated with positive acidified s. (HEMPAS)
- s. hormone transport
- s. 25-hydroxyvitamin D
- s. iron level
- s. methylmalonic acid
- s. osmolality
- s. paralysis
- s. protein electrophoresis (SPEP)
- s. reaction
- s. sickness
- s. sodium concentration
- s. therapy
- s. thyroid-stimulating hormone
- s. thyroid-stimulating hormone assay
- s. total thyroxine
- s. transaminase level elevation
- s. triiodothyronine
- s. vitamin B_{12}

service
- AIDS Clinical Trials Information S. (ACTIS)
- care s.'s
- Corporation for National S. (CNS)
- HIV/AIDS Treatment Information S. (ATIS)
- Indian Health S. (IHS)
- National Association for Practical Nurse Education and S.'s (NAPNES)
- National Health S. (England) (NHS)
- Public Health S. (PHS)
- The Centers for Medicare and Medicaid S.'s

United States Public Health S. (USPHS)

Serzone

sesamoid

sesamoiditis

sessile

sestamibi
- technetium-99m s.
- s. test

set
- enteral feeding s.
- LifeGuard enteral feeding s.

seton procedure

setting
- assisted living s.
- primary care s.
- S. Priorities for Retirement Years (SPRY)
- S. Priorities for Retirement Years Foundation

setting-sun sign

settlement
- claim s.

seven
- subtract serial s.'s

seven-day fever

severe
- s. aplastic anemia (SAA)
- s. chronic hepatitis
- s. combined immunodeficiency syndrome (SCIDS)
- s. malabsorption symptoms
- s. persistent asthma

severely disabled

severity

sex
- s. hormone
- s. hormone-binding globulin (SHBG)

sex-linked hypochromatic anemia of Rundles and Falls

sextan

sexual
- s. asphyxia
- s. aversion disorder
- s. desire disorder
- s. dimorphism
- s. dwarfism
- s. history
- s. infantilism
- s. intercourse
- s. misconduct
- s. pain
- s. potency
- s. precocity
- s. response cycle

sexually transmitted disease (STD)

SF-36
Medical Outcomes Study SF-36
MOS SF-36
SGOT
serum glutamic oxaloacetic transaminase
SGPT
serum glutamic pyruvic transaminase
SH
serum hepatitis
SH renal disease
shake
smelter's s.'s
shallow breathing
shampoo
Capitrol s.
coal tar s.
shankapulshpi
shared epitope
sharing
United Network for Organ S.
(UNOS)
shark cartilage
sharp touch
shave excisional biopsy
Shaver disease
shawl-sign rash
SHBG
sex hormone-binding globulin
shear
shearing force
sheath
neurovascular s.
rectus s.
Sheehan
S. disease
S. syndrome
Sheehy syndrome
Shekelton aneurysm
Sheldon catheter
shellfish poison
Shenton line
SHHH
Self Help for Hard of Hearing People,
Inc.
Shibley sign
shift
s. change
fluid s.
internal fluid s.
microbial antigenic phase s.
transcellular potassium s.
transcellular water s.

shifting dullness
Shiga bacillus
Shigella
S. flexneri
S. infection
S. sonnei
shigelloides
Aeromonas s.
shigellosis
Shiley tracheotomy tube
shimamushi disease
shin
s. bone fever
s. splints
s. spot
shingles
ship
s. beriberi
s. fever
Shirodkar procedure cerclage
SHMO
social health maintenance organization
shock
burn s.
cardiac s.
cardiogenic s.
direct-current s.
distributive s.
electric s.
gut-derived infectious toxic s.
(GITS)
hemorrhagic s.
hypoglycemic s.
hypovolemic s.
s. index
insulin s.
irreversible s.
s. lung
nitroid s.
obstructive s.
postoperative s.
septic s.
toxic s.
traumatic s.
vasodilatory s.
venovasodilatory s.
wet s.
shock-like
electric s.-l.
shock-wave lithotripsy
shoddy fever

NOTES

shoe
    Darco s.
    Nike s.
shop typhus
short
    s. cosyntropin stimulation test
    s. incubation hepatitis
    s. leg cast
    S. Portable Mental Status
    Questionnaire (SPMSQ)
    s. tandem repeat
short-acting
    s.-a. beta agonist
    s.-a. insulin analog
short-bowel syndrome
short-colon examination
shortening
Short-Form Geriatric Depression Scale
shortness of breath (SOB)
short-term
    s.-t. followup
    s.-t. insomnia
    s.-t. institutional respite care
    s.-t. memory (STM)
shortwave
    s. diathermy
    s. treatment
Shoshin disease
shot
    cortical s.
shotgun prescription
shotty node
shoulder
    s. arthritis
    dislocated s.
    frozen s.
    s. girdle
    Head & S.'s
    Milwaukee s.
    s. pain
show
    scleral s.
Shulman syndrome
shunt
    arteriovenous s.
    bidirectional Glenn s.
    bilateral Glenn s.
    classic Glenn s.
    s. fraction
    Glenn s.
    LeVeen s.
    palliative s.
    s. patency
    portacaval s.
    portosystemic s.
    Scribner s.
    ventriculoperitoneal s.
    Waterston s.

shunting
    arteriovenous s.
shuttle-walking distance
Shwachman-Diamond syndrome
Shwachman syndrome
Shy-Drager syndrome
SI
    sacroiliac
    SI joint
SIADH
    syndrome of inappropriate secretion of
    antidiuretic hormone
sialadenitis
    acute suppurative s.
sialectasis
sialidosis
sialoadenitis
sialoaerophagy
sialoangiitis
sialogastrone
sialogram
sialolithiasis
sialometaplasia
sialorrhea pancreatica
sialosemiology
Siberian
    S. ginseng
    S. tick typhus
sibilant
    expiratory s.
    s. rale
sibilus
sibirica
    Rickettsia s.
sibutramine hydrochloride
sicca
    cholera s.
    s. complex
    keratoconjunctivitis s.
    pharyngitis s.
sicchasia
Sichel disease
sick
    s. building syndrome
    s. euthyroid syndrome
    s. sinus syndrome (SSS)
sickening
sickle
    s. cell
    s. cell anemia
    s. cell anemia test (SCAT)
    s. cell C disease
    s. cell crisis
    s. cell dactylitis
    s. cell nephropathy
    s. cell test
    s. cell-thalassemia disease
    s. cell trait
sicklemia

sickness
 acute African sleeping s.
 aerial s.
 African sleeping s.
 air s.
 altitude s.
 balloon s.
 black s.
 caisson s.
 car s.
 cave s.
 chronic African sleeping s.
 chronic mountain s.
 decompression s.
 East African sleeping s.
 green s.
 green tobacco s.
 high-altitude s.
 S. Impact Profile (SIP)
 Indian s.
 Jamaican vomiting s.
 milk s.
 motion s.
 mountain s.
 radiation s.
 sea s.
 serum s.
 sleeping s.
 space s.
 West African sleeping s.
Sidbury syndrome
side effect
siderans
 pestis s.
sideremic anemia
sideroachrestic process
sideroblast
sideroblastic anemia
sideropenic anemia
siderosilicosis
siderosis
 pulmonary s.
siderotica
 granulomatosis s.
 pneumoconiosis s.
 splenogranulomatosis s.
siderotic splenomegaly
Sidler-Huguenin endothelioma
SIDS
 sudden infant death syndrome
Siegert sign

sig
 sigmoidoscopy
  flex sig
   flexible sigmoidoscopy
sigmoid colon
sigmoidoscopy (sig)
 flexible s. (flex sig)
 flexible fiberoptic s. (FFS)
Sigmund gland
sign
 Aaron s.
 Abadie s.
 Abrahams s.
 accessory s.
 antecedent s.
 assident s.
 Auerbrugger s.
 Aufrecht s.
 Babinski s.
 Baccelli s.
 Ballance s.
 Ballet s.
 Barré s.
 Bassler s.
 Bastedo s.
 Becker s.
 Bèhier-Hardy s.
 Biederman s.
 Biernacki s.
 Biot breathing s.
 Bird s.
 Blumberg s.
 Boston s.
 Bouchard s.
 bowstring s.
 Bozzolo s.
 Brudzinski s.
 burning drops s.
 Burton s.
 Cantelli s.
 cardinal s.
 Carnett s.
 Carvallo s.
 Chilaiditi s.
 Chvostek and Trousseau s.'s
 Clark s.
 Claybrook s.
 cogwheel s.
 Comby s.
 commemorative s.
 Cope s.
 Corrigan s.

NOTES

sign *(continued)*
Courvoisier s.
Cowen s.
Cruveilhier s.
Cruveilhier-Baumgarten s.
Cullen s.
Dalrymple s.
Dance s.
de Musset s.
de Mussy s.
d'Espine s.
Dixon Mann s.
doll's eye s.
drawer s.
Duchenne s.
Duckworth s.
Durkan s.
Enroth s.
Erb s.
fabere s.
Faget s.
fat pad s.
Federici s.
Fischer s.
focal neurologic s.
Forchheimer s.
frontal release s.
Gilbert s.
Goggia s.
Gorlin s.
Graefe s.
Grey Turner s.
Grocco s.
groove s.
Gubler s.
Gunn s.
Guyon s.
Hamman s.
Heberden s.
Homans s.
Hoover s.
Horn s.
Hoyne s.
Huchard s.
Jaccoud s.
Jellinek s.
Jendrassik s.
Joffroy s.
jugular s.
Kehr s.
Kernig s.
Knies s.
Kocher s.
Kussmaul s.
Lennhoff s.
Lhermitte s.
Livierato s.
local s.
long-tract s.

Lorenz s.
Lovibond profile s.
Lucas s.
Magnus s.
Mann s.
Marañón s.
Marfan s.
Marie s.
McBurney s.
Means s.
Mirchamp s.
Möbius s.
Morquio s.
Moschcowitz s.
Mosler s.
Müller s.
Murphy s.
Myerson s.
Nikolsky s.
Nothnagel s.
objective s.
obturator s.
Ortolani s.
Osler s.
Parkinson s.
Pastia s.
Payr s.
Pemberton s.
Perez s.
Pfuhl s.
Phalen s.
physical s.
Plummer s.
prodromic s.
pseudo-Graefe s.
psoas s.
puddle s.
Quant s.
Queckenstedt s.
Quincke s.
raccoon s.
Ramond s.
Ransohoff s.
Raynaud s.
red, white, and blue s.
Reusner s.
Riesman s.
Ripault s.
Robertson s.
Romberg s.
Rommelaere s.
Rosenbach s.
Rovsing s.
Rumpel-Leede s.
Rust s.
setting-sun s.
Shibley s.
Siegert s.
Simon s.

Skoda s.
Snellen s.
soft s.
spinal s.
Spurling s.
Steinberg thumb s.
Stellwag s.
Sternberg s.
Stierlin s.
Strauss s.
subjective s.
Suker s.
Sumner s.
ten Horn s.
Thomson s.
Tinel s.
Toma s.
Topolanski s.
Traube s.
Tresilian s.
Troisier s.
Trousseau s.
Turner s.
Unschuld s.
Vipond s.
vital s.
von Graefe s.
Wilder s.
Winterbottom s.
wrist s.
Yergason s.
signal transduction
signet ring cell
significance
    atypical squamous cell of
        undetermined s. (ASCUS)
significantly impaired
significant other (SO)
siguatera
Sigvaris stocking
SIL
    squamous intraepithelial lesion
Silastic implant
sildenafil
silent
    s. coronary heart disease
    s. myocardial infarction
    s. neoplasia
    s. nociceptor
    s. thyroiditis
    s. tumor

silicate pneumoconiosis
silicatosis
silicoanthracosis
siliconoma
silicoproteinosis
silicosiderosis
silicosis
    accelerated s.
    acute s.
    chronic s.
silicotic granuloma
silicotuberculosis
Silipos pad
silo-filler's
    s.-f. disease
    s.-f. lung
Silon Dual-Dress wound dressing
Silvadene
silver
    Centrum S.
    s. fork deformity
    s. poisoning
    s. sulfadizine dressing
simethicone
similar
    law of s.'s
similia similibus curantur
similimum
Simmonds
    S. disease
    S. syndrome
Simon
    S. disease
    S. Foundation for Continence
    S. sign
simple
    s. acid-base disorder
    s. cystometry
    s. eosinophilic pneumonia
    s. mastectomy
    s. necrosis
    s. obesity
    s. pulmonary eosinophilia
simplex
    adiposis tuberosa s.
    herpes s.
    icterus s.
    labial herpes s.
    lichen chronicus s.
    purpura s.
    scarlatina s.

S

NOTES

simplex *(continued)*
    toxoplasmosis, other infections,
        rubella, cytomegalovirus infection,
        herpes s. (TORCH)
SimpliRED
    S. D-dimer test
    S. D-dimer testing
simulation
simultagnosia
simultaneous
simvastatin
sincalide
sinciput, pl. **sinciputs, sincipita**
Sindbis fever
Sine-Aid
Sinemet
sinensis
    Clonorchis s.
Sinequan
single
    s. dual-beam photon absorptiometry
    s. thyroid nodule
    s. toxic nodule
single-photon
    s.-p. absorptiometry
    s.-p. emission computed
        tomography (SPECT)
    s.-p. emission computed
        tomography method
    s.-p. emission computed
        tomography scan
    s.-p. planar imaging
singlet
singultus
sinister
    oculus s. (OS)
sinistrocardia
sinistrocerebral
sinoatrial (SA)
    s. exit block
    s. node
sinobronchial
sinopulmonary system
sinus
    s. bradycardia
    s. culture
    draining s.
    infected pilonidal s.
    s. infection
    lymph s.
    marginal s.
    medullary s.
    s. nodal reentry
    s. node
    pilonidal s.
    s. rhythm (SR)
    s. tachycardia
    traumatic s.
    s. trephination

s. tumor
s. of Valsalva
s. of Valsalva aneurysm
s. venosus
s. venous defect
s. x-ray
sinusitis
    acute s.
    chronic s.
    ethmoid s.
    maxillary s.
    mucormycosis s.
    sphenoid s.
SIP
    Sickness Impact Profile
Sipple syndrome
Sippy diet
siriasis
sirolimus
SIRS
    systemic inflammatory response
        syndrome
site
    cancer with unknown primary s.
    primary s.
    s. specific
    unknown primary s.
situ
    carcinoma in s. (CIS)
    ductal carcinoma in s. (DCIS)
    in s.
    lobular carcinoma in s.
situational syncope
sitz bath
sixth disease
size
    weight-for-frame s.
Sjögren
    S. disease
    S. syndrome
Skelaxin
Skene gland
skill
    cognitive coping s.
    coping s.
    technical s.
    visuospatial s.
skilled
    s. care
    s. nursing facility (SNF)
skin
    abraded s.
    bronzed s.
    s. caliper
    s. cancer
    dry s.
    elastic s.
    s. fragility
    glabrous s.

s. infection
s. inflammation
s. integrity
s. lesion
s. prick test
s. puncture test
senile s.
The S. Cancer Foundation
s. ulcer
skinfold thickness
skipping
Skoal chewing tobacco
Skoda
S. rale
S. sign
S. tympany
skodaic resonance
skodique
bruit s.
SKSD
streptokinase streptodornase
skull
natiform s.
SKY epidural pain control system
slaty anemia
SLC-90
Symptom Checklist 90
SLE
systemic lupus erythematosus
SLE-like syndrome
sleep
s. apnea
s. architecture alteration
s. center
s. deprivation
s. diary
s. disruption
disturbance in maintaining s.
(DIMS)
s. efficiency
s. enuresis
s. hygiene
inadequate s.
s. latency
s. mask
s. myoclonus
nonrestorative s.
s. offset
s. onset
s. phase disorder
rapid eye movement s.
REM s.

s. schedule
slow-wave s.
stage 4 s.
s. structure
s. study
s. terror
sleep-disordered breathing
sleep-enhancing behavioral technique
sleepiness
daytime s.
sleeping
s. pill
s. sickness
sleep-wake cycle
sleepwalking
sleeve
Bell-Horn knee s.
Reid s.
SLI
splenic localization index
sliding
s. hiatal hernia
s. scale
slime fever
Slim Fast
sling
s. procedure
pulmonary artery s.
Slinky balloon catheter
slippage
slippery elm
slit-lamp examination
Slo-bid
Slo-Niacin
Slo-phyllin
S.-p. GG
slough
sloughed
sloughing
tissue s.
slow
S. Fe
s. fever
s. paroxysmal atrial tachycardia
(SPAT)
s. virus disease
slow-channel blocker
Slow-K
Slow-Mag
slow-transit constipation
slow-wave sleep

S

NOTES

363

SLR
straight leg raising
Sluder neuralgia
sludge
biliary s.
SMA-20
sequential multiple analysis-20
SMAC
Sequential Multiple Analyzer Computer
small
s. bowel obstruction
s. bowel x-ray
s. cell
s. intestinal bacterial overgrowth
s. intestine
s. intestine function
s. neck incisional hernia
Small-Carrion penile prosthesis
small-cell lung cancer (SCLC)
small-intestinal lymphoma
small-intestine resection
smallpox
confluent s.
discrete s.
fulminating s.
hemorrhagic s.
malignant s.
modified s.
s. vaccination
West Indian s.
small-vessel vasculitis
smear
abnormal Pap s.
liver s.
Pap s.
Papanicolaou smear
Papanicolaou s. (Pap smear)
peripheral blood s.
Tzanck s.
smearing
smegma preputii
smell disorder
smelter's
s. chills
s. fever
s. shakes
Smith-Lemli-Opitz syndrome
Smith-Strang disease
smoke inhalation
smokeless tobacco
smoking
s. cessation
s. cessation counseling
smoldering
s. multiple myeloma
s. myeloid leukemia
smooth
s. diet
s. muscle

smooth-muscle relaxant
smudging
SN
SeniorNet
snail fever
snake bite
snap
opening s.
Snellen
S. eye chart
S. sign
SNF
skilled nursing facility
snoring
apneic spell associated with
loud s.
heroic s.
loud s.
snout reflex
SNRI
serotonin-norepinephrine reuptake
inhibitor
snub-nose dwarfism
snuffbox
SO
significant other
SO$_4$
sulfate
soak
Domeboro s.
soaked cotton pledget 4%
SOAP
subjective, objective, assessment, and
plan
soap
super-fatted s.
soapsuds enema
SOB
shortness of breath
social
s. cognition
s. disinhibition
s. health maintenance organization
(SHMO)
s. medicine
s. phobia
S. Security
S. Security Administration (SSA)
s. worker
socialization
socialized medicine
society
American Cancer S. (ACS)
American Geriatrics S. (AGS)
Delta S.
Fellow of the Royal S. (Canada)
(FRSC)
International Hearing S.
League of Red Cross s.'s

Leukemia and Lymphoma S., Inc. (LLS)
National Multiple Sclerosis S. (NMSS)
S. for Neuroscience
North American Menopause S. (NAMS)

sociodemographic group
socioeconomic factor
sociomedical
sock
    Creative diabetic s.'s
sodium
    s. balance
    carbenicillin indanyl s.
    s. cellulose
    cerivastatin s.
    s. chloride (NaCl)
    s. cromoglycate
    cromolyn s.
    danaparoid s.
    s. depletion
    enoxaparin s.
    fluvastatin s.
    s. intake
    levothyroxine s.
    nedocromil s.
    nitroprusside s.
    s. pump
    rabeprazole s.
    s. reabsorption
    risedronate s.
    S. Sulamyd
    s. valproate
sodoku
soft
    s. corn
    s. mechanical diet
    s. sign
    s. tissue infection
    s. tissue mass
    s. tissue rheumatism
    s. tissue sarcoma
Sof-Tact glucose monitor
softener
    fecal s.
SOH
    sympathetic orthostatic hypotension
sokosho
Solaquin Forte
solar
    s. elastosis

    s. fever
    s. keratosis
    s. lentigo
    s. purpura
    s. therapy
    s. treatment
    s. urticaria
Solaraze
soldier's heart
sole
    Visco S.'s
soleus muscle
solid tumor
solis
    ictus s.
solitary
    s. plasmacytoma
    s. pulmonary nodule (SPN)
    s. rectal ulcer
solium
    taeniasis s.
Solomon 7-Minute Mental Status Battery
solubilization
    cholesterol s.
Solu-Cortef
Solu-Medrol
solute gain
solution
    Cortisporin Otic S.
    high-osmolarity s.
    Lotrimin s.
    Reminyl Oral S.
    Synalar s.
Soma
somasthenia
somata
    neuronal s.
somatalgia
somatasthenia
somatic
    s. complaint
    s. death
    s. mutation theory
    s. pain
    s. pudendal nerve
    s. symptom
    s. teniasis
somatization
somatocrinin
somatoform disorder
somatoliberin

NOTES

somatomammotropin
  human chorionic s. (hCS)
somatome
somatomedin
  s. C
  s. C test
  plasma s. C
somatopathic
somatopathy
somatopause
somatoscopy
somatosensory
  s. cortex
  s. pathway
somatosexual
somatostatin
somatotherapy
somatotropic hormone (STH)
somatotropin release-inhibiting factor (SRIF)
somatotropin-releasing factor (SRF)
somatotype
somnambulance
somnambulism
somni
  hora s. (h.s.)
    at bedtime
  quaque hora s. (q.h.s.)
somnolence
somnolent and obtunded
Somogyi
  S. effect
  S. phenomenon
  S. reflex
  S. units
Sonata
Songo fever
Sonicator
  MEDCO S.
Sonne-Duval bacillus
sonnei
  Shigella s.
sonogram
sonorous rale
sophisticate
soporific
sorbitol
sordes
sore
  bed s.
  Delhi s.
  Lahore s.
  natal s.
  pressure s.
soroche
  chronic s.
SOT
  Sensory Organization Test
sotalol

Soto syndrome
souffle
  mammary s.
  splenic s.
soufflet
  bruit de s.
sound
  amphoric voice s.
  anvil s.
  aortic second s. (A_2)
  auscultatory s.
  bell s.
  bowel s.
  cavernous voice s.
  cracked-pot s.
  crunching s.
  first heart s. (S_1)
  fourth heart s. (S_4)
  friction s.
  heart s.
  hippocratic succussion s.
  Korotkoff s.
  muscle s.
  percussion s.
  posttussis suction s.
  respiratory s.
  Santini booming s.
  second s.
  second heart s. (S_2)
  succussion s.
  tambour s.
  third heart s. (S_3)
  van Buren s.
  voice s.
  water-whistle s.
  xiphisternal crunching s.
source
  gastrointestinal bleeding from an unknown s.
south
  S. African tick-bite fever
  S. African-type porphyria
  S. American blastomycosis
  S. American trypanosomiasis
southeast Asian ovalocytosis
southern
  S. blot analysis
  S. blot hybridization
  S. blotting
SP
  suprapubic
S/P
  status post
spa
space
  s. adaptation syndrome
  cavitary s.
  intercostal s.
  s. medicine

pars s.
Retzius s.
s. sickness
subarachnoid s.
Traube semilunar s.
space-occupying lesion
spacer
Ellipse compact s.
span
adult life s.
life s.
Spanish influenza
Spansules
Ornade S.
sparfloxacin
sparganosis
Sparine
spasm
concomitant esophageal s.
diaphragmatic s.
diffuse esophageal s.
epidemic transient diaphragmatic s.
esophageal s.
hemifacial s.
pedal s.
piriformis muscle s.
tonic reflex s.
spasmodic asthma
spasmus nutans
spastic
s. ileus
s. motility disorder
spastica
cholepathia s.
spasticity
SPAT
slow paroxysmal atrial tachycardia
spatial orientation
spear
special
s. hospital
s. nurse
specialist
mental health s.
neurologic s.
psychiatric s.
specialization
specialize
specialty
species
Haemophilus s., *Actinobacilus actinomycetemcomitans,*

Cardiobacterium hominis,
Eikenella corrodens, Kingella s.
s. tolerance
specific
age s.
s. cause
s. disease
gender s.
s. gravity
gut s.
site s.
s. therapy
specificity
specimen
spun s.
SPECT
single-photon emission computed
tomography
SPECT scan
spectacle
cataract s.
hemianopic prism s.'s
Spectazole
spectral telescopic system
spectrum, pl. **spectra**
fortification s.
speculum
Graves s.
Pederson s.
vaginal s.
virginal s.
speech
s. discrimination testing
s. and language pathology
s. therapist
s. therapy
speed
gait s.
spell
apneic s.
Spenco
S. metatarsal pad
S. Polysorb Orthotics
SPEP
serum protein electrophoresis
spermatocele
spermatorrhea
spermatozoon, pl. **spermatozoa**
SPF
sun protective factor
sphenoid sinusitis

NOTES

S

sphere
    affective s.
spherocyte
spherocytic
    s. anemia
    s. hereditary elliptocytosis
spherocytosis
    hereditary s.
spherule
sphincter
    artificial s.
    s. control
    s. electromyography
    esophageal s.
    hypertensive lower esophageal s.
    lower esophageal s. (LES)
    s. of Oddi
    upper esophageal s. (UES)
sphincterotomy
sphingolipidosis
    cerebral s.
sphingolipodystrophy
sphygmomanometer
    aneroid s.
    mercury s.
spica splint
spicule
spider
    s. angioma
    s. bite
    s. telangiectasia
Spiegler-Fendt sarcoid
Spielmeyer-Sjögren disease
Spielmeyer-Vogt disease
spiff
    dobutamine s.
spigelian line
spike
    M s.
    monoclonal s.
spike-like glycoprotein
spina, pl. **spinae**
    s. bifida
    s. bifida occulta
    erector spinae
    s. ventosa
spinach stool
spinal
    s. catheter
    s. cord
    s. cord compression
    s. cord conduction
    s. cord dysfunction
    s. cord injury
    s. cysticercosis
    s. disorder
    s. fluid loss headache
    s. lesion
    s. manipulation

    s. sign
    s. stenosis
    s. stroke
    s. tumor
spine
    anterior superior iliac s. (ASIS)
    s. of scapula
spinnbarkeit
spinocerebellar ataxia
spinothalamic
spinous process
spiral
    s. computed tomography
    s. reconstruction
spirillum fever
spirochetal
    s. icterus
Spirochetes
spirochetosis
    bronchopulmonary s.
spirochetotic
spirogram
spirometer
spirometry
    incentive s.
spirometry-defined OAD
spironolactone test
Spirozide
Spitzer Quality of Life Index
splanchnic
    s. artery aneurysm
    s. ischemia
splanchnolith
splanchnomicria
splanchnopathy
spleen
    accessory s.
    Gandy-Gamna s.
    lardaceous s.
splenadenoma
splenalgia
splenatrophy
splenauxe
splenectasis
splenectomize
splenectomy
splenelcosis
splenemia
splenemphraxis
splenetic
splenic
    s. anemia
    s. artery aneurysm
    s. circulation
    s. flexure
    s. flexure syndrome
    s. localization index (SLI)
    s. mycosis
    s. neutropenia

s. sequestration
s. sequestration crisis
s. souffle
s. vein thrombosis
splenicterus
splenitis
spodogenous s.
splenocolic
splenocyte
splenodynia
splenogenous
splenogram
splenogranulomatosis siderotica
splenography
splenohepatomegaly
splenokeratosis
splenolymphatic
splenolysin
splenolysis
splenoma
splenomalacia
splenomedullary leukemia
splenomegalic polycythemia
splenomegaly
choluric hemolytic icterus with s.
Gaucher s.
hemolytic s.
hypercholesterolemic s.
hyperreactive malarious s.
myelophthisic s.
Niemann s.
siderotic s.
spodogenous s.
tropical s.
splenometry
splenomyelogenous leukemia
splenomyelomalacia
splenonephric
splenonephroptosis
splenoparectasis
splenopathy
splenophrenic
splenoptosis
splenorrhagia
splenosis
splenotoxin
splenulus
splint
air s.
Capener s.
cock-up wrist s.
Futura wrist s.

outrigger s.
shin s.'s
spica s.
sugar tong s.
ulnar gutter s.
splinter hemorrhage
splinting
split-night sleep study
split S_2
splitting
fixed s.
paradoxic s.
physiologic s.
reversed s.
SPMSQ
Short Portable Mental Status
Questionnaire
SPN
solitary pulmonary nodule
spodogenous
s. splenitis
s. splenomegaly
spondylarthritis
spondylitis
ankylosing s.
Bekhterev-Strümpell s.
Marie-Strümpell s.
von Bekhterev-Strümpell s.
spondyloarthropathy
enteropathic s.
seronegative s.
spondyloepiphysial dysplasia
spondylolisthesis
spondylolysis
spondylosis
ankylosis s.
cervical s.
spondylotomy
spongioblastoma
spontanea
dactylolysis s.
spontaneous
s. gas gangrene
s. hypoglycemia
s. necrosis
spooning
sporadic
s. Alzheimer disease
s. medullary thyroid cancer
Sporanox
sporotrichosis
sporotrichotic

S

NOTES

Sporotrichum schenckii
sport
> Center for the Study of
> Aging/International Association of
> Physical Activity, Aging, and S.'s
> (IAPAAS)
> s.'s medicine
> President's Council on Physical
> Fitness and S.'s (PCPFS)

spot
> Bitot s.
> café au lait s.
> cherry-red s.
> cotton wool s.
> epigastric s.
> Janeway s.
> Koplik s.
> mulberry s.
> rose s.
> Roth s.
> shin s.
> trigger s.

spotted fever
spousal abuse
sprain
> ankle s.
> back s.
> knee s.

spray
> Flonase nasal s.
> Miacalcin nasal s.
> nicotine nasal s.
> PreSun S.

spread
> hematogenous s.

Sprengel deformity
sprue
> celiac s.
> collagenous s.
> nontropical s.
> refractory s.
> tropical s.

SPRY
> Setting Priorities for Retirement Years
> SPRY Foundation

spun specimen
spur
> s. cell
> s. cell anemia
> heel s.

spuria
> melena s.

spurious
> s. hyperkalemia
> s. polycythemia

Spurling sign
spurring
> hypertrophic s.

sputum, pl. **sputa**

s. aerogenosum
currant jelly s.
s. examination
green s.
prune-juice s.
purulent s.
rusty s.

SQ
> subcutaneous (*See also* subq)

squamocolumnar junction
squamous
> s. cell carcinoma (SCC)
> s. cell hyperplasia
> s. dysplasia
> s. intraepithelial lesion (SIL)
> s. metaplasia

squared
> meters s. (m^2)

squeezing
SR
> sinus rhythm
> > Calan SR
> > Indocin SR
> > Procan SR

SRF
> somatotropin-releasing factor

SRI
> serotonin reuptake inhibitor

SRIF
> somatotropin release-inhibiting factor

SSA
> Social Security Administration

SSPE
> sclerosing panencephalitis

SSRI
> selective serotonin reuptake inhibitor

SSS
> sick sinus syndrome

ST
> ST segment
> ST segment elevation
> ST and T wave

St.
> St. Anthony disease
> St. Anthony fire
> St. John's wort
> St. Jude prosthetic valve
> St. Vitus dance

stabbing
stability
> endemic s.
> enzootic s.

stabilization
stabilizer
> mood s.

stable
> s. hypertension

stably
stachybotryotoxicosis

stadiometer
stadium
Stadol
staff
    s. of Aesculapius
    attending s.
    consulting s.
    house s.
    paramedical s.
stage
    algid s.
    cold s.
    defervescent s.
    end s.
    eruptive s.
    s. III lung cancer
    s. I–IV breast cancer
    s. I–IV Hodgkin disease
    incubative s.
    s. of invasion
    latent s.
    prodromal s.
    s. 4 sleep
    Tanner s. (I–V)
staghorn calculus
staging
    cancer s.
    Tanner s. (I–V)
    TNM s.
    tumor, node, metastasis s.
    s. workup
stagnant anoxia
stain
    acid-fast s.
    chromatin s.
    eosin s.
    Giemsa s.
    Gram s.
    hematoxylin s.
    iodine-fixed crystal violet s.
    port-wine s.
    Wright s.
stainable iron
staining
    fluorescein s.
Stamm gastroplasty
standard
    s. deviation
    gold s.
standing test
stapedectomy
stapes

staphylococcal
    s. pneumonia
    s. scalded skin syndrome
staphylococci (*pl. of* staphylococcus)
staphylococcosis
Staphylococcus
    S. aureus pneumonia
    S. epidermidis
    S. food poisoning
    S. hominis
    S. warneri
staphylococcus, pl. **staphylococci**
starch blocker
stare
    reptilian s.
Stargardt syndrome
Starling equilibrium
Starlix
startle test
starvation
    s. acidosis
    s. diabetes
starve
stasis
    intestinal s.
    s. syndrome
    s. ulcer
    venous s.
stat., STAT
    at once
    statim
Statak suture
state
    anxiety s.
    catabolic s.
    contractile s.
    eunuchoid s.
    fasting s.
    s. hospital
    hyperadrenergic s.
    hypercoagulable s.
    hyperosmolar nonketotic s.
    hyperserotonergic s.
    hypoadrenergic s.
    hypometabolic s.
    inotropic s.
    International Classification of
      Diseases, Adapted for Use in the
      United S.'s (ICDA)
    meningococcal carrier s.
    nonketotic s.
    nutritional s.

S

NOTES

state *(continued)*
    postictal s.
    Profile of Mood S.'s (POMS)
    steady s.
Statham transducer
static
    s. air mattress
    s. symptom
statim (stat., STAT)
statin therapy
stationary
statistic
    National Center for Health S.'s
      (NCHS)
    vital s.'s
statistically
stature
    brittle hair, impaired intelligence,
      decreased fertility, short s.
      (BIDS)
status
    altered mental s.
    s. arthriticus
    s. asthmaticus
    s. calcifames
    cardiovascular risk s.
    s. choleraicus
    cognitive s.
    s. degenerativus
    DNH s.
    DNR s.
    do-not-hospitalize s.
    do-not-resuscitate s.
    economic s.
    s. epilepticus
    excellent functional s.
    fluctuating mental s.
    functional s.
    health s.
    Karnofsky s.
    s. lymphaticus
    marital s.
    mental s.
    nutrition s.
    nutritional s.
    oral health s.
    s. parathyroprivous
    s. post (S/P)
    s. praesens
    psychophysical health s.
    s. thymicolymphaticus
    s. thymicus
Staub-Traugott
    S.-T. effect
    S.-T. phenomenon
    S.-T. test
stavudine

stay
    hospital s.
    length of s.
STD
    sexually transmitted disease
steady state
stealing
    pathological s.
steal syndrome
steam-fitter's asthma
stearrhea
steatohepatitis
    alcoholic s.
    nonalcoholic s.
steatorrhea
    biliary s.
    intestinal s.
    pancreatic s.
steatosis
    drug-induced s.
Steell murmur
steering wheel injury
stegnosis
stegnotic
Steinberg thumb sign
Steinbrinck anomaly
Steinert disease
Stein-Leventhal syndrome
Steinmann pin
Stelazine
ST-elevation myocardial infarction
stellate
    s. ganglion blockade
    s. laceration
    s. telangiectasia
Stellwag
    S. brawny edema
    S. sign
stem
    s. cell leukemia
    s. cell transplant
stenocardia
stenosis, pl. stenoses
    anastomotic s.
    aortic valvular s.
    aqueductal s.
    artery s.
    bilateral foraminal s.
    calcific aortic s.
    carotid s.
    cervical spinal s.
    congenital pulmonary valve s.
    congenital valvular aortic s.
    coronary s.
    foraminal s.
    hypertrophic s.
    idiopathic hypertrophic subaortic s.
     (IHSS)
    infundibular s.

mitral s.
pulmonary artery s.
pulmonary valve s.
pulmonic valvular s.
pyloric s.
renal artery s.
spinal s.
subaortic s.
supravalvular aortic s.
vaginal s.
valvular s.
stenostenosis
stenotic
s. renal angiography
s. renal artery
Stensen canal
stent
Belgium Netherlands s.
(BENESTENT)
stenting
endoluminal s.
step care
step-down
s.-d. care
step-down approach
stephanion
steppage
stepped-care hypertensive regimen
step-up approach
sterane
stercoraceous vomiting
stercoral
s. appendicitis
s. colic
s. ulcer
stercoralis
Strongyloides s.
stercorous
stercus
stereognosis
stereoscopic fundus photography
stereotactic
sterid
sterilely
sterile NaCl
sterilisans
therapia magna s.
sterility
aspermatogenic s.
dysspermatogenic s.
male s.
normospermatogenic s.

Steri-Strip
sternal heart border
Sternberg
S. disease
S. giant cell
S. sign
Sternberg-Reed cell
sternoclavicular subluxation
sternocleidomastoid (SCM)
s. muscle
sternomanubrial
sternotomy
sternum nudge
steroid
adrenal s.
adrenocortical s.
s. diabetes
s. fever
s. injection
intranasal s.
s. withdrawal syndrome
steroidal
steroid-induced
s.-i. glaucoma
s.-i. osteoporosis
steroidogenesis
steroidogenic diabetes
steroid-resistant rejection
stertor
stertorous
s. breathing
s. respiration
stethoscope
binaural s.
Bowles type s.
differential s.
stethoscopic
stethoscopy
Stevens-Johnson syndrome
Stewart-Morel syndrome
STH
somatotropic hormone
sthenia
sthenic habitus
Stierlin sign
stiffening
arterial s.
stiffer gait
stiffness
stigma, pl. **stigmata**
malpighian s.
stigmatic

S

NOTES

373

stigmatism
stigmatization
stillbirth
stillborn
Still-Chauffard syndrome
Still disease
stimulant
    central nervous system s.
    s. laxative
    thermogenic s.
stimulation
    beta-adrenergic s.
    electrical s.
    nerve root s.
    percutaneous on-surface s. (POSS)
    programmed ventricular s.
    s. test
    transcranial magnetic s.
    transcutaneous electrical nerve s.
      (TENS)
stimulator
    dorsal column s.
    long-acting thyroid s. (LATS)
stimulus, pl. **stimuli**
    noxious s.
    osmotic s.
    provocative s.
    warm or cold s.
sting
    scorpion s.
STM
    short-term memory
stochastic
stocking
    s. distribution
    elastic s.
    Jobst s.
    pressure-graded s.
    Sigvaris s.
    TED s.
    thromboembolic disease s.
stoicism
Stokes
    S. amputation
    S. basket
    S. collar
Stokes-Adams attack
stoma
stomach
    s. ache
    s. pump
    upset s.
    watermelon s.
stomachalgia
stomachal vertigo
stomachodynia
stomatitis
    acute necrotizing s.
    allergic s.

    angular s.
    aphthobullous s.
    s. aphthosa
    aphthous s.
    bismuth s.
    catarrhal s.
    contact s.
    denture s.
    epidemic s.
    epizootic s.
    erythematopultaceous s.
    s. exanthematica
    fusospirochetal s.
    gangrenous s.
    gonococcal s.
    gonorrheal s.
    herpetic s.
    infectious s.
    s. intertropica
    lead s.
    s. medicamentosa
    membranous s.
    mercurial s.
    mycotic s.
    necrotizing ulcerative s.
    s. nicotina
    nonspecific s.
    s. prosthetica
    recurrent aphthous s.
    s. scarlatina
    s. scorbutica
    syphilitic s.
    traumatic s.
    tropical s.
    ulcerative s.
    uremic s.
    s. venenata
    vesicular s.
    Vincent s.
    vulcanite s.
stomatocyte
stomatocytosis
    acquired s.
stomatodynia
stomatonecrosis
stomocephalus
stone
    black s.
    brown s.
    calcium apatite s.
    cystine s.
    struvite s.
    uric acid s.
    xanthine s.
stonemason's disease
stool
    black, tarry s.
    butter s.
    s. color

fatty s.
s. guaiac
rice-water s.
spinach s.
tarry s.
Trélat s.
storage
s. disorder
s. pool disease
storm
thyroid s.
STP
serenity-tranquility-peace
STP pill
strabismus
Strachan-Scott syndrome
Strachan syndrome
straight
s. cane
s. leg raising (SLR)
s. leg raising test
strain
back s.
neck s.
straining
strangulation
strangury
strata (*pl. of* stratum)
strategy
genome replication s.
stratification
risk s.
stratified
s. care
s. squamous epithelium
stratiform
stratum, pl. **strata**
s. corneum
Strauss sign
strawberry tongue
streak
fibrotic s.
stream
force of s.
Life S.
strength
motor s. 5+/5+
strengthen
strepitus
streptocerciasis
streptococcal
s. empyema

s. group A, B, G
s. pneumonia
s. soft tissue infection
s. toxic shock syndrome
streptococci (*pl. of* streptococcus)
streptococcosis
Streptococcus
S. agalactiae
S. bovis
S. constellatus
S. faecalis
S. faecium
S. milleri
S. pneumoniae
S. pneumoniae vaccine
S. viridans infection
streptococcus, pl. **streptococci**
alpha-hemolytic s.
group A, B, G s.
streptodornase
streptokinase s. (SKSD)
streptogramin
streptokinase streptodornase (SKSD)
streptolysin O
streptomycin
streptothrichosis, streptotrichiasis
streptozocin
streptozyme test
stress
chronic s.
s. factor
s. fracture
s. incontinence
s. management
s. myocardial perfusion imaging
orthostatic s.
s. polycythemia
pressor s.
s. test
stress-induced angina
stress-related disorder
Stresstabs
stretch syncope
stria, pl. **striae**
striatonigral degeneration
stricture
biliary s.
peptic s.
stride length reduction
strident
stridor
inspiratory s.

NOTES

S

375

strip
- Accu-Chek Comfort Curve test s.'s
- glucometer s.
- glucose test s.
- Micral urine test s.

stripper's asthma

strobila

stroke
- atherosclerotic s.
- atherothrombic s.
- brainstem s.
- cardioembolic s.
- classic heat s.
- dysphagic s.
- embolic s.
- s. in evolution
- exertional heat s.
- heat s.
- hemorrhagic s.
- ischemic s.
- National Institute of Neurological Disorders and S. (NINDS)
- s. rehabilitation
- spinal s.
- sun s.
- thrombotic s.
- s. volume
- s. volume index (SVI)
- Wallenberg s.

stroking

stroma, pl. **stromata**

stromal hyperplasia

Strong bacillus

Strongyloides stercoralis

strongyloidiasis disorder

strongyloidosis

structural
- s. alteration
- s. heart disease
- s. modification

structure
- hepatic s.
- sleep s.
- supraglottic s.

struma, pl. **strumae**
- s. basedowificata
- Hashimoto s.
- s. lymphomatosa
- s. medicamentosa
- s. ovarii
- Riedel s.

strumipriva
- cachexia s.

Strümpell disease

strut

struvite stone

Stryker collar

Stryker-Halbeisen syndrome

ST-segment depression

ST-T
- ST-T abnormality
- ST-T wave change

Stuart-Bras
- S.-B. disease
- S.-B. syndrome

Stuart factor

stuartii
- *Providencia s.*

student nurse

study, pl. **studies**
- acoustogram s.
- adenosine thallium s.
- Alpha-Tocopherol Beta-Carotene S.
- Atherosclerosis Risk in Communities S.
- bone mineral density s.
- carotid Doppler s.
- case control s.
- *cis*-retinoic acid s.
- cohort s.
- cross-sectional s.
- diachronic s.
- domperidone s.
- Doppler s.
- double blind s.
- drug s.
- Early versus Later L-DOPA s.
- ELLDOPA s.
- esophageal manometry s.
- esophageal motility s.
- fluorourodynamic s. (FUDS)
- Framingham Heart S.
- isotretinoin drug s.
- longitudinal s.
- Medical Outcomes S. (MOS)
- National Health and Nutrition Examination Follow-Up S.
- nerve conduction s.
- neuroimaging s.
- nonrandomized s.
- observational s.
- perindopril (Aceon) protection against recurrent stroke s. (PROGRESS)
- platelet function s.
- pressure-flow s.
- Pulseless Electrical S. (PEA)
- sleep s.
- split-night sleep s.
- synchronic s.
- thyroid function studies
- transurethral ultrasound-guided laser-induced s.
- troglitazone Sankyo s.
- TULIP s.
- urodynamic s.

videofluoroscopic swallowing s. (VSS)

virologic s.

Stühmer disease

stupor

anergic s.

benign s.

Cairns s.

catatonic s.

stuporous

Sturge disease

Sturge-Weber-Dimitri disease

Sturge-Weber syndrome

styloid process

Stypven time

subacromial

subacute

s. bacterial endocarditis (SBE)

s. care

s. cerebellar degeneration

s. cortical cerebellar degeneration (SCCD)

s. cutaneous lupus erythematosus

s. endocarditis

s. hepatitis

s. inflammation

s. lymphocyte thyroiditis

s. myeloid leukemia

s. rehabilitation

s. rheumatism

s. sclerosing panencephalitis

subalimentation

subaortic stenosis

subarachnoid

s. hemorrhage (SAH)

s. neurocysticercosis

s. space

subareolar

subastragalar

subcapital hip fracture

subcarinal lymphadenopathy

subchondral bone

subclavian

s. steal syndrome

s. vein

subclinical

s. coccidioidomycosis

s. Cushing syndrome

s. diabetes

s. hyperthyroidism

s. hypothyroidism

subconjunctival hemorrhage

subcortical infarct

subcostal

subcostalgia

subcrepitant rale

subcrepitation

subcurative

subcutaneous (SQ, subq)

s. bursitis

s. calcification

s. emphysema

s. enoxaparin

s. insulin delivery

s. wound

subcuticular

subdermal progestin

subdiaphragmatic pyopneumothorax

subdural

s. empyema

s. hematoma

subendocardial infarction

subependymal

suberosis

subicteric

subintrant

subitum

exanthema s.

subjective

s. fremitus

s., objective, assessment, and plan (SOAP)

s. sign

s. symptom

s. vertigo

sublethal

subleukemic leukemia

subliminal thirst

sublimis

sublingual

s. nitroglycerin

subluxation

atlantoaxial s.

sternoclavicular s.

submandibular

submassive hepatic necrosis

submental node

subnasal

subnormal

subnormality

suboptimal

subpapillary

subperiosteal

subphrenic abscess

S

NOTES

subpial
subq
    subcutaneous
subscale
    Alzheimer Disease Assessment
      Scale-Cognitive S. (ADAS-cog)
subscapular
subscription
subserous
subsibilant
subsistence diet
subspecialty
substance
    s. abuse
    S. Abuse and Mental Health
      Services Administration
      (SAMSHA)
    autocoid s.
    exophthalmos-producing s. (EPS)
    s. P
    s. P inhibitor
    s. P of Lewis
    s. withdrawal delirium
substance-induced delirium
substance-intoxication delirium
substernal goiter
substitution therapy
substitutive therapy
substrate
substrate-1
    insulin receptor s.-1 (IRS-1)
subtalar arthritis
subtentorial lesion
subtest
    Digit Symbol S.
subtilis
    Bacillus s.
subtilisin
subtotal colectomy
subtract serial sevens
subtrochanteric fracture
subungual toe abscess
subunit
    beta-human chorionic
      gonadotropin s.
subvirile
subxiphoid
succedaneum
successful aging
succinate
    metoprolol s.
    sumatriptan s.
succorrhea
succuss
succussed
succussion
    hippocratic s.
    s. sound
sucrose lysis test

sucrosemia
suction
    posttussive s.
suctioning
    airway s.
Sudafed
sudden
    s. cardiac death
    s. distention
    s. infant death syndrome (SIDS)
    s. unexplained death syndrome
      (SUDS)
Sudeck
    S. atrophy
    S. disease
Sudeck-LeRiche syndrome
sudomotor
    s. dysfunction
    s. function test
sudor anglicus
sudoresis
SUDS
    sudden unexplained death syndrome
suffusion
sugar
    blood s. (BS)
    fasting blood s. (FBS)
    fingerstick blood s. (FSBS)
    postprandial blood s. (PPBS)
    random blood s. (RBS)
    s. test
    s. tong splint
suggestive therapeutics
suicidal
    s. ideation
    s. intent
suicide
    assisted s.
    physician-assisted s.
suis
    Brucella s.
Suker sign
Sulamyd
    Sodium S.
Sular
sulbactam
sulcus
sulfacetamide
Sulfamethoprim
sulfamethoxazole
sulfapyridine
sulfasalazine
sulfate (SO$_4$)
    abacavir s.
    chondroitin s.
    dehydroepiandrosterone s. (DHEAS)
    ferrous s. (FeSO)
    glucosamine s.
    hyglucosamine s.

indinavir s.
L-hyoscyamine s.
morphine s.
penbutolol s.
quinine s.
sulfatide lipidosis
sulfatidosis
sulfhemoglobinemia
sulfhydryl group
sulfisoxazole
sulfobromophthalein
sulfonamide antibiotic
sulfonylurea
s. agent
s. assay
bedtime insulin, daytime s. (BIDS)
daytime s.
sulfur dioxide poisoning
sulindac
sumatriptan succinate
summary
Mental Component S. (MCS)
Physical Component S. (PCS)
summation
summer
s. asthma
s. diarrhea
Sumner sign
Sumycin
sun
s. protective factor (SPF)
s. stroke
sunburn
sundowning
sundown syndrome
superacidity
superacute
superalimentation
superciliary
super-fatted soap
superficial
s. frostbite
s. phlebitis
s. pneumonia
s. spreading melanoma
s. thrombophlebitis
superficialis
colitis cystica s.
supergeneric drug
superinfection
superior
s. axis

s. hemorrhagic polioencephalitis
s. vena cava
s. vena cava syndrome
superius
tuberculum thyroideum s.
supernumerary
supernutrition
superoxide
supersaturated potassium iodide
superscription
supervene
supine position
supplement
Arginaid dietary s.
dietary s.
fiber s.
ginkgo s.
vitamin s.
supplementary medical insurance
supplementation
appropriate nutritional s.
calcium s.
fiber s.
macronutrient s.
micronutrient s.
mineral s.
phosphate s.
support
advanced cardiac life s. (ACLS)
advanced life s.
basic life s.
s. group
s. hose
nutritional s.
suppository
urethral s.
suppressant
cough s.
suppressed breathing
suppression
adrenal s.
appetite s.
bone marrow s.
s. of replication
viral s.
suppuration
intracranial s.
suppurativa
hidradenitis s.
suppurative
s. arthritis
s. pneumonia

S

NOTES

suppurative (*continued*)
    s. synovitis
    s. thrombophlebitis
supraclavicular
supracondylar
    s. femoral fracture
supraglottic structure
suprahyoid accessory thyroid gland
supranuclear palsy
suprapatellar
suprapubic (SP)
suprarenale
    melasma s.
suprarenal gland
suprarenalis
    macrogenitosomia praecox s.
suprasellar
supraspinatus
suprasternal notch
supratentorial lesion
supravalvular aortic stenosis
supraventricular tachycardia (SVT)
supravital
Suprax
sura
suralimentation
sural nerve conduction
suramin
surdocardiac syndrome
Sure Dose insulin syringe
surface
    s. area
    s. thermometer
    ulcerative s.
Surfak
surge
    early morning s.
surgeon
    American Academy of
      Orthopedic S.'s
    American College of S.'s (ACS)
surgery
    s. Academy of Otolaryngology-
      Head and Neck Surgery (AAO-
      HNS)
    ambulatory s.
    antireflux s.
    breast-conserving s.
    CABG s.
    cardiac s.
    clitoral s.
    coronary artery bypass graft s.
    cytoreductive s.
    glaucoma filtration s.
    lung volume reduction s. (LVRS)
    Master of S. (MC)
    mitral valve s.
    Mohs micrographic s.
    refractive s.

    selective transsphenoidal s.
    transsphenoidal s.
    video-assisted thoracoscopic s.
surgical
    s. abdomen
    s. abortion
    s. debridement
    s. infection
    s. menopause
    s. repair
Surmontil
surrogate
    s. decision-maker
    s. decision-making
surveillance
    S., Epidemiology, and End Results
      (SEER)
    S., Epidemiology, and End Results
      cancer registry
survey
    National Health and Nutrition
      Examination S. (NHANES)
survival
    s. rate
    s. time
survivin
Susac syndrome
susceptibility cassette
suspended animation
suspension
    Isophane insulin s.
Sustacal
sustained
    s. release
    s. ventricular tachycardia
sustained-release
    s.-r. morphine
    s.-r. oxycodone
Sustaire
sustentaculum tali
susurrus
Sutton-Rendu-Osler-Weber syndrome
suture
    Dupuytren s.
    Ethilon s.
    Statak s.
    Vicryl s.
SVI
    stroke volume index
SVT
    supraventricular tachycardia
swallow
    barium s.
swallowing
    s. evaluation
    fiberoptic endoscopic examination
      of s. (FEES)
Swan-Ganz catheter

sway
   body s.
swaying
sweat
   s. chloride determination
   night s.'s
   s. test
sweet clover
swelling
   hunger s.
   objective s.
   salivary gland s.
   scrotum s.
Swift disease
swimmer's
   s. ear
   s. view
swine
   Battey avian s.
swineherd's disease
Swyer syndrome
Sydenham chorea
Sydney
   S. crease
   S. line
Sylvest disease
Sylvian fissure
symballophonc
Syme amputation
Symmers disease
Symmetrel
symmetric asphyxia
sympathectomy
sympathetic
   s. block
   s. ganglion
   s. nervous system
   s. orthostatic hypotension (SOH)
   s. postganglionic neuron
   s. symptom
sympathicotonic orthostatic hypotension
sympathoadrenal system
sympathochromaffin
sympatholytic
   s. agent
   centrally acting s.
sympathomimetic
   s. agent
   s. amine
symphysis, pl. symphyses
   s. pubis

symptom
   abstinence s.'s
   accessory s.
   accidental s.
   acute on chronic s.
   assident s.
   behavioral s.
   Bolognini s.
   Buerger s.
   cardinal s.
   Charcot triad of s.'s
   S. Checklist 90 (SLC-90)
   s. complex
   concomitant s.
   consecutive s.
   constellation of s.'s
   constitutional s.
   dearth of s.'s
   deficiency s.
   depressive s.
   direct s.
   equivocal s.
   factitious s.
   first rank s. (FRS)
   s. group
   Huchard s.
   incarceration s.
   induced s.
   Jellinek s.
   local s.
   localizing s.
   s. magnification
   malabsorption s.
   negative s.
   nocturnal s.
   objective s.
   pathognomonic s.
   Pel-Ebstein s.
   premonitory s.
   presenting s.
   psychotic s.
   rational s.
   reflex s.
   Rogcr s.
   severe malabsorption s.'s
   somatic s.
   static s.
   subjective s.
   sympathetic s.
   systemic s.
   vasomotor s.
   withdrawal s.'s

NOTES

symptomatic
- s. cholelithiasis
- s. fever
- s. hypotonicity
- s. improvement
- s. partial epilepsy
- s. pharmacotherapy
- s. porphyria
- s. pruritus
- s. purpura
- s. treatment

symptomatica
- porphyria cutanea tarda s.
- purpura s.

symptomatology
symptomatolytic, symptomolytic
symptosis
Synalar-HP
Synalar solution
Synalgos-HP
synandrogenic
synapse
synapsis
synaptic
synaptopodin
Synarel
synarthrosis
synchondrosis
synchronic study
synchronous colonic neoplasia
syncopal attack
syncope
- s. angiosa
- carotid sinus s.
- cough s.
- defecation s.
- deglutition s.
- effort s.
- heat s.
- hypoxic s.
- micturition s.
- neurocardiogenic s.
- postmicturition s.
- posttussive s.
- situational s.
- stretch s.
- tussive s.
- vasodepressor s.
- vasovagal s.

syncytium, pl. **syncytia**
syndactyly
syndesmophyte
syndesmosis
syndrome
- Aarskog s.
- Abercrombie s.
- Abt-Letterer-Siwe s.
- acetaldehyde s.
- Achard-Thiers s.

acquired immune deficiency s. (AIDS)
acquired immunodeficiency s. (AIDS)
acquired long QT s.
acute chest s.
acute coronary s.
acute HIV infection s.
acute respiratory distress s. (ARDS)
acute urethral s.
Adamantiades-Behçet s.
Adams-Stokes s.
addisonian s.
adiposogenital s.
adrenal cortical s.
adrenal virilizing s.
adrenogenital s. (AGS)
adult respiratory distress s. (ARDS)
afferent loop s.
Ahumada-Del Castillo s.
Aicardi s.
Alagille s.
Alajouanine s.
Albright s.
alcohol withdrawal s. (AWS)
Aldrich s.
Aldrich-Wiskott s.
Alice in Wonderland s.
Alport s.
Alström s.
anaerobic-cavitary pneumonia s.
Andersen s.
Andrade s.
Angelman s.
anorectal s.
anterior chest wall s.
antibody deficiency s.
antiphospholipid antibody s.
Anton-Babinski s.
Arnold nerve reflex cough s.
articular s.
Ascher s.
Ascholl s.
Asherman s.
asplenia s.
Ayerza s.
Baastrup s.
Baber s.
Babinski s.
Babinski-Fröhlich s.
Baelz s.
Bakwin-Elger s.
Balint s.
Ballantyne-Runge s.
Bannwarth s.
Banti s.
Bar s.
Bárány s.

Barlow s.
Barrett s.
Bàrsony-Polgàr s.
Barter-Schwartz s.
Bartter s.
Basedow s.
Bassen-Kornzweig s.
battered child s.
battered spouse s.
Bayer s.
Bearn-Kunkel s.
Bearn-Kunkel-Slater s.
Beau s.
Beckwith s.
Beckwith-Wiedemann s.
Behçet s.
Behr s.
Benedikt s.
Beradinelli s.
Bernard-Homer s.
Bernard-Sergent s.
Bernard-Soulier s.
Bing-Neel s.
Blackfan-Diamond s.
Blatin s.
blind loop s.
blood pressure dysregulation s.
blue toe s.
Bodian-Schwachman s.
Boerhaave s.
Bonnevie-Ullrich s.
Börjeson-Forssman-Lehmann s.
Bouillaud s.
bowel bypass s.
Brennemann s.
Brock s.
Brown-Seĝuard s.
Brugada s.
Budd s.
Budd-Chiari s.
Bürger-Grütz s.
Burnett s.
calcinosis cutis, Raynaud
  phenomenon, esophageal
  dysfunction/hypermotility,
  sclerodactyly, telangiectasia s.
Cannon s.
Caplan s.
carcinoid s.
cardiac denervation s.
cardiofacial s.
carotid sinus s.

carpal tunnel s. (CTS)
Carpenter s.
Cassidy s.
Cassidy-Scholte s.
cauda equina s.
Ceelen-Gellerstedt s.
celiac s.
cellular immunity deficiency s.
central cord s. (CCS)
cervical rib s.
cervical root s.
cervical sympathetic s.
chancriform s.
Chauffard s.
Chauffard-Still s.
Chédiak-Higashi s.
Chiari s.
Chiari-Arnold s.
Chiari-Budd s.
Chinese restaurant s. (CRS)
Christian s.
chronic alcohol s. (CAS)
chronic fatigue s. (CFS)
chronic fatigue immune
  deficiency s. (CFIDS)
chronic hyperventilation s.
chronic pelvic pain s.
chubby puffer s.
Churg-Strauss s.
chylomicronemia s.
Clarke-Hadfield s.
Cogan s.
Cogan-Reese s.
Cohen s.
colonic polyposis s.
comalike s.
compartment s.
congenital long QT s.
Conn s.
contiguous gene s.
coronary s.
Costen s.
costochondritis s.
costoclavicular s.
Cowden s.
Crandall s.
CREST s.
cri-du-chat s.
Crigler-Najjar s.
Crouzon s.
Cruveilhier-Baumgarten s.
cryoglobulin s.

S

NOTES

syndrome (*continued*)

Curtius s.
Cushing s.
cutaneomucouveal s.
cutaneous paraneoplastic s.
cystic acne s.
Danbolt-Closs s.
Dandy-Walker s.
dead-in-bed s.
Debré-Sémélaigne s.
Degos s.
Del Castillo s.
delirium s.
de Morsier s.
de Morsier-Gauthier s.
dengue shock s.
Dennie-Marfan s.
de Quervain s.
dermatitis-arthritis s.
dermatitis-arthritis-tenosynovitis s.
diabetes insipidus, diabetes mellitus,
  optic atrophy, deafness s.
dialysis disequilibrium s.
dialysis encephalopathy s.
Diamond-Blackfan s.
Dieulafoy s.
DiGeorge s.
Di Guglielmo s.
DIMOAD s.
Diogenes s.
distal intestinal obstructive s.
disuse s.
Donath-Landsteiner s.
Dorfman-Chanarin s.
Down s.
Dresbach s.
Dressler s.
dry eye s.
Dubin-Johnson s.
dumping s.
Duncan s.
dysmyelopoietic s.
Eaton-Lambert s.
ectopic ACTH s.
ectopic adrenocorticotropic
  hormone s.
egg-white s.
Ehlers-Danlos s.
Eisenmenger s.
EMG s.
empty sella s.
envenomation s.
epidermal nevus s.
Erdheim s.
euthyroid sick s.
Evans s.
exomphalos, macroglossia, and
  gigantism s.
extrapyramidal s.

Faber s.
Fabry s.
failed back s.
Fanconi s.
Farber s.
Felty s.
fetal alcohol s. (FAS)
fibromyalgia s.
Fiessinger-Leroy-Reiter s.
Fitz s.
Fitz-Hugh-Curtis s.
Forbes-Albright s.
fragile X s.
Franceschetti-Valerio s.
Frey s.
Frey-Baillarger s.
Friderichsen-Waterhouse s.
Fröhlich s.
frontal abulic s.
frontal disinhibition s.
frontal opercular s.
Fukuyama s.
functional prepubertal castration s.
Gaisböck s.
Gardner s.
gastrojejunal loop obstruction s.
Gerstmann s.
Gilbert s.
Gilles de la Tourette s.
Gitelman s.
Gjessing s.
glucagonoma s.
Goodpasture s.
Gordon s.
Gradenigo s.
Greenfield s.
Guillain-Barré s.
Gulf War s.
Günther s.
Hadfield-Clarke s.
Hand s.
hand-and-foot s.
Hand-Schüller-Christian s.
Hanot s.
Hanot-Chauffard s.
Hartnup s.
Haven s.
Hawes-Pallister-Landor s.
Hayem-Widal s.
Heberden s.
Hedinger s.
heel spur s.
Heerfordt s.
hemolytic uremic s. (HUS)
hemophagocytic s.
hemorrhagic fever with renal s.
Henoch-Schönlein s.
hepatopulmonary s.
hepatorenal s.

HIV wasting s.
Holt-Oram s.
Horner s.
Horton s.
Houssay s.
Houssay-Biasotti s.
Hughes s.
hungry bone s.
Hunter s.
Hurler s.
hydralazine s.
17-hydroxylase deficiency s.
hyperaldosteronism s.
hypereosinophilic s.
hyper-IgE s.
hyperimmunoglobulin E s.
hyperventilation s.
hypometabolic s.
hypoparathyroidism s.
Imerslund s.
immotile cilia s.
immune complex-like s.
s. of inappropriate antidiuretic
  hormone secretion
inappropriate antidiuretic hormone
  secretion s.
s. of inappropriate secretion of
  antidiuretic hormone (SIADH)
inspissated s.
irritable bowel s. (IBS)
Ivemark s.
Jaccoud s.
Jakob-Creutzfeldt s.
Jansky-Bielschowsky s.
Jervell and Lange-Nielsen s.
jet lag s.
Job s.
Kallmann s.
Kartagener s.
Katayama s.
Kawasaki s.
Kiloh-Nevin s.
Kimmelstiel-Wilson s.
Kleine-Levin s.
Klinefelter s.
Klippel-Trenaunay s.
Klüver-Bucy s.
Kniest s.
Kocher-Debré-Sémélaigne s.
Koenig s.
König s.
Krabbe s.

Kunkel s.
Labbé s.
Lady Windemere's s.
Lambert-Eaton myasthenic s.
Laron s.
late lupus s.
Launois s.
Launois-Cléret s.
Laurence-Biedl s.
Laurence-Moon s.
Laurence-Moon-Biedl s.
Lawrence-Seip s.
Lejeune s.
Lemierre s.
Lennox-Gastaut-Dravet s.
lentigines, electrocardiographic
  abnormalities, ocular hypertelorism,
  pulmonary stenosis, abnormalities
  of genitalia, retardation of
  growth, deafness s.
LEOPARD s.
Lépine-Froin s.
Leriche s.
Lesch-Nyhan s.
Lhermitte s.
Libman-Sacks s.
Liddle s.
Li-Fraumeni s.
Lignac s.
Lignac-Fanconi s.
liver kidney s.
Lloyd s.
Löffler s.
Löfgren s.
long QT s.
Lorain-Lévi s.
Lowe s.
Lowe-Terrey-MacLachlan s.
low-salt s.
Luft s.
lumbar disk s.
lupuslike s.
lymphoproliferative s.
Macleod s.
macronutrient deficiency s.
Madelung s.
Mad Hatter s.
malabsorption s.
malignant carcinoid s.
malignant hyperthermia s.
Mallory-Weiss s.
Marchiafava-Bignami s.

S

NOTES

syndrome *(continued)*

Marchiafava-Micheli s.
Marfan s.
Marie s.
Marie-Robinson s.
Marie-Strümpell s.
marker X s.
Maroteaux-Lamy s.
Marshall s.
Martin-Bell s.
massive bowel resection s.
Mauriac s.
McArdle s.
McCune-Albright s.
medication rebound s.
Meigs s.
Mendelson s.
Ménière s.
Menkes s.
mesenteric artery s.
metabolic s.
metastatic carcinoid s.
Meyer-Betz s.
Mibelli s.
middle lobe s.
Mikulicz-Radecki s.
Mikulicz-Sjögren s.
milk-alkali s.
minimal-change nephrotic s.
Minkowski-Chauffard s.
mitral leaflet s.
Möbius s.
Mondor s.
Monge s.
Moore s.
Morel s.
Morel-Wildi s.
Morgagni s.
Morquio s.
Morquio-Brailsford s.
Morquio-Ullrich s.
Morris s.
Mosse s.
moving toes, painful leg s.
Muckle-Wells s.
mucocutaneous lymph node s.
 (MLNS)
mucocutaneous ocular s.
multiple cholesterol emboli s.
multiple endocrine deficiency s.
multiple glandular deficiency s.
multiple lentigines s.
multiple organ dysfunction s.
Münchausen by proxy s.
muscular pain-fasciculation s.
myasthenic s.
myelodysplastic s. (MDS)
myofascial pain s.
Naegeli s.

nail patella s.
Nelson s.
nephritic s.
nephrotic s.
nerve root s.
Nettleship s.
night eating s.
non-A s.
nonketotic hyperosmolar s.
Nonne-Milroy-Meige s.
nonthyroidal illness s.
Noonan s.
Norman-Wood s.
Nothnagel s.
obesity hypoventilation s.
obstructive sleep apnea s. (OSAS)
oculobuccogenital s.
oculocerebrorenal s.
oculosympathetic s.
Ogilvie s.
Oldfield s.
Omenn s.
Opitz s.
organic brain s. (OBS)
Osler s. II
Osler-Weber-Rendu s.
overlap s.
overuse s.
Paget-von Schroetter s.
pancreatorenal s.
paraneoplastic s.
Parinaud s.
Parkes-Weber s.
Parkinson s.
Paterson s.
Paterson-Brown-Kelly s.
Paterson-Kelly s.
Pellizzi s.
Pendred s.
Pepper s.
pericolic membrane s.
peripheral nerve root s.
Persian Gulf s.
pertussis s.
pertussis-like s.
Peutz-Jeghers s.
Pfaundler-Hurler s.
pharyngeal pouch s.
Pick s.
pickwickian s.
Pierre Robin s.
Plummer-Vinson s.
POEMS s.
Poland s.
polyangiitis overlap s.
polycystic ovary s. (PCOS)
polyendocrine deficiency s.
polyglandular endocrine s.
polyneuritis s.

polyneuropathy, organomegaly, endocrinopathy, monoclonal gammopathy, skin change s.
polyposis coil s.
popliteal artery entrapment s.
portopulmonary s.
Posner-Schlossman s.
postadrenalectomy s.
postconcussive s.
posterior interosseous s.
postfall s.
postgastrectomy s.
postphlebitic s.
postpolio s.
postthrombotic s.
postviral s.
Pott s.
Potter s.
Prader-Willi s.
Prader-Willi-Angelman s.
precordial catch s.
premenstrual dysphoric s. (PMDS)
primary headache s.
primary immunodeficiency s. (PIS)
prolonged QT s.
prune belly s.
pseudo-Cushing s.
pulmonary aspiration s.
pulmonary-renal s.
punchdrunk s.
purple toe s.
quiescent migrainous s.
Quincke I s.
radiation s.
Ramsay Hunt s.
Ramsay Hunt s. type 1
Raynaud s.
reactive airways dysfunction s.
red man s.
Reese s.
refeeding s.
Refetoff s.
Refsum s.
Reichmann s.
Reifenstein s.
Reiter s.
Rendu-Osler-Weber s.
reset osmostat s.
respiratory distress s. (RDS)
restless legs s. (RLS)
Reye s.
Richards-Rundle s.

Richner-Hanhart s.
Rieger s.
Riley-Day s.
Roberts s.
Romberg-Paessler s.
Rosenbach s.
Rosenthal s.
Rot-Bielschowsky s.
Rothmann-Makai s.
Rotor s.
Rud s.
Rundles-Falls s.
Russell s.
Rust s.
Rutherford s.
salt depletion s.
salt-losing s.
Samter s.
Sanfilippo s.
SAPHO s.
scalded skin s.
scalenus anticus s.
Schafer s.
Schaumann s.
Scheie s.
Scheuthauer-Marie-Sainton s.
Schmidt s.
Schönlein-Henoch s.
Schwachman s.
Schwartz-Bartter s.
sciatic nerve s.
Scott s.
Seip-Lawrence s.
selenium toxicity s.
Sclyc adaptation s.
Senear-Usher s.
sepsis s.
septic shock s.
serotonin s.
Sertoli-cell-only s.
severe combined immunodeficiency s. (SCIDS)
Sheehan s.
Sheehy s.
short-bowel s.
Shulman s.
Shwachman s.
Shwachman-Diamond s.
Shy-Drager s.
sick building s.
sick euthyroid s.
sick sinus s. (SSS)

S

NOTES

syndrome *(continued)*
    Sidbury s.
    Simmonds s.
    Sipple s.
    Sjögren s.
    SLE-like s.
    Smith-Lemli-Opitz s.
    Soto s.
    space adaptation s.
    splenic flexure s.
    staphylococcal scalded skin s.
    Stargardt s.
    stasis s.
    steal s.
    Stein-Leventhal s.
    steroid withdrawal s.
    Stevens-Johnson s.
    Stewart-Morel s.
    Still-Chauffard s.
    Strachan s.
    Strachan-Scott s.
    streptococcal toxic shock s.
    Stryker-Halbeisen s.
    Stuart-Bras s.
    Sturge-Weber s.
    subclavian steal s.
    subclinical Cushing s.
    sudden infant death s. (SIDS)
    sudden unexplained death s.
      (SUDS)
    Sudeck-LeRiche s.
    sundown s.
    superior mesenteric artery s.
    superior vena cava s.
    surdocardiac s.
    Susac s.
    Sutton-Rendu-Osler-Weber s.
    Swyer s.
    synovitis, acne, pustulosis,
      hyperostosis, osteitis s.
    systemic capillary leak s.
    systemic inflammatory response s.
      (SIRS)
    systemic lupus erythematosus-like s.
    Takayasu s.
    tarsal tunnel s.
    temporomandibular joint s.
    Terry s.
    testicular feminization s.
    thalamic s.
    thalassemia s.
    Thiemann s.
    third and fourth pharyngeal
      pouch s.
    Thompson s.
    thoracic outlet s. (TOS)
    thoracic outlet compression s.
    Thorn s.
    Tietze s.

    time-zone change s.
    TMJ s.
    Tommaselli s.
    TORCH s.
    Tourette s.
    toxic s.
    toxicity s.
    toxic shock s. (TSS)
    toxoplasmosis, other infections,
      rubella, cytomegalovirus infection,
      herpes simplex s.
    Treacher-Collins s.
    trisomy 20 s.
    Troisier s.
    Troisier-Hanot-Chauffard s.
    tropical splenomegaly s.
    Trousseau s.
    tumor humoral s.
    tumor lysis s.
    Turcot s.
    Turner s.
    Ullrich-Turner s.
    Ulysses s.
    ureteral bowel s.
    urethrooculosynovial s.
    uveoencephalitic s.
    vanishing lung s.
    vasculocardiac s.
    Verner-Morrison s.
    Vernet s.
    Vinson s.
    von Hippel-Lindau s.
    von Mikulicz s.
    Waardenburg s.
    Waldenström s.
    Walker s.
    Wallenberg s.
    wasting s.
    Waterhouse-Friderichsen s.
    watery diarrhea, hypokalemia,
      achlorhydria s.
    WDHA s.
    Weber-Christian s.
    Weil s.
    Weinstein s.
    Werlhof s.
    Wermer s.
    Werner s.
    Wernicke s.
    Wernicke-Korsakoff s.
    Whipple s.
    white coat s.
    Widal s.
    Widal-Abrami s.
    Wiedemann s.
    Willebrand-Jërgens s.
    Williams s.
    Wiskott-Aldrich s.
    Wissler s.

withdrawal s.
Wolff-Parkinson-White s.
Wolfram s.
Wright s.
XO s.
XXY s.
XYZ s.
Young s.
yo-yo s.
Zieve s.
Zollinger-Ellison s.
syndromic
synechia, pl. **synechiae**
synergetic
synergia
synergic
synergism
bacterial s.
synergist
synergistic
s. effect
s. system
synergy
synidrosis
synkinesia
synophrys
synostosis
synovia
synovial
s. fluid examination
s. membrane
synovioma
synovitis
s., acne, pustulosis, hyperostosis,
osteitis (SAPHO)
s., acne, pustulosis, hyperostosis,
osteitis syndrome
crystal-induced s.
leukemic s.
pigmented villonodular s.
purulent s.
suppurative s.
villonodular s.
syntax
synthesis, pl. **syntheses**
DNA s.
hormone s.
protein s.
synthetase
carbamoyl phosphate s. (CAPS)
uroporphyrin s.
synthetic

Synthroid
syntropic
syntropy
inverse s.
syphilis
benign s.
cardiovascular s.
congenital s.
s. d'emblée
early s.
early latent s.
endemic s.
gummatous s.
s. hereditaria
s. hereditaria tarda
late benign s.
late latent s.
latent s.
meningovascular s.
nonvenereal s.
primary s.
quaternary s.
secondary s.
tertiary s.
syphilitic
s. cirrhosis
s. hepatitis
s. stomatitis
syphilitic aortitis
syphiloid
syphilologist
syphilology
Syriac ulcer
syringe
hypodermic s.
insulin s.
MediSense Precision Sure Dose
insulin s.
Precision Sure Dose insulin s.
Sure Dose insulin s.
syringomyelia
lumbar s.
syrinx
syrup
ipecac s.
Pancof HC s.
system
Activa Parkinson's Control
Therapy S.
adaptive immune s.
Behavioral Risk Factor
Surveillance S. (BRFSS)

S

NOTES

system (*continued*)
blood glucose monitoring s.
cardiovascular s.
central nervous s. (CNS)
continuous insulin delivery s.
(CIDS)
Cordis Checkmate S.
diabetes control s.
endocrine s.
ErecAid vacuum s.
Fast Take blood glucose
monitoring s.
Glucometer DEX s.
glucose monitoring s.
hexaxial reference s.
His-Purkinje s.
home access s.
immune s.
In Charge diabetes control s.
InDuo s.
injection s.
insulin delivery s.
insulin injection s.
intrarenal renin angiotensin s.
kallikrein-kinin s.
Medical Literature Analysis and
Retrieval S. (MEDLARS)
medicated urethral s.
MediSense Precision Q-I-D blood
glucose monitoring s.
mesolimbic dopamine s.
needle-free injection s.
needle management s.
Novoste Beta-Cath S.
personal emergency response s.
(PERS)
Precision Q-I-D blood glucose
monitoring s.
Q 103 needle management s.
renin-angiotensin s. (RAS)
renin-angiotensin-aldosterone s.
sinopulmonary s.
SKY epidural pain control s.
spectral telescopic s.

sympathetic nervous s.
sympathoadrenal s.
synergistic s.
TD Glucose monitoring s.
transdermal delivery s.
vestibular s.
Vitajet-3 needle-free injection s.
systemic
s. anterior motion (SAM)
s. arterial hypertension
s. arteriole
s. autoimmune disease
s. blastomycosis
s. capillary leak syndrome
s. corticosteroid
s. embolization
s. febrile disease
s. fungal infection
s. hemangiomatosis
s. inflammatory response syndrome
(SIRS)
s. lupus erythematosus (SLE)
s. lupus erythematosus-like
syndrome
s. mastocytosis
s. mycosis
s. proliferating
angioendotheliomatosis
s. rheumatoid vasculitis
s. sclerosis
s. sclerosis sine scleroderma
s. symptom
s. therapy
systole
end s.
systolic
apical s.
s. blood pressure (SBP)
s. dysfunction
s. ejection murmur (SEM)
s. heart murmur
s. hypertension
systolic/diastolic angiography
systolic-diastolic hypertension (SDH)

T₄
    thyroxine
        free T₄
        plasma free T4
        total T4
T₃
    triiodothyronine
        free T₃
        T3 resin uptake
        T3 resin uptake test
        T3 suppression test
        total T3
T&A
    tonsillectomy and adenoidectomy
tabardillo
tabes
        diabetic t.
        t. dorsalis
        t. mesenterica
tabetic
table
        examining t.
        Gaffky t.
        life t.
        tilt t.
tablet
        Calciferol t.'s
        Omniflox t.'s
        pantoprazole delayed-release t.
tabourka
        bruit de t.
tabs
        Berocca Plus t.
        Glynase Pres T.
        Senna T.
Tac
tachistoscope
tachyarrhythmia
        paroxysmal t.
        ventricular t.
tachycardia
        antidromic t.
        atrial t.
        atrial ectopic t. (AET)
        atrioventricular junctional t.
        atrioventricular nodal reentrant t.
        AV nodal reentrant t.
        bundle-branch reentrant
            ventricular t.
        ectopic atrial t.
        idiopathic ventricular t.
        junctional t.
        left septal ventricular t.
        long R-P t.
        monomorphic ventricular t.

        multifocal atrial t. (MAT)
        narrow-complex t.
        nodal t.
        nonparoxysmal atrioventricular
            junctional t.
        nonspecific t.
        nonsustained ventricular t. (NSVT)
        orthodromic reciprocating t.
        pacemaker-mediated t.
        paroxysmal atrial t.
        paroxysmal nodal t. (PNT)
        paroxysmal supraventricular t.
            (PSVT)
        paroxysmal ventricular t.
        postoperative supraventricular t.
        pulseless ventricular t.
        reciprocating t.
        recurrent sustained ventricular t.
        resting t.
        septal ventricular t.
        sinus t.
        slow paroxysmal atrial t. (SPAT)
        supraventricular t. (SVT)
        sustained ventricular t.
        ventricular t. (V-tach)
        wide-complex t. (WCT)
tachygastria
tachyphylaxis
tachypnea
tacrine hydrochloride
tacrolimus ointment
Tacticon device
tactile fremitus
TAD
        thoracic asphyxiant dystrophy
        thrombin activation device
Taekwondo
Taenia
taeniasis
        t. saginata
        t. solium
TAF
        tissue angiogenesis factor
        tumor angiogenesis factor
Tagamet
tagged red blood cell scanning
TAH
        total abdominal hysterectomy
tai
        t. chi
        t. chi chuan
Taiwan acute respiratory (TWAR)
Takahara disease
Takayasu
        T. arteritis

Takayasu *(continued)*
    T. pulseless disease
    T. syndrome
Talacen
talar navicular
talcosis
    pulmonary t.
talc poudrage
tali (*pl. of* talus)
talipedic
talipes
Tallerman treatment
Talma disease
talocrural joint
talus, pl. **tali**
    sustentaculum tali
Talwin
Tambocor
tambour
    bruit de t.
    t. sound
Tamiflu
tamoxifen
tamponade
    balloon t.
    cardiac t.
tamsulosin
tanapox
tandem ICON
Tangier disease
tangle
    neurofibrillary t.
tank
    Hubbard t.
Tanner
    T. growth chart
    T. stage (I–V)
    T. staging (I–V)
TAO
    thromboangiitis obliterans
Tapazole
taped
    buddy t.
tapeworm infestation
tarda
    hyperphosphatasemia t.
    osteogenesis imperfecta t.
    porphyria cutanea t.
    rachitis t.
    syphilis hereditaria t.
tardive
    t. akathisia
    t. dyskinesia
    t. dystonia
    forme t.
tardus
    hyperkinetic t.

target
    t. cell anemia
    t. organ
Tarlov cyst
tarry stool
tarsal
    t. tunnel
    t. tunnel syndrome
tarsometatarsal
tarsorrhaphy
tarsotomy
tartrate
    tolterodine t.
taste
    t. deficiency
    t. disorder
    t. perversion
tattoo
    amalgam t.
tau
taurine
Tavist-1
Tavist-D
taxis
Tay-Sachs disease
tazarotene
tazobactam
    piperacillin and t.
TB
    tuberculosis
TBE
    tick-borne encephalitis
TBG
    thyroid-binding globulin
TBI
    thyroid-binding index
TBII
    thyroid-binding inhibitory
     immunoglobulin
T_4-binding globulin level
Tc
    cytotoxic T-cell
TCA
    tricyclic antidepressant
T-cell
    T-c. anergy
    cytotoxic T-c. (Tc)
    lymphoid precursor T-c.
    T-c. lymphoma
    T-c. therapy
TCSG
    The Center for Social Gerontology
Td
    tetanus-diphtheria
    Td booster
TD Glucose monitoring system
tea
    bananas, rice, applesauce, toast, t.
    (BRATT)

chamomile t.
Lacey LeBeau t.
teaching hospital
Teale amputation
tear
anterior cruciate ligament t.
artificial t.
Bion T.'s
ligamentous t.
Mallory-Weiss t.
meniscal t.
teardrop fracture
tearing
meniscal t.
teaspoonful
technetium-99m sestamibi
technical skill
technician
patient care t. (PCT)
technique
behavioral t.
distraction t.
provocative t.
relaxation t.
Seldinger t.
sleep-enhancing behavioral t.
transseptal t.
T-tube t.
technology
medical t.
tectum
optic t.
TED
thromboembolic disease
TED hose
TED stocking
Tedral
TEE
thermic effect of exercise
transesophageal echocardiogram
transesophageal echocardiography
TEF
thermic effect of food
Tegaderm
Tegison
tegmen, pl. **tegmina**
Tegopen
Tegretol
teichoic acid
teicoplanin
telalgia

telangiectasia
calcinosis, Raynaud phenomenon,
esophageal motility disorders,
sclerodactyly, t. (CREST)
cyanosis, redness, scleroderma, t.
(CRST)
hereditary hemorrhagic t.
spider t.
stellate t.
telangiectasis
telangiitis
telangion
telangiosis
telediagnosis
telemedicine
telemetry
teleroentgenogram
teleroentgentherapy
telescope
Bioptic t.
teletherapy
Telfa dressing
tellurism
telmisartan
telogen
telognosis
telomerase enzyme
temafloxacin
temazepam
Tembid
Isordil T.
Temovate Cream
temozolomide
temperament
temperature
axillary t.
basal body t.
core body t.
t., pulse, respiration (TPR)
rectal t.
tympanic t.
template
temporal
t. arteritis
t. lobe epilepsy
t. muscle wasting
temporomandibular
t. joint (TMJ)
t. joint syndrome
tenacious
tenant
locum t.

T

NOTES

Tenckhoff catheter
tender
    t. incarceration
    markedly t.
tenderness
    costovertebral angle t.
    CVA t.
    diffuse lumbosacral t.
    parotid t.
    pencil t.
    rebound t.
    t. and rebound (T&R)
tendinitis, tendonitis
    Achilles t.
    calcific t.
    posterior tibial t.
tendinous xanthoma
tendo Achillis
tendon
    Achilles t.
    t. rupture
    t. xanthoma
tendonitis (*var. of* tendinitis)
tenecteplase
tenens
    locum t.
tenesmic
tenesmus
Tenex
ten Horn sign
teniasis
    somatic t.
teniposide
tennis elbow
Tenoretic
Tenormin
tenosynovitis
    de Quervain t.
    flexor t.
    infectious flexor t.
TENS
    transcutaneous electrical nerve
    stimulation
    TENS unit
Tensilon test
tension
    carbon monoxide t.
    t. headache
tension-type headache
tensor
tent
    oxygen t.
Tenuate Dospan
tenuous
Tequin
teratogen
teratogenic
teratoma
teratospermia

Terazol
terazosin
terbinafine
terbutaline inhaler
terminal
    t. cancer
    t. dribbling
    t. ileus
    t. infection
    t. interphalangeal (TIP)
    t. pneumonia
Terramycin
terrazzo
terror
    sleep t.
Terry
    T. nail
    T. syndrome
tertian
    double t.
    t. fever
    t. malaria
tertiary
    t. aging
    t. disease
    t. hyperparathyroidism
    t. hypothyroidism
    t. medical care
    t. prevention
    t. syphilis
Teslac
Tessalon Perles
test
    abnormal screening t.
    acetowhite t.
    acid perfusion t.
    acid reflux t.
    ACTH stimulation t.
    Adamkiewicz t.
    adrenocorticotropic hormone
       stimulation t.
    Albarran t.
    alcohol screening t.
    Allen t.
    alpha-fetoprotein t.
    Anderson-Collip t.
    animal-naming t.
    apnea t.
    arginine t.
    autonomic function t.
    Balke-Ware t.
    BEI t.
    Békésy t.
    belt t.
    Berg balance t.
    Bernstein t.
    blood t.
    bromocriptine suppression t.
    bromsulphalein t.

Broth dilution t.
butanol-extractable iodine t.
CAGE t.
CAMP t.
capillary fragility t.
capillary resistance t.
Casoni intradermal t.
Casoni skin t.
cellophane tape t.
Christie-Atkins-Munch-Petersen t.
Chymex t.
CK t.
clock completion t.
clock drawing t.
coin t.
cold pressor t.
conglutinating complement
  absorption t.
Coombs t.
corticotropin-releasing hormone t.
corticotropin stimulation t.
Cortrosyn stimulation t.
cough t.
C peptide suppression t.
creatine kinase t.
Delayed Word Recall T.
dexamethasone suppression t. (DST)
diabetes t.
diagnostic t.
discontinuation t.
doll's eye t.
edrophonium t.
Ellsworth-Howard t.
Epsilometer t. (E-test)
estrogen receptor assay t.
exercise stress t.
exercise treadmill t. (ETT)
fall screen t.
fecal occult blood t. (FOBT)
finger-to-nose t.
Finkelstein t.
flip t.
FR t.
free T$_4$ t.
fructosamine t.
functional reach t.
Galveston Orientation and
  Amnesia T. (GOAT)
get-up-and-go t.
GlucoProtein t.
glucose insulin tolerance t. (GITT)
glucose suppression t.

glucose tolerance t. (GTT)
glycosylated hemoglobin t.
gonadotropin-releasing hormone t.
Göthlin t.
growth hormone-releasing factor t.
Hanger-Rose skin t.
head-up tilt t.
head-up tilt-table t.
heel-to-shin t.
Hemoccult t.
heterophile t.
Hickey-Hare t.
high-dose dexamethasone
  suppression t.
HIV t.
Hodgkinson Mental T.
Hoesch t.
Hoover t.
indirect hemagglutination t.
iodine-I-131 uptake t.
17-ketogenic steroid assay t.
Kveim-Siltzbach t.
latex agglutination t.
leishmanin t.
levodopa t.
lift-off t.
liver function t. (LFT)
low-dose dexamethasone
  suppression t.
Maclagan thymol turbidity t.
McMurray t.
t. meal
Meltzer-Lyon t.
metyrapone t.
Michigan alcohol screening t.
Miller-Fisher t.
Monospot t.
Montenegro t.
Moschcowitz t.
motor coordination t. (MCT)
Neer t.
nontreponemal t.
number connection t. (NCT)
Ober t.
occult blood t.
oculocephalic t.
oral glucose tolerance t. (OGTT)
OraSure t.
overnight dexamethasone
  suppression t.
palmin t.
pancreatic function t.

NOTES

test *(continued)*
pancreozymin-secretin t.
Pap t.
Papanicolaou t.
Patrick t.
Persantine-thallium stress t.
Perthes t.
Pfeiffer t.
Phalen t.
phentolamine t.
phrenic pressure t.
pinprick t.
pituitary function t.
polymerase chain reaction t.
polyuria t.
pregnancy t.
provocative t.
pull t.
pulmonary function t. (PFT)
Quick t.
radioactive iodine uptake t.
radioallergosorbent t.
radioallergosorbent assay t. (RAST)
range of motion t.
rapid strep-antigen t.
recall t.
renal function t.
rheumatoid arthritis t.
rheumatoid factor t.
Rinne t.
Romberg t.
Rubin t.
Rumpel-Leede t.
Sabin-Feldman dye t.
Schilling t.
Schirmer t.
Schwartz t.
screening t.
secretin t.
Sensory Organization T. (SOT)
sestamibi t.
short cosyntropin stimulation t.
sickle cell t.
sickle cell anemia t. (SCAT)
SimpliRED D-dimer t.
skin prick t.
skin puncture t.
somatomedin C t.
spironolactone t.
standing t.
startle t.
Staub-Traugott t.
stimulation t.
straight leg raising t.
streptozyme t.
stress t.
sucrose lysis t.
sudomotor function t.
sugar t.

sweat t.
Tensilon t.
Thomas t.
three-item recall t.
thyroid antibody t.
thyroid function t. (TFT)
thyroid laboratory t.
thyroid suppression t.
thyrotropin-releasing hormone
  stimulation t.
tilt t.
time and change t.
timed up and go t.
tourniquet t.
treadmill t.
treponemal t.
Treponema pallidum
  immobilization t.
T3 resin uptake t.
triiodothyronine uptake t.
troponin I t.
T3 suppression t.
tuberculin skin t.
TUG t.
tuning fork t.
Tzanck t.
urine t.
urine pregnancy t. (UPT)
urodynamic t.
vestibular t.
vitamin C t.
Volhard t.
Wassermann t.
Weber t.
Werner t.
Western blot t.
whisper t.
Widal t.
Word Fluency T.
testalgia
testicular
  t. cancer
  t. disorder
  t. dysgenesis
  t. feminization
  t. feminization syndrome
  t. torsion
testing
  allergen challenge t.
  breath t.
  cognitive t.
  colonic transit t.
  D-dimer t.
  electropharmacologic t.
  electrophysiologic t.
  fecal occult blood t.
  genetic t.
  hypothesis t.
  invasive t.

light touch t.
Mantoux t.
noninvasive cardiac t.
pharmacologic stress t.
quantitative sensory t. (QST)
radioallergoabsorbent t.
secretory t.
serial t.
SimpliRED D-dimer t.
speech discrimination t.
tilt table t.
treadmill t.
urodynamic t.
Testoderm patch
testoid hyperthecosis
testosterone
t. gel
t. level
t. patch
plasma t.
t. production
prolactin t.
t. replacement
tetanoid
tetanus
diphtheria, pertussis, t. (DPT)
neonatal t.
t. neonatorum
tetanus-diphtheria (Td)
tetanus-diphtheria toxoid
tetany
t. of alkalosis
gastric t.
hyperventilation t.
hypoparathyroid t.
infantile t.
latent t.
parathyroid t.
parathyroprival t.
phosphate t.
postoperative t.
rheumatic t.
thyroprival t.
tetraacetate
tetrabenazine
tetracycline antibiotic
tetrad
tetradic
tetraethyl poisoning
tetralogy of Fallot
tetramere

tetranitrate
erythrityl t.
pentaerythritol t.
TFT
thyroid function test
TG
triglyceride
TGF-beta
transforming growth factor beta
TH-1, -2
thalamic
t. column neurostimulation
t. syndrome
t. syndrome of Déjérine and
Roussy
thalamotomy
thalamus
thalassemia
t. major
t. minor
t. syndrome
t. trait
thalassotherapy
thalidomide
Thalitone
thallium
t. 201
exercise t.
t. poisoning
t. scintigraphy
thallotoxicosis
thanatognomonic
thanatography
thanatoid
thanatology
thanatophoric
Thaysen disease
The
T. Centers for Medicare and
Medicaid Services
T. Center for Social Gerontology
(TCSG)
T. Dana Alliance for Brain
Initiative
T. Skin Cancer Foundation
theaism
thecoma
Theelin injection
theinism
thelalgia
thelarche
thenar eminence

NOTES

Theo-24
Theochron
Theo-Dur
Theolair
theophylline
    t. anhydrous
    t. toxicity
theorem
theory
    Cannon t.
    cell-aging t.
    endocrine t.
    free radical t.
    Frerichs t.
    immune t.
    t. of medicine
    neuroendocrine t.
    scientific t.
    somatic mutation t.
    wear-and-tear t.
theotherapy
Thera-Band exercise
Theragran
therapeusis
therapeutic
    t. abortion
    t. anesthesia
    t. community
    t. drug monitoring
    t. electrode
    t. fever
    t. index
    t. nihilism
    t. optimism
    t. pessimism
    t. rehabilitation
    suggestive t.'s
therapeutic-to-toxic ratio
therapeutist
therapia magna sterilisans
therapist
    low-vision rehabilitation t.
    occupational t. (OT)
    physical t. (PT)
    rehabilitation t.
    speech t.
therapy
    ablation t.
    Activa Parkinson's Control T.
    adoptive cellular t.
    aerosol t.
    alkali t.
    alternative cancer t.
    aminoglycoside t.
    ancillary t.
    androgen-deprivation t.
    antimicrobial t.
    antiplatelet t.
    antipyretic t.

antireflux t.
antiretroviral t.
antiviral t.
aquatic t.
behavioral t.
bicarbonate t.
bladder relaxant t.
blood component t.
burst of t.
cancer t.
catheter-directed thrombolytic t.
chelation t.
CI t.
cognitive behavior t.
constraint-induced movement t.
cytoreductive t.
cytotoxic t.
depot t.
diuretic t.
electroconvulsive t. (ECT)
electrolyte t.
endoscopic hemostatic t.
endovascular t.
enteral nutritional t.
enterostomal t. (ET)
estrogen replacement t. (ERT)
etidronate t.
external beam radiation t. (EBRT)
fever t.
first-line pharmacologic t.
fluorohydrocortisone t.
fluoroquinolone t.
gene t.
geriatric t.
group t.
growth hormone t.
hemostatic t.
heparin t.
herbal t.
high-dose diuretic t.
highly active antiretroviral t.
  (HAART)
home nutrition t.
hormonal ablation t.
hormone t.
hormone replacement t. (HRT)
hyperbaric oxygen t.
insulin t.
insulin coma t. (ICT)
interferon alpha t.
intralesional t.
iron chelation t.
irradiation t.
laser t.
light t.
lipid-lowering t.
long-term RBC transfusion t.
luteal phase t.
macrolide t.

magnet t.
maintenance drug t.
massage t.
medicated urethral system for
  erection t.
microwave t.
movement t.
MUSE t.
neuroprotective t.
nicotine replacement t. (NRT)
nonpharmacologic t.
nutritional t.
occupational t. (OT)
open-loop pump t.
oral rehydration t. (ORT)
orthomolecular t.
oxygen t.
pain t.
parenteral t.
pharmacologic t.
photodynamic t.
physical t. (PT)
plasma t.
postural drainage t.
psoralen ultraviolet A-range t.
pulse t.
PUVA t.
radioactive iodine t.
radiofrequency catheter ablative t.
recombinant human replacement t.
reflex t.
rehydration t.
renal replacement t.
reperfusion t.
replacement t.
salvage t.
serum t.
solar t.
specific t.
speech t.
statin t.
substitution t.
substitutive t.
systemic t.
T-cell t.
thrombolytic t.
thyroid t.
transfusion t.
thermal
  t. bird
  t. burn
thermatology

thermic
  t. effect
  t. effect of exercise (TEE)
  t. effect of food (TEF)
  t. fever
thermica
  myalgia t.
thermoablation
thermogenic stimulant
thermography
thermometer
  axilla t.
  axillary t.
  clinical t.
  surface t.
thermopenetration
thermophore
thermoplegia
thermoregulation
thermoregulatory
thermotherapy
thesaurismosis
thesaurismotic
thesaurosis
theta activity
Thezac-Porsmeur method
thiabendazole
thiamine
  t. deficiency
  t. HC
thiazide
  t. diabetes
  t. diuretic
thiazolidinedione
thickening
  breast t.
thick-handled cutlery
thickness
  Breslow t.
  intimal-medial t. (IMT)
  skinfold t.
thick and thin preparation
Thiemann
  T. disease
  T. syndrome
Thiersch graft
thimerosal
thin basement membrane disease
thin-walled cyst
thioguanine
thionamide
thioridazine

NOTES

thiotepa
thiothixene
thiouracil
thiourea
third
t. disease
t. and fourth pharyngeal pouch syndrome
t. heart sound (S_3)
t. party payer
third-degree
t.-d. atrioventricular block
t.-d. burn
thirst
false t.
t. fever
insensible t.
morbid t.
subliminal t.
true t.
thistle
milk t.
Thomas test
Thompson syndrome
Thomson sign
thoracalgia
thoracentesis
thoraces (*pl. of* thorax)
thoracic
t. asphyxiant dystrophy (TAD)
t. goiter
t. outlet compression syndrome
t. outlet syndrome (TOS)
t. pain
t. zygomycosis
thoracodynia
thoracolumbar
thoracometer
thoracomyodynia
thoracopathy
thoracoscopic biopsy
thoracoscopy
thoracotomy
thorax, pl. **thoraces**
barrel-shaped t.
Thorazine
Thorn syndrome
THR
total hip replacement
three-day
t.-d. fever
t.-d. measles
three-item recall test
three times a day (t.i.d.)
thresher's lung
threshold percussion
thrill
hydatid t.
thrive
failure to t.
throat
t. clearing
t. culture
ears, nose, t. (ENT)
head, ears, eyes, nose, t. (HEENT)
throbbing
thrombasthenia
Glanzmann t.
thrombi (*pl. of* thrombus)
thrombin
t. activation device (TAD)
autologous t.
thromboangiitis obliterans (TAO)
thrombocyst
thrombocytasthenia
thrombocythemia
essential t.
thrombocytic
thrombocytopathic
thrombocytopathy
thrombocytopenia
drug-induced immune t.
gestational t.
heparin-induced t.
HIV-associated t.
idiopathic t.
immune t.
thrombocytopenic purpura
thrombocytopoiesis
thrombocytopoietic
thrombocytosis
reactive t.
thromboembolic
t. disease (TED)
t. disease hose
t. disease stocking
t. disorder
t. pulmonary hypertension
thromboembolism
acute t.
venous t.
thrombogenic
thrombohemolytic microangiopathy
thromboid
thrombolysis
thrombolytic
t. agent
t. therapy
thrombolytica
purpura t.
thrombopathy
constitutional t.
thrombopenia
thrombopenic
t. anemia
t. purpura

thrombophilia
  inherited t.
thrombophlebitis
  cavernous sinus t.
  deep vein t.
  iliofemoral t.
  intracranial t.
  postpartum iliofemoral t.
  purulent t.
  t. saltans
  septic intracranial t.
  superficial t.
  suppurative t.
thromboplastin
thrombose
thrombosed external hemorrhoid
thrombosis
  agonal t.
  arterial t.
  atrophic t.
  calf vein t.
  cardiac t.
  creeping t.
  deep vein t. (DVT)
  deep venous t. (DVT)
  idiopathic deep vein t.
  isolated calf vein t.
  marantic t.
  mesenteric venous t.
  microvascular t.
  ovarian vein t.
  pelvic vein t.
  portal vein t.
  renal vein t.
  in situ t.
  splenic vein t.
  upper extremity t.
  vein t.
  venous t.
thrombotic
  t. microangiopathic hemolytic
    anemia
  t. stroke
  t. thrombocytopenic purpura (TTP)
  t. thrombohemolytic purpura
thrombus, pl. **thrombi**
  t. formation
  marantic t.
  mural t.
  traumatic t.
**through-and-through myocardial
  infarction**

thrush
thudding
thumbprinting
thump
  chest t.
thunderclap headache
thymectomy
thymelcosis
thymi (*pl. of* thymus)
thymic
  t. hypoplasia
  t. involution
  t. medullary hyperplasia
thymica
  mors t.
thymicolymphaticus
  status t.
thymicus
  status t.
thymidine kinase (TK)
thymine
Thymoglobulin
thymokinetic
thymolipoma
thymoma
thymopathy
thymoprival
thymus, pl. **thymi, thymuses**
  congenital aplasia of t.
  t. gland
  t. treatment
thyroaplasia
thyrocalcitonin
thyrocardiac
thyrocele
thyrogenic
thyroglobulin antibody
thyroglossal
thyroid
  aberrant t.
  accessory t.
  t. adenoma
  t. antibody test
  Armour T.
  t. bruit
  t. cancer
  t. crisis
  t. deficiency
  desiccated t.
  t. disease
  t. dysfunction
  ectopic t.

T

NOTES

thyroid *(continued)*
  free t.
  t. function
  t. function studies
  t. function test (TFT)
  t. gland
  Hashimoto t.
  t. hormone
  t. hormone-binding index
  t. hormone resistance
  t. infantilism
  t. insufficiency
  intrathoracic t.
  t. laboratory test
  lingual t.
  t. lobectomy
  t. lymphoma
  t. malignant neoplasia
  t. microsomal antibody
  t. nodule
  retrosternal t.
  t. storm
  t. suppression test
  t. therapy
  t. toxicosis
  t. ultrasonography
thyroid-binding
  t.-b. globulin (TBG)
  t.-b. index (TBI)
  t.-b. inhibitory immunoglobulin
    (TBII)
thyroidea
  cachexia t.
thyroidectomy
  chemical t.
  medical t.
thyroidism
thyroiditis
  autoimmune t.
  chronic autoimmune t.
  chronic fibrosing t.
  chronic fibrous t.
  chronic lymphadenoid t.
  chronic lymphocytic t.
  de Quervain t.
  fibrosing t.
  fibrous t.
  giant follicular t.
  Hashimoto t.
  ligneous t.
  lymphadenoid t.
  lymphocytic t.
  parasitic t.
  postpartum t.
  Riedel t.
  silent t.
  subacute lymphocyte t.
thyroidology

thyroid-stimulating
  t.-s. hormone (TSH)
  t.-s. hormone deficiency
  t.-s. hormone-mediated
    hyperthyroidism
  t.-s. hormone overproduction
  t.-s. hormone-releasing factor (TSH-
    RF)
  t.-s. immunoglobulin (TSI)
thyrointoxication
Thyrolar-2
thyroliberin
thyromegaly
  discrete t.
thyropathy
thyrophyma
thyropriva
  cachexia t.
thyroprival tetany
thyroprivia
thyroprivic
thyroprotein
thyrotoxic
  t. coma
  t. crisis
  t. ophthalmoplegia
thyrotoxicosis
  acute t.
  apathetic t.
  t. ectopia
  t. factitia
  t. medicamentosa
  trophoblastic t.
thyrotoxin
thyrotropic hormone
thyrotropin, thyrotrophin
thyrotropin-releasing
  t.-r. factor (TRF)
  t.-r. hormone (TRH)
  t.-r. hormone stimulation test
thyroxine (T_4)
  t. clearance
  serum total t.
  t. toxicosis
TIA
  transient ischemic attack
tiagabine hydrochloride
Tiazac
TIBC
  total iron-binding capacity
tibia
tibial
  t. plateau fracture
  posterior t. (PT)
  t. tuberosity
tic
  t. douloureux
  motor t.
  phonic t.

ticarcillin-clavulanic acid
tick
- t. bite
- deer t.
- t. typhus

tick-bite fever
tick-borne encephalitis (TBE)
Ticlid
ticlopidine HCl
t.i.d.
- three times a day

tidal volume
Tietze
- T. disease
- T. syndrome

Tigan
Tilade
TILS
- tumor-infiltrating lymphocyte

tilt
- t. table
- t. table testing
- t. test

time
- activated partial thromboplastin t. (APTT, aPTT)
- capillary refill t.
- t. and change test
- lead t.
- leisure t.
- median survival t.
- mortality rate doubling t.
- partial prothrombin t. (PPT)
- partial thromboplastin t. (PTT)
- pro t.
- prolonged activated partial thromboplastin t.
- prolonged prothrombin t.
- prothrombin t. (pro time, PT)
- reaction t.
- Stypven t.
- survival t.
- tincture of t.

Timecaps
- Levsinex T.

timed
- t. up and go (TUG)
- t. up and go test

Timentin
time-zone change syndrome
timing
Timolide

timolol
Timoptic
Tinactin cream
tinctorial
tincture of time
tine
tinea
- t. barbae
- t. capitis
- t. corporis
- t. cruris
- t. faciei
- t. manus
- t. manuum
- t. pedis
- t. unguium
- t. versicolor

Tinel sign
tingling
tinnitus
- t. aurium
- clicking t.
- Leudet t.
- nervous t.
- objective t.
- vibratory t.

Tinver lotion
TIP
- terminal interphalangeal

tires
tiring
tirofiban
Tiselius apparatus
tissue
- adipose t.
- t. angiogenesis factor (TAF)
- body adipose t.
- devitalized t.
- fibrovascular t.
- gross examination of t.
- t. perfusion
- t. plasminogen activator (TPA, tPA, t-PA)
- t. preparation
- t. proteinosis
- t. roundworm
- t. sloughing
- t. tin concentration
- t. typing

tissue-damaging process
titer
- antistreptolysin-O t.

NOTES

T

titer (continued)
 ASO t.
 CMV t.
 cytomegalovirus t.
 EBV t.
 Epstein-Barr virus t.
 Lyme t.
 TWAR t.
 viral t.
Titralac Plus Liquid
titrate
titubation
tizanidine hydrochloride
TK
 thymidine kinase
TKR
 total knee replacement
TLC
 total lung capacity
TLE
 total life expectancy
TM
 tympanic membrane
TMJ
 temporomandibular joint
 TMJ syndrome
TNF-alpha
 tumor necrosis factor-alpha
TNKase
TNM
 tumor, necrosis, metastasis
 TNM staging
TNTC
 too numerous to count
to-and-fro oscillation
toast
 bananas, rice, applesauce, t.
 (BRAT)
 bananas, rice cereal, applesauce, t.
 (BRAT)
tobacco
 t. abuse
 Skoal chewing t.
 smokeless t.
tobaccoism
Tobia fever
tobramycin
Tobrex
tocainide
tocolysis
tocolytics
tocopherol
Todd cirrhosis
toe
 mallet t.
toenail
 ingrown t.
Tofranil

together
 Generations T. (GT)
toilet
 pulmonary t.
toileting
 scheduled t.
toilet-seat angina
tolazamide
tolbutamide
Tolectin DS
tolerability
tolerance
 cross t.
 t. dose
 drug t.
 exercise t.
 genotypic t.
 glucose t. (GT)
 impaired glucose t. (IGT)
 individual t.
 oral glucose t.
 species t.
tolerant
tolerate
Tolinase
tolnaftate
tolterodine tartrate
tomaculous
Toma sign
Tommaselli
 T. disease
 T. syndrome
tomogram
tomographic
tomography
 adrenal computerized t.
 automated computerized axial t.
 (ACAT)
 computed t. (CT)
 computed axial t. (CAT)
 contrast agent-enhanced spiral
 computed t.
 electron beam computed t. (EBCT)
 gated single-proton emission
 computed t.
 high-resolution computed t. (HRCT)
 positron emission t. (PET)
 single-photon emission computed t.
 (SPECT)
 spiral computed t.
 xenon computed t.
tone
 t. decay
 heart t.
 vasomotor t.
tongue
 amyloid t.
 antibiotic t.
 baked t.

bald t.
black hairy t.
choreic t.
coated t.
furred t.
geographic t.
hairy t.
magenta t.
parrot t.
raspberry t.
red strawberry t.
Sandwith bald t.
strawberry t.
tonic
bitter t.
t. reflex spasm
t. seizure
tonic-clonic seizure
tonicity
muscle t.
tonin
Tonocard
tonoclonic
tonometry
applanation t.
tonsil
tonsillar
t. crypt
t. ulcer
tonsillectomy and adenoidectomy (T&A)
tonsillitis
tonsillopharyngitis
tool
decision-support t.'s
too numerous to count (TNTC)
tooth, pl. **teeth**
t. abscess
t. decay
tophaceous gout
tophus, pl. **tophi**
gouty tophi
topica
topical
t. antibiotic
t. corticosteroid
t. estrogen
MetroGel T.
t. penile minoxidil
Topicort gel
topiramate
topoisomerase inhibitor
Topolanski sign

topopathogenesis
topophylaxis
Toprol XL
Toradol injection
TORCH
toxoplasmosis, other infections, rubella,
cytomegalovirus infection, herpes
simplex
TORCH syndrome
torcular Herophili
Torecan
tori (*pl. of* torus)
tormina
Tornalate
torsades de pointes
torsemide
torsion
fallopian tube t.
testicular t.
torticollis
flexible t.
tortuosity
tortuous
Torulopsis glabrata
torulosis
torulus
torus, pl. **tori**
tori palatinus
TOS
thoracic outlet syndrome
total
t. abdominal hysterectomy (TAH)
t. bilirubin
t. hip replacement (THR)
t. incontinence
t. iron-binding capacity (TIBC)
t. knee replacement (TKR)
t. life expectancy (TLE)
t. lung capacity (TLC)
t. mastectomy
t. parenteral hyperalimentation
t. parenteral nutrition (TPN)
t. parenteral nutrition cholestasis
t. peripheral parenteral nutrition
(TPPN)
t. T3
t. T4
t. triiodothyronine
t. urinary gonadotropin (TUG)
touch
light t.

NOTES

T

405

touch (*continued*)
    royal t.
    sharp t.
Tourette syndrome
tourniquet
    t. paralysis
    t. poditis
    t. test
toxemia
toxemic
    t. pneumonia
toxic
    t. amblyopia
    t. cirrhosis
    t. cyanosis
    t. delirium
    t. encephalitis
    t. epidermal necrolysis
    t. inhalant
    t. liver disease
    t. methemoglobinemia
    t. multinodular goiter
    t. nephrosis
    t. neuropathy
    t. nodule
    t. paralytic anemia
    t. shock
    t. shock syndrome (TSS)
    t. shock syndrome toxin-1 (TSST-1)
    t. syndrome
toxicity
    acetaminophen t.
    acid t.
    alkaline t.
    amphetamine t.
    antidepressant t.
    barbiturate t.
    benzodiazepine t.
    beta-adrenergic antagonist t.
    calcium channel antagonist t.
    cardiac t.
    cardiovascular t.
    clozapine t.
    cocaine t.
    cyclic antidepressant t.
    diethylene glycol t.
    digitalis t.
    digoxin t.
    drug t.
    ethanol t.
    ethylene glycol t.
    gamma-hydroxybutyrate t.
    gastrointestinal t.
    halothane t.
    hydrocarbon t.
    isopropyl alcohol t.
    lithium t.
    liver t.

    methanol t.
    3,4-methylenedioxymethamphetamine t.
    neuroleptic t.
    olanzapine t.
    opioid t.
    organophosphate t.
    overdose t.
    oxygen t.
    phencyclidine t.
    renal t.
    salicylate t.
    selective serotonin reuptake inhibitor t.
    t. syndrome
    theophylline t.
toxicosis
    endogenic t.
    exogenic t.
    thyroid t.
    thyroxine t.
    triiodothyronine t.
toxignomic
toxin
    botulinum t.
    Clostridium difficile t.
    uremic t.
toxin-1
    toxic shock syndrome t.-1 (TSST-1)
toxin-mediated infection
Toxocara canis
toxocariasis disorder
toxoid
    diphtheria-tetanus t. (dT)
    Infanrix diphtheria and tetanus t.
    tetanus-diphtheria t.
Toxoplasma
toxoplasmosis
    acquired t.
    ocular t.
    t., other infections, rubella, cytomegalovirus infection, herpes simplex (TORCH)
    t., other infections, rubella, cytomegalovirus infection, herpes simplex syndrome
TP
    trigger point
    TP segment
TPA, tPA
    tissue plasminogen activator
TPI
    trigger point injection
TPN
    total parenteral nutrition
TPPN
    total peripheral parenteral nutrition

TPR
  temperature, pulse, respiration
T&R
  tenderness and rebound
trabecular
  t. bone
  t. meshwork cell
trabeculation
trabeculoplasty
trace
  t. ankle edema
  t. occult blood
  t. positive
trachea
tracheitis
trachelagra
tracheobronchial aspiration
tracheobronchitis
tracheophony
tracheostomy
trachoma
trachomatis
  Chlamydia t.
tracing boundary
tract
  aerodigestive t.
  t. axon
  flow t.
  lower respiratory t.
  respiratory t.
  right ventricular outflow t.
  upper respiratory t.
  urinary t.
  urothelial t.
  vestibulospinal t.
traction
  Cotrel t.
  t. headache
  vitreoretinal t.
trade-off hypothesis
tragus
training
  autogenic t.
  balance-and-gait t.
  bladder t.
  gait t.
trait
  alpha-thalassemia-1, -2 t.
  sickle cell t.
  thalassemia t.
tramadol

tramadol/acetaminophen
trance
  death t.
Trandate
trandolapril
transaminase
  serum glutamic oxaloacetic t.
    (SGOT)
  serum glutamic pyruvic t. (SGPT)
transbronchial needle aspiration
transcellular
  t. potassium shift
  t. water shift
transcobalamin II deficiency
transcortical
  motor aphasia t.
transcranial
  t. Doppler ultrasound
  t. magnetic stimulation
transcriptional profile
transcriptionist
  certified medical t. (CMT)
  medical t.
transcutaneous
  t. electrical nerve stimulation
    (TENS)
  t. electrical nerve stimulation unit
transdermal
  t. delivery system
  estradiol t.
  t. estrogen
  t. fentanyl
  t. nicotine
transdermic
Transderm Scopolamine
transduce
transducer
  Statham t.
transduction
  cochlear t.
  signal t.
transesophageal
  t. echocardiogram (TEE)
  t. echocardiography (TEE)
trans **fatty acid**
transfer
  Camitz t.
  cell-to-cell t.
transferase
  adenine phosphoribosyl t. (APRT)
  gamma glutamyl t. (GGT)

· **NOTES**

T

transferrin
transforming growth factor beta (TGF-beta)
transfusion
    autologous t.
    emergency RBC t.
    emergency red blood cell t.
    granulocyte t.
    t. hepatitis
    massive t.
    platelet t.
    t. reaction
    red blood cell t.
    t. therapy
transfusional hemosiderosis
transfusion-associated graft-versus-host disease
transfusion-related acute lung injury
transgenerational violence
transient
    t. bacteremia
    t. diabetes insipidus
    t. hyperphenylalaninemia
    t. hyperthyroidism
    t. incontinence
    t. insomnia
    t. ischemic attack (TIA)
    t. monocular blindness
    t. neutropenia
    t. period of breathing cessation
    t. weakness
transilluminate
transit
    colonic t.
transitional zone
transition zone
translocation
    robertsonian t.
transmissible
transmission
    GABAergic t.
    iatrogenic t.
    perinatal HIV t.
transmural myocardial infarction
transmyocardial laser revascularization
transperineal route
transplant
    allogeneic stem cell t.
    autologous stem cell t.
    bilateral lung t.
    bilobar t.
    bone marrow t.
    heart t.
    heart-lung t.
    liver t.
    living donor bilobar t.
    lung t.
    t. malignancy
    t. medicine

    organ t.
    t. rejection
    renal t.
    stem cell t.
transplant-associated nephropathy
transplantation
    allogeneic marrow t.
    bone marrow t.
    cardiac t.
    heart-lung t.
    hematopoietic stem cell t.
    renal t.
transport
    deranged water and electrolyte t.
    serum hormone t.
transportation
    Department of T. (DOT)
transposition
    congenitally corrected t.
transposon
transseptal technique
transsphenoidal surgery
transtentorial herniation
transthermia
transthoracic
    t. echocardiogram
    t. echocardiography (TTE)
    t. needle aspiration
    t. needle biopsy
    t. two-dimensional echocardiography
transtracheal
    t. aspiration
    t. needle
transtubular potassium concentration gradient
transudate
transudative
    t. ascites
    t. pleural effusion
transurethral
    t. electrovaporization of prostate (TUEVP)
    t. incision of prostate (TUIP)
    t. needle ablation (TUNA)
    t. resection (TUR)
    t. resection of prostate (TURP)
    t. ultrasound-guided laser-induced prostatectomy (TULIP)
    t. ultrasound-guided laser-induced prostatectomy study
Trans-Ver-Sal
transverse
    t. colon
    t. myelopathy
Tranxene
tranylcypromine
trapeze
trapezius

trapping
    air t.
trastuzumab
Traube
    T. bruit
    T. dyspnea
    T. semilunar space
    T. sign
trauma, pl. **traumata, traumas**
    head t.
    ocular t.
traumatic
    t. amenorrhea
    t. brain injury
    t. delirium
    t. fever
    t. headache
    t. hemolytic anemia
    t. pneumonia
    t. shock
    t. sinus
    t. spinal cord injury
    t. stomatitis
    t. thrombus
traumatica
    folliculitis barbae t.
traumatopnea
traumatopyra
traumatotherapy
travel
    airplane t.
traveler's diarrhea
trazodone
Treacher-Collins syndrome
treadmill
    scaler t.
    t. test
    t. testing
treatment
    active t.
    aftercare t.
    Allen t.
    antimicrobial t.
    Brehmer t.
    carbon dioxide laser t.
    causal t.
    conservative t.
    dietetic t.
    empiric t.
    expectant t.
    Fab AV t.
    gold t.

    hyperbaric oxygen t.
    infrared t.
    isoserum t.
    life-sustaining t.
    light t.
    meal-related t.
    medical t.
    microwave diathermy t.
    Nauheim t.
    palliative t.
    Paul t.
    pharmacologic t.
    t. plan
    preventive t.
    prophylactic t.
    t. protocol
    Prussian blue t.
    psoralen ultraviolet A-range t.
     (PUVA)
    t. refusal
    Schott t.
    shortwave t.
    solar t.
    symptomatic t.
    Tallerman t.
    thymus t.
    Weir Mitchell t.
    Yeo t.
treatment-related emergency
tree
    biliary t.
Trélat stool
trematode infection
trematodiasis
tremens
    delirium t. (DT)
tremor
    action t.
    arsenic t.
    coarse t.
    essential t.
    flapping t.
    intention t.
    pill-rolling t.
    postural t.
    primary writing t.
    rest t.
    resting t.
tremulous
tremulousness
trench fever
Trendelenburg position

NOTES

Trental
trephination
  sinus t.
trephine
Treponema
  T. pallidum
  T. pallidum immobilization test
treponemal test
treponematosis
  nonvenereal t.
treponemiasis
trepopnea
Tresilian sign
tretinoin gel
TRF
  thyrotropin-releasing factor
TRH
  thyrotropin-releasing hormone
triad
  Andersen t.
  Basedow t.
  Beck t.
  Charcot t.
  disease t.
  Falta t.
  female athlete t.
  Hutchinson t.
  Kartagener t.
  Merseburg t.
  Osler t.
  Saint t.
  Virchow t.
  Whipple t.
triaditis
triage
trial
  BENESTENT Study Group T.
  CARE t.
  Cholesterol and Recurrent Events t.
  European/Australian Stroke
    Prevention in Reversible
    Ischaemia T. (ESPRIT)
  MULTIFIT t.
  PROGRESS t.
  randomized t.
triamcinolone acetonide
Triaminic
triamterene
triangle
  cardiohepatic t.
  color t.
  crural t.
  Garland t.
  Grocco t.
  Kiesselbach t.
  paravertebral t.
triatriatum
  cor t.
Triavil

triazolam
tribade
triceps reflex
trichalgia
trichiasis
Trichinella
trichinelliasis
trichinellosis
trichiniasis
trichinosis
trichinous polymyositis
trichloroacetaldehyde
trichobezoar
trichocephaliasis
Trichocephalus
trichomonad
Trichomonas
  T. hominis
  T. vaginalis
trichomoniasis
trichophytid
trichophytin
trichophytobezoar
Trichophyton
  T. mentagrophytes
  T. rubrum
trichorrhexis nodosa
trichotillomania
trichuriasis
Trichuris
tricuspid
  t. atresia
  t. regurgitation
  t. valve
  t. valve disease
Tri-Cyclen
  Ortho T.-C.
tricyclic
  anticholingeric t.
  t. antidepressant (TCA)
Tridesilon cream
trifascicular
trifid
trifluoperazine
trifluorinated corticosteroid
trigeminal neuralgia
trigeminy
trigger
  t. point (TP)
  t. point injection (TPI)
  t. spot
triglyceride (TG)
trigone
  retromolar t.
trigonitis
trigonum
  os t.
trihydroxy bile acid

trihydroxyestrin
triiodothyronine (T$_3$)
    resin t. (RT$_3$)
    resin sponge uptake of t.
    serum t.
    total t.
    t. toxicosis
    t. uptake test
Trilafon
Tri-Levlen
Trilisate
trimeclizine
trimethoprim
trimethoprim-sulfamethoxazole
Trimox
Trimpex
Trinalin
Tri-Norinyl
Trinsicon
triolein-T
triolet
    bruit de t.
triorthocresyl phosphate polyneuritis
triose-phosphate isomerase deficiency
  anemia
triphasic diabetes insipidus
Triphasil
5′-triphosphate
    inosine 5-t. (ITP)
Tripier amputation
triple
    t. quartan
    t. symptom complex
tripsis
triptan
triquetrum
trisalicylate
    choline magnesium t.
trismus
trisomy 20 syndrome
Tritec
tritiated water
tritici
    farina t.
Trivora
Trizivir
trochanteric bursitis
trochanter roll
troche
    Mycelex t.
trochlea
troglitazone Sankyo study

Troisier
    T. ganglion
    T. node
    T. sign
    T. syndrome
Troisier-Hanot-Chauffard syndrome
Trombicula
    T. akamushi
    T. deliensis
trombiculiasis
tromethamine
    ketorolac t.
trophedema
trophoblastic
    t. neoplasm
    t. thyrotoxicosis
trophozoite
tropica
    frambesia t.
    myositis purulenta t.
tropical
    t. anemia
    t. bubo
    t. diarrhea
    macrocytic anemia t.
    t. measles
    t. medicine
    t. myositis
    t. pulmonary eosinophilia
    t. pyomyositis
    t. splenomegaly
    t. splenomegaly syndrome
    t. sprue
    t. stomatitis
    t. typhus
tropicum
    granuloma t.
tropism
troponin
    cardiac-specific t.
    t. I
    t. I test
    t. T
trough of dosage
trousers
    medical antishock t. (MAST)
Trousseau
    T. phenomenon
    T. sign
    T. syndrome
trovafloxacin
trovafloxacin-alatrofloxacin

T

NOTES

TRP
   tubular reabsorption phosphate
true
   t. dwarfism
   t. reactive hypoglycemia
   t. thirst
truncal
truncate
truncation
truncus arteriosus
Trusopt
Trypanosoma
trypanosome fever
trypanosomiasis
   acute t.
   African t.
   American t.
   chronic t.
   Cruz t.
   East African t.
   Gambian t.
   Rhodesian t.
   South American t.
   West African t.
trypsinogen
tryptophan
tryptophanuria with dwarfism
T-score
tsetse fly
TSH
   thyroid-stimulating hormone
TSH-displacing antibody
TSH-RF
   thyroid-stimulating hormone-releasing
      factor
TSI
   thyroid-stimulating immunoglobulin
TSS
   toxic shock syndrome
TSST-1
   toxic shock syndrome toxin-1
tsutsugamushi
   t. disease
   t. fever
   Rickettsia t.
TTE
   transthoracic echocardiography
TTP
   thrombotic thrombocytopenic purpura
T-tube technique
TT virus
t-type calcium channel blocker
tubam
   per t.
tube
   Dobbhoff t.
   endotracheal t.
   t. enterostomy
   eustachian t.

fallopian t.
t. feeding
nasogastric t.
nasojejunal t.
NG t.
NJ t.
PEG t.
percutaneous endoscopic
   gastrostomy t.
Shiley tracheotomy t.
Wangensteen t.
tubercle
   Farre t.
tubercular
tuberculin skin test
tuberculitis
tuberculocele
tuberculoid myocarditis
tuberculosis (TB)
   active t.
   adult t.
   aerogenic t.
   anthracotic t.
   arrested t.
   attenuated t.
   atypical t.
   basal t.
   childhood type t.
   enteric t.
   extrapulmonary t.
   exudative t.
   generalized t.
   genitourinary t.
   healed t.
   inactive t.
   t. infection
   miliary t.
   multidrug-resistant t.
   Mycobacterium t. (MTB)
   open t.
   pericardial t.
   peritoneal t.
   pleural t.
   postprimary t.
   primary t.
   t. prophylaxis
   pulmonary t.
   reinfection t.
   renal t.
   secondary t.
tuberculostatic
tuberculotic
tuberculous
   t. arthritis
   t. bronchopneumonia
   t. enteritis
   t. lymphadenopathy
   t. meningitis
   t. myocarditis

t. peritonitis
t. pneumonia
tuberculum
t. thyroideum inferius
t. thyroideum superius
tuberoeruptive xanthoma
tuberosity
omental t.
tibial t.
tuberosum
xanthoma t.
tuberous
t. angioma
t. xanthoma
tuboovarian
tubotympanic
tubotympanum
tubular
t. adenoma
t. atrophy
t. necrosis
t. proteinuria
t. reabsorption
t. reabsorption phosphate (TRP)
t. respiration
tubule
seminiferous t.
tubulointerstitial disease
tubulointestinal disease
TUEVP
transurethral electrovaporization of prostate
TUG
timed up and go
total urinary gonadotropin
TUG test
Tuinal
TUIP
transurethral incision of prostate
tularemia
glandular t.
oculoglandular t.
pulmonary t.
pulmonic t.
typhoidal t.
tularemic pneumonia
tularensis
t. agglutinin
Pasteurella t.

TULIP
transurethral ultrasound-guided laser-induced prostatectomy
TULIP study
tumefaction
tumescence
nocturnal penile t. (NPT)
tumor
adrenocorticotropic hormone-secreting t.
AIDS-related t.
t. angiogenesis factor (TAF)
brain t.
t. burden
Burkitt t.
cardiac t.
t. cell
central nervous system t.
chest wall t.
deoxycorticosterone-producing t.
desmoid t.
endocrine t.
esophageal t.
estrogen receptor-positive t.
fungating t.
germ cell t.
Grawitz t.
growth hormone-secreting pituitary t.
hematologic t.
hepatic t.
t. humoral syndrome
Hürthle cell t.
hypervascular t.
hypopharyngeal t.
hypothalamic t.
inherited cardiac t.
intestinal t.
t. invasion
islet cell t.
t. lysis syndrome
t. marker
metastatic brain t.
metastatic cardiac t.
mixed-tissue t.
mucinous t.
müllerian mixed t.
t. necrosis factor
t. necrosis factor inhibitor
t., necrosis, metastasis (TNM)
neuroendocrine t.
t., node, metastasis staging

NOTES

tumor *(continued)*
    nonislet cell t.
    nonresponsive t.
    oropharyngeal t.
    Pancoast t.
    pancreatic t.
    paranasal sinus t.
    pineal t.
    pituitary t.
    polypeptide-secreting t.
    primary benign cardiac t.
    primary cardiac t.
    primary malignant cardiac t.
    prolactin-secreting pituitary t.
    radiocurable t.
    radioresistant t.
    radiosensitive t.
    t. registry
    renin-secreting t.
    responsive t.
    salivary gland t.
    sellar t.
    serous t.
    silent t.
    sinus t.
    solid t.
    spinal t.
    vasoactive intestinal polypeptide t.
    (VIPoma)
    Wilms t.
    Zollinger-Ellison t.
tumorigenesis
tumor-induced osteomalacia
tumor-infiltrating lymphocyte (TILS)
TUNA
    transurethral needle ablation
tunable dye laser
tunica, pl. **tunicae**
    t. albuginea
tuning fork test
tunnel
    t. anemia
    t. disease
    tarsal t.
Tuohy needle
TUR
    transurethral resection
turbinate
    nasal t.
Turcot syndrome
turgor
turista
turkey gobbler neck
Turner
    T. mosaic
    T. sign
    T. syndrome
turnover
    bone t.

TURP
    transurethral resection of prostate
turpentine enema
Tuss-Delay
tussigenic
Tussionex
Tussi-Organidin
tussive
    t. fremitus
    t. syncope
Tuss-Ornade
TWAR
    Taiwan acute respiratory
    TWAR titer
T wave
T-wave abnormality
twice a day [L. *bis in die*] (b.i.d., bis in die)
twin
    dizygotic t.
    monozygotic t.
twisting
twitching
    fascicular t.
two-dimensional
    t.-d. echocardiogram
    t.-d. transthoracic echocardiography
two-envelope glycoprotein
two-point discrimination
tylectomy
Tylenol
    Extra-Strength T.
    T. No. 3
tyloma
tylosis
Tylox
tympanal
tympania
tympanic
    t. membrane (TM)
    t. resonance
    t. temperature
tympanicity
tympanism
tympanites
    false t.
tympanitic
    t. abdomen
    t. membrane
    t. resonance
tympanitis
tympanogram
tympanous
tympanum
tympany
    Skoda t.
type
    buffalo t.
    t. 1, 2 diabetes

t. 1, 2 diabetes mellitus
t. 1–7 glycogenosis
t. II, III, IV, VI, VII glycogen
storage disease
Landouzy t.
t. IH mucopolysaccharidosis
t. IS mucopolysaccharidosis
t. II mucopolysaccharidosis
t. III mucopolysaccharidosis
t. IVA mucopolysaccharidosis
t. IVB mucopolysaccharidosis
t. V mucopolysaccharidosis
t. VI mucopolysaccharidosis
t. VII mucopolysaccharidosis
Pepper t.
Runeberg t.
senile dementia of Alzheimer t.
(SDAT)

typhi
Rickettsia t.
Salmonella t.

typhimurium
Salmonella enterica subsp. *t.*

typhinia
typhlitis
typhoid
abdominal t.
ambulatory t.
apyretic t.
bilious t.
t. cholera
t. fever
latent t.
t. pellagra
t. pleurisy
t. pneumonia
provocation t.
walking t.

typhoidal tularemia
typhoides
icterus t.

typhomania

typhosa
Salmonella t.

typhous
typhus
Australian tick t.
endemic t.
epidemic t.
European t.
exanthematous t.
t. fever
flea-borne t.
Indian tick t.
louse-borne t.
Manchurian t.
Mexican t.
mite t.
mite-born t.
t. mitior
murine t.
North Queensland tick t.
prison fever t.
Queensland tick t.
recrudescent t.
São Paulo t.
scrub t.
shop t.
Siberian tick t.
tick t.
tropical t.
urban t.

typing
tissue t.

tyramine
tyremesis
tyrosinemia
tyrosinosis
tyrosis
Tzanck
T. cell
T. smear
T. test

NOTES

T

UA
　　urinalysis
ubiquitous
UC
　　ulcerative colitis
UES
　　upper esophageal sphincter
UFC
　　urinary free cortisol
UGI
　　upper gastrointestinal
UGIS
　　upper gastrointestinal series
ulcer
　　　　aphthous u.
　　　　Barrett u.
　　　　chiclero u.
　　　　corneal u.
　　　　Curling u.
　　　　cutaneous u.
　　　　decubitus u.
　　　　diabetic foot u.
　　　　duodenal u.
　　　　foot u.
　　　　infected pressure u.
　　　　ischemic u.
　　　　leg u.
　　　　malleolus stasis u.
　　　　Meleney chronic undermining u.
　　　　Palmer acid test for peptic u.
　　　　Parrot u.
　　　　peptic u.
　　　　perforated peptic u.
　　　　pressure u.
　　　　pyloric channel u.
　　　　rectal u.
　　　　rodent u.
　　　　serpiginous corneal u.
　　　　skin u.
　　　　solitary rectal u.
　　　　stasis u.
　　　　stercoral u.
　　　　Syriac u.
　　　　tonsillar u.
ulcera (*pl. of* ulcus)
ulcera penetrans
ulceration
　　　　bulb u.
　　　　corneal u.
ulcerative
　　　　u. colitis (UC)
　　　　u. disease
　　　　u. ileojejunitis
　　　　u. keratitis
　　　　u. proctocolitis

　　　　u. stomatitis
　　　　u. surface
ulcerogenic
ulceromembranous angina
ulcus, pl. **ulcera**
Ullrich-Turner syndrome
ulna
ulnar
　　　　u. gutter splint
　　　　u. nerve entrapment
ulnocarpal joint
ULQ
　　upper left quadrant
ultimate
Ultracet
ultradian
Ultralente
Ultram
Ultrase
ultrashortwave diathermy
ultrasonography
　　　　abdominal u.
　　　　carotid u.
　　　　endoscopic u.
　　　　renal u.
　　　　thyroid u.
ultrasound
　　　　abdominal u.
　　　　carotid u.
　　　　Doppler u.
　　　　gallbladder u.
　　　　pelvic u.
　　　　transcranial Doppler u.
Ultravate
ultraviolet radiation
Ulysses syndrome
umbilicus, pl. **umbilici**
unabated
Unasyn
**unbound thyroxine-binding globulin
　　(UTBG)**
unciform pancreas
uncinariasis
uncinate
uncompensated acidosis
uncompetitive inhibition
uncomplicated cystitis
unconjugated hyperbilirubinemia
unconsciousness
unconscious patient
underactivity
　　　　detrusor u.
underestimated
underlying disease
undermedicated

U

417

undernutrition
protein-energy u.
underwear
HipSaver protective u.
protective u.
Underwood disease
undiagnosed pleural effusion
undifferentiated
u. cell leukemia
u. connective tissue disease
u. large-cell carcinoma
u. type fever
Undritz anomaly
undulans
febris u.
undulant fever
undulating fever
unfractionated heparin
unguis, pl. **ungues**
incarnatio u.
unguium
tinea u.
ungula
Uni-Decon
Uni-Dur
unilateral
u. hyperhidrosis
u. leg edema
u. nasal obstruction
u. pneumonia
u. retroperitoneal fibrosis
u. salpingo-oophorectomy (USO)
u. weakness (UW)
unimodal
union
primary u.
secondary u.
uniparental
Uniphyl
unipolar
Unisom
unit
ambulatory care u. (ACU)
basic multicellular u. (BMU)
centimeter-gram-second u.
CGS u.
coronary care u. (CCU)
critical care u. (CCU)
intensive care u. (ICU)
intermediate medical care u.
 (IMCU)
International U. (IU)
medical intensive care u. (MICU)
MicroSpacer u.
million international u.'s (MIU)
motor u.
Somogyi u.'s
TENS u.

transcutaneous electrical nerve
 stimulation u.
united
U. Network for Organ Sharing
 (UNOS)
U. Seniors Health Council (USHC)
U. States Public Health Service
 (USPHS)
U. Way of America
Univasc
universal
u. infantilism
u. precautions
universalis
adiposis u.
calcinosis u.
unknown
u. cause
u. primary site
unmask
unmyelinated
Unna boot
UNOS
United Network for Organ Sharing
unplanned pregnancy
unresectable
unresolved pneumonia
unsanitary
Unschuld sign
unstable
u. angina
u. hemoglobin hemolytic anemia
unsustained effort
untreatable
"up and go" screen
upper
u. airway disease
u. airway obstruction
u. bound estimate
u. esophageal sphincter (UES)
u. extremity thrombosis
u. eyelid
u. gastrointestinal (UGI)
u. gastrointestinal biopsy
u. gastrointestinal bleeding
u. gastrointestinal endoscopy
u. gastrointestinal series (UGIS)
u. GI
u. left quadrant (ULQ)
u. motor neuron
u. pole of kidney
u. respiratory infection (URI)
u. respiratory tract
u. respiratory tract infection
u. right quadrant (URQ)
u. urinary tract obstruction
upset stomach
UPT
urine pregnancy test

uptake
    24-hour RAI u.
    peak oxygen u.
    radioactive iodine u.
    radioiodine u. (RIU)
    resin sponge u.
    resin triiodothyronine u.
    RT$_3$ u.
    T3 resin u.
UR
    urinary
urachal
uracil
urate nephropathy
Urbach-Wiethe disease
urban typhus
urea
    u. frost
    u. kinetics
    u. nitrogen
urealyticum
    Mycoplasma u.
    Ureaplasma u.
Ureaplasma urealyticum
urease
Urecholine
ureidopenicillin
urelcosis
uremia
uremic
    u. acidosis
    u. amaurosis
    u. amblyopia
    u. bleeding
    u. breath
    u. colitis
    u. osteodystrophy
    u. pneumonia
    u. polyneuropathy
    u. stomatitis
    u. toxin
ureteral
    u. bowel syndrome
    u. colic
    u. duplication
    u. ectopy
ureter cancer
ureterectasia
ureteric vesical junction obstruction
ureterocele
ureterolithiasis

ureteroneocystostomy
ureteropathy
ureteropelvic
ureterorenal reflux
ureterovesical
    u. junction (UVJ)
    u. junction obstruction
urethra
    hypospadiac u.
urethral
    u. closure pressure
    u. diverticulum
    u. fever
    u. obstruction/incompetence
    u. pressure profilometry
    u. suppository
    u. valve
urethritica
    arthritis u.
urethritis
    gonococcal u.
    gouty u.
    herpetic u.
    senile u.
urethrocele
urethrooculosynovial syndrome
urethropexy
    laparoscopic retropubic u.
urethrotrigonitis
urethrovesical
URF
    uterine relaxing factor
urge incontinence
urgency
    hypertensive u.
    urinary u.
urgent
    u. care
    u. care clinic
URI
    upper respiratory infection
uric acid stone
uricemia
uricosuria
uricosuric drug
uridine diphosphate-glucuronosyltransferase
uridrosis crystallina
Urimar-T
urinalysis (UA)
    clean-catch u.

U

NOTES

urinalysis *(continued)*
    screening u.
    u. showed trace protein
urinary (UR)
    u. antimuscarinic
    u. antiseptic
    u. bladder
    u. catheter
    u. concentration
    u. continence
    u. crystal
    u. fever
    u. free cortisol (UFC)
    u. incontinence
    u. retention
    u. schistosomiasis
    u. tract
    u. tract cancer
    u. tract infection (UTI)
    u. tract infection and pregnancy
    u. tract obstruction
    u. urgency
urine
    clean-catch u.
    u. concentration
    u. dipstick
    u. flowmetry
    u. flow rate
    u. for 5-HIAA
    honey u.
    incontinence of u.
    u. ketone
    maple syrup u.
    u. osmolality
    u. oxalate
    postprostate massage u.
    u. pregnancy test (UPT)
    u. reflux
    u. tandem ICON
    u. test
    u. volume
Urised
Urispas
uroanthelone
urobilinemia
urobilin icterus
urobilinogen
urobilinogenemia
urobilinuria
Urocit-K
urocrisia
urocrisis
urodynamic
    u. study
    u. test
    u. testing
    video u.'s
uroenterone
uroflowmetry

urogastrone
urogonadotropin
urogram
urography
    excretory u.
urogynecology
urolithiasis
urology
uropathy
    microobstructive u.
uroporphyrin synthetase
urosepsis
    catheter-associated u.
urothelial tract
urotoxicity
URQ
    upper right quadrant
ursodeoxycholic acid
ursodiol
urticaria
    acute u.
    cholinergic u.
    cold u.
    febrile u.
    solar u.
urticarial fever
USA
    Catholic Charities USA (CCUSA)
use
    caffeine u.
    chronic steroid u.
USHC
    United Seniors Health Council
USO
    unilateral salpingo-oophorectomy
USPHS
    United States Public Health Service
ustilaginism
usual interstitial pneumonia
UTBG
    unbound thyroxine-binding globulin
uteri (*pl. of* uterus)
uterine
    u. bleeding
    u. cancer
    u. colic
    u. corpus malignancy
    u. disease
    u. fibroid
    u. myonecrosis
    u. prolapse
    u. relaxing factor (URF)
uteroglobin-adducin
uterovesical
uterque
    oculus u. (OU)
uterus, pl. **uteri**
    cervix uteri

UTI
    urinary tract infection
utilization reviewer
utricle
uveitis
      hypopyon u.
uveoencephalitic syndrome
uveomeningitis
UVJ
    ureterovesical junction
      UVJ obstruction
uvula, pl. **uvuli**

uvulectomy
UW
    unilateral weakness
U wave
Uzbekistan hemorrhagic fever

NOTES

U

VA
Department of Veterans Affairs
vaccination (*See also* vaccine)
smallpox v.
vaccine (*See also* vaccination)
acellular pertussis v.
AN-1792 v.
bacille Calmette-Guérin v.
bacillus Calmette-Guérin v.
BCG v.
Calmette-Guérin v.
Haemophilus influenzae v.
Havrix v.
hepatitis A v.
hepatitis B v.
influenza v.
Japanese encephalitis v.
Lyme disease v.
measles and rubella v.
meningococcal conjugate v.
meningococcal polysaccharide v.
MR v.
mumps v.
pneumococcal-CRM197 conjugate v.
pneumococcal polysaccharide v.
pneumonia v.
poliomyelitis v.
polysaccharide v.
rubella v.
Streptococcus pneumoniae v.
vaccinia-rabies glycoprotein v.
23-valent pneumococcal v.
varicella v.
varicella-zoster virus v.
vaccinia
v. gangrenosa
v. virus
vaccinia-rabies glycoprotein vaccine
vacuolar nephrosis
vacuole
vacuolization phenomenon
vacuum
v. constriction device
v. joint phenomenon
vagally mediated
vagina cancer
vaginal
v. birth after cesarean section
(VBAC)
v. bleeding
v. cone
v. cream
v. discharge
v. erosion
v. introitus

v. lesion
v. lubricant
v. ring
v. speculum
v. stenosis
vaginalis
Trichomonas v.
vaginismus
vaginitis
atrophic v.
vaginosis
bacterial v. (BV)
cytolytic v.
Vagisil
vagotomy
vagovagal
valacyclovir
valerian root
valetudinarian
valetudinarianism
valga
coxa v.
valgus
genu v.
hallux v.
validity
valine acid
Valisone
Valium
vallecula, pl. **valleculae**
valley
v. fever
lily of the v.
valproate
sodium v.
valproic acid
Valrelease
Valsalva
V. maneuver
sinus of V.
valsartan
Valsuani disease
Valtrex
value
anthropometric v.
baseline v.
homing v.
2-hour postchallenge v.
negative predictive v.
positive predictive v.
predictive v.
valve
aortic v.
bicuspid aortic v.
Bjork-Shiley v.

V

valve *(continued)*
    cardiac v.
    heart v.
    mechanical heart v.
    mitral v.
    porcine v.
    posterior urethral v.
    v. prolapse
    prosthetic heart v.
    pulmonic v.
    v. replacement
    St. Jude prosthetic v.
    tricuspid v.
    urethral v.
valvular
    v. heart disease
    v. heart disease in pregnancy
    v. insufficiency
    v. perforation
    v. regurgitation
    v. stenosis
valvuloplasty
    percutaneous balloon aortic v.
valvulotomy
    mitral v.
van
    v. Buren sound
    v. Heuven anatomical classification
    v. Heuven anatomical classification
        of diabetic retinopathy
vanadium
vanadiumism
Vancenase
Vanceril inhaler
vancomycin
vancomycin-resistant *Enterococcus* **(VRE)**
vanishing
    v. lung
    v. lung syndrome
Vantin
VAP
    ventilator-associated pneumonia
Vaqta
variability
variable
variant
variation
    seasonal v.
variceal
    v. bleeding
    v. hemorrhage
    v. ligation
varicella vaccine
varicella-zoster
    v.-z. virus
    v.-z. virus vaccine
varices (*pl. of* varix)
varicocele
varicose vein

variegated
variegate porphyria
Varilux lens
variocele
variola
    v. benigna
    v. hemorrhagica
    v. major
    v. maligna
    v. miliaris
    v. minor
    v. pemphigosa
    v. sine eruptione
    v. vera
    v. verrucosa
variolar
variolation
variolic
varioliform
varioliformis
    pityriasis lichenoides et v.
variolization
varioloid
variolosa
    orchitis v.
    purpura v.
variolous
Varivax
varix, pl. **varices**
    esophageal v.
    gastric v.
    ileal v.
varum
    genu v.
varus
    adductus primus v.
    metatabus primus v.
vasa vasorum
vascula (*pl. of* vasculum)
vascular
    v. biology
    v. catheter
    v. defect
    v. dementia
    v. headache
    v. hemophilia
    v. hepatic disease
    v. hypertension
    v. hypotension
    v. lesion
    v. medicine
    v. parkinsonism
    v. purpura
    v. rings anomaly
    v. septal defect (VSD)
vascularization
vasculature
    pulmonary v.

vasculitis
cutaneous v.
granulomatous v.
leukocytoclastic v.
necrotizing v.
small-vessel v.
systemic rheumatoid v.
vasculocardiac
v. syndrome
v. syndrome of hyperserotonemia
vasculopathy
coronary allograft v.
vasculum, pl. **vascula**
v. aberrans
vas deferens
Vaseretic
vasoactive
v. agent
v. intestinal polypeptide (VIP)
v. intestinal polypeptide tumor
(VIPoma)
Vasocon-A
vasoconstriction
hypoxic pulmonary v.
pulmonary alveolar hypoxic v.
(PAHVC)
v. thrombus formation
vasodepression
vasodepressor syncope
Vasodilan
vasodilatation
vasodilating nitric oxide
vasodilation
vasodilator
direct-acting v.
oral v.
parenteral v.
vasodilatory shock
vasoganglion
vasomotor
v. angina
v. symptom
v. tone
vasomotoricity
vasoneuropathy
vasoocclusive pain crisis
vasopeptidase inhibitor
vasopressin (VP)
arginine v. (AVP)
8-lysine v.
vasopressin-resistant diabetes
vasopressor

vasoreactivity
vasorum
vasa v.
vasospasm
cerebral v.
cold-induced v.
coronary v.
Vasosulf
Vasotec
vasotocin
vasotrophic
vasovagal syncope
vastus
Vater
ampulla of V.
V. papilla
VBAC
vaginal birth after cesarean section
V-Cillin K
VD
venereal disease
VDRL
Venereal Disease Research Laboratory
vector
frontal plane v.
vectorcardiography
VEDA
Vestibular Disorders Association
Veetids
vegan diet
vegetans
pemphigus v.
vegetarian diet
vegetarianism
vegetation
cardiac v.
vegetatious clot
veiled puff
Veillonella
vein
basilic v.
Boyd communicating perforation v.
brachiocephalic v.
Cockett communicating
perforating v.
pial v.
portal v.
pulmonary v. (Ppv)
subclavian v.
v. thrombosis
varicose v.
Velban

V

NOTES

Velcro rale
velocity
    conduction v.
    contractile v.
velopharyngeal
Velpeau deformity
VEN
    venlafaxine
vena, pl. venae
    v. cava
venenata
    stomatitis v.
venenation
venerea
    lues v.
venereal
    v. bubo
    v. disease (VD)
    V. Disease Research Laboratory
      (VDRL)
    v. lymphogranuloma
venereum
    lymphogranuloma v.
    malum v.
Venezuelan equine encephalitis
venipuncture
venisection
venlafaxine (VEN)
venoclysis
venoconstriction
venodilation
venogram V
venography
    magnetic resonance v. (MRV)
venoocclusive
    v. disease
    v. disease of liver
venostasis
venosus
    sinus v.
venous
    v. claudication
    v. disease
    v. hyperemia
    v. hypertension
    v. insufficiency
    v. lake
    v. limb gangrene
    v. pressure
    v. stasis
    v. stasis change
    v. thromboembolism
    v. thrombosis
venovasodilatory shock
ventilation
    intermittent positive-pressure v.
      (IPPV)
    inverse ratio v.
    lung-protective pressure-targeted v.

    maximum voluntary v. (MVV)
    mechanical v.
    minute v.
    noninvasive positive pressure v.
    partial liquid v.
    pressure-support v.
ventilation/perfusion (V/Q)
    v. inequality
    v. lung scan
    v. mismatch
ventilator-associated
    v.-a. lung injury
    v.-a. pneumonia (VAP)
ventilator management
ventilatory
    v. control disorder
    v. failure
Ventolin
ventosa
    spina v.
ventral
    v. decubitus
    v. pallidum receptor
ventricle
    left v. (LV)
    right v. (RV)
ventricular
    v. arrhythmia
    v. asystole
    v. cardiomyopathy
    v. ectopic beat
    v. ectopy
    v. ependyma
    v. free wall rupture
    v. hypertrophy
    v. irritability
    left v. (LV)
    v. mechanoreceptor
    v. parasystole
    v. preexcitation
    v. premature beat (VPB)
    v. pseudoaneurysm
    v. rate
    right v. (RV)
    v. septal defect (VSD)
    v. septal rupture
    v. tachyarrhythmia
    v. tachycardia (V-tach)
ventriculogram
ventriculography
    left v.
    right v.
ventriculomegaly
ventriculoperitoneal shunt
ventriculophasic sinus arrhythmia
ventriculotomy
ventriculus, pl. ventriculi
    filtrum ventriculi
Venturi mask

vera
    melena v.
    polycythemia rubra v.
    rubra v.
    variola v.
verapamil
verbal
    v. fluency
    v. scale
Verelan
vergae
    cavum v.
verge
    anal v.
vermicular colic
verminous
    v. appendicitis
    v. ileus
Vermox
Verner-Morrison syndrome
Vernet
    V. paralysis
    V. syndrome
vernix
verruca, pl. **verrucae**
    v. peruana
    plana v.
    v. vulgaris
verruciform
verrucosa
    variola v.
verrucous
verruga peruana
Versed
versicolor
    depigmented rash of tinea v.
    pityriasis v.
    tinea v.
Verstraeten bruit
vertebra, pl. **vertebrae**
    H-shaped v.
vertebral
    v. body
    v. compression
    v. compression fracture
    v. foramina
    v. fracture
    v. osteomyelitis
vertebrobasilar
    v. insufficiency
    v. migraine
vertex, pl. **vertices**

vertiginous
vertigo
    abrupt attack of v.
    arteriosclerotic v.
    benign paroxysmal positional v.
     (BPPV)
    benign paroxysmal postural v.
    benign positional v. (BPV)
    cardiac v.
    cardiovascular v.
    disabling positional v.
    essential v.
    paroxysmal positional v.
    physiologic v.
    positional v.
    posttraumatic v.
    postural v.
    stomachal v.
    subjective v.
    vestibular v.
verumontanum
very
    v. high density lipoprotein (VHDL)
    v. low density lipoprotein (VLDL)
    v. low density lipoprotein-
     triglyceride (VLDL-TG)
vesical
vesicle
vesicoureteral reflux
vesicular
    v. breathing
    v. murmur
    v. rale
    v. resonance
    v. respiration
    v. rickettsiosis
    v. stomatitis
vesiculation
vesiculobronchial
vesiculocavernous respiration
vesiculopapular
vesiculoprostatitis
    compulsive v.
vesiculotubular
vesiculotympanic resonance
vesiculotympanitic resonance
vesnarinone
vessel
    conductance v.
    v. lumen
vestibular
    v. disease

NOTES

vestibular *(continued)*
 V. Disorders Association (VEDA)
 v. migraine
 v. neuronitis
 v. system
 v. test
 v. vertigo
vestibulitis
 chronic vulvar v.
vestibulocerebellar abnormality
vestibuloocular
vestibulospinal tract
vestibulotoxic drug
veteran
 V.'s Administration hospital
 Disabled American V.'s (DAV)
 V.'s Health Administration (VHA)
Vexol
VH
 viral hepatitis
VHA
 Veterans Health Administration
VHC
 Oxipor VHC
VHDL
 very high density lipoprotein
Viagra
vibex, pl. **vibices**
Vibramycin
Vibra-Tabs
vibration
 chest wall v.
 v. sense
vibratory tinnitus
Vibrio
 V. parahaemolyticus
 V. parahaemolyticus infection
 V. vulnificus
 V. vulnificus infection
vicarious menstruation
vicious circle
Vicodin
Vicon-C
Vicryl suture
victimization
video-assisted
videodisc
videofluoroscopic swallowing study
 (VSS)
videoscope
 Olympus v.
video urodynamics
Videx
view
 coned-down v.
 swimmer's v.
vigabatrin
villi (*pl. of* villus)
villoglandular

villonodular synovitis
villose
villous
 v. adenoma
 v. duct cancer
villus, pl. **villi**
VIN
 vulvar intraepithelial neoplasia
vinblastine
Vincent
 V. angina
 V. stomatitis
vincristine
Vinson syndrome
vinyl chloride
Vioform
Viokase
violaceous
violence
 domestic v.
 transgenerational v.
violet
 crystal v.
 Gard V.
Vioxx
VIP
 vasoactive intestinal polypeptide
VIPoma
 vasoactive intestinal polypeptide tumor
Vipond sign
viral
 v. airway hyperactivity
 v. arthritis
 v. conjunctivitis
 v. diarrhea
 v. dysentery
 v. encephalitis
 v. enteritis
 v. gastroenteritis
 v. genome
 v. hemorrhagic fever
 v. hepatitis (VH)
 v. hepatitis type A, B, C, E
 v. infection
 v. load
 v. meningitis
 v. pericarditis
 v. pneumonia
 v. resistance
 v. serology
 v. suppression
 v. thymidine kinase
 v. titer
Virchow
 V. angle
 V. triad
viremia
vires
virginal speculum

viricidal
viridans
    icterus v.
virile
virilism
    adrenal v.
    prosopopilary v.
virility
virilization
virilizing hyperplasia
virion
viripotent
virologic study
virologist
virology
    quantitative v.
virulence factor
virulent bubo
virus
    v. A, B, C hepatitis
    Andes v.
    attenuated mumps v.
    blood-borne v.
    Bolivian hemorrhagic fever v.
    Chandipura v.
    chronic Epstein-Barr v. (CEBV)
    croup-associated v. (CAV)
    cytomegalic inclusion v. (CMV)
    delta v.
    Ebola v.
    Epstein-Barr v. (EBV)
    Hanta v.
    v. hepatitis
    hepatitis A v. (HAV)
    hepatitis B v. (HBV)
    hepatitis C v. (HCV)
    hepatitis delta v.
    herpes simplex v. (HSV)
    herpes-type v. (HTV)
    herpes varicella-zoster v.
    herpes zoster v. (HZV)
    human immunodeficiency v. (HIV)
    human T-cell lymphotropic v.
      (HTLV)
    human T-cell lymphotropic v. III
      (HTLV-III)
    Jeryl-Lynn v.
    Lassa v.
    lymphadenopathy-associated v.
      (LAV)
    lymphotropic v.
    molluscum contagiosum v.

    nonenveloped v.
    Norwalk-like agent v.
    Oropouche v.
    parainfluenza v.
    pharyngoconjunctival fever v.
    respiratory syncytial v. (RSV)
    Rift Valley fever v.
    Rous-associated v. (RAV)
    Schwartz leukemia v.
    TT v.
    vaccinia v.
    varicella-zoster v.
viscera (*pl. of* viscus)
visceral
    v. angiitis
    v. hypersensitivity
    v. larva migrans
    v. leishmaniasis
    v. pain
visceralgia
visceromegaly
visceromotor, viscerimotor
visceroptosis
viscerosensory reflex
viscerotrophic
viscerotropic
viscidosis
Viscoheel cushion
vis conservatrix
viscosity
Visco Soles
viscosupplementation
viscous
    V. Xylocaine
viscus, pl. **viscera**
vision
    blurry v.
    impaired v.
    v. screen
visit
    ambulatory v.
visiting
    v. nurse
    V. Nurse Association of America
      (VNAA)
Vistaril
visual
    v. acuity
    v. analogue scale
    v. blurring
    v. disturbance

V

NOTES

visual (*continued*)
    v. field
    v. rehabilitation
visuospatial
    v. distortion
    v. functioning
    v. skill
Vitajet-3 needle-free injection system
vital
    v. capacity
    v. index
    v. sign
    v. statistics
Vitallium
vitam
    intra v.
vitamin
    v. A deficiency
    v. B_{12}
    v. B_{12} deficiency
    v. C test
    v. D deficiency
    v. deficiency
    v. D malabsorption
    v. D-resistant rickets
    v. E
    free radical-scavenging v.
    v. K deficiency
    v. K replacement
    v. supplement
vitiation
vitiligo
vitium
    v. conformationis
vitrectomy
    pars plana v.
vitreoretinal
    v. traction
vitreoretinopathy
    proliferative v. (PVR)
vitreous
vitro
    in v.
Vitron-C
Vivactil
Vivarin
vivax
    v. fever
    v. malaria
    Plasmodium v.
Vivelle
vividiffusion
vivo
    in v.
VLDL
    very low density lipoprotein
VLDL-TG
    very low density lipoprotein-triglyceride

VNAA
    Visiting Nurse Association of America
vocal
    v. cord
    v. cord paralysis
    v. fremitus
    v. resonance (VR)
Vogt-Spielmeyer disease
voice
    amphoric v.
    bronchial v.
    cavernous v.
    v. sound
voiding
volar wrist flexion crease
Volhard test
Volkmann contracture
Volmax
voltage
    QRS v.
Voltaren
volume
    cell v.
    v. depletion
    v. of distribution
    end-systolic v.
    forced expiratory v. (FEV)
    lung v.
    mean corpuscular v. (MCV)
    normal extracellular fluid v.
    v. overload
    postvoid residual v.
    v. regulation
    residual v. (RV)
    stroke v.
    tidal v.
    urine v.
voluntary hospital
volvulus
vomer
vomit
    Barcoo v.
    bilious v.
    black v.
    coffeeground v.
vomiting
    cerebral v.
    cyclic v.
    dry v.
    epidemic v.
    explosive v.
    fecal v.
    hysterical v.
    nausea and v. (N&V)
    periodic v.
    pernicious v.
    projectile v.
    psychogenic v.
    recurrent v.

retention v.
stercoraceous v.
vomition
vomiturition
vomitus
coffeeground v.
v. cruentes
v. marinus
v. matutinus
v. niger
von
v. Bekhterev-Strümpell spondylitis
v. Gierke disease
v. Graefe sign
v. Hippel-Lindau syndrome
v. Jaksch anemia
v. Mikulicz disease
v. Mikulicz syndrome
v. Recklinghausen disease
v. Recklinghausen neurofibromatosis
v. Willebrand disease
v. Willebrand factor
VoSol
vox choleraica
VP
vasopressin
VPB
ventricular premature beat
V/Q
ventilation/perfusion
V/Q scan
VR
vocal resonance
VRE
vancomycin-resistant *Enterococcus*

VSD
vascular septal defect
ventricular septal defect
V-sign rash
VSS
videofluoroscopic swallowing study
V-tach
ventricular tachycardia
vulcanite stomatitis
vulgaris
acne v.
pemphigus v.
Proteus v.
verruca v.
vulnificus
Vibrio v.
vulva, pl. **vulvae**
v. cancer
kraurosis v.
pruritus v.
vulval dystrophy
vulvar
v. dermatosis
v. intraepithelial neoplasia (VIN)
v. irritation
v. lesion
v. malignancy
v. pruritus
vulvovaginal candidiasis
vulvovaginitis
acute herpetic v.
bacterial v.
candidal v.
V1, V2 receptor
V wave

NOTES

V

w-3 polyunsaturated fatty acid
Waardenburg syndrome
waddling
waist circumference
wakefulness
wakening
    early w.
Waldenström
    W. hyperglobulinemic purpura
    W. macroglobulinemia
    W. syndrome
Waldeyer ring
walker
    wheeled w.
Walker syndrome
walk-in clinic
walking
    w. aid
    w. pneumonia
    w. typhoid
wall
    peptidoglycan rigid cell w.
Wallenberg
    W. stroke
    W. syndrome
Walthard islet
wandering pneumonia
Wangensteen tube
ward
warehousemen's itch
warfarin and aspirin
warm
    w. antibody autoimmune hemolytic
      anemia
    w. or cold stimulus
    W. and Form corset
warneri
    Staphylococcus w.
wart
    genital w.
    Peruvian w.
    plantar w.
Wartenberg
    W. disease
    W. neuralgia
wartpox
warty excrescence
Wassermann test
wasting
    muscle w.
    salt w.
    w. syndrome
    temporal muscle w.
water
    w. balance

w. bed
w. brash
w. canker
deuterated w.
w. diuresis
extracellular w.
w. intake
w. intoxication
intracellular w.
w. loss
tritiated w.
waterhammer pulse
Waterhouse-Friderichsen syndrome
Waterlow classification
watermelon stomach
watershed
Waterston shunt
Waters view x-ray
water-whistle sound
watery
    w. diarrhea, hypokalemia,
      achlorhydria (WDHA)
    w. diarrhea, hypokalemia,
      achlorhydria syndrome
wave
    A w.
    delta w.
    F w.
    fluid w.
    ST and T w.
    T w.
    U w.
    V w.
    X descent w.
    Y descent w.
waxy flexibility
WBC
    white blood cell
WCT
    wide-complex tachycardia
WDHA
    watery diarrhea, hypokalemia,
      achlorhydria
    WDHA syndrome
WDLL
    well-differentiated lymphocytic
      lymphoma
WDWN
    well-developed, well-nourished
weak flow rate
weakness
    muscle w.
    neuromuscular w.
    opponens w.
    pelvic floor w.

W

weakness *(continued)*
    transient w.
    unilateral w. (UW)
wean
weaning
wear-and-tear theory
weaver's cough
webbed neck
Weber-Christian
    W.-C. disease
    W.-C. syndrome
Weber test
Wechsler
    W. Adult Intelligence Scale-Revised
    W. Memory Scale (WMS)
wedge resection
WEE
    Western equine encephalitis
weekend hospital
weekly
    Prozac W.
Wegener
    W. disease
    W. granulomatosis
Wehdryl
weight
    w. bearing joint
    body w.
    w. cycling
    dry w.
    w. loss
weightbearing exercise
weight-for-frame size
Weil
    W. disease
    W. syndrome
Weil-Felix reaction
Weinstein syndrome
Weir
    W. Mitchell disease
    W. Mitchell treatment
weird
Welchol
welder's lung
well-being
Wellbutrin
well-developed, well-nourished (WDWN)
well-differentiated lymphocytic lymphoma (WDLL)
well-nourished
    w.-n. female (WNF)
    w.-n. man (WNM)
    well-developed, w.-n. (WDWN)
Well Spouse Foundation (WSF)
Wenckebach
    W. arrhythmia
    W. block

Werdnig-Hoffman
    W.-H. disease
    W.-H. paralysis
Werlhof
    W. disease
    W. syndrome
Wermer
    W. disease
    W. syndrome
Werner
    W. syndrome
    W. test
Wernicke
    W. aphasia
    W. disease
    W. encephalopathy
    W. syndrome
Wernicke-Korsakoff
    W.-K. encephalitis
    W.-K. psychosis
    W.-K. syndrome
Wertheim operation
Wesselsbron
    W. disease
    W. fever
west
    W. African fever
    W. African sleeping sickness
    W. African trypanosomiasis
    W. Indian smallpox
    W. Nile fever
Westcort
Westergren
    W. method
    W. sedimentation rate
western
    W. blot
    W. blot assay
    W. blot test
    W. equine encephalitis (WEE)
Westphal-Strümpell
    W.-S. disease
    W.-S. pseudosclerosis
wet
    w. age-related macular degeneration
    w. AMD
    w. lung
    w. nurse
    w. pack
    w. shock
wet-to-dry dressing
Wetzel grid
Wharton duct
wheal
wheat product antibody
wheeled walker
wheeze
    asthmatoid w.
    end-expiratory w.

expiratory w.
forced end-expiratory w.
inspiratory w.
wheezing
whiff
whiplash
Whipple
W. disease
W. operation
W. syndrome
W. triad
whipworm infection
whirlpool bath
whispered
w. bronchophony
w. pectoriloquy
whisper test
whistling rale
white
w. bile
w. blood cell (WBC)
w. blood cell count
w. clover
w. coat syndrome
w. matter
w. pneumonia
w. willow bark
white-coat
w.-c. hypertension
w.-c. normotension
whitepox
whitlow
herpetic w.
Whitman operation
Whitmore bacillus
WHO
World Health Organization
whole bowel irrigation
whoop
whooping cough
whorl
Widal
W. syndrome
W. test
Widal-Abrami syndrome
wide-complex tachycardia (WCT)
Wiedemann syndrome
Wigraine
Wilder
W. diet
W. sign
Wilkie disease

Wilkins disease
will
living w.
Willebrand
W. disease
W. factor
Willebrand-Jërgens syndrome
Williams
W. flexion
W. syndrome
Willis
W. antrum
circle of W.
W. disease
W. pancreas
willow bark
Wills anemia
Wilms tumor
Wilson
W. disease
W. nodule
window
aortopulmonary w.
Winkler disease
Winslow pancreas
Winterbottom sign
winter itch
wire
iridium w.
wiring
jaw w.
Wirsung duct
Wiskott-Aldrich syndrome
Wissler syndrome
withdrawal
alcohol w.
cocaine w.
drug w.
gradual w.
heroin w.
opioid w.
w. seizure
w. symptoms
w. syndrome
withholding
within normal limits (WNL)
Witts anemia
Wladimiroff-Mikulicz amputation
WMS
Wechsler Memory Scale
WNF
well-nourished female

NOTES

435

WNL
within normal limits
WNM
well-nourished man
Woillez disease
Wolff-Chaikoff
W.-C. block
W.-C. effect
wolffian duct
Wolff-Parkinson-White (WPW)
W.-P.-W. syndrome
Wolfram syndrome
Wolman
W. disease
W. xanthomatosis
women's medicine
wooden resonance
Woods
W. light
W. light examination
woolsorter's
w. disease
w. pneumonia
word
w. descriptor scale
W. Fluency Test
work
w. hardening
w. stabilization program
worker
National Association of
Social W.'s (NASW)
social w.
workup
staging w.
World Health Organization (WHO)

wormian bone
wort
St. John's w.
wound
w. culture
w. dressing
w. fever
w. infection
septic w.
subcutaneous w.
WPW
Wolff-Parkinson-White
wrap
Ace w.
Elastoplast w.
Wright
W. maneuver
W. peak flow
W. stain
W. syndrome
wrist
w. arthrocentesis
w. sign
wrist-drop
writhe
wrote memory
wry neck
WSF
Well Spouse Foundation
Wuchereria bancrofti **infection**
wuchereriasis
Wycillin IM
Wygesic
Wytensin

Xanax
xanomeline
xanthelasma
xanthene
xanthine stone
xanthinuria, xanthiuria
xanthinuric
xanthochromia
xanthofibroma
xanthogranulomatosis
xanthogranulomatous
xanthoma
    diabetic x.
    x. diabeticorum
    eruptive x.
    generalized plane x.
    palmar x.
    planar x.
    x. striatum palmare
    tendinous x.
    tendon x.
    tuberoeruptive x.
    x. tuberosum
    tuberous x.
xanthomatosis
    biliary x.
    cerebrotendinous x.
    chronic idiopathic x.
    familial hypercholesteremic x.
    Wolman x.
xanthosis
    x. diabetica
    x. diabeticorum
xanthurenic
    x. acid
    x. aciduria
xanthuria
X descent wave
Xenical
xenogeneic
xenon
    x. arc
    x. computed tomography

xerocytosis
xeroderma
    Kaposi x.
    x. pigmentosum
Xeroform
xerophagia
xerosis
xerostomia
xerotic dermatitis
xinafoate
    salmeterol x.
xiphisternal crunching sound
xiphoidalgia
xiphoiditis
xiphoid process
Xi-scan
XL
    Ditropan XL
    Glucotrol XL
    Lescol XL
    Procardia XL
    Toprol XL
X-linked
    X-l. cardiomyopathy
    X-l. disorder
    X-l. mental retardation
XO syndrome
XO/XY mosaicism
XR
    Effexor XR
x-ray
    x-r. anemia
    chest x-r. (CXR)
    sinus x-r.
    small bowel x-r.
    Waters view x-r.
XXY syndrome
xylene
Xylocaine
    Viscous X.
XYZ syndrome

X

yabapox
YAG
> yttrium, argon, garnet

Yangtze Valley fever
yaw
> mother y.

yawn
Y descent wave
year
> Setting Priorities for
> Retirement Y.'s (SPRY)

yeast
yellow
> y. atrophy
> y. atrophy of liver
> y. fever

yellow-brown serous ascites
Yeo treatment
Yergason sign
Yersinia
> *Y. enterocolitica*
> *Y. enterocolitica* infection
> *Y. pseudotuberculosis*

yersiniosis
> nonplague y.
> pseudotubercular y.

YMCA
> Young Men's Christian Association

Yocon
yoga
yohimbe
yohimbine
young
> maturity-onset diabetes of the y.
> (MODY)
> Y. Men's Christian Association
> (YMCA)
> Y. rule
> Y. syndrome
> Y. Women's Christian Association
> (YWCA)

yo-yo
> y.-y. dieting
> y.-y. syndrome

yttrium, argon, garnet (YAG)
YWCA
> Young Women's Christian Association

zafirlukast
Zagam
zalcitabine
zaleplon
zanamivir
Zantac
Zaroxolyn
Z-Bec
Zeasorb
Zecril
Zeis
    sebaceous gland of Z.
Zemuron
Zenker
    Z. diverticulum
    Z. fixative
zero stool since birth (ZSB)
Zestoretic
Zestril
Zetran
Ziac
zidovudine
Zieve syndrome
zileuton
Zimmerlin atrophy
Zinacef
zinc
    z. colic
    z. deficiency
    z. fume fever
Zincon
ziprasidone
Zithromax
Zocor
Zoladex
Zollinger-Ellison
    Z.-E. syndrome
    Z.-E. tumor
zolmitriptan
Zoloft
zolpidem
Zomax
zona, pl. zonae
    z. fasciculata
    z. glomerulosa
    z. reticularis

zonal
Zonalon
zonary
zone
    dependent z.
    Head z.
    z. of hyperalgesia
    large loop excision of transition z.
      (LLETZ)
    Looser z.
    prostate-specific antigen transition z.
      (PSA-TZ)
    secondary X z.
    transition z.
    transitional z.
ZORprin
zoster
    herpes z. (HZ)
    z. sine herpete
zosteriform
Zostrix
Zosyn
Zovirax
Z-Pak
Z-plasty
ZSB
    zero stool since birth
Z-tract injection
Zubrod scale
Zung Self-Rating Depression Scale
zwieback
Zyflo
zygapophysis
zygomycosis
    abdominopelvic z.
    cutaneous z.
    rhinocerebral z.
    thoracic z.
Zyloprim
zymolysis
zymosan
zymotic
    z. disease
    z. papilloma
Zyrtec
Zyrtec-D

Z

Appendix 1
Anatomical Illustrations

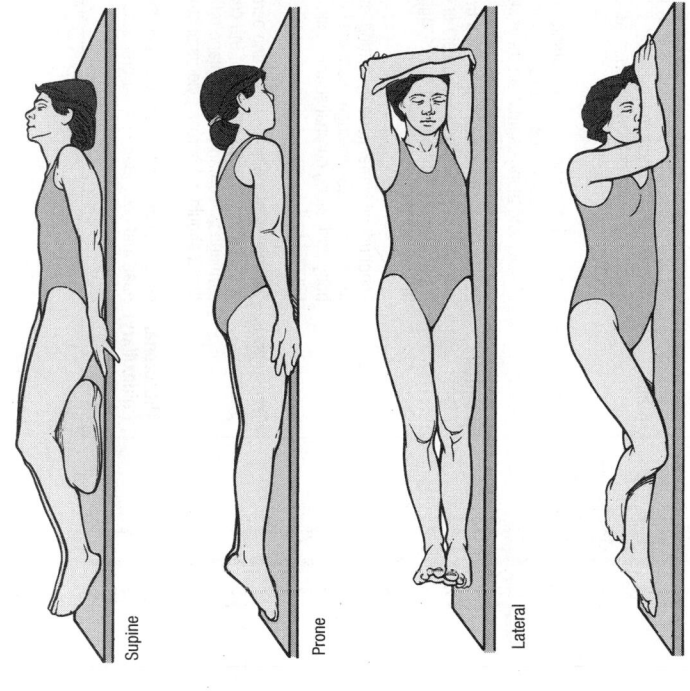

Supine

Prone

Lateral

Oblique

Figure 2. Patient positions.

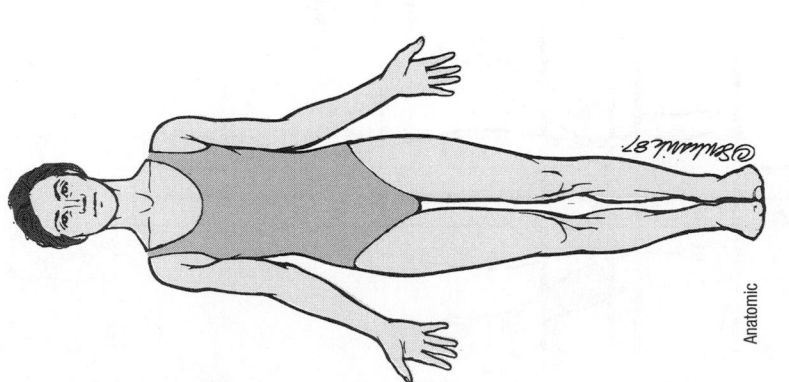

Anatomic

Figure 1. Patient position.

Figures 1–4, created by Mikki Senkarik, for *Stedman's Medical Dictionary, 27th Edition*, Baltimore, Lippincott Williams & Wilkins, 2000, B1–3, appear here with permission and courtesy of Lippincott Williams & Wilkins.

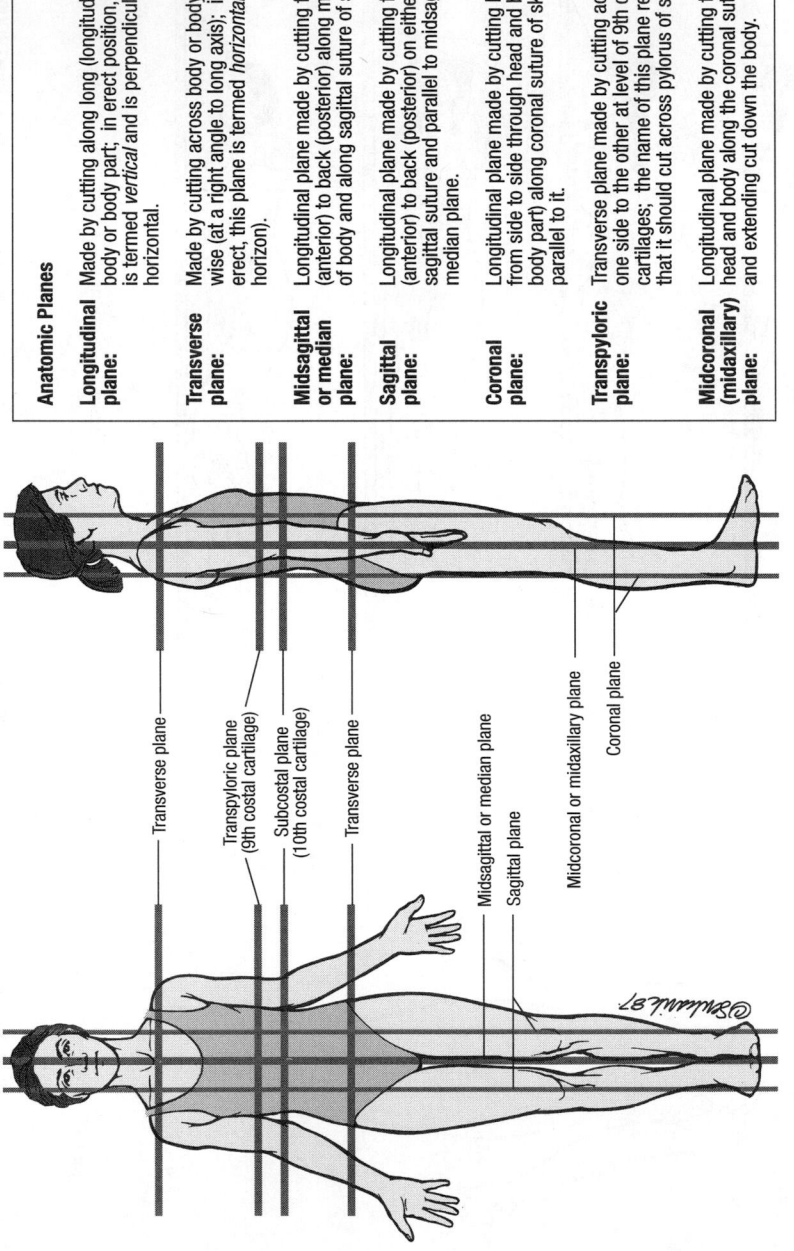

Figure 3. Terms of relationship. Anatomic planes.

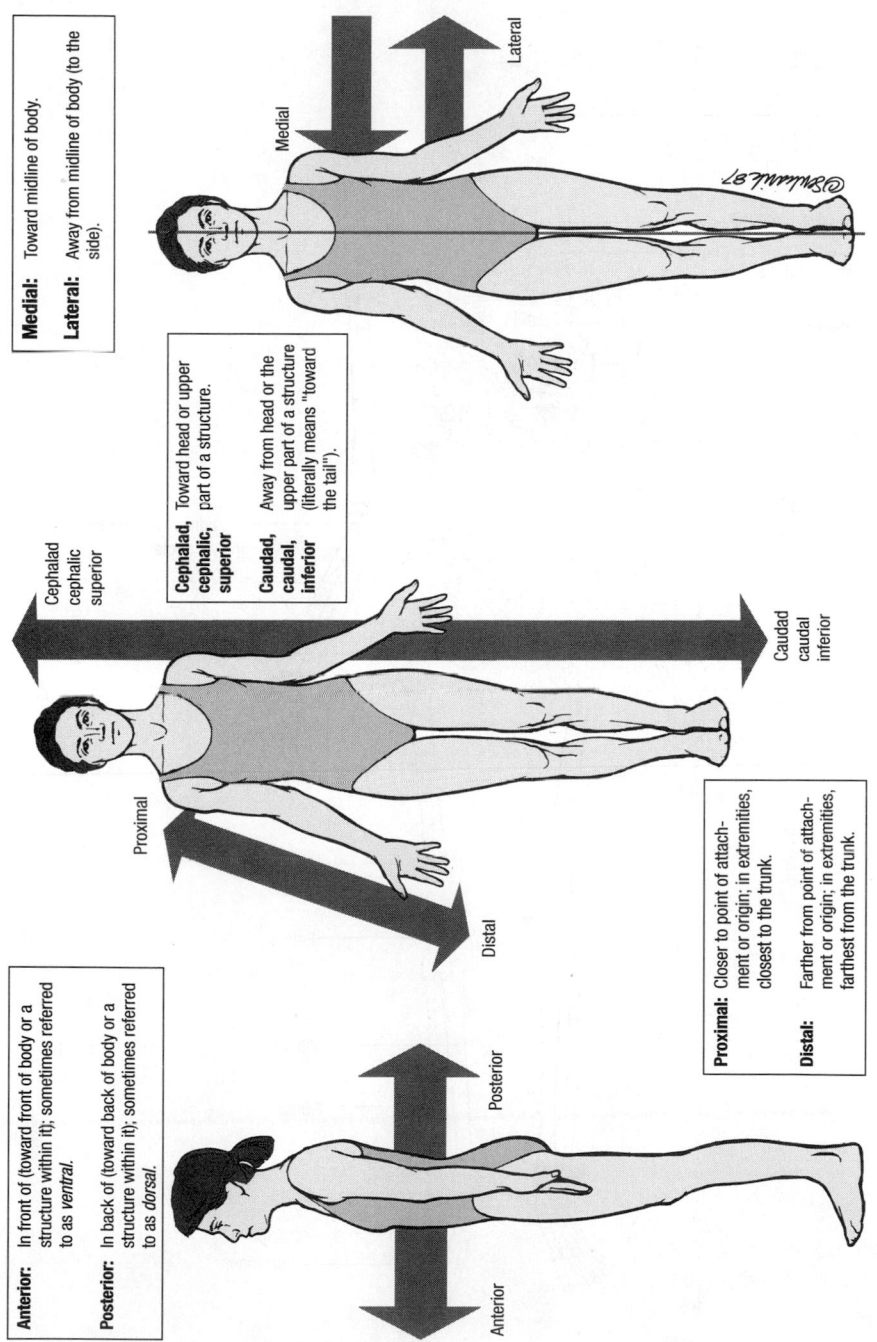

Medial: Toward midline of body.

Lateral: Away from midline of body (to the side).

Cephalad, cephalic, superior Toward head or upper part of a structure.

Caudad, caudal, inferior Away from head or the upper part of a structure (literally means "toward the tail").

Proximal: Closer to point of attachment or origin; in extremities, closest to the trunk.

Distal: Farther from point of attachment or origin; in extremities, farthest from the trunk.

Anterior: In front of (toward front of body or a structure within it); sometimes referred to as *ventral*.

Posterior: In back of (toward back of body or a structure within it); sometimes referred to as *dorsal*.

Figure 4. Terms of relationship. Body part terminology.

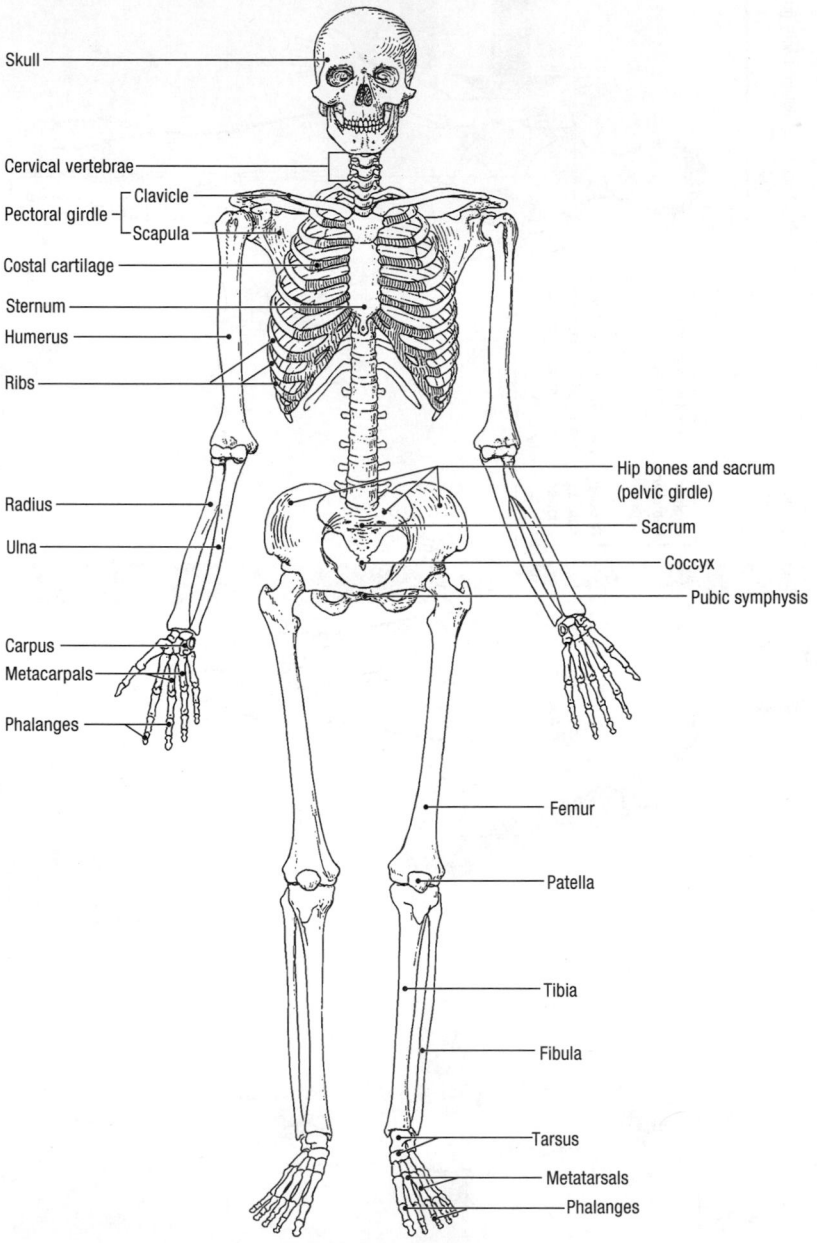

Skull

Cervical vertebrae

Pectoral girdle — [Clavicle
                  [Scapula

Costal cartilage

Sternum

Humerus

Ribs

Radius

Ulna

Carpus

Metacarpals

Phalanges

Hip bones and sacrum
(pelvic girdle)

Sacrum

Coccyx

Pubic symphysis

Femur

Patella

Tibia

Fibula

Tarsus

Metatarsals

Phalanges

Figure 5. Skeleton, adult, anterior view.

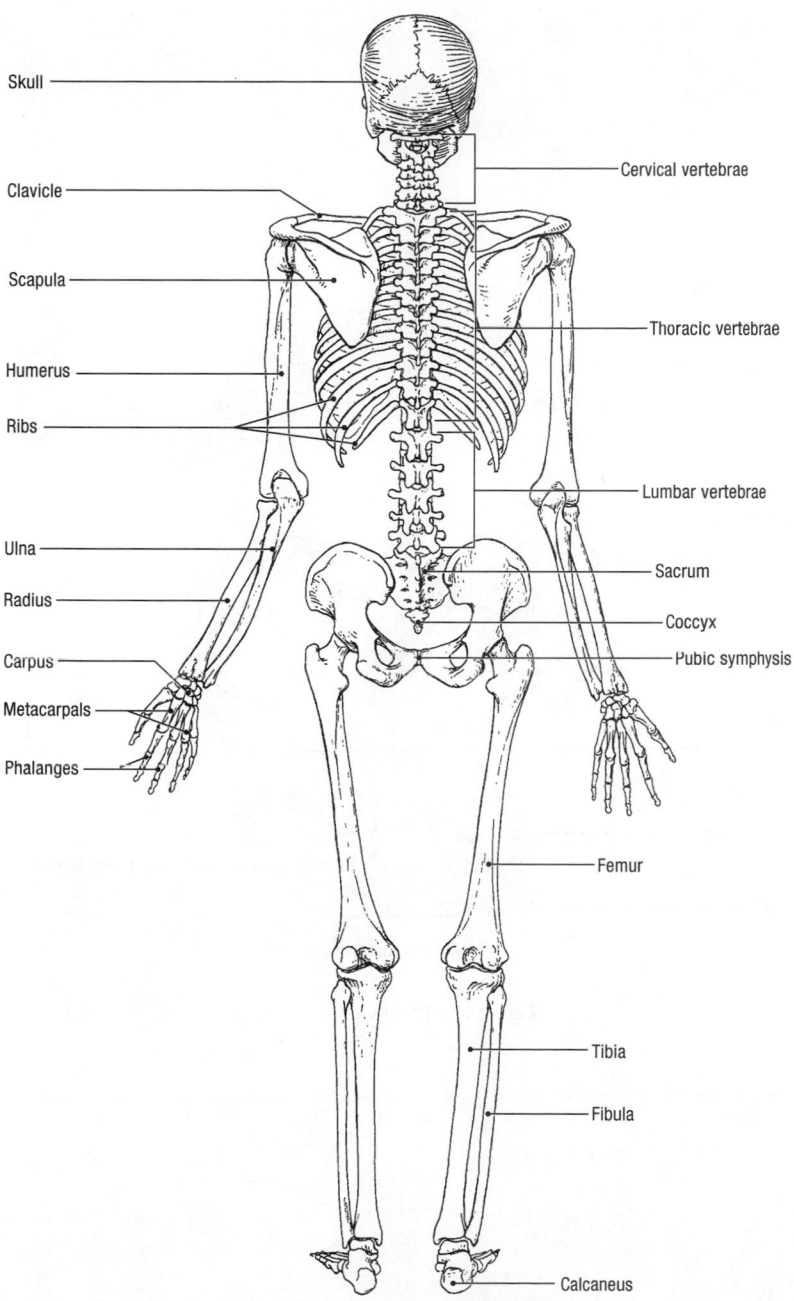

Skull

Clavicle

Scapula

Humerus

Ribs

Ulna

Radius

Carpus

Metacarpals

Phalanges

Cervical vertebrae

Thoracic vertebrae

Lumbar vertebrae

Sacrum

Coccyx

Pubic symphysis

Femur

Tibia

Fibula

Calcaneus

Figure 6. Skeleton, adult, posterior view.

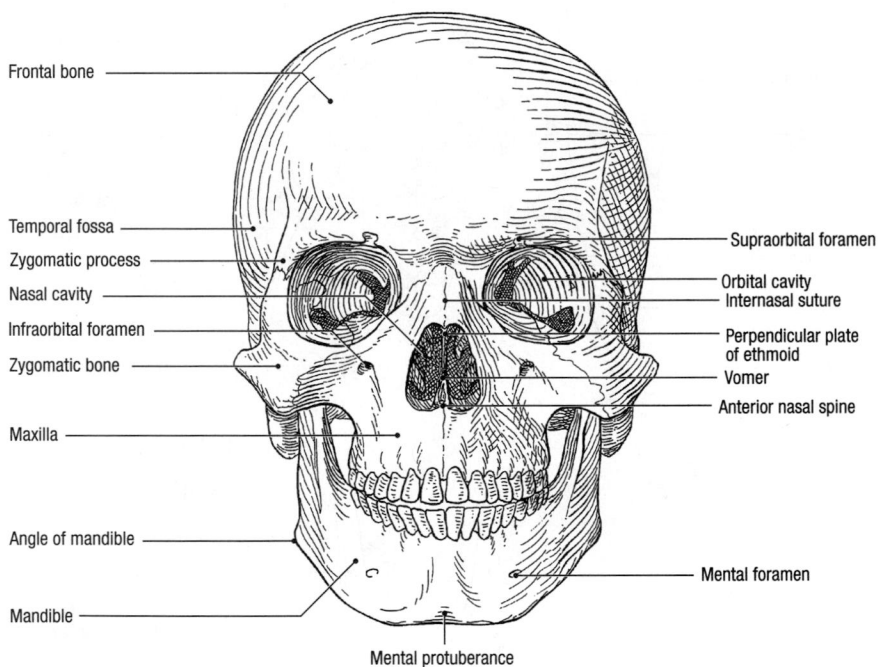

Figure 7. Front view of skull.

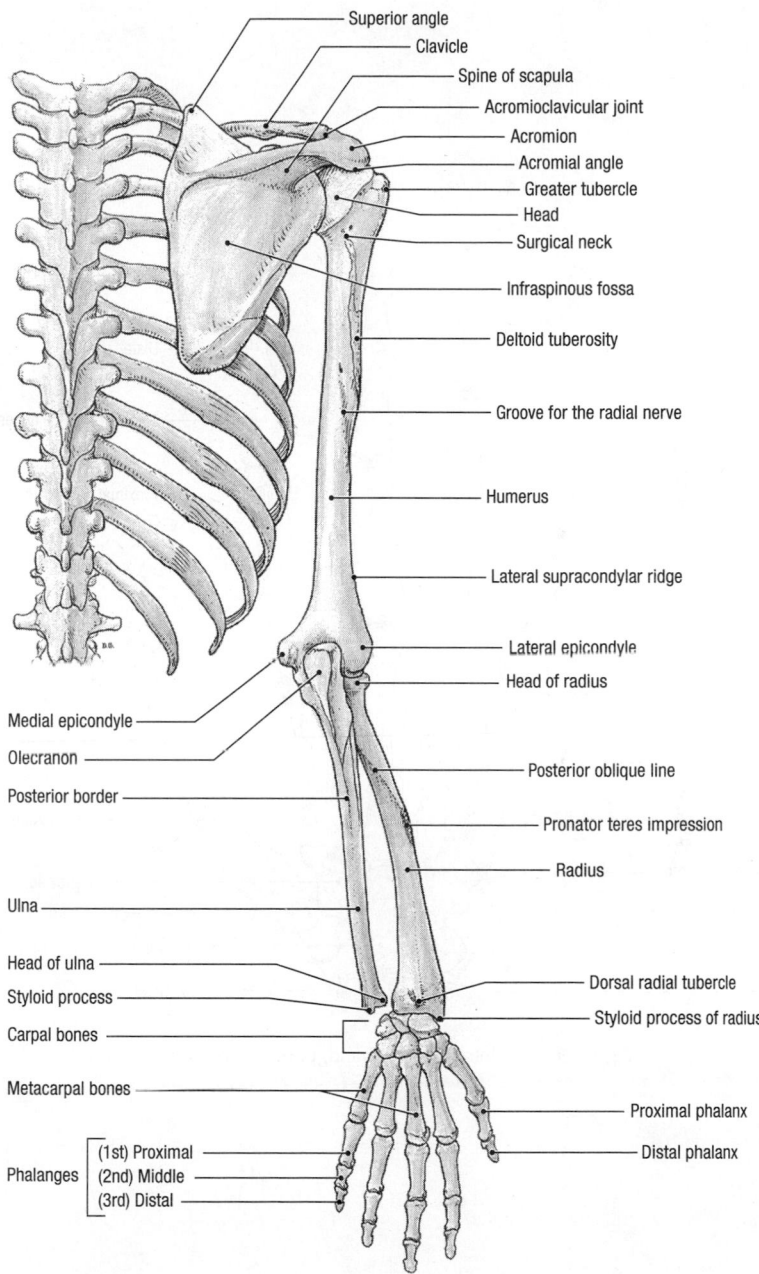

Superior angle
Clavicle
Spine of scapula
Acromioclavicular joint
Acromion
Acromial angle
Greater tubercle
Head
Surgical neck
Infraspinous fossa
Deltoid tuberosity
Groove for the radial nerve
Humerus
Lateral supracondylar ridge
Lateral epicondyle
Head of radius
Medial epicondyle
Olecranon
Posterior oblique line
Posterior border
Pronator teres impression
Radius
Ulna
Head of ulna
Dorsal radial tubercle
Styloid process
Styloid process of radius
Carpal bones
Metacarpal bones
Proximal phalanx
Distal phalanx
Phalanges (1st) Proximal
(2nd) Middle
(3rd) Distal

Figure 8. Bones of upper limb, posterior view.

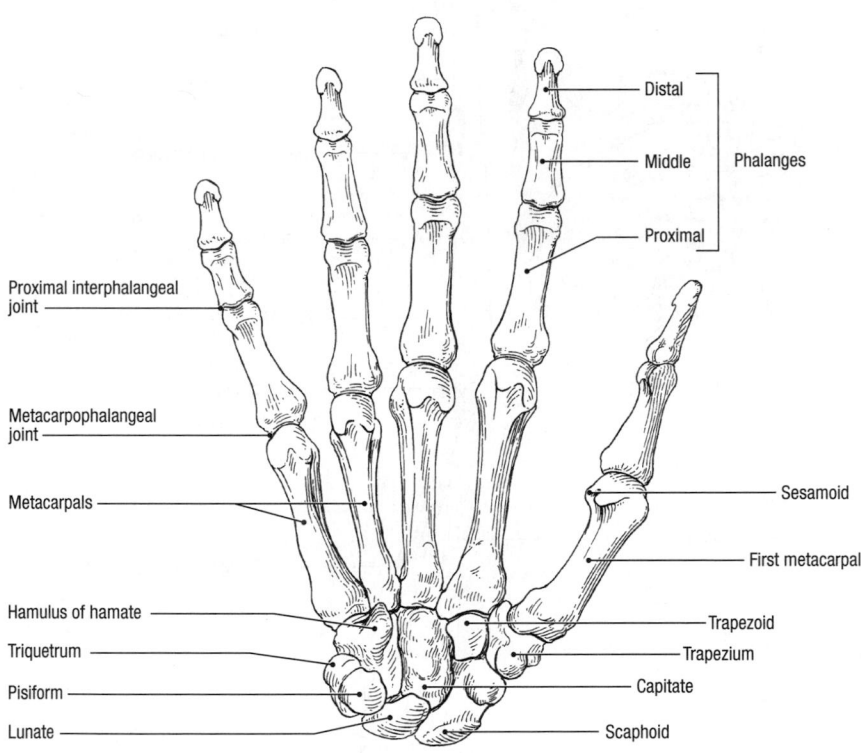

Figure 9. Skeleton of right hand, palmar (anterior) view.

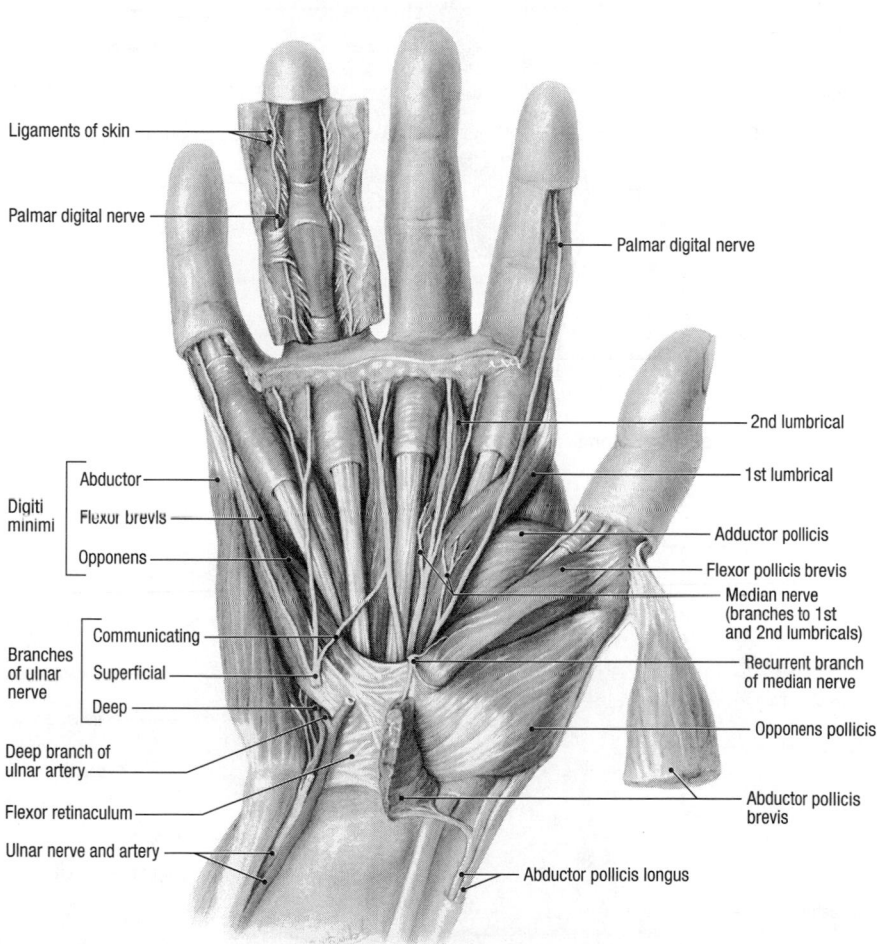

Ligaments of skin

Palmar digital nerve

Palmar digital nerve

2nd lumbrical

1st lumbrical

Digiti minimi
- Abductor
- Flexor brevis
- Opponens

Adductor pollicis

Flexor pollicis brevis

Median nerve (branches to 1st and 2nd lumbricals)

Branches of ulnar nerve
- Communicating
- Superficial
- Deep

Recurrent branch of median nerve

Opponens pollicis

Deep branch of ulnar artery

Flexor retinaculum

Ulnar nerve and artery

Abductor pollicis brevis

Abductor pollicis longus

Figure 10. Superficial dissection of palm, ulnar and median nerves, palmar (anterior) view.

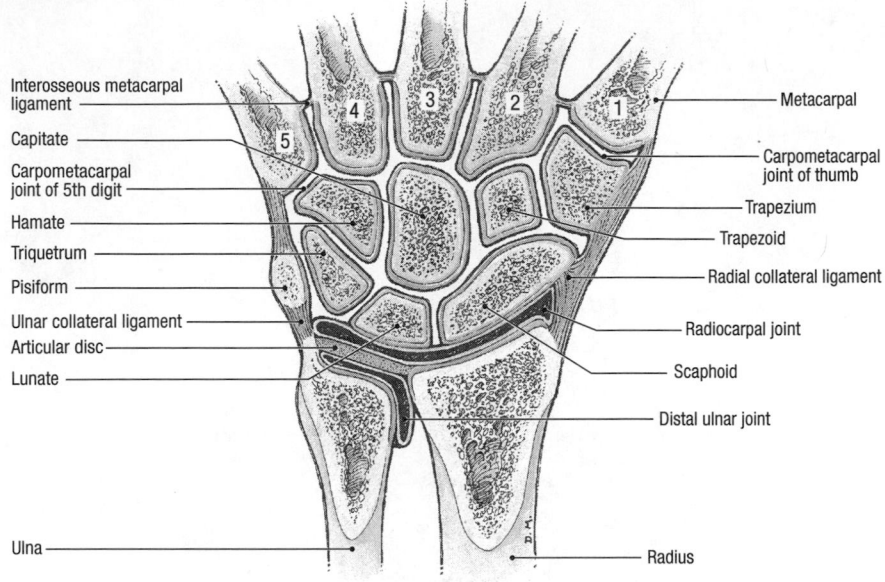

Interosseous metacarpal ligament

Capitate

Carpometacarpal joint of 5th digit

Hamate

Triquetrum

Pisiform

Ulnar collateral ligament

Articular disc

Lunate

Ulna

Metacarpal

Carpometacarpal joint of thumb

Trapezium

Trapezoid

Radial collateral ligament

Radiocarpal joint

Scaphoid

Distal ulnar joint

Radius

Figure 11. Coronal section of wrist and hand, palmar (anterior) view.

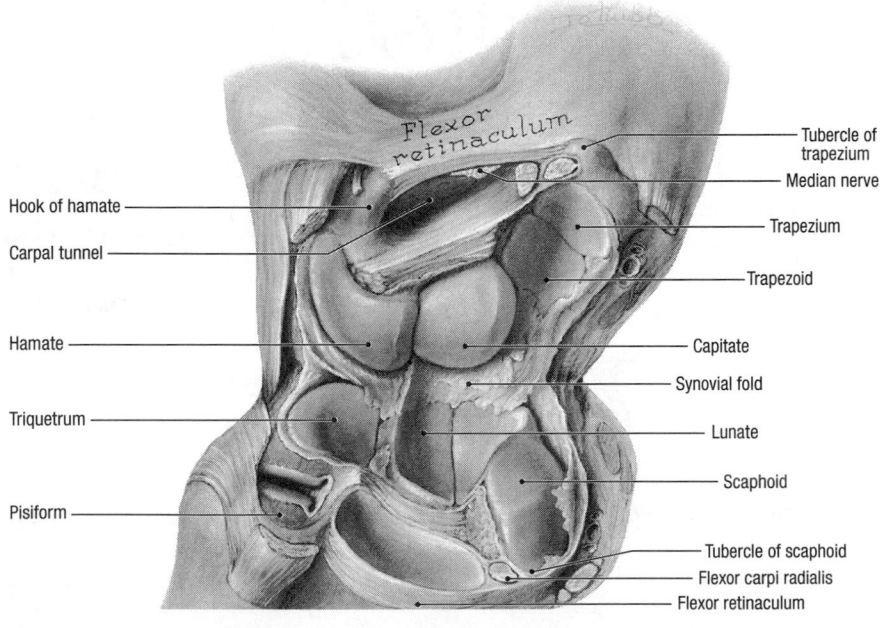

Flexor retinaculum

Hook of hamate

Carpal tunnel

Hamate

Triquetrum

Pisiform

Tubercle of trapezium

Median nerve

Trapezium

Trapezoid

Capitate

Synovial fold

Lunate

Scaphoid

Tubercle of scaphoid

Flexor carpi radialis

Flexor retinaculum

Figure 12. Surfaces of midcarpal (transverse carpal) joint, opened anteriorly.

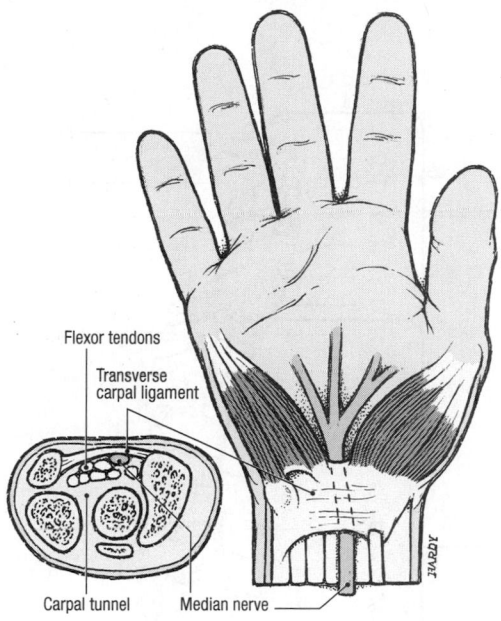

Figure 13. The carpal tunnel contains the median nerve and the flexor tendons of the fingers and thumb.

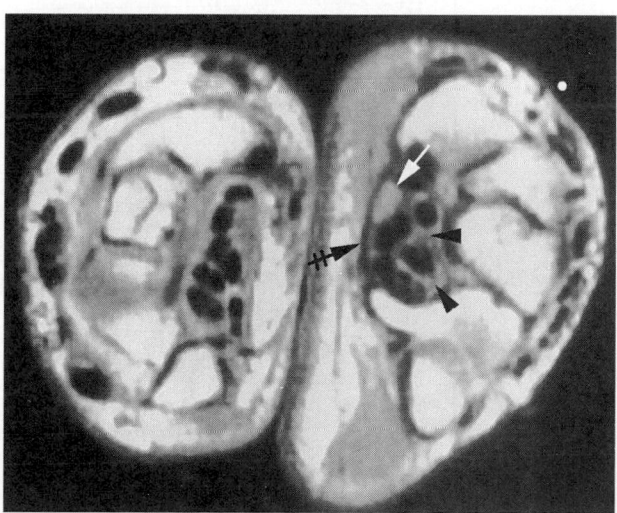

Figure 14. Carpal tunnel syndrome. MRI of both wrists. Swelling of the right median nerve (white arrow), increased fluid between flexor tendons within tunnel (black arrowheads), and slight bowing of the flexor retinaculum (crossed arrow). This image, from Brant WE & Helms CA, *Fundamentals of Diagnostic Radiology, 2nd Edition,* Baltimore, Williams & Wilkins, 1999, appears here with permission and courtesy of Lippincott Williams & Wilkins.

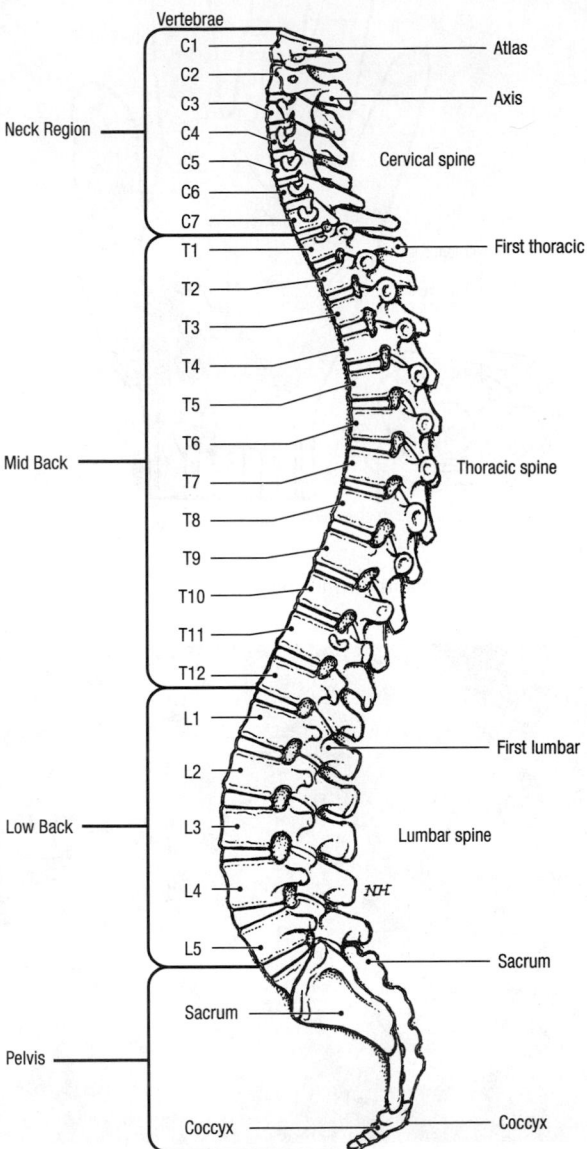

Figure 15. Vertebral column, lateral view.

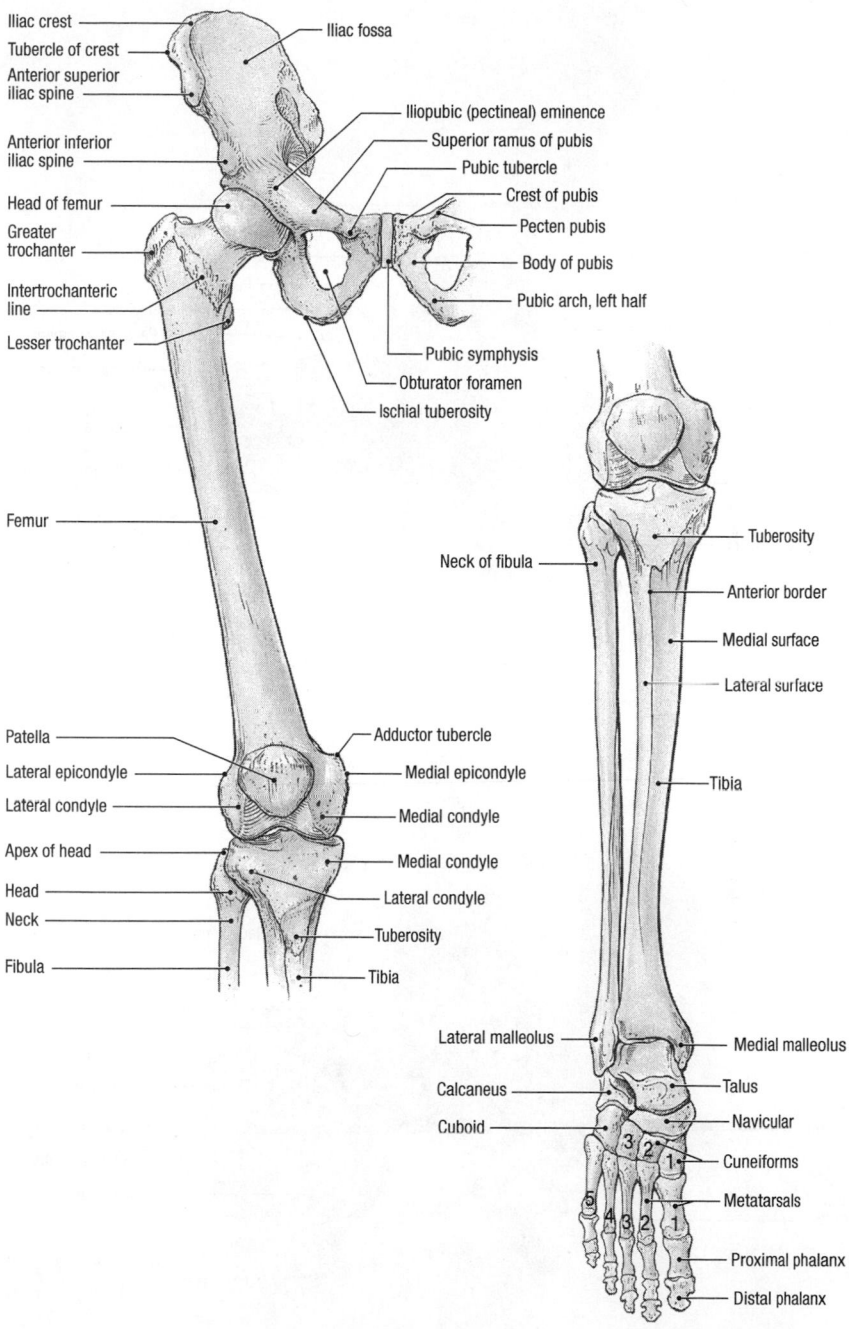

Figure 16. Bones of the lower limb, anterior view.

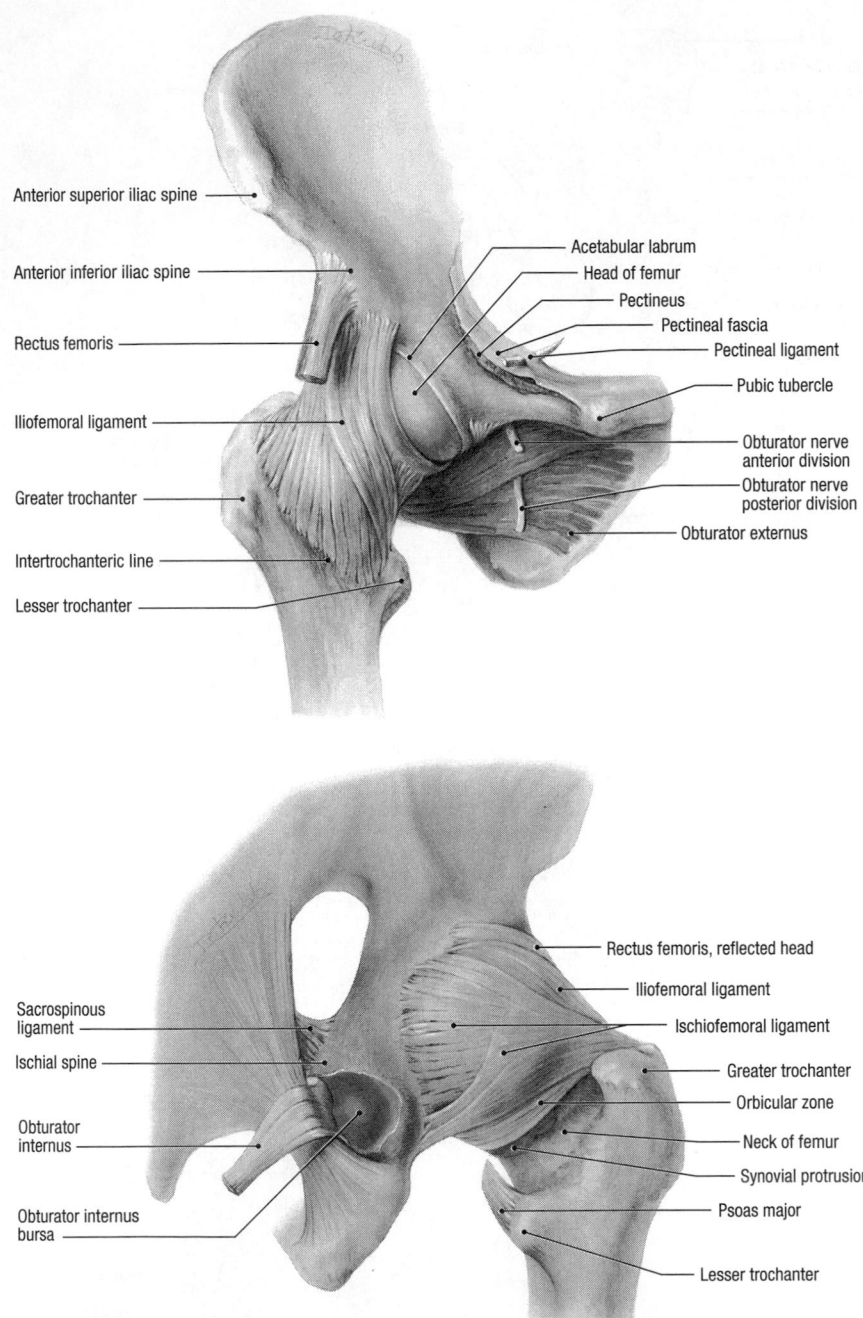

Anterior superior iliac spine

Anterior inferior iliac spine

Rectus femoris

Iliofemoral ligament

Greater trochanter

Intertrochanteric line

Lesser trochanter

Acetabular labrum

Head of femur

Pectineus

Pectineal fascia

Pectineal ligament

Pubic tubercle

Obturator nerve anterior division

Obturator nerve posterior division

Obturator externus

Sacrospinous ligament

Ischial spine

Obturator internus

Obturator internus bursa

Rectus femoris, reflected head

Iliofemoral ligament

Ischiofemoral ligament

Greater trochanter

Orbicular zone

Neck of femur

Synovial protrusion

Psoas major

Lesser trochanter

Figure 17. Hip joint. Anterior view (top), posterior view (bottom).

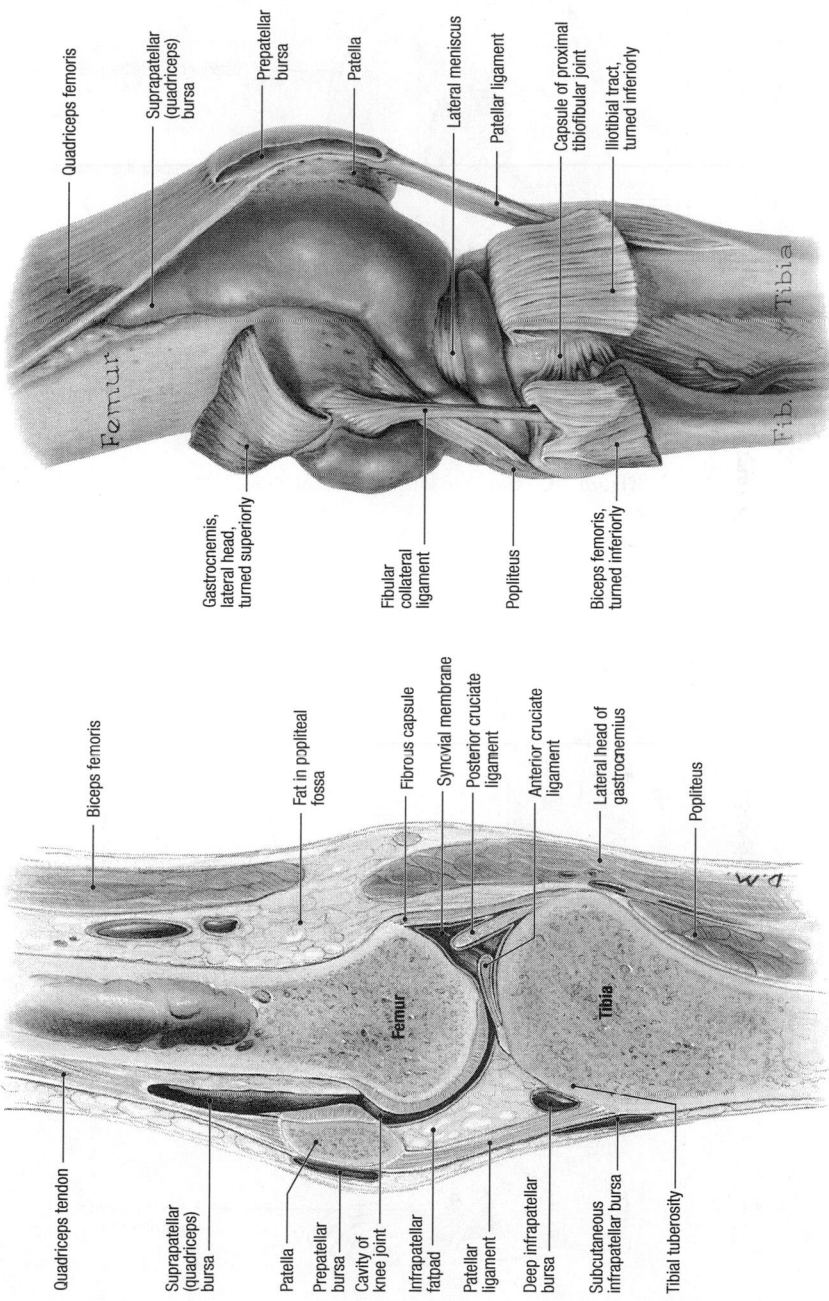

Quadriceps femoris

Suprapatellar (quadriceps) bursa

Prepatellar bursa

Patella

Lateral meniscus

Patellar ligament

Capsule of proximal tibiofibular joint

Iliotibial tract, turned inferiorly

Femur

Fib. Tibia

Gastrocnemius, lateral head, turned superiorly

Fibular collateral ligament

Popliteus

Biceps femoris, turned inferiorly

Figure 19.   Distended knee joint, lateral view.

Biceps femoris

Fat in popliteal fossa

Fibrous capsule

Synovial membrane

Posterior cruciate ligament

Anterior cruciate ligament

Lateral head of gastrocnemius

Popliteus

Femur

Tibia

p.m.

Quadriceps tendon

Suprapatellar (quadriceps) bursa

Patella

Prepatellar bursa

Cavity of knee joint

Infrapatellar fatpad

Patellar ligament

Deep infrapatellar bursa

Subcutaneous infrapatellar bursa

Tibial tuberosity

Figure 18.   Sagittal section of knee.

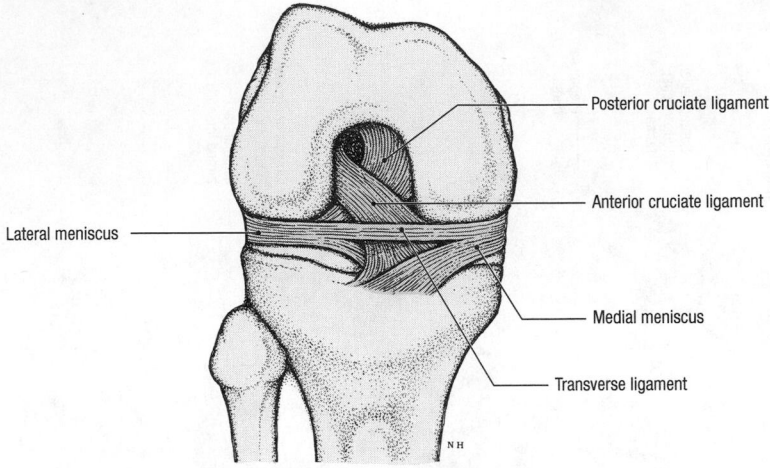

Figure 20. Cruciate ligaments of the knee.

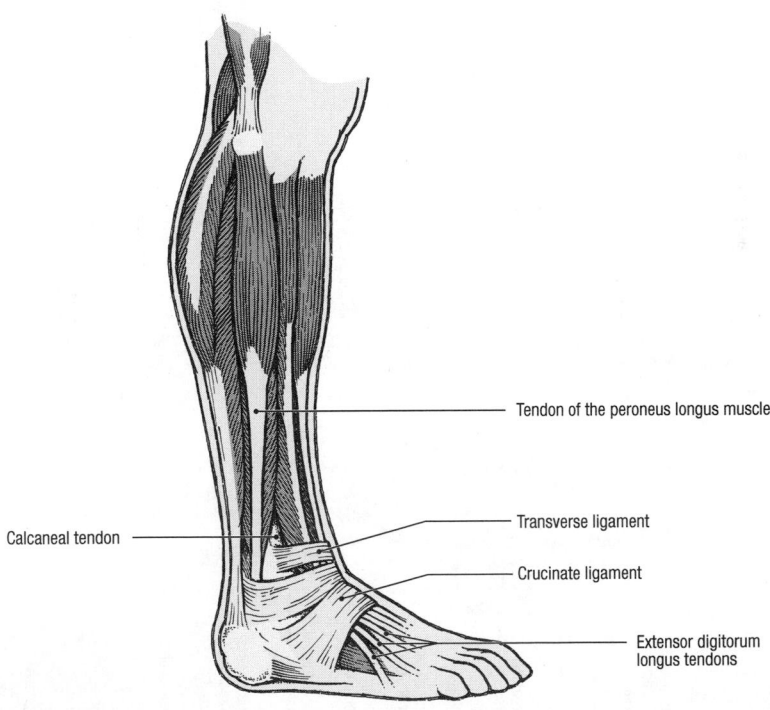

Figure 21. Tendons and ligaments of the lower leg, lateral view.

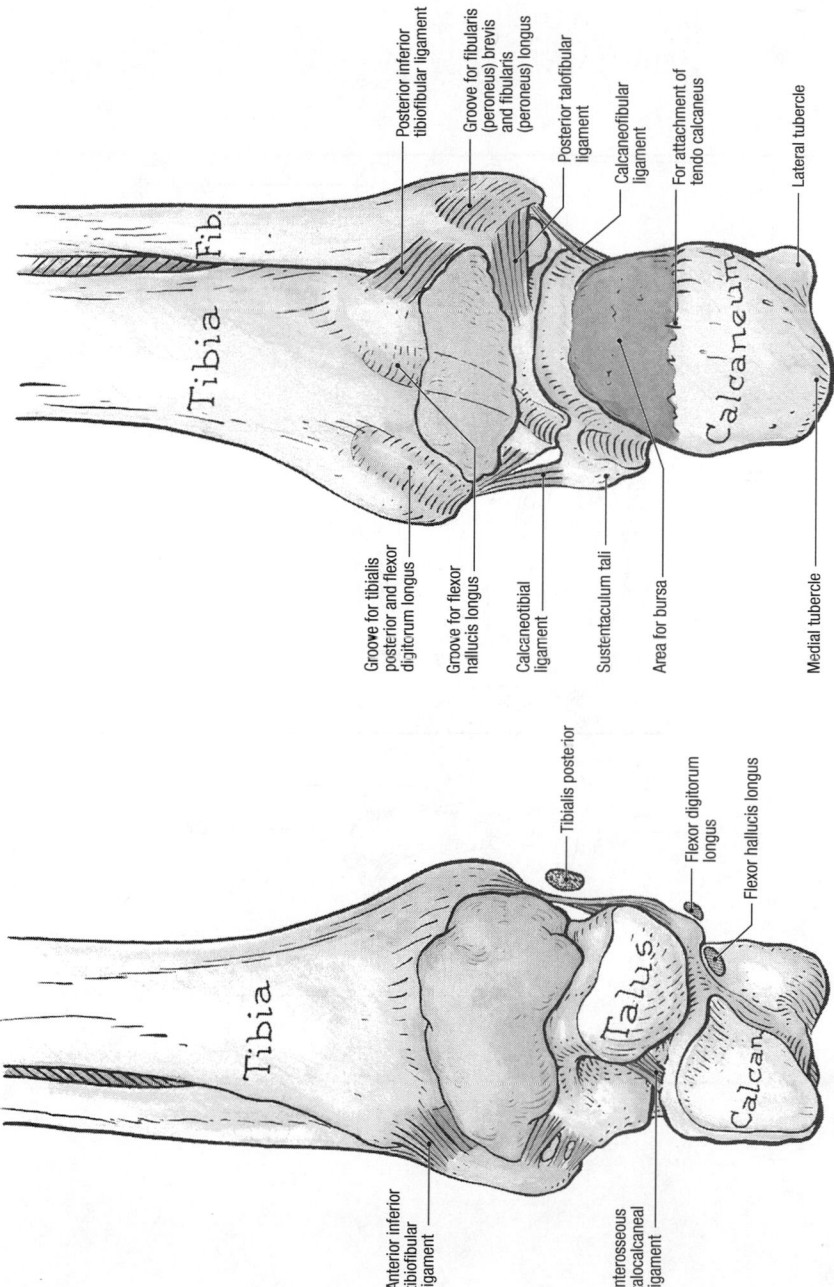

Figure 22. Distended ankle joint. Anterior view (left), posterior view (right).

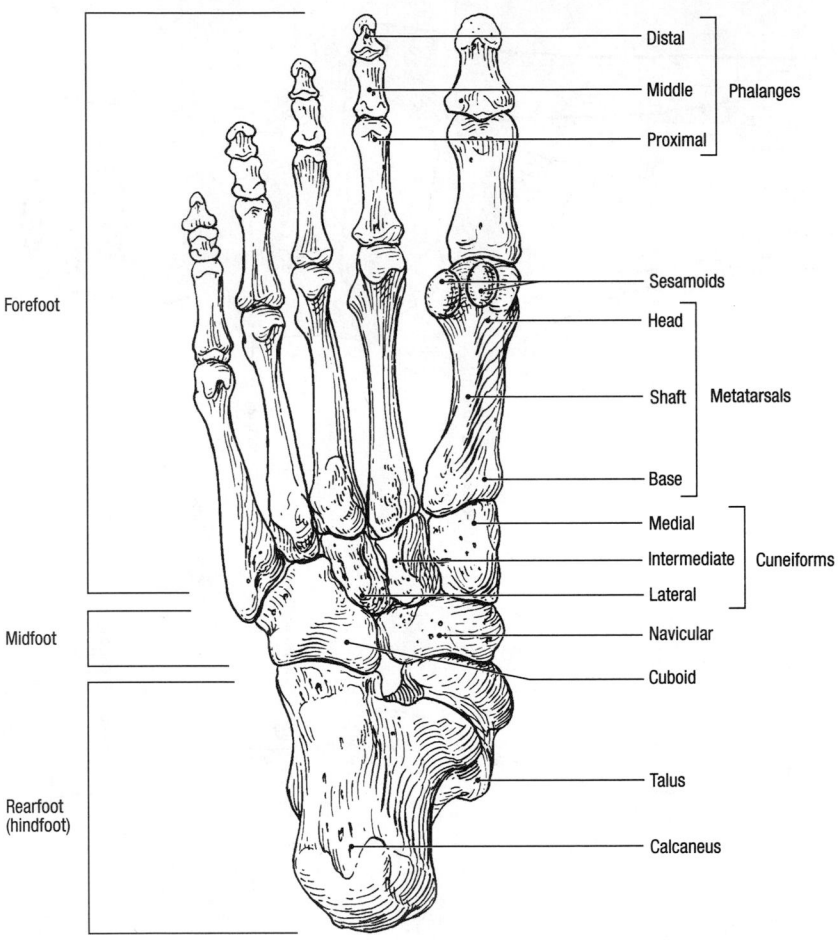

Figure 23. Skeleton of foot, plantar view.

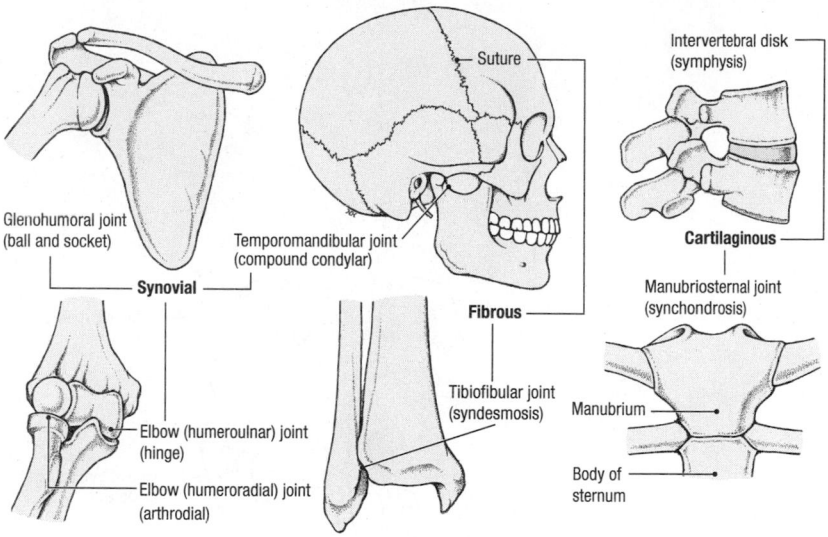

Figure 24. Types of joints.

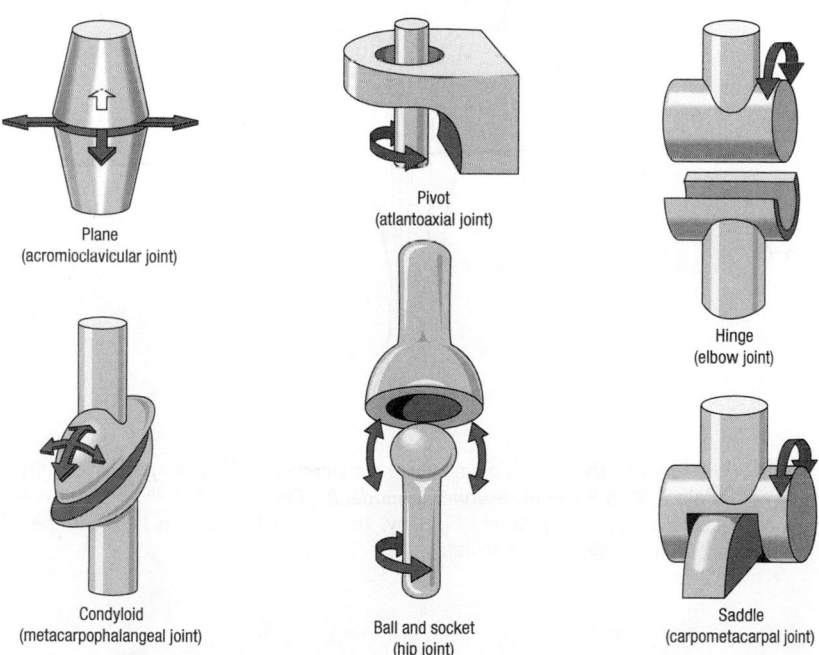

Figure 25. Illustrations of different types of movements of joints as demonstrated by mechanical models.

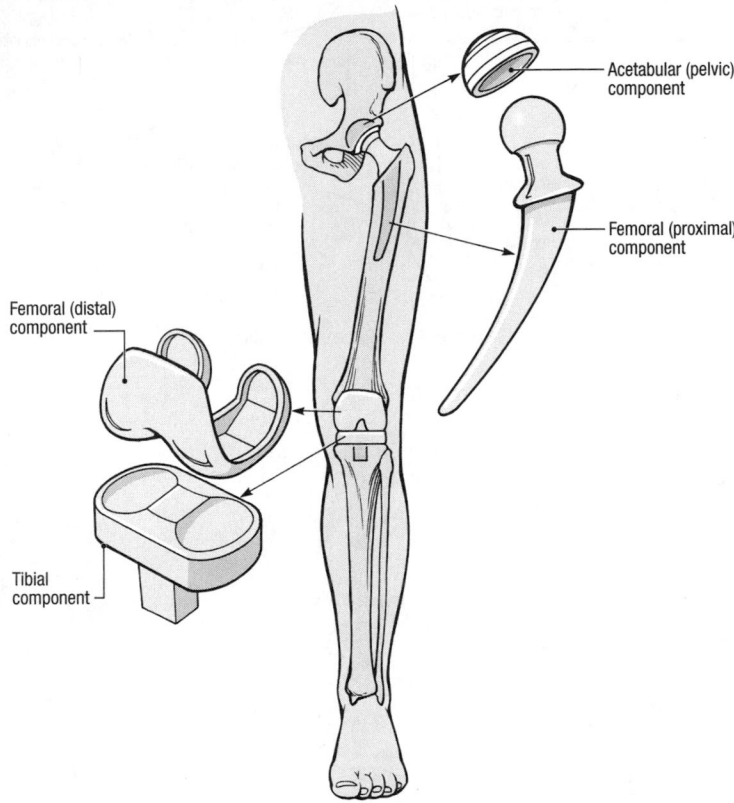

Figure 26. Arthroplasty, showing hip and knee replacements. This image, created by Mikki Senkarik, for Smeltzer SC & Bare GB, *Brunner & Suddarth's Textbook of Medical Surgical-Nursing, 8th Edition,* Philadelphia, J.B. Lippincott Company, 1996, fig. 62.9, appears here with permission and courtesy of Lippincott Williams & Wilkins.

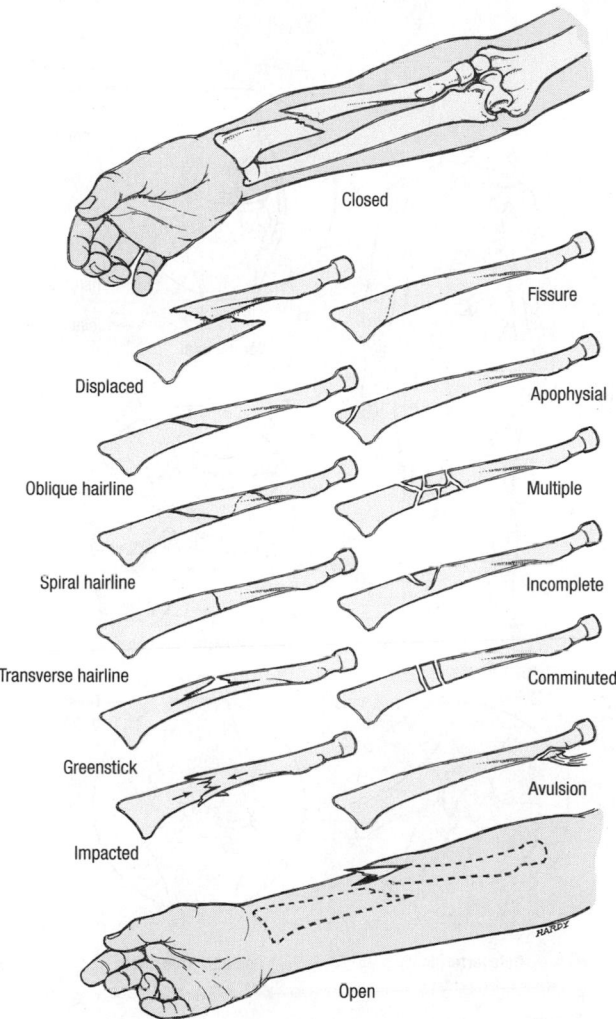

Closed

Fissure

Displaced

Apophysial

Oblique hairline

Multiple

Spiral hairline

Incomplete

Transverse hairline

Comminuted

Greenstick

Avulsion

Impacted

Open

Figure 27. Types of fractures.

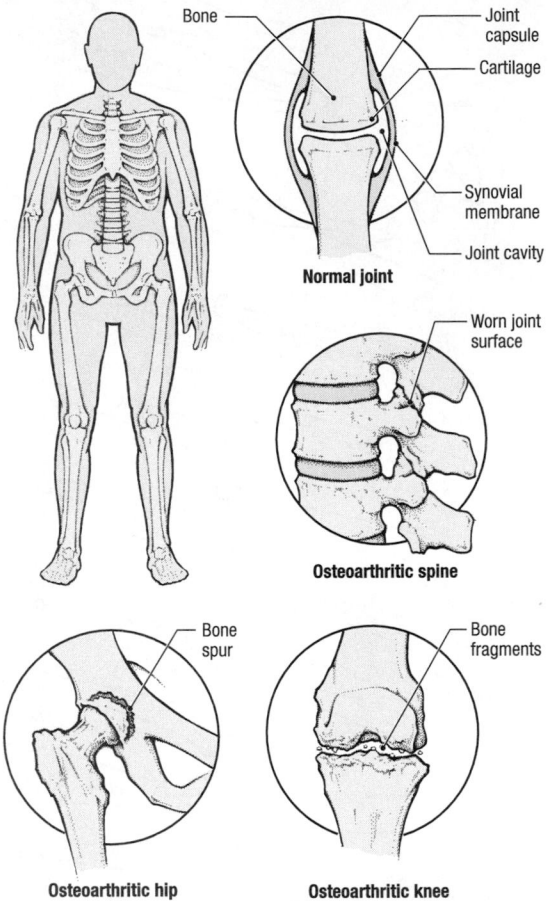

Figure 28. Osteoarthritis. Problems associated with osteoarthritis and some sites where they commonly occur. This image, created by Duckwall Productions, for *Stedman's Medical Dictionary, 27th Edition,* Baltimore, Lippincott Williams & Wilkins, 2000, p. 1282, appears here with permission and courtesy of Lippincott Williams & Wilkins.

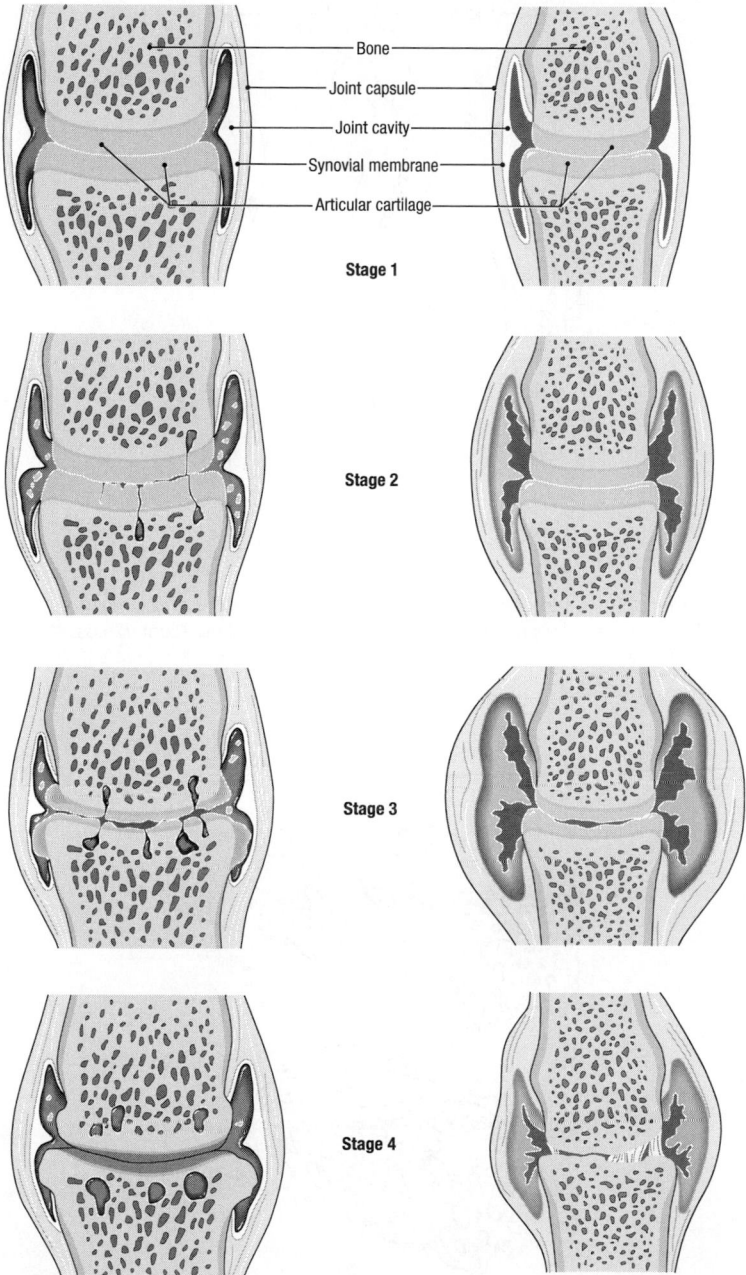

Figure 29. Cross-sections of synovial joints showing the progression of osteoarthritis (left) and rheumatoid arthritis (right) in four stages.

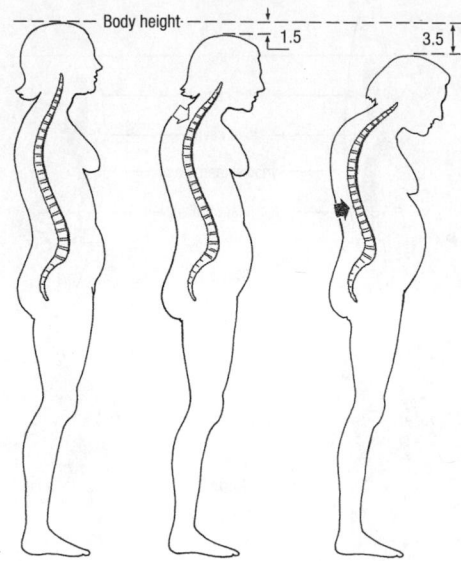

Figure 30. Osteoporosis and aging. Spinal column within outline of a woman at 10 years postmenopause (left). Changes (loss of height) at 15 years postmenopause (center). Loss at 25 years postmenopause (right).

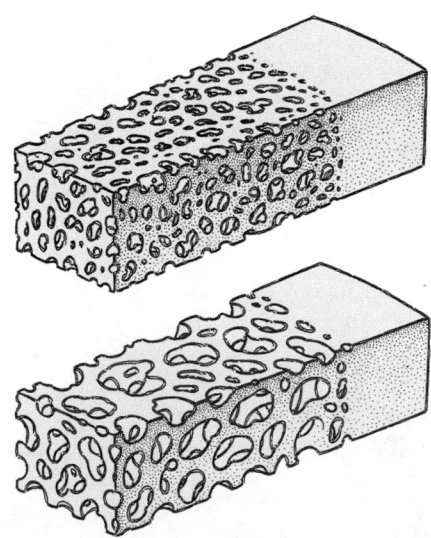

Figure 31. Osteoporosis. Normal bone (top), osteoporotic bone (bottom).

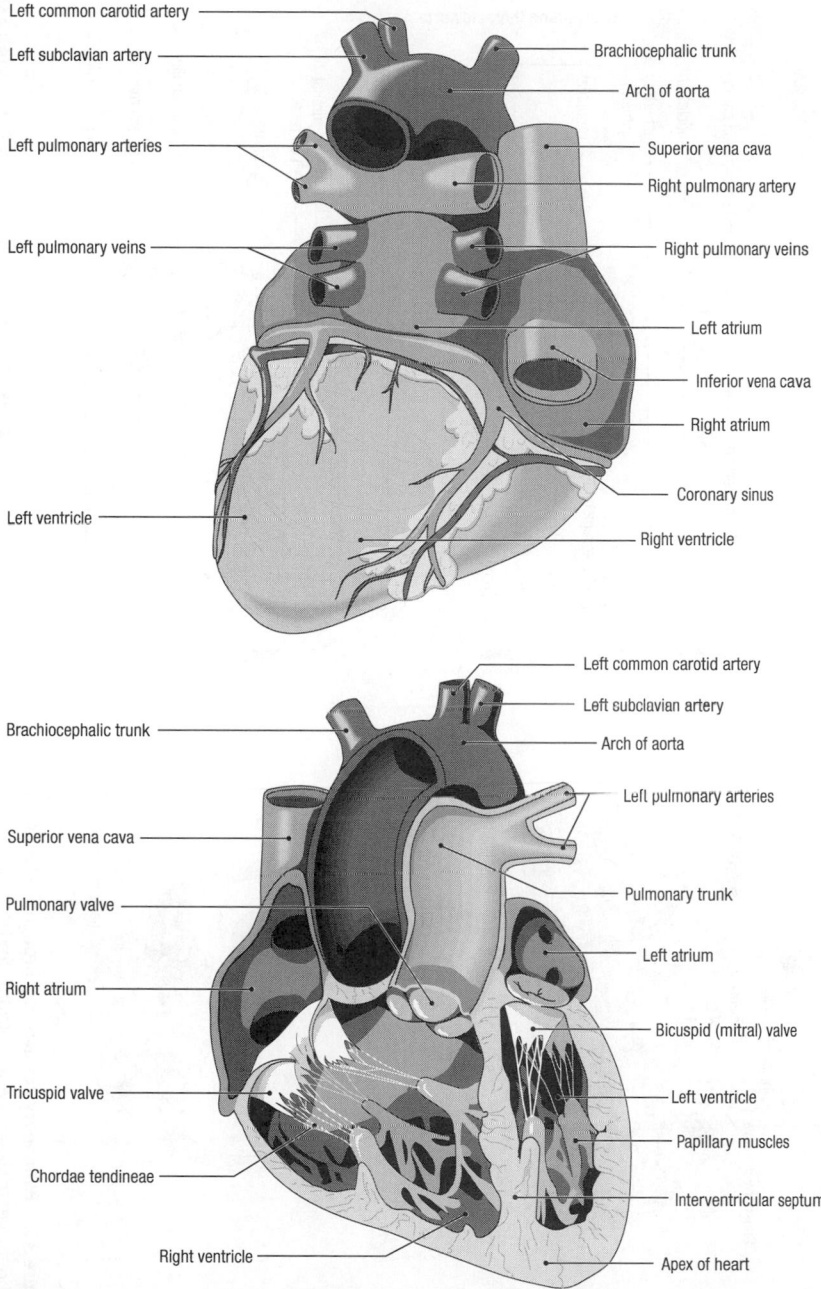

Figure 32. The relationship of the great vessels of the heart. Posterior view (top), coronal view (bottom).

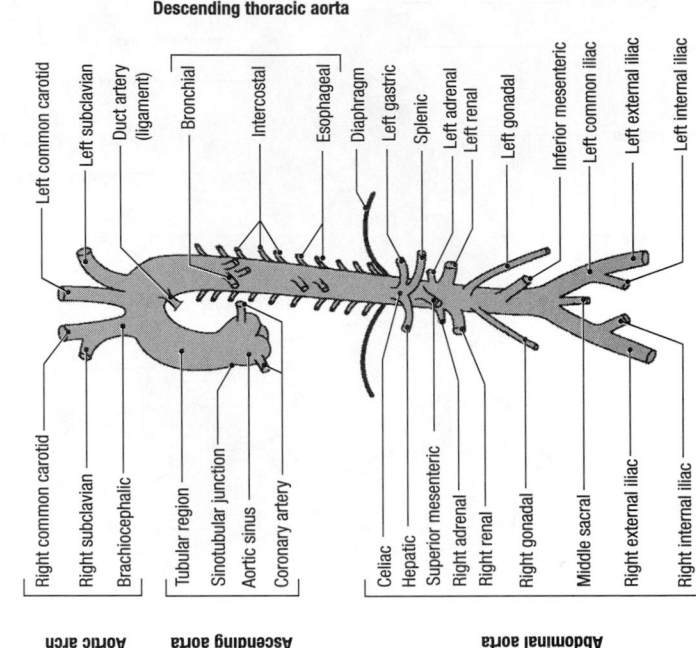

Figure 34. Systemic arteries, shown schematically. The aorta consists of ascending, arch, descending thoracic, and abdominal regions.

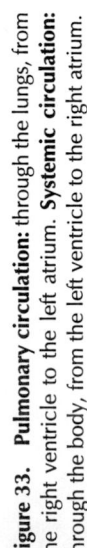

Figure 33. **Pulmonary circulation:** through the lungs, from the right ventricle to the left atrium. **Systemic circulation:** through the body, from the left ventricle to the right atrium.

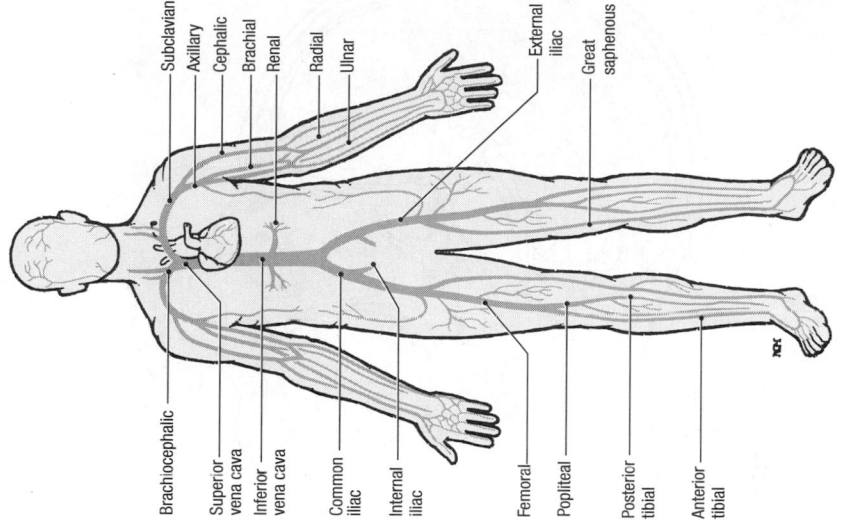

Figure 36. Major veins of the body.

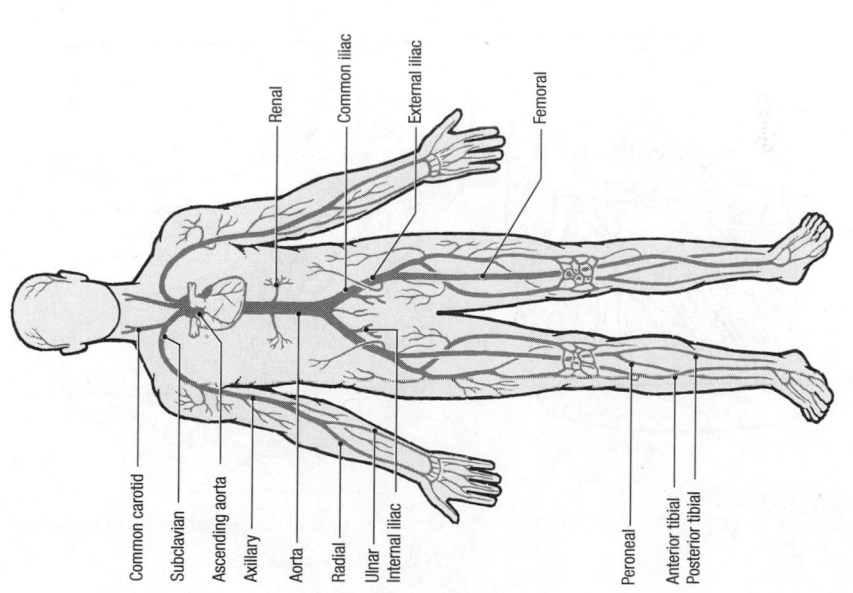

Figure 35. Major arteries of the body.

A27

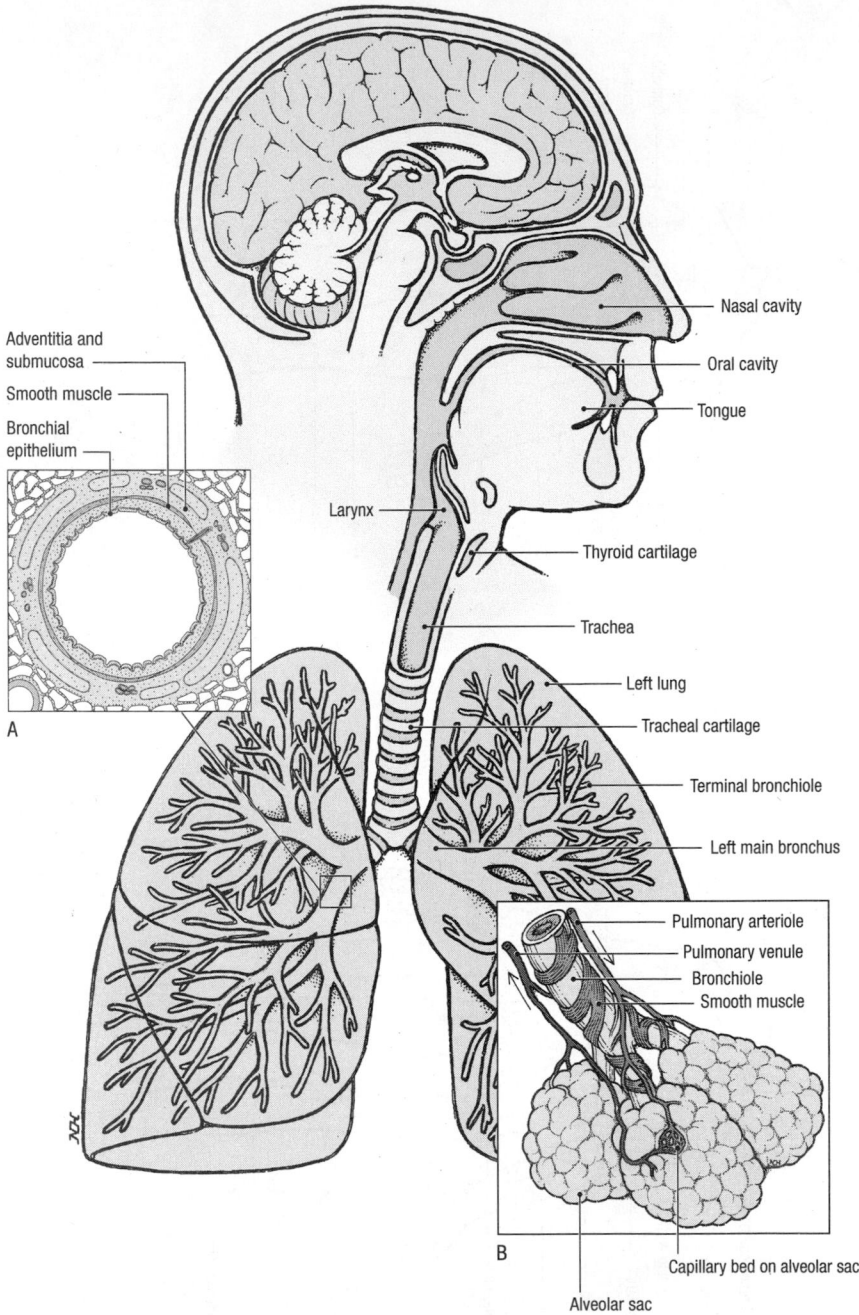

Figure 37. Lungs and respiratory anatomy. (A) Intrapulmonary bronchus. (B) Pulmonary alveolus.

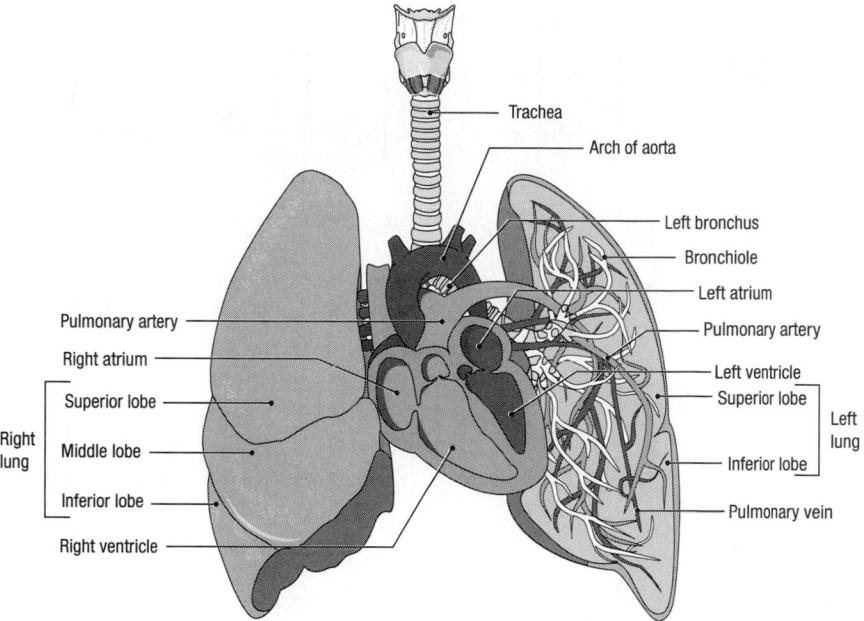

Trachea

Arch of aorta

Left bronchus

Bronchiole

Left atrium

Pulmonary artery

Pulmonary artery

Right atrium

Left ventricle

Superior lobe

Superior lobe

Right lung

Middle lobe

Left lung

Inferior lobe

Inferior lobe

Pulmonary vein

Right ventricle

Figure 38. Cardiopulmonary system shown with cutaway of heart and left lung revealing internal anatomy.

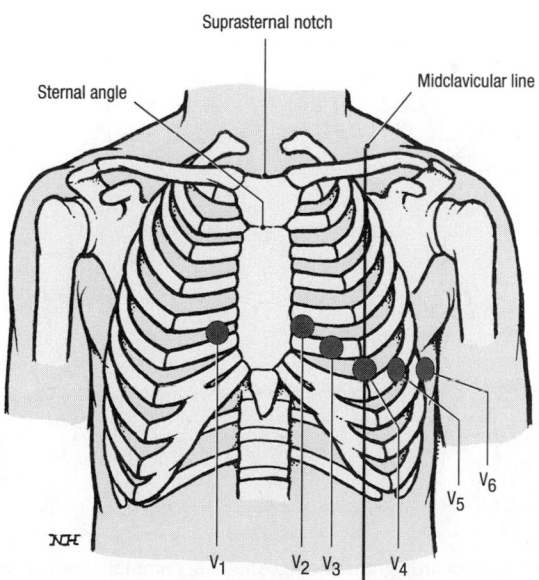

Suprasternal notch

Sternal angle

Midclavicular line

V_6

V_5

V_1 V_2 V_3 V_4

Figure 39. Electrocardiogram (ECG) lead placement. Landmarks for chest lead placement.

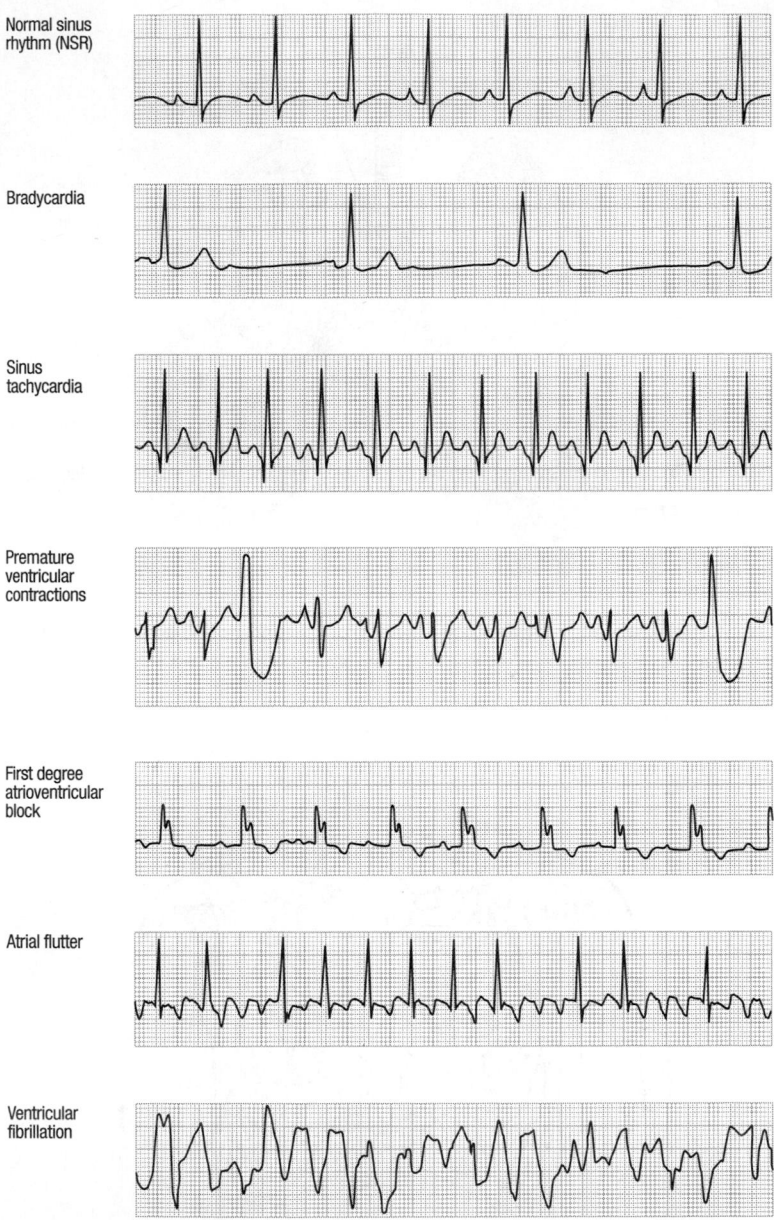

Normal sinus
rhythm (NSR)

Bradycardia

Sinus
tachycardia

Premature
ventricular
contractions

First degree
atrioventricular
block

Atrial flutter

Ventricular
fibrillation

Figure 40. Rhythm. Electrocardiogram tracings showing common types of arrhythmia. This image, from Willis MC, *Medical Terminology: The Language of Health Care,* Baltimore, Williams & Wilkins, 1996, fig. 7.9, appears here with permission and courtesy of Lippincott Williams & Wilkins.

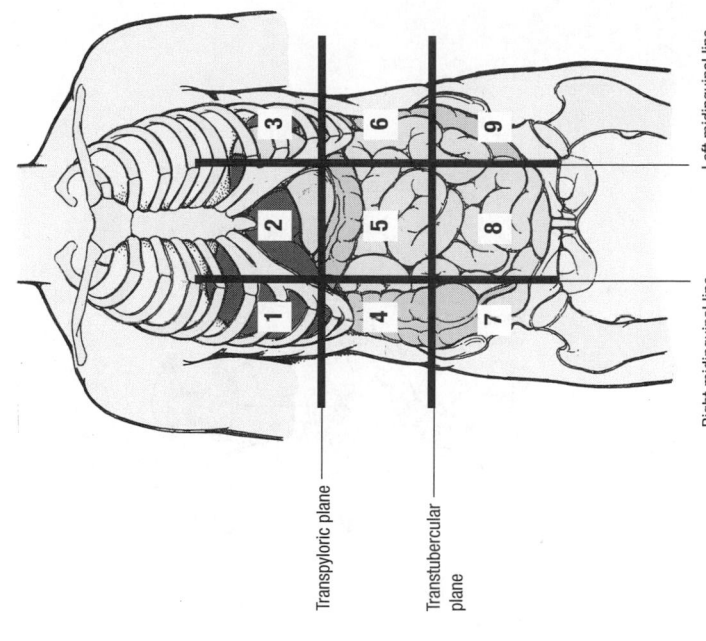

Figure 42. Abdominal regions. (1) Right hypochondriac. (2) Epigastric. (3) Left hypochondriac (4) Right lateral (lumbar). (5) Umbilical. (6) Left lateral (lumbar). (7) Right iliac. (8) Hypogastric (suprapubic). (9) Left iliac.

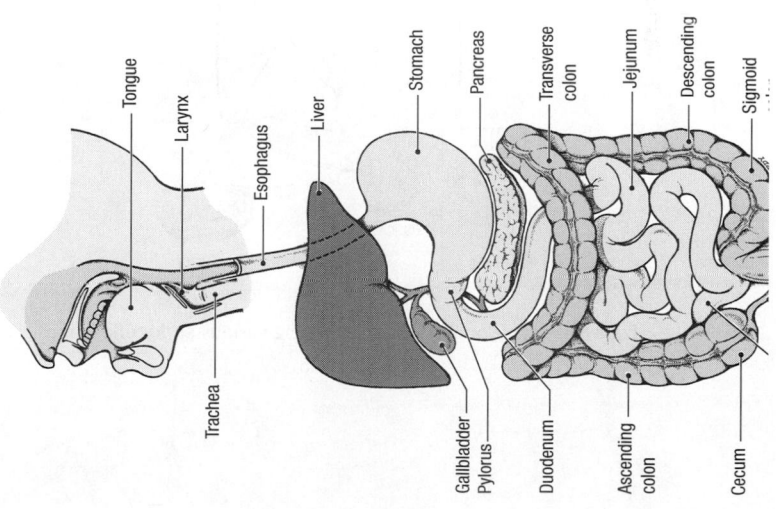

Figure 41. Digestive organs and associated structures.

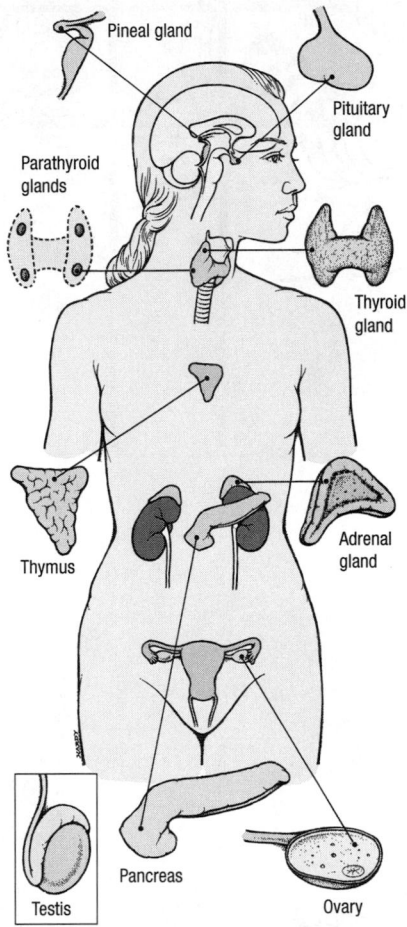

Figure 43. Endocrine system, showing various endocrine glands.

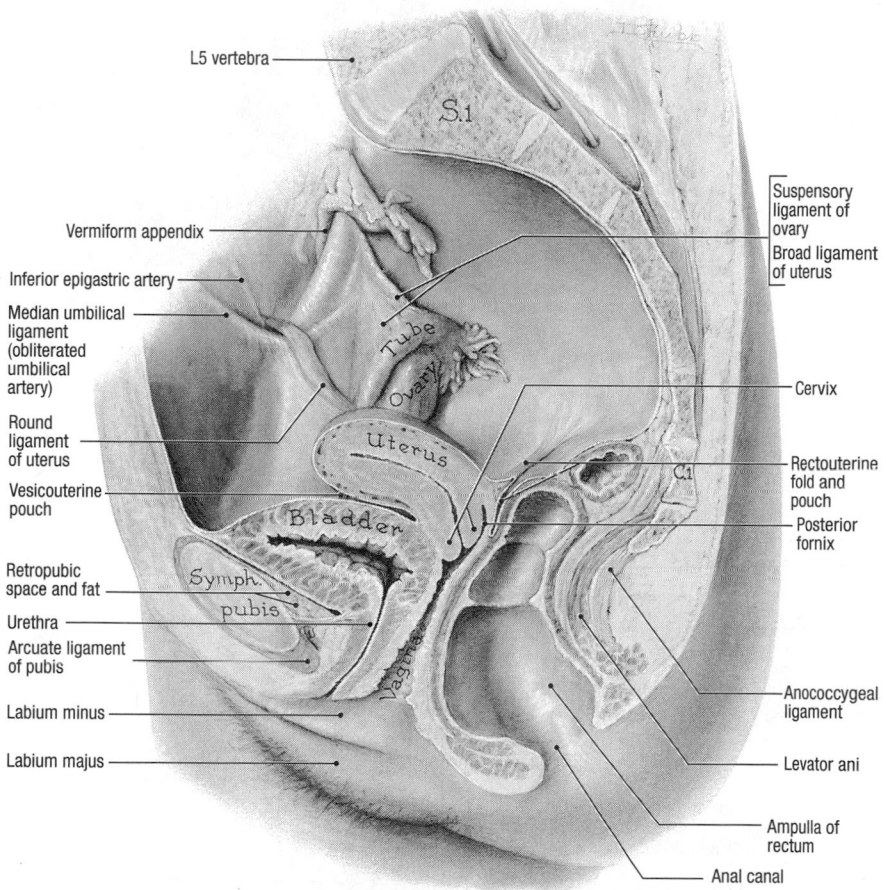

L5 vertebra

S.1

Suspensory ligament of ovary

Broad ligament of uterus

Vermiform appendix

Inferior epigastric artery

Median umbilical ligament (obliterated umbilical artery)

Round ligament of uterus

Vesicouterine pouch

Retropubic space and fat

Urethra

Arcuate ligament of pubis

Labium minus

Labium majus

Tube

Ovary

Uterus

Bladder

Symph. pubis

Vagina

C.1

Cervix

Rectouterine fold and pouch

Posterior fornix

Anococcygeal ligament

Levator ani

Ampulla of rectum

Anal canal

Figure 44.   Female pelvis, median section.

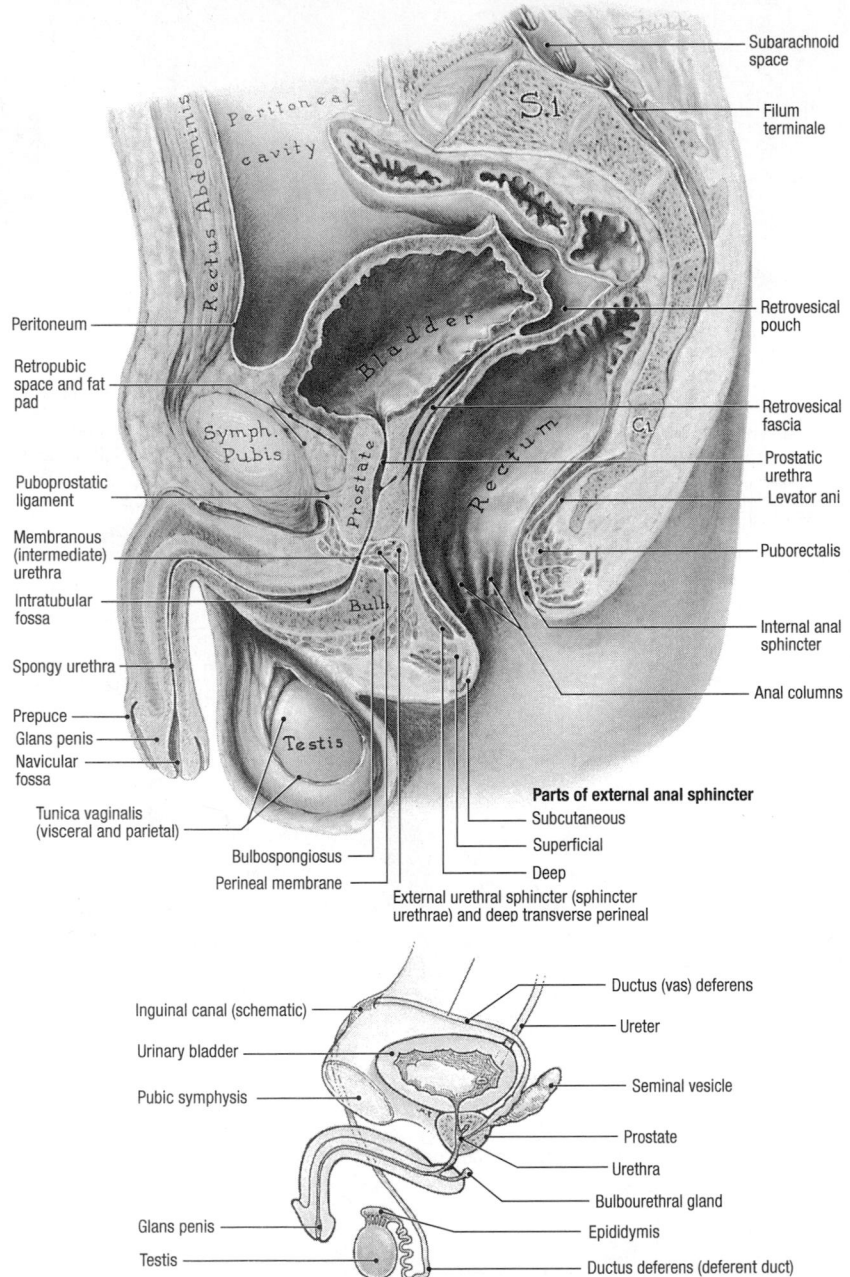

Figure 45. Male pelvis. Median section (top). Overview of urogenital system, median section (bottom).

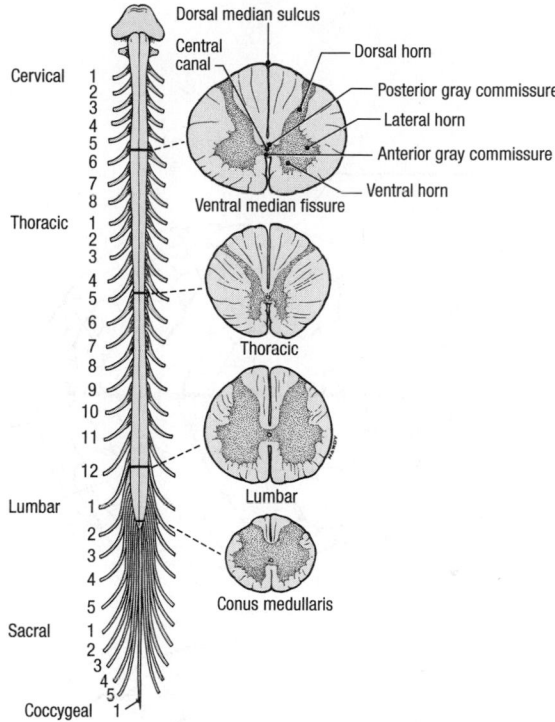

Figure 46. Spinal cord with transverse views showing regional variations in the gray matter.

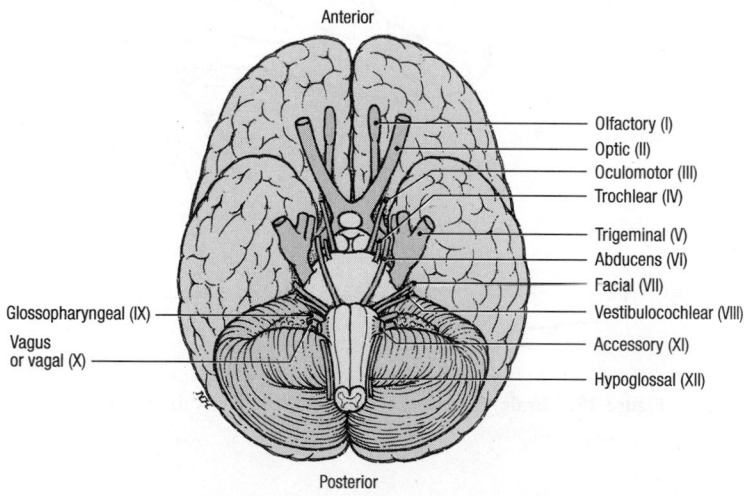

Figure 47. Cranial nerves, inferior view.

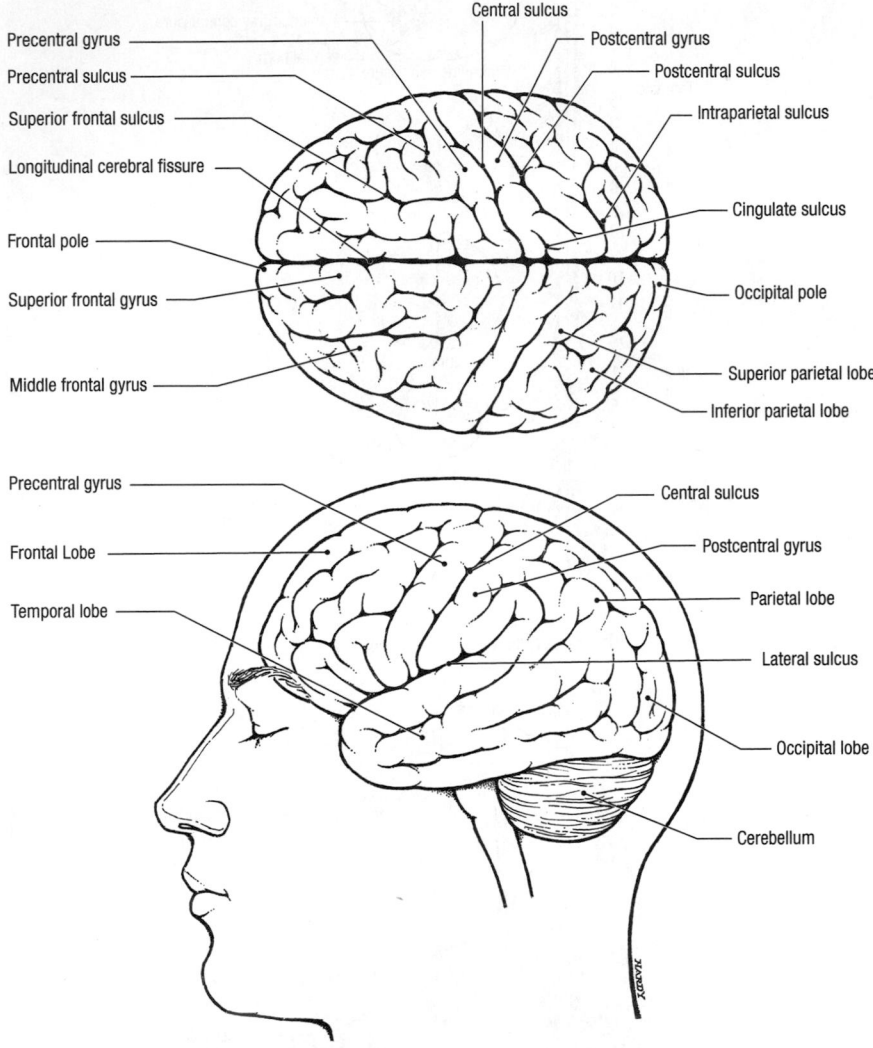

Figure 48. Brain. Superior view (top), lateral view (bottom).

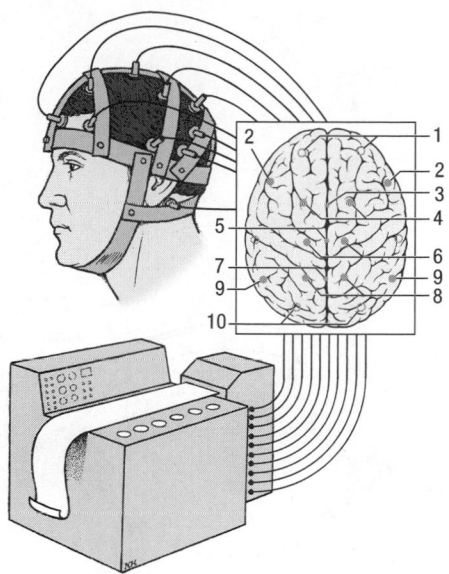

Figure 49. Electroencephalography, insert shows leads used. (1) Frontal. (2) Temporal (front). (3) Bregma. (4) Precentral. (5) Vertex. (6) Central. (7) Lambda. (8) Parietal. (9) Temporal (rear). (10) Occipital.

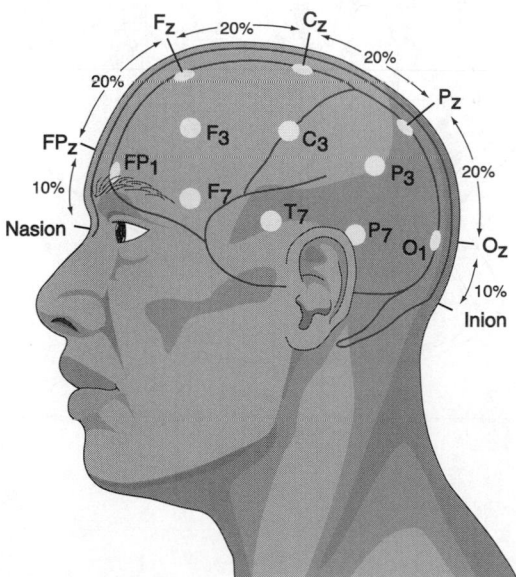

Figure 50. Lateral view of male head showing proper EEG electrode placement.

A37

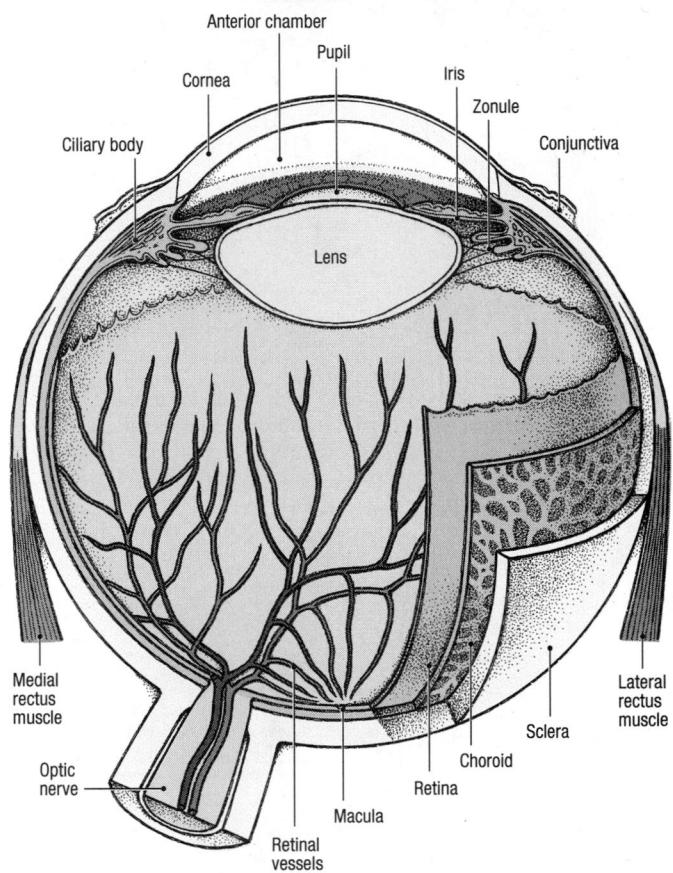

Figure 51. Eye.

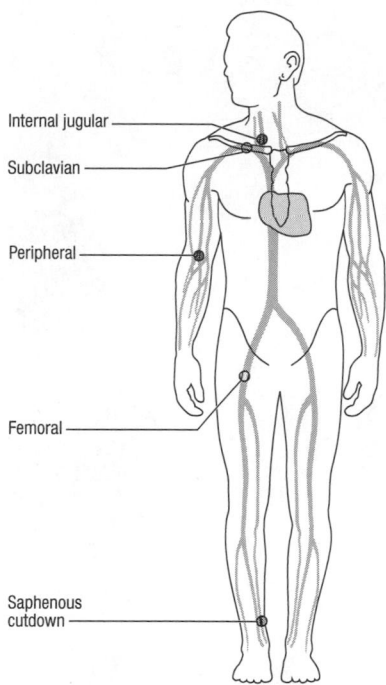

Internal jugular

Subclavian

Peripheral

Femoral

Saphenous
cutdown

Figure 52. Adult IV sites.

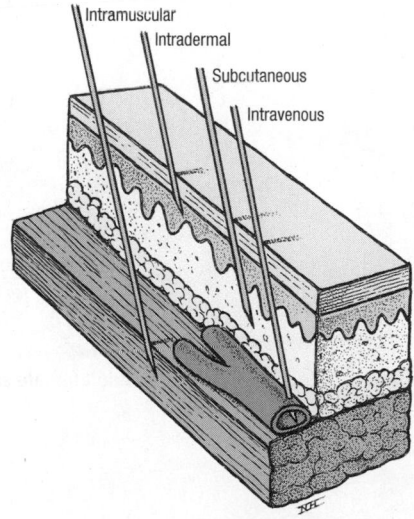

Intramuscular

Intradermal

Subcutaneous

Intravenous

Figure 53. Injection.

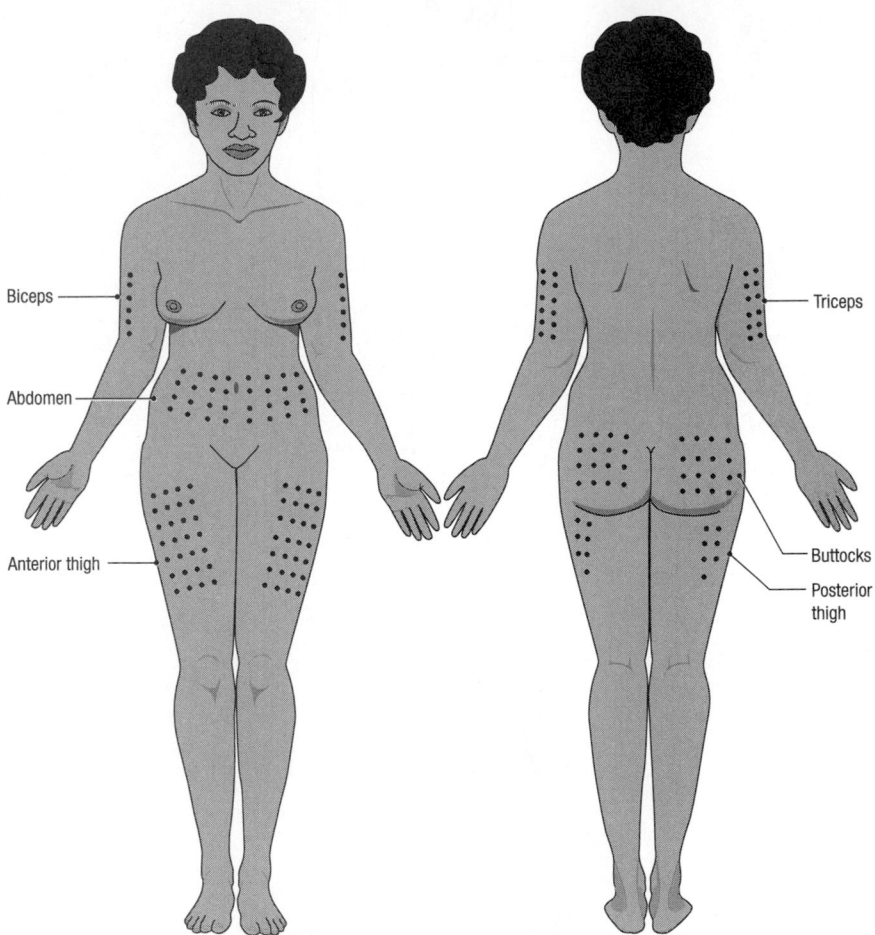

Figure 54. Anterior (left) and posterior (right) views of adult female showing multiple sites for insulin injection.

Appendix 2
Abbreviations Commonly Used in Internal Medicine and Geriatrics

Abbreviation	Expansion
AAA	abdominal aortic aneurysm
Ab	antibody
ABG	arterial blood gas
ABO	blood group system
a.c.	*ante cibum,* before meals
AC	acromioclavicular
ACE	angiotensin-converting enzyme
ACEI	angiotensin-converting enzyme inhibitor
ACTH	adrenocorticotropic hormone
AD	*auris dextra,* right ear; Alzheimer disease
ad lib	*ad libitum,* freely, as desired
ADH	antidiuretic hormone
ADHD	attention deficit hyperactivity disorder
ADL	activities of daily living
ADP	adenosine 5'-diphosphate
AEA, A-E	above-elbow amputation
AF	atrial fibrillation; atrial flutter
AFB	acid-fast bacillus
AFP	alpha-fetoprotein
AHF	antihemophilic factor
AIDS	acquired immunodeficiency syndrome
AKA, A-K	above-knee amputation
ALD	adrenoleukodystrophy
ALL	acute lymphocytic leukemia
ALT	alanine aminotransferase
AML	acute myelogenous leukemia
ANA	antinuclear antibody
ANS	autonomic nervous system
APA	antipernicious anemia (factor)
A-P-C	adenoidal-pharyngeal-conjunctival (virus)
APS	antiphospholipid antibody syndrome
APTT	activated partial thromboplastin time
ARDS	adult respiratory distress syndrome
ARF	acute renal failure
AS	*auris sinistra,* left ear
ASA	acetylsalicylic acid

ASCUS	abnormal squamous cells of undetermined significance
ASCVD	atherosclerotic cardiovascular disease
ASHD	arteriosclerotic heart disease
ASO	antistreptolysin O
AST	aspartate aminotransferase
AU	*auris utraque,* each ear, both ears
AV, A-V	arteriovenous
AVN	atrioventricular node
AZT	azidothymidine
BAER	brainstem auditory-evoked response
BBB	blood-brain barrier; bundle-branch block
BCG	bacille Calmette-Guérin (vaccine)
BE	barium enema
BEA	below-elbow amputation
b.i.d.	*bis in die,* twice a day
BiPAP	bilevel positive airway pressure
BKA	below-knee amputation
BM	bowel movement
BMD	bone mineral density
BMI	body mass index
BMT	bone marrow transplant
BP	blood pressure
BPH	benign prostatic hyperplasia
BRAT	banana, rice, applesauce, toast (diet)
BT	bleeding time
BUN	blood urea nitrogen
BUS	Bartholin glands, urethra, Skene glands
Bx, BX	biopsy
C	Celsius
CA	cancer; carcinoma; cardiac arrest
CABG	coronary artery bypass graft
CAPD	continuous ambulatory peritoneal dialysis
CBC	complete blood (cell) count
C1-C7	cervical vertebrae one through seven
CC	chief complaint
cc	cubic centimeter
CCK	cholecystokinin
CCU	coronary care unit; critical care unit
CDC	Centers for Disease Control and Prevention
CEA	carcinoembryonic antigen
CF	cystic fibrosis
CG	chorionic gonadotropin

CHF	congestive heart failure
CIS	carcinoma in situ
CLL	chronic lymphocytic leukemia
cm	centimeter
CML	chronic myelogenous leukemia
CMV	controlled mechanical ventilation; cytomegalovirus
CNS	central nervous system
CO_2	carbon dioxide
CoA	coenzyme A
COLD	chronic obstructive lung disease
COPD	chronic obstructive pulmonary disease
CP	cerebral palsy
CPAP	continuous positive airway pressure
CPK-MB	myocardial band enzymes of creatine phosphokinase
CPPB	continuous positive-pressure breathing
CPR	cardiopulmonary resuscitation
CRD	chronic respiratory disease
CRH	corticotropin-releasing hormone
CRP	cross-reacting protein
C&S	culture and sensitivity
CSF	cerebrospinal fluid
CT	computed tomography
CTR	cardiothoracic ratio
CTS	carpal tunnel syndrome
CV	cardiovascular
CVA	cerebrovascular accident
CVP	central venous pressure
CXR	chest x-ray
DC, d/c	discontinue
D&C	dilation and curettage; dilatation and curettage
DDAVP, dDAVP	desmopressin acetate
DDD	degenerative disk disease
DEXA	dual-energy x-ray absorptiometry
DHEA	dehydro-3-epiandrosterone
DHHS	Department of Health and Human Services
DIP	distal interphalangeal (joint)
DJD	degenerative joint disease
DKA, DK	diabetic ketoacidosis
DLCO	diffusing capacity of lung for carbon monoxide
DMSO	dimethyl sulfoxide
DNA	deoxyribonucleic acid
DNR	do not resuscitate
DOA	dead on arrival

DPT	diphtheria, pertussis, tetanus (vaccine)
DT	delirium tremens; duration of tetany
DUB	dysfunctional uterine bleeding
DVT	deep venous thrombosis; deep vein thrombosis
D_5W	dextrose 5% in water
EBV	Epstein-Barr virus
ECF	extracellular fluid
ECG, EKG	electrocardiogram
EEG	electroencephalogram
EGD	esophagogastroduodenoscopy
EIA	enzyme immunoassay
ELISA	enzyme-linked immunosorbent assay
EMC	encephalomyocarditis (virus)
EMG/NCV	electromyogram/nerve conduction velocity
EMS	emergency medical services
ENG	electroneurography
EOM	external otitis media
EOMI	extraocular movements intact
ERCP	endoscopic retrograde cholangiopancreatography
ESR	erythrocyte sedimentation rate
ESRD	end-stage renal disease
ETOH, EtOH	ethyl alcohol
F	Fahrenheit
FB	foreign body
FBS	fasting blood sugar
FEF	forced expiratory flow
$FeSO_4$	ferrous sulfate
FEV	forced expiratory volume
FIO_2	fraction of inspired oxygen
FNA	fine-needle aspiration
FSH	follicle-stimulating hormone
5-FU	5-fluorouracil
FUO	fever of unknown origin
FVC	forced vital capacity
Fx	fracture
g	gram
GE	gastroesophageal
GERD	gastroesophageal reflux disease
GGT	gamma-glutamyl transferase
GI	gastrointestinal
GTT	glucose tolerance test
gtt.	*guttae,* drops
GU	genitourinary

h.s.	*hora somni,* at bedtime
HAV	hepatitis A virus
HbA_{1c}	glycosylated hemoglobin
HB_cAg	hepatitis B core antigen
HB_sAb	hepatitis B surface antibody
HB_sAg	hepatitis B surface antigen
HBV	hepatitis B virus
HCG, hCG	human chorionic gonadotropin
HCT, Hct	hematocrit
HCTZ	hydrochlorothiazide
HDL	high-density lipoprotein
HGB, Hgb	hemoglobin
H&H	hemoglobin and hematocrit
5-HIAA	5-hydroxyindoleacetic acid
HIV	human immunodeficiency virus
HMO	health maintenance organization
H&P	history and physical (examination)
HPI	history of present illness
HPV	human papilloma virus
^{123}I	iodine-123 (radioisotope)
^{125}I	iodine-125 (radioisotope)
^{131}I	iodine-131 (radioisotope)
IBS	irritable bowel syndrome
ICF	intracellular fluid
ICU	intensive care unit
ID	infectious disease
I&D	incision and drainage
IDDM	insulin-dependent diabetes mellitus
IgG	immunoglobulin G
IM	internal medicine; intramuscular
INR	international normalized ratio
I&O	intake and output
IPPB	intermittent positive-pressure breathing
ITP	idiopathic thrombocytopenia purpura
IU	International Unit
IUCD	intrauterine contraceptive device
IV	intravenous
IVP, IV_P	intravenous push (dose)
J	joule
JVD(P)	jugular venous distension (pressure)
KCl	potassium chloride
KOH	potassium hydroxide
KUB	kidneys, ureters, bladder

L	liter
LDH, LD	lactate dehydrogenase
LDL	low-density lipoprotein
LE	lupus erythematosus
LEEP	loop electrosurgical excision procedure
LFT	liver function test
LH	luteinizing hormone
L1-L5	lumbar vertebrae one through five
LLL	left lower lobe
LLQ	left lower quadrant
LML	left middle lobe
LMP	last menstrual period
LUL	left upper lobe
LUQ	left upper quadrant
LVH	left ventricular hypertrophy
MAOI	monoamine oxidase inhibitor
mcg, μg	microgram
MCH	mean corpuscular hemoglobin
MCHC	mean corpuscular hemoglobin concentration
MCV	mean corpuscular volume
MDI	metered-dose inhaler
mEq	milliequivalent
MI	myocardial infarction
mL, ml	milliliter
mm	millimeter
MMPI	Minnesota Multiphasic Personality Inventory
MMR	measles, mumps, rubella (vaccine)
MRI	magnetic resonance imaging
MS	multiple sclerosis
ms, msec	millisecond
MUGA	multiple-gated acquisition (imaging)
NAD	no acute distress
NIDDM	non–insulin-dependent diabetes mellitus
NIH	National Institutes of Health
NKA	no known allergies
nm	nanometer
NPO	*non per os,* nothing by mouth
NSAID	nonsteroidal antiinflammatory drug
NSR	normal sinus rhythm
OC	oral contraceptive
OCD	obsessive-compulsive disorder
OD	*oculus dexter,* right eye; overdose
OP	outpatient

O&P	ova and parasites
OR	operating room
OS	*oculus sinister,* left eye
OSHA	Occupational Safety and Health Administration
OT	occupational therapy
OTC	over the counter
OU	*oculus uterque,* each eye, both eyes
oz	ounce
p	pico-
PAO_2	partial pressure of arterial oxygen
PCO_2, PCO_2	partial pressure of carbon dioxide
PE	pulmonary embolus
PEEP	positive end-expiratory pressure
PEG	percutaneous endoscopic gastrostomy
PERRLA	pupils equal, round, reactive to light and accommodation
PET	positron emission tomography
PFT	pulmonary function test
pH	hydrogen ion concentration
PICC	peripherally inserted central catheter
PID	pelvic inflammatory disease
PKU	phenylketonuria
PMI	point of maximum impulse
PMS	premenstrual syndrome
PND	paroxysmal nocturnal dyspnea; postnasal drip
p.o.	*per os,* by mouth
PO_2, PO_2	partial pressure of oxygen
PPBS	postprandial blood sugar
PPD	purified protein derivative (of tuberculin)
p.r.	*per rectum,* by way of rectum
p.r.n.	*pro re nata,* as needed
PSA	prostate-specific antigen
PSBO	partial small bowel obstruction
PT	physical therapy; prothrombin time
PTA	prior to admission
PTCA	percutaneous transluminal coronary angioplasty
PTH	parathyroid hormone
PTU	propylthiouracil
PUD	peptic ulcer disease
PVC	premature ventricular contraction
q.d.	*quaque die,* every day
q.i.d.	*quarter in die,* four times a day
q.s.	*quantum satis,* as much as is enough

R/O	rule out
RA	rheumatoid arthritis
RAST	radioallergosorbent test
RBC	red blood (cell) count
RBS	random blood sugar
RDA	recommended daily allowance
RDS	respiratory distress syndrome
RLL	right lower lobe
RLQ	right lower quadrant
RML	right middle lobe
RNA	ribonucleic acid
ROM	range of motion
RRR	regular rate and rhythm
RSD	reflex sympathetic dystrophy
RSV	respiratory syncytial virus; Rous sarcoma virus
RUL	right upper lobe
RUQ	right upper quadrant
RVH	right ventricular hypertrophy
Rx	*recipe,* take; prescription
S-A	sinoatrial
SBE	subacute bacterial endocarditis
SC	subcutaneous; sternoclavicular
SDAT	senile dementia, Alzheimer type
SGOT	serum glutamic-oxaloacetic transaminase
SGPT	serum glutamic-pyruvic transaminase
SIADH	syndrome of inappropriate antidiuretic hormone
SK	streptokinase
SLE	systemic lupus erythematosus
SLR	straight leg raising
SMA-20	sequential multiple analysis of 20 chemical constituents
SMAC	Sequential Multiple Analyzer Computer
SOAP	subjective (data), objective (data), assessment, and plan
SOB	short(ness) of breath
S/P, SP	status post
SPECT	single photon emission computed tomography
SPF	sun protection factor
S1-S5	sacral vertebrae one through five
SSRI	selective serotonin reuptake inhibitor
SSS	sick sinus syndrome
stat., STAT	*statim,* immediately, at once
STD	sexually transmitted disease

SVT	supraventricular tachycardia
T$_3$	3,5,3'-triiodothyronine
T$_4$	tetraiodothyronine (thyroxine)
T-7	free thyroxine factor
T&A	tonsillectomy and adenoidectomy
TAHBSO	total abdominal hysterectomy and bilateral salpingo-oophorectomy
TB	tuberculosis
T&C	type and crossmatch
TED	thromboembolic disease (hose)
TEE	transesophageal echocardiography
TENS	transcutaneous electrical nerve stimulation
THR	total hip replacement
TIA	transient ischemic attack
TIBC	total iron-binding capacity
t.i.d.	*ter in die,* three times a day
TKR	total knee replacement
TMJ	temporomandibular joint
TOS	thoracic outlet syndrome
TSH	thyroid-stimulating hormone
TSS	toxic shock syndrome
T1-T12	thoracic vertebrae one through twelve
TTP	thrombotic thrombocytopenic purpura
TTS	tarsal tunnel syndrome
TURBT	transurethral resection of bladder tumor
TURP	transurethral resection of prostate
UA	urinalysis
URI	upper respiratory infection
US	ultrasound
UTI	urinary tract infection
VDRL	Venereal Disease Research Laboratory (test)
VHDL	very-high-density lipoprotein
VLDL	very-low-density lipoprotein
V/Q	ventilation/perfusion ratio
WBC	white blood (cell) count
WDWN	well-developed, well-nourished
WPW	Wolff-Parkinson-White (syndrome)
YAG	yttrium-aluminum-garnet (laser)

Appendix 3

Common Tests with Descriptions

NAME/SYNONYMS	INDICATION(S)	DESCRIPTION/SPECIMEN
Abdominal aorta sonogram; ultrasonography	To detect and measure suspected abdominal aortic aneurysm	Ultrasound waves sent into the body with a small transducer; sound waves are transformed into a visual display on a monitor
Acid-fast bacilli (AFB)	To identify mycobacteria in sputum specimens	Sputum that is sent for Gram stain
Adrenocorticotropic hormone (ACTH); corticotropin	To evaluate adrenal cortical dysfunction	Blood sample
Alanine aminotransferase (ALT); formerly serum glutamic-pyruvic transaminase (SGPT)	To monitor liver damage	Blood sample
Aldosterone	To diagnose primary and secondary aldosteronism	Blood and urine samples
Alkaline phosphatase (ALP)	To measure serum levels of alkaline phosphatase, an enzyme that is increased in bone growth, liver disease, biliary obstruction, osteogenic sarcoma, or breast or prostate cancer with metastases to the bone	Blood sample
Allergen-specific IgE antibody; radioallergosorbent test (RAST); allergy screen	To test for allergies to allergens	Blood sample
Alpha-fetoprotein (AFP)	To test for neural tube defects in the fetus such as spina bifida and anencephaly	Blood sample
Ambulatory electrocardiography; ambulatory monitoring; event monitoring; Holter monitoring	To monitor electrical activity of the heart and to detect arrhythmias which occur sporadically	Electrodes are applied to the skin, monitor and case are positioned, and the recorder is turned on

Test	Description	Sample
Ammonia	To assess for accumulation of ammonia in the bloodstream	Blood sample
Amylase	To assess for pancreatitis, diabetic ketoacidosis, cirrhosis, hepatitis, cholelithiasis, hyper-thyroidism, or other conditions	Blood or urine sample
Angiotensin-converting enzyme (ACE); serum angiotensin-converting enzyme	To assess for diabetic retinopathy, Gaucher disease, hyperthyroidism, liver disease, or sarcoidosis	Blood sample
Anion gap	To determine causes of metabolic acidosis including those associated with renal failure, diabetic ketoacicosis, or lactic acidosis	Blood sample
Anti-DNA antibody test	Detects presence of antibodies to native or double-stranded DNA, indicating some type of autoimmune disease	Blood sample
Antinuclear antibody test (ANA)	Used to rule out systemic lupus erythematosus, endocarditis, cirrhosis, connective tissue diseases, and chronic autoimmune hepatitis	Blood sample
Arterial blood gas (ABG) analysis; blood gases	For information regarding the acid-base status of the patient	Blood sample
Arteriography of the lower extremities; lower extremity angiography	Visualization of blood vessels	Contrast dye is injected through a catheter into an artery; radiographic films are then taken of the artery
Arthrocentesis; synovial fluid analysis	To diagnose arthritis, to investigate joint effusion, or to remove excess fluid from the joint	Synovial fluid sample

continued

NAME/SYNONYMS	INDICATION(S)	DESCRIPTION/SPECIMEN
Arthrogram	To assess for joint damage and/or cartilage tears	Injection of radiopaque dye or air into the joint; radiographs are taken as the joint is manipulated
Arthroscopy	To directly visualize joint structures and to perform biopsy and simple repairs	The arthroscope is inserted into the joint spaces; the joint is manipulated as it is visualized
Aspartate aminotransferase (AST); formerly serum glutamic oxaloacetic transaminase (SGOT)	To assess for heart muscle damage as in myocardial infarction; to assess for liver damage	Blood sample
Barium enema; large bowel study; lower GI series	Fluoroscopic examination of the large intestines for lower abdominal pain, changes in bowel habits, stools containing blood or mucus, visualizing polyps, diverticula or tumors	The entire intestine is filled from the rectum to the ileocecal valve; the area is observed on a fluoroscopic screen with films taken periodically
Barium swallow; esophageal radiography; esophagography	To evaluate dysphagia or regurgitation, hiatal hernia, diverticula, achalasia, esophagitis, polyps, and/or strictures	Patient swallows a thick barium mixture for fluoroscopic exam of the pharynx and esophagus; part of upper GI series
Bilirubin, direct (conjugated); indirect bilirubin (unconjugated); total bilirubin	To assess for choledocholithiasis, cirrhosis, hepatitis, myocardial infarction, pernicious anemia, and/or septicemia	Blood sample
Bleeding time; aspirin tolerance test; Duke bleeding time; ivy bleeding time; modified ivy; template bleeding time	To screen for disorders involving platelet function and vascular defects that interfere with clotting	A standard skin incision is made usually just below the crease of the elbow; blood drops are blotted every 30 seconds; time is stopped when bleeding ceases
Blood alcohol; ethanol; ethyl alcohol (ETOH)	To screen for alcohol ingestion	Blood sample
Blood culture and sensitivity	To screen for bacteria in the blood	Blood sample

Test	Purpose	Specimen/Procedure
Blood smear; peripheral blood smear; red blood cell smear (RBC smear)	Examines cells in terms of size, shape, color, and structure	Blood sample
Blood typing; ABO typing; ABO red cell groups; blood groups; Rh typing; type and crossmatch (T&C); type and screen	To determine an individual's blood type, Rh factors in the blood, and compatibility in donor blood	Blood sample
Bone marrow biopsy; bone marrow aspiration	To screen for cancer, depressed hematopoiesis, granuloma, infection, iron-deficiency anemia, leukemia, multiple myeloma, polycythemia vera, or thalassemia	A large-bore needle is advanced through the subcutaneous tissue cortex of bone to aspirate a sample of bone marrow
Bone scan	To detect metastatic cancer of the bone and monitor the progression of degenerative bone disorders; to detect fractures in patients with continued pain when x-rays have been negative	A radionuclide is injected intravenously; scintillation camera takes radioactivity reading from the body and transforms them into two-dimensional pictures of the skeleton
Brain scan (cerebral blood flow)	To assess for brain abscess, tumors, contusions, hematomas or cerebrovascular accidents (CVAs); interruption of the blood-brain barrier	A radionuclide is injected intravenously; scintillation camera takes radioactivity reading from the head and transforms them into two-dimensional pictures of the brain
Breast biopsy	To assess for malignancy	Needle biopsy: a sample of tissue is aspirated into a syringe for examination Open biopsy: an excision is made over the breast mass, which is excised in its entirety for testing
Bronchoscopy	To visualize abnormalities found on radiography, obtain sputum specimens, remove foreign bodies, conduct endobronchial radiation, or obliterate neoplastic obstruction	The bronchoscope is introduced through the mouth or nose; the anatomy of the trachea and bronchi are inspected

continued

NAME/SYNONYMS	INDICATION(S)	DESCRIPTION/SPECIMEN
CA 15–3, CA 19–9, CA-125, tumor markers/antigens	To assess for the presence of cancer	Blood sample
Calcitonin; thyrocalcitonin	To assess for hypercalcemia	Blood sample
Calcium	To assess calcium level	Blood or urine sample
Candida antibody test	To assess for *Candida* infection	Blood sample
Carboxyhemoglobin; carbon monoxide (CO)	To assess for carbon monoxide poisoning	Blood sample
Carcinoembryonic antigen (CEA)	To assess carcinoembryonic antigen levels for malignancy	Blood sample
Cardiac catheterization; angiocardiography, coronary angiography; coronary arteriography; heart catheterization	Visualization of the blood vessels to assess for heart size, structure, movement, wall thickness, blood flow, valve motion, and/or coronary vasculature	A catheter is inserted through an artery into the correct position and dye is inserted; radiographic films are taken of the artery
Carotid duplex scanning; carotid phono-angiography (CPA)	To assess for plaque, stenosis, or partial occlusion of arteries	A transducer is placed on the skin; sound waves are transformed into a visual display on a monitor
Cerebral angiography; cerebral arteriography	To detect cerebrovascular abnormalities such as aneurysm or arteriovenous malformation, to study vascular displacement, or to evaluate postoperative status of blood vessels	A catheter is inserted through an artery into the correct position and dye is inserted; radiographic films are taken of the artery
Cerebrospinal fluid (CSF) analysis; cisternal puncture; lumbar puncture (LP); spinal tap; ventricular puncture	To assist in the diagnosis of a wide variety of central nervous system diseases, including infectious diseases	A sample of cerebrospinal fluid is collected using a spinal needle

Chemistry profile	To assess multiple organ systems to determine overall health and wellness	May include alanine aminotransferase (ALT); alkaline phosphatase (ALP); aspartate aminotransferase (AST); bilirubin; calcium; carbon dioxide; chloride; cholesterol; creatinine kinase (CK); creatinine; gamma-glutamyl transferase (GGT); glucose; lactic dehydrogenase (LDH); phosphorus; potassium; protein; sodium; triglycerides; urea nitrogen; and uric acid tests
Chest x-ray (CXR); chest radiography	To identify abnormalities of the lungs and other structures of the thorax including heart, ribs, and diaphragm	X-ray of the chest
Chlamydia	To assess for *Chlamydia trachomatis* or trachoma	Titer: Blood sample; Eye culture: Swab of inner canthus or lower conjunctiva; Cervical culture: Swab of the cervix
Chloride	To evaluate the chloride level in the blood or kidneys	Blood or urine sample
Cholecystography; gallbladder radiography; gallbladder series; oral cholecystogram	To assess for gallbladder disease	After ingestion of a contrast medium, films are taken of the right upper quadrant in three positions
Cholesterol	To evaluate LDL and HDL and risk potential for atherosclerosis and heart disease	Blood sample
Clostridium difficile (*C. difficile*) toxin assay; clostridial toxin assay	To evaluate for pseudomembranous colitis	Stool specimen
Coagulation factor assay; factor assay; clotting factors	To assess for congenital or acquired deficiency of blood clotting factor	Blood sample

continued

NAME/SYNONYMS	INDICATION(S)	DESCRIPTION/SPECIMEN
Coagulation studies	To evaluate coagulation disorders	Include antithrombin III; bleeding time; clot retraction; coagulation factors; D-dimer; euglobulin lysis time; fibrin degradation; fibrinogen; partial thromboplastin time; plasminogen; protein C; protein S; prothrombin time; and thrombin clotting time tests
Colonoscopy	To assess lower GI bleeding, change in bowel habits, high risk for colon cancer due to polyps, or ulcerative colitis or history	Direct visualization of the large intestine through the use of a flexible fiberoptic endoscope
Colposcopy; endometrial biopsy	To identify the area of cellular dysplasia	Direct visualization of the cervix and vagina with a colposcope with magnifying lens and light
Complete blood cell count with differential (CBC with diff)	To evaluate red blood counts, white blood counts, and platelets	Includes blood smear; hematocrit; hemoglobin; platelets; RBC count; RBC indices (MCV, MCH, MCHC); WBC count; and differential
Computed tomography (CT) of the abdomen; CT scan of the abdomen; computerized axial tomography (CAT) of the abdomen	To diagnose pathologic conditions of the abdominal organs including inflammation, cysts, tumors of the liver, gallbladder, pancreas, spleen, kidneys, and pelvic organs	Contrast dye is given by IV injection; films are taken in the body scanner
Computed tomography (CT) of the brain; CT scan of the head; computerized axial tomography (CAT) of the head	To diagnose pathologic conditions such as neoplasms, cerebral infarctions, aneurysm, and intracranial hemorrhage	Contrast dye is given by IV injection; films are taken in the body scanner
Computed tomography (CT) of the chest; CT scan of the chest; computerized axial tomography (CAT) of the chest	To diagnose pathologic conditions, including inflammation, cysts, and tumors of the lungs, esophagus, and lymph nodes	Contrast dye is given by IV injection; films are taken in the body scanner

Test	Description	Specimen
Coombs test, direct; direct antiglobulin test; red blood cell (RBC) antibody screen	To assess if antibodies are attached to the red blood cells, indicating infectious mono-nucleosis or systemic lupus erythematosus; to detect red blood cell sensitization to drugs or blood transfusions	Blood sample
Coombs test, indirect; antibody screening test	To detect unexpected circulating antibodies that may react against transfused red blood cells, other than those of the ABO groups	Blood sample
Cortisol	To assess for normal function of the anterior pituitary gland	Blood or urine sample
C-reactive protein test (CRP)	To assess for inflammatory process	Blood sample
Creatine kinase (CK) and isoenzymes; formerly creatine phosphokinase (CPK)	To assess for myocardial infarction	Blood sample
Creatinine; creatinine clearance	To evaluate renal function	Blood and/or urine sample
Cystometry; cystometrography (CMG)	To evaluate detrusor instability and cause of bladder dysfunction	Instillation of fluid and/or air into the bladder, assessment of neurologic and muscular responses to this filling, and assessment of patient's voiding for abnormalities
Cystourethrography	To evaluate chronic urinary tract infections (UTIs)	Instillation of contrast medium into the bladder through a urethral catheter; x-ray films are taken as the bladder fills and as the patient voids

continued

A57

NAME/SYNONYMS	INDICATION(S)	DESCRIPTION/SPECIMEN
Cystourethroscopy; cystoscopy; urethroscopy	Calculi removal, diagnosis; therapeutic procedures other than calculi removal: obstruction, urothelial carcinoma, filling defects, unilateral gross hematuria, malignant cytology, surveillance, passage of ureteral catheter for obstruction of fistula, foreign body, resection/fulguration of selected tumors, and dilation/incision of strictures	Passing of cystoscope into the bladder to visualize the urinary tract
Disseminated intravascular coagulation screening (DIC screening)	To assess when both clotting and bleeding occur at abnormally high levels	See coagulation studies
Doppler study; Doppler ultrasonography	To evaluate blood flow in the major veins and arteries of the legs, arms, and neck	Ultrasound waves are sent into the body with a small transducer pressed against the skin
Echocardiography; echo; heart sonogram	To assess heart chambers, valves, blood flow or muscle	Ultrasound waves are sent into the body with a small transducer pressed against the skin
Electrocardiography, electrocardiogram (ECG, EKG)	To record the electrical current generated by the heart	Monitoring electrodes are placed on the body
Electroencephalography (EEG)	To record the electrical activity of the brain	Monitoring electrodes are placed on the scalp
Electromyography, electromyelography (EMG)	To record the electrical activity in the skeletal muscle groups	Insertion of needle electrodes into the muscle
Electroneurography, electromyoneurography (ENG)	To assess for peripheral nerve disease or injury	Electrodes over a nerve initiate electrical impulse at the proximal site; time is recorded for the impulse to reach a distal site on the same nerve

Test	Purpose	Description
Endoscopic retrograde cholangiopancreatography (ERCP)	To assess for obstructive jaundice, cancer, calculi, or stenosis	Radiographic viewing of the pancreatic ducts and hepatobiliary tree through an endoscope
Erythrocyte sedimentation rate (ESR), sedimentation rate (sed rate); Westergren; Wintrobe	To assess for inflammatory and necrotic conditions	Blood sample
Esophageal manometry; acid reflux test; Bernstein test; esophageal function studies	To assess the esophagus for normal contractile activity	Manometric catheter is placed at various levels in the esophagus; baseline pressure measurements are taken as the patient swallows
Esophagogastroduodenoscopy (EGD); esophagoscopy; gastroscopy; upper gastrointestinal (GI) endoscopy	To assess the esophagus, stomach, and upper duodenum via direct visualization	The endoscope is inserted through the mouth to inspect anatomy, remove tissue specimen, and/or remove foreign bodies
Estradiol receptor and progesterone receptor (ER/PR) in breast cancer; ER/PR assay	To assess whether breast cancer tissue would respond to treatment to reduce the hormone level	Specimen of breast tissue is removed by excision or needle biopsy
Estrogen; estrogen total; estrogen fractions; estradiol; estriol	To evaluate adrenal cortex, ovaries, and testes function	Blood sample
Evoked potential studies (EP studies); evoked responses; auditory brainstem-evoked potentials; somatosensory evoked potentials; visual evoked potentials	To diagnose lesions of the nervous system by evaluating integrity of the visual, somatosensory, and auditory nerve pathways	Electrodes are placed in appropriate positions and recordings measured
Exercise electrocardiography (exercise ECG); graded exercise tolerance test; stress testing; treadmill test	Measures the efficiency of the heart during physical activity	Electrocardiography and blood pressure monitoring while the patient walks a treadmill; pharmacological stress through adenosine, dipyridamole and dobutamine rather than exercise
Fecal fat	To evaluate for steatorrhea in Crohn disease, cystic fibrosis, or Whipple disease	Stool samples for three days

continued

NAME/SYNONYMS	INDICATION(S)	DESCRIPTION/SPECIMEN
Ferritin	To evaluate the size of iron storage compartments; to diagnose anemia	Blood sample
Folic acid; folate	To diagnose macrocytic anemia	Blood sample
Follicle-stimulating hormone (FSH)	To diagnose hypogonadism, infertility, menstrual disorders, or precocious puberty	Blood sample
Free erythrocyte protoporphyrin (FEP)	To detect iron-deficiency anemia	Blood sample
Gallbladder scan; hepatobiliary imaging; HIDA scan	To assess for cholecystitis or obstruction of the cystic duct	Injection of a radionuclide compound; visualization of the biliary system using a scintillation camera
Gallium scan; body scan	To detect primary neoplasms, metastatic lesions, and inflammatory processes	Injection of radioactive gallium citrate; a scintillation camera is used to scan the entire body
Gamma-glutamyl transferase (GGT); gamma-glutamyl transpeptidase (GGTP)	To assist in the diagnosis of liver problems	Blood sample
Glucose tolerance test (GTT); oral glucose tolerance test (OGTT)	To assess the rate at which glucose is removed from the bloodstream	Blood and urine sample
Glucose, postprandial; 2-hour postprandial blood sugar (2-hour PPBS); 2-hour p.c. glucose	To assess response of the body to ingestion of a meal with a standard amount of carbohydrates; to assess for effectiveness of insulin therapy	Blood sample
Glucose; blood sugar; fasting blood sugar (FBS); fasting plasma glucose (FPG)	To assess for problems with glucose metabolism	Blood sample
Glycosylated hemoglobin (G-Hb); glycated Hgb; glycohemoglobin; hemoglobin A_{1c} (HbA_{1c}, $HgbA_{1c}$)	To determine the average blood glucose level for the previous two to three months	Blood sample

Gonorrhea culture	To test for *Neisseria gonorrhoeae*	Endocervical culture: swab of cervical mucus Urethral culture: swab from 2–3 cm within the urethra Rectal culture: swab from 1 inch within the anal canal Oral culture: swab of the pharynx and tonsillar crypts
Heart scan; cardiac nuclear scanning; multiple gated acquisition (MUGA) scan; myocardial scan; nitroglycerin scan; pyrophosphate (PYP) heart scan; thallium scan; thallium stress testing	To assess for occurrence, extent, and prognosis of myocardial infarction; to monitor effectiveness of angioplasty coronary artery grafts; to assess myocardial wall abnormalities; to assess effect of nitroglycerin on ventricular function	Injection of radiopharmaceutical followed by nuclear imaging
Hematocrit (Hct); crit; packed cell volume (PCV)	To assess the extent of blood loss and of normal hydration levels	Blood sample
Hemoglobin electrophoresis (Hgb electrophoresis)	To identify abnormal types or amounts of hemoglobin	Blood sample
Hepatitis antigens and antibodies; hepatitis A; hepatitis B; hepatitis C; Deltavirus	To assess for inflammation of the liver caused by virus, bacteria, or toxic substance	Blood sample
Herpes simplex antibody; herpes genitalis; herpes simplex virus (HSV); herpesvirus	To assess for the herpes simplex virus	Blood sample
High-density lipoprotein (HDL)	To assess for high-density lipoprotein in the blood	Blood sample
Human immunodeficiency virus (HIV) testing; acquired immunodeficiency syndrome (AIDS) test; AIDS serology; ELISA for HIV and antibody; HIV antibody test; Western blot for HIV and antibody	To assess for human immunodeficiency virus	Blood sample

continued

NAME/SYNONYMS	INDICATION(S)	DESCRIPTION/SPECIMEN
Human leukocyte antigen test (HLA test); HLA typing; tissue typing	To determine tissue compatibility (organ transplantation) and paternity testing	Blood sample
5-Hydroxyindoleacetic acid (5-HIAA)	To identify the presence of carcinoid tumors of the intestine	Urine sample
Immunoelectrophoresis; antibodies; gamma globulins; immunoglobulins (IgA, IgD, IgE, IgG, IgM)	To measure immunoglobulins in the blood	Blood sample
Immunoglobulin light chain; Bence Jones protein	To assess for multiple myeloma and amyloidosis	Urine sample
Insulin; insulin assay; serum insulin	To assess the level of insulin in the serum	Blood sample
Iron (Fe)	To assess for anemia	Blood sample
Kidneys, ureters, and bladder (KUB) radiography; flat plate x-ray of the abdomen; scout film	To provide an overall view of the lower abdomen; to assess for renal enlargement or displacement, congenital anomalies, renal or ureteral calculi, or ascites and gas in the intestine	X-ray film
Lactic acid; blood lactate	To assess for liver disease	Blood sample
Lactic dehydrogenase and isoenzymes; lactate dehydrogenase (LDH, LD)	To assess for myocardial infarction, biliary obstruction, bone metastases, cancer of prostate, hepatitis, liver damage, macrocytic anemia, pneumonia, muscular dystrophy, shock, or trauma	Blood sample
Lactose tolerance test	To assess for lactose intolerance	Blood sample
Laparoscopy; gynecologic laparoscopy; pelvic endoscopy; pelviscopy; peritoneoscopy	To assess pelvic pain for carcinoma, ectopic pregnancy, endometriosis, pelvic inflammatory disease (PID), and pelvic masses; to view fallopian tubes; to perform lysis of adhesions, ovarian biopsy and tubal ligation	Insertion of a laparoscope through a small subumbilical incision for visualization and performance of procedures

Lipase	To assess abdominal pain	Blood sample
Lipid profile	To evaluate coronary heart disease risk	Usually includes high-density lipoprotein cholesterol, low-density lipoprotein cholesterol, triglycerides, and total cholesterol tests
Liver and pancreatobiliary system ultrasonography; gallbladder and biliary system sonogram; liver sonogram; pancreas sonogram	To assess for jaundice, hepatomegaly, abdominal trauma, cholecystectomy, metastatic tumors of the liver, or pancreatic carcinoma; to guide needle biopsy	Ultrasound waves are sent into the body with a small transducer pressed against the skin
Liver biopsy; percutaneous liver biopsy; percutaneous needle biopsy of the liver	To assess for disease of the liver, elevated liver enzymes, jaundice, hepatomegaly, or possible rejection of a transplanted liver	An aspirated sample of liver tissue
Low-density lipoprotein (LDL)	To assess for low-density lipoprotein in the blood	Blood sample
Lung biopsy	To determine malignancy of a lung mass	An aspirated sample of lung mass tissue
Lung scan; lung perfusion scan; lung ventilation scan; ventilation/perfusion scanning	To detect pulmonary emboli and assess arterial perfusion of the lungs	Perfusion: A radiopharmaceutical is injected; scintillation camera is positioned over the chest Ventilation: Radioactive gas is inhaled through a face mask and the chest is scanned
Lupus erythematosus test (LE test); LE cell prep	To assess for lupus erythematosus	Blood sample
Luteinizing hormone (LH)	To determine whether ovulation occurred; to assess amenorrhea and infertility	Blood sample
Lyme disease antibody test	To evaluate for Lyme disease	Blood sample
Lymphangiography; lymphography	To detect and stage lymphomas and assist in diagnosis	Injection of contrast medium, fluoroscopic visualization, and radiographic films

continued

NAME/SYNONYMS	INDICATION(S)	DESCRIPTION/SPECIMEN
Magnesium	To assess magnesium level in the blood	Blood sample
Magnetic resonance imaging (MRI)	To evaluate cerebral infarct, abnormalities of the brain and spine, knee injuries, arteriovenous malformation, congenital heart disease, dementia, glomerulonephritis, hydronephrosis, multiple sclerosis, osteomyelitis, seizures, or spinal cord injuries	Imaging while in the MRI cylinder
Mammography	Routine screening for tumors	X-ray film of the breast
Mediastinoscopy	To assess for lymphoma, sarcoidosis, staging of lung cancer	Direct visualization of the contents of the mediastinum via a mediastinoscope inserted at the suprasternal notch
Mononucleosis test; Epstein-Barr virus (EBV) antibody test; heterophil antibody titer (HAT); infectious mononucleosis testing; Monospot test	To assess for infectious mononucleosis	Blood sample
Myelography	To assess the subarachnoid space of the spinal column for tumors, bone structure changes, or herniations of intervertebral disks	Injection of contrast dye; visualization via fluoroscopy
Osmolality; serum/urine osmolality	To assess fluid and electrolyte imbalance, fluid requirements, urine concentration, and antidiuretic hormone (ADH) secretion, and for toxicology workups	Blood or urine sample
Oximetry; ear oximetry; pulse oximetry; oxygen saturation (SaO_2)	To monitor the oxygen saturation of arterial blood	A sensor emits beams of light through the skin tissue; rate and amount of absorption is converted to percentage of oxygen saturation present in the blood and is shown on monitor

Test	Purpose	Description
Papanicolaou smear (Pap smear); exfoliative cytologic study; Pap test	To detect cervical cancer	Vaginal speculum is used to collect secretions from the cervix and endocervical canal
Paracentesis; abdominal paracentesis; abdominal tap; peritoneal fluid analysis; peritoneal tap	To determine cause of ascites or to remove ascites; to check for abdominal bleeding	Sample of fluid obtained through incision or needle
Parathyroid hormone (PTH); parathormone	To assist in differential diagnosis of parathyroid disorder	Blood sample
Partial thromboplastin time (PTT); activated partial thromboplastin time (APTT)	To detect bleeding disorders	Blood sample
Phosphorus (P); phosphate (PO_4)	To assess phosphorus level	Blood sample
Platelet count; thrombocyte count	To assess for thrombocytopenia, thrombocytosis, and platelet production	Blood sample
Pleural biopsy	To determine the nature of pleural tissue	Pleural tissue aspirated through a needle
Positron emission tomography (PET); single photon emission computed tomography (SPECT)	To study blood flow and metabolic changes in organs or regions of body tissues	A radionuclide is administered via IV or inhalation while the patient is in the PET scanner
Potassium, blood/urine	To assess potassium level in the blood	Blood or urine sample
Pregnancy test; human chorionic gonadotropin (hCG)	To determine pregnancy	Blood sample
Proctosigmoidoscopy; anoscopy; proctoscopy; sigmoidoscopy	To assess lower abdominal pain, change in bowel habits, and passage of blood, mucus, or pus in the stool	The sigmoidoscope is inserted into the anus and advanced into the distal sigmoid colon; the sigmoid colon, rectum, and anus are visualized
Progesterone	To assess the level of progesterone in the blood	Blood sample

continued

NAME/SYNONYMS	INDICATION(S)	DESCRIPTION/SPECIMEN
Prostate-specific antigen (PSA)	To assess for prostate cancer, monitor its progression, or monitor response to prostate cancer treatment	Blood sample
Protein C (PC)	To evaluate severe thrombosis	Blood sample
Protein electrophoresis; serum protein electrophoresis (SPEP)	To evaluate albumin and each of the globulins	Blood sample
Protein; total protein (TP); albumin; alpha globulins; beta globulins; gamma globulins	To assess level of protein in the blood	Blood sample
Prothrombin time (PT); PT ratio/INR; pro time	To evaluate the coagulation process	Blood sample
Pulmonary function tests (PFTs); spirometry	To measure pulmonary volume and capacity	Mouth-breathing into a spirometer as directed for readings of lung capacity and volume
Pyruvate kinase (PK)	To assess the level of pyruvate kinase in the blood; to assess for hemolytic anemia	Blood sample
Red blood cell count (RBC count); erythrocyte count	To measure the number of red blood cells per cubic millimeter of blood	Blood sample
Red blood cell indices (RBC indices); blood indices; mean corpuscular hemoglobin (MCH); mean corpuscular hemoglobin concentration (MCHC); mean corpuscular volume (MCV)	To determine normal size and amount of red blood cells	Blood sample
Renal biopsy; kidney biopsy	To assist in diagnosis of renal parenchymal disease	Renal tissue sample obtained through surgical incision or needle aspiration
Renal scan; kidney scan	To detect renal infarct, renal arterial atherosclerosis, renal trauma, renal tumor or cyst, or primary renal disease	Radiopharmaceutical administered by injection; scintillation camera is positioned over the right upper quadrant
Reticulocyte count (retic count)	To assist in differential diagnosis of anemia	Blood sample

Test	Purpose	Description
Retrograde pyelography; pyelography	To assess for bladder tumor, hydronephrosis, polycystic kidney disease, ureteral calculi, or renal cysts	Radiopaque iodine-based contrast medium is injected through a catheter into each kidney; radiographic films are taken of the ureters
Rheumatoid factor (RF); rheumatoid arthritis (RA) factor	To assess for rheumatoid arthritis	Blood test
Scrotal ultrasound; ultrasound of testes	To assess for scrotal masses and infection; to evaluate scrotal pain; to locate undescended testicles	A transducer is placed on the skin and moved as needed to provide visualization of the scrotal contents
Semen analysis; seminal cytology; sperm count	Used in fertility workup	Semen specimen
Skeletal x-ray; bone x-ray; sella turcica x-ray; skeletal radiography; skull x-ray; spinal x-ray; vertebral x-ray	To assess for bone deformities, fractures, dislocations, tumors, or metabolic abnormalities	Radiographic films of specific area
Sodium	To assess sodium level in the blood	Blood or urine sample
Sputum culture and sensitivity (sputum C&S)	To diagnose bacterial, fungal, or nonbacterial lower respiratory tract pneumonia	Sputum sample
Stool culture; stool for ova and parasites	To identify pathogens in the GI tract	Stool sample
Stool for occult blood; Hematest; Hemoccult (guaiac)	To identify blood in the GI tract	Stool sample
Syphilis serology; fluorescent treponemal antibody absorption (FTA-ABS); micro-hemagglutination-*Treponema pallidum* (MHA-TP); rapid plasma reagin (RPR); Venereal Disease Research Laboratory (VDRL)	To assess for *Treponema pallidum*	Blood sample

continued

A67

NAME/SYNONYMS	INDICATION(S)	DESCRIPTION/SPECIMEN
T- and B-cell lymphocyte counts; acquired immunodeficiency syndrome (AIDS) T-lymphocyte cell markers; CD4 marker; T- and B-cell lymphocyte surface markers	To assess for Graves disease, viral infection, human immunodeficiency virus (HIV) infection, risk of AIDS, measles, or Hodgkin disease	Blood sample
Testosterone	To assess testosterone level in blood	Blood sample
Thoracentesis; pleural fluid analysis; pleural tap	To determine the cause of fluid production in the lungs	Aspiration of pleural fluid via a needle
Throat culture and sensitivity	To assess for pathogens	Swab of the tonsillar area and posterior pharynx
Thyroid scan	To assess size, shape, position, and function of the thyroid gland	IV administration of radioactive trace; scanning with scintillation camera
Thyroid-stimulating hormone (TSH); thyrotropin	To assess thyroid hormone levels	Blood sample
Thyroxine (T_4); total T_4	To assess thyroid hormone levels	Blood sample
Thyroxine, free; free T_4 (FT_4)	To assess thyroid hormone levels	Blood sample
Total carbon dioxide content; carbon dioxide content (CO_2 content)	To assess carbon dioxide level in the blood	Blood sample
Total iron-binding capacity (TIBC)	To assess the maximum amount of iron that can be bound to transferrin	Blood sample
Toxicology screen; drug screen	To determine cause of drug toxicity, monitor compliance, and detect presence of drugs for employment or legal purposes	Blood or urine specimen
Transesophageal echocardiography (TEE)	To evaluate thoracic, aortic, and cardiac disorders	Gastroscope introduced into the mouth and advanced to the level of the right atrium of the heart; sound waves from the transducer on the gastroscope are transformed into a visual display

Test	Purpose	Sample
Transferrin; iron-binding protein; siderophilin	To assess the level of transferrin	Blood sample
Triglycerides	To assess triglyceride levels	Blood sample
Triiodothyronine (T_3); total T_3	To assess thyroid hormone levels	Blood sample
Triiodothyronine uptake test (T_3 uptake); T_3 resin uptake	To assess thyroid hormone levels	Blood sample
Tuberculin (TB) skin test; Mantoux test; purified protein derivative (PPD) skin test; tine test	To screen for previous infection by tubercle bacillus	Intradermal injection of purified protein derivatives (PPDs)
Upper gastrointestinal and small bowel series; gastric radiography; small bowel study; stomach x-ray; upper GI series	To assess dysphagia, regurgitation, burning epigastric pain, hematemesis, melena, or weight loss	Barium is ingested while fluoroscopic films are taken of the esophagus, stomach, and small intestine
Urea nitrogen; blood urea nitrogen (BUN); urinary urea nitrogen	To assess the level of urea nitrogen	Blood or urine sample
Uric acid	To assess for uric acid	Blood or urine sample
Urinalysis (UA); routine urinalysis	Routine screening in physical examination, preoperative testing, hospital admission for diagnosis of infection of the kidneys and urinary tract, and diseases unrelated to the urinary system	Urine sample
Urine culture and sensitivity (urine for C&S)	To identify the specific bacterial organism present in the urine	Urine sample
Uroflowmetry; urine flow studies; urodynamic studies	To detect dysfunctional voiding patterns	Urination into a flowmeter to measure duration, amount, and rate
Urography; infusion pyelogram; intravenous pyelogram (IVP)	To demonstrate normal anatomy and wide range of abnormalities involving the urinary tract	IV administration of contrast material, which is excreted by the kidneys; radiographs are exposed for evaluation of the morphology and function of the urinary tract

continued

NAME/SYNONYMS	INDICATION(S)	DESCRIPTION/SPECIMEN
Vanillylmandelic acid and catecholamines (VMA); dopamine; epinephrine; norepinephrine; metanephrine; normetanephrine	To assess for neuroblastoma, stress, idiopathic orthostatic hypertension, and pheochromocytoma	Urine sample
Vitamin B_{12}; cyanocobalamin; extrinsic factor	To assess for macrocytic anemia	Blood sample
White blood cell (WBC) count and differential; basophil count; eosinophil count; leukocyte count; lymphocyte count; monocyte count; neutrophil count	To assess the total number of white blood cells and percentage of differentiation	Blood sample
Wound culture and sensitivity	To identify the specific bacterial organism present in the wound	Swab of the wound site

Normal Lab Values

Tests	Conventional Units	SI Units
*alanine aminotransferase (ALT, SGPT), serum		
male	13–40 U/L (37°C)	0.22–0.68 μkat/L (37° C)
female	10–28 U/L (37°C)	0.17–0.48 μkat/L (37° C)
albumin, serum, adult	3.5–5.2 g/dL	35–52 g/L
adult >60 y	3.2–4.6 g/dL	32–46 g/L
*aldolase, serum	1.0–7.5 U/L (30° C)	0.02–0.13 μkat/L (30° C)
ammonia, plasma (heparin)	9–33 μmol/L	9–33 μmol/L
*amylase		
serum	27–131 U/L	0.46–2.23 μkat/L
urine	1–17 U/h	0.017–0.29 μkat/h
*aspartate aminotransferase (AST, SGOT), serum	10–59 U/L (37°C)	0.17–1.00 −2 to +3 kat/L (37°C)
bicarbonate, serum (venous)	22–29 mmol/L	22–29 mmol/L
*bilirubin, serum, total	0.2–1.3 mg/L	3–22 μmol/L
blood urea nitrogen (BUN), serum	6–20 mg/dL	2.1–7.1 mmol urea/L
calcium, serum	8.6–10.0 mg/dL	2.15–2.50 mmol/L
carbon dioxide content, total, serum or plasma (heparin)	22–28 mmol/L	22–28 mmol/L
carotene, serum	10–85 μg/dL	0.19–1.58 μmol/L
*cell counts, adult		
RBC		
male	4.7–$6.1 \times 10^6/\mu L$	4.7–$6.1 \times 10^{12}/L$
female	4.2–$5.4 \times 10^6/\mu L$	4.2–$5.4 \times 10^{12}/L$
WBC (leukocytes)		
total	4.8–$10.8 \times 10^3/\mu L$	4.8–$10.8 \times 10^6/L$
differential	*Percentage*	
myelocytes	0	
neutrophils – bands (bands, stabs)	3–5	
neutrophils – segmented (segs)	54–62	
lymphocytes (lymphs)	23–33	
monocytes (monos)	3–7	
eosinophils (eos)	1–3	
basophils (basos)	0–1	
platelets	130–$400 \times 10^3/\mu L$	130–$400 \times 10^9/L$
reticulocytes	0.5–1.5% red cells	0.005–0.015 of RBC

continued

Tests	Conventional Units	SI Units
chloride, serum or plasma	98–107 mEq/L	98–107 mmol/L
cholesterol, serum, adult		
desirable	<200 mg/dL	<5.2 mmol/L
borderline	200–239 mg/dL	5.2–6.2 mmol/L
high risk	≥240 mg/dL	≥6.2 mmol/L
*creatinine, serum or plasma		
male	0.7–1.3 mg/dL	62–115 μmol/L
female	0.6–1.1 mg/dL	53–97 μmol/L
ferritin, serum		
male	20–150 ng/mL	20–250 μg/L
female	10–120 ng/mL	10–120 μg/L
Note: Ferritin values of <20 ng/mL (20 μg/L) have been reported to be generally associated with depleted iron stores.		
*folate, serum	3–20 ng/mL	7–45 nmol/L
glucose (fasting)		
blood	65–95 mg/dL	3.5–5.3 mmol/L
plasma or serum	74–106 mg/dL	4.1–5.9 mmol/L
glucose, 2 h postprandial, serum	<120 mg/dL	<6.7 mmol/L
HDL-cholesterol (HDL-C), serum or plasma (EDTA), adult		
desirable	>40 mg/dL	>1.04 mmol/L
borderline	35–40 mg/dL	0.78–1.04 mmol/L
high risk	<35 mg/dL	<0.78 mmol/L
hematocrit		
male	42–52%	0.42–0.52
female	37–47%	0.37–0.47
hemoglobin		
male	14.0–18.0 g/dL	2.17–2.79 mmol/L
female	12.0–16.0 g/dL	1.86–2.48 mmol/L
*iron, serum		
male	65–175 μg/dL	11.6–31.3 μmol/L
female	50–170 μg/dL	9.0–30.4 μmol/L
iron binding capacity, total (TIBC), serum	250–425 μg/dL	44.8–71.6 μmol/L
iron saturation, serum		
male	20–50%	0.2–0.5
female	15–50%	0.15–0.5

continued

Tests	Conventional Units	SI Units
*isoenzymes, serum by agarose gel electrophoresis		
fraction 1	14–26% of total	0.14–0.26 fraction of total
fraction 2	29–39% of total	0.29–0.39 fraction of total
fraction 3	20–26% of total	0.20–0.26 fraction of total
fraction 4	8–16% of total	0.08–0.16 fraction of total
fraction 5	6–16% of total	0.06–0.16 fraction of total
*lactate dehydrogenase (LDH), total, serum, adult	100–190 U/L	1.7–3.2 μkat/L
adult >60 y	110–210 U/L	1.9–3.6 μkat/L
LDL-cholesterol (LDL-C), serum or plasma (EDTA), adult		
desirable	<130 mg/dL	<3.37 mmol/L
borderline	130–159 mg/dL	3.37–4.12 mmol/L
high risk	≥ 160 mg/dL	≥ 4.13 mmol/L
*lipase, serum	23–300 U/L (37°C))	0.39–5.1 μkat/L (37°C)
magnesium		
serum	1.3–2.1 mEq/L	0.65–1.07 mmol/L
	1.6–2.6 mg/dL	16–26 mg/L
urine	6.0–10.0 mEq/24 h	3.0–5.0 mmol/24 h
osmolality		
serum	275–295 mOsm/kg serum water	275–295 mmol/kg serum water
urine	50–1200 mOsm/kg water	50–1200 mmol/kg water
ratio, urine/serum	1.0–3.0	1.0–3.0
	3.0–4.7 after 12 h fluid restriction	3.0–4.7 after 12 h fluid restriction
partial thromboplastin time, activated (APTT)	<35 sec	<35 sec
*phosphatase, alkaline, total, serum	38–126 U/L (37°C)	0.65–2.14 μkat/L
phosphorus, inorganic, serum, adult	2.7–4.5 mg/dL	0.87–1.45 mmol/L
potassium		
plasma (hep)	3.5–4.5 mEq/L	3.5–4.5 mmol/L
serum	3.5–5.1 mEq/L	3.5–5.1 mmol/L
*protein, total, serum	6.4–8.3 g/dL	64–83 g/L
*prothrombin time (pro time, PT)	12–14 sec	12–14 sec
sodium, serum or plasma (heparin), adult	136–145 mEq/L	136–145 mmol/L

continued

Tests	Conventional Units	SI Units
specific gravity, urine	1.002–1.030	1.002–1.030
*thyroid-stimulating hormone (TSH), serum	0.4–4.2 μU/mL	0.4–4.2 mU/L
thyroxine (T_4), serum	5–12 μg/dL (varies with age)	65–155 nmol/L (varies with age)
triglycerides, serum, fasting		
desirable	<250 mg/dL	<2.83 mmol/L
borderline high	250–500 mg/dL	2.83–5.67 mmol/L
hypertriglyceridemic	>500 mg/dL	>5.65 mmol/L
*uric acid		
serum, enzymatic		
male	4.5–8.0 mg/dL	0.27–0.47 mmol/L
female	2.5–6.2 mg/dL	0.15–0.37 mmol/L

*Test values are method dependent.

Appendix 5
Sample Reports and Dictation

ADMISSION SUMMARY

DATE OF ADMISSION: 06/01/02

HISTORY OF PRESENT ILLNESS: This is a 64-year-old black male who was transferred to us status post respiratory failure secondary to cardiac arrest and pneumonia, status post thoracic aortic aneurysm repair, chronic renal failure, insulin-dependent diabetes mellitus, and congestive heart failure. This patient was admitted to an outside hospital to the cardiothoracic service 1 day prior to repair of his aortic arch aneurysm. The patient had reported intermittent episodes of shortness of breath which were relieved with rest. His condition has worsened over the past 2 years. He had a cardiac catheterization done which revealed normal left ventricular flow, mild coronary artery disease, mild aortic insufficiency, and an ascending aortic aneurysm measuring 6.8 cm. An echocardiogram that same month revealed a dilated aortic root, mild aortic insufficiency with marked concentric left ventricular hypertrophy, and an ejection fraction of 50%. The patient reported no chest pain at that time.

The patient underwent surgery and was diagnosed with annuloaortic ectasia with ascending aortic aneurysm. There was an aortic insufficiency. Procedure performed was a Tyrone David aortic valve resuspension and aortic root replacement utilizing a 28-mm Hemashield Dacron tube graft combined with ascending aortic replacement. This was done on cardiopulmonary bypass with moderate hypothermia. The patient was weaned post surgery, extubated.

Hemodialysis was also begun on his first postoperative day without complications. On the third and fourth postoperative days, he developed a decrease in his mental status and became febrile and had increased respiratory distress. He was started on tobramycin and blood cultures were taken, as well as sputum and urinary cultures. On the fifth postoperative day, the patient suffered a cardiac arrest, from which he was successfully resuscitated. This required approximately 5 minutes of cardiopulmonary resuscitation and multiple pressure support and re-intubation.

Since then, the patient has had a very rocky intensive care unit course. This included multiple treatments for pneumonia and continued respiratory failure, also requiring tracheostomy placement. He continued to require hemodialysis three times per week. This was also complicated by failure of his atrioventricular shunt in his left forearm, which required him to undergo a Quinton catheter replacement. He had a gastrojejunostomy tube placed on the 22nd postoperative day. A CAT scan done on the 20th postoperative day revealed global atrophy and age-related changes; no sign of hemorrhage or infarction was noted. The patient also developed a fever and was started on IV antibiotics. He was cultured positive for Serratia in his sputum. This would be continued into this hospitalization.

PAST MEDICAL HISTORY: Positive for aortic insufficiency, aortic arch aneurysm, insulin-dependent diabetes mellitus, diabetic retinopathy, congestive heart failure, end-stage renal disease, and blindness of his right eye.

PAST SURGICAL HISTORY: Removal of bladder cyst. Left atrioventricular shunt for dialysis.

PSYCHOSOCIAL HISTORY: The patient apparently lives with family. He does not smoke cigarettes or drink alcohol.

ALLERGIES: No known allergies.

MEDICATIONS ON TRANSFER: Heparin flush for his arterial line; Nystatin 10 cc t.i.d. swish and swallow; Prilosec 20 mg via tube q.d.; Nu-Iron 150 mg p.o. b.i.d.; Diflucan 100 mg per tube q.d.; NPH insulin 40 units subq q.a.m.; NPH insulin 40 units subq q.p.m.; Amphojel 90 cc/L with tube feedings; sliding scale insulin q.4h.; Haldol 2 to 5 mg IV q.2h. p.r.n. agitation; calcium chloride 10 mg/kg IV if calcium less than 2.0; Amphojel 30 cc per NG tube q.6h. p.r.n. for pH less than 5 or positive guaiacs; KCl 40 mEq q.d.; Artificial Tears both eyes p.r.n.; Senokot 10 cc via J-tube q.d.; Colace 100 mg per J-tube b.i.d.; trach care every shift; cefepime 500 mg IV q.d. to be given immediately after dialysis Monday, Wednesday, and Friday; lactulose 30 cc per J-tube q.6h.; deflate rectal balloons q.4h.; calcitonin 200 IU subq q.12h.; and tube feedings at 40 cc/hr.

TRANSFER LABS: WBC 5.6, hematocrit 36.2, platelets 192. BUN 26, creatinine 6.6.

PHYSICAL EXAMINATION: This is a large black man who is not responding to verbal stimuli and appears to be in no acute distress. HEENT: No nodes or masses are noted. The patient has an opaque right pupil and opacity also noted of left pupil. The trachea is midline. The patient has fair dentition. He is n.p.o. No JVD is noted. Chest: Bilateral breath sounds are equal; rhonchi bilaterally. Tan secretions. He is on assist control of 8, tidal volume 800, PEEP of +5, FiO_2 50%. Bilateral chest excursion is equal. Atrial and ventricular pacemaker wires are noted and insulated at this time. Midsternal incision is well healed. There is a left subclavian triple-lumen catheter noted which is two days old. No drainage noted. Cardiovascular: S_1, S_2, S_4, occasional PVCs. Apical pulse and radial pulse are not equal. The patient is on dopamine 8 mcg/kg per minute and epinephrine 0.01 mcg/kg per minute. Unable to get O_2 saturations. A right radial A-line is intact and correlates with his cuff blood pressure. Abdomen: Large and soft. Positive bowel sounds. A Moss tube is noted with some granulation tissue. No tube feedings at this time. Extremities: Cool. An old AV shunt is noted in the left forearm, but there is no bruit or thrill noted. There is a new left femoral Quinton catheter in place. He has 1+ pedal pulses. Skin: Skin is extremely dry with tenting. Buttocks and sacral area are excoriated. A stage II noted. Foley to straight gravity drainage with amber urine. There is also a rectal tube intact with large amounts of green diarrhea. Neurologic: The patient responds to painful and some tactile stimuli but does not follow commands.

IMPRESSIONS
1. Respiratory failure secondary to cardiac arrest and pneumonia.
2. Congestive heart failure.
3. Chronic renal failure.
4. Insulin-dependent diabetes mellitus.
5. Status post thoracic aortic aneurysm repair.
6. Serratia pneumonia.
7. Malnutrition.
8. Right eye blindness.
9. Hypercalcemia.

PLAN
1. Continue ventilatory support at this time and evaluate for weaning.
2. Possible neurologic evaluation.
3. Dialysis 3 times per week.
4. Continue IV antibiotics.
5. PT and OT evaluations.
6. Monitor labs.
7. Check A-line and check ulnar pulse.
8. Check fluid status.
9. Wound care to sacral area.
10. Monitor calcium, phosphate, and magnesium levels.

CARDIAC ULTRASOUND

PATIENT: **CHART #:**   **DATE:**

REFERRING PHYSICIAN: **TAPE #:**

SEX: **AGE:**   **DOB:**   **HEIGHT:** ' "   **WEIGHT:** lbs.

REASONS FOR REFERRAL: Atrial fibrillation, history of stroke, TIA.

MEASUREMENTS (2-D/M-MODE)

LEFT VENTRICLE:
   9 IVSD (8–11 mm)
   6 LVPW (8–11 mm)
   40 LVEDD (<57 mm)
   21 LVESD
   45% Fractional Shortening (>25%)
   77% Ejection Fraction, 69% by volume studies

RIGHT VENTRICLE:
   5 RV Free Wall
   36 RV Dimension

LEFT ATRIUM:
   38 AP diam. (<40 mm)

   21 Area   (<18 cm^2)
RIGHT ATRIUM:

   19 Area (<18 cm^2)
AORTA:
   25 AP diam (<35 mm)

IVC:
   Collapsibility Index

INTERPRETATION

Parasternal imaging reveals normal aortic root. Left atrium is 21 cm^2 in the apical view, 38 mm by M-mode. Septum is 9 mm. Posterior wall is 6 mm. Left ventricular end-diastolic dimension is 40 mm. End-systolic dimension is 21 mm. Ejection fraction is 77% by volume studies.

In the apical view, left ventricular function is normal with good symmetrical wall motion. There is very mild mitral regurgitation. There is 1+ tricuspid regurgitation. Right ventricular systolic pressure is 34 mm. There is no apparent thrombus in the left atrium or left ventricle.

IMPRESSIONS

1. Mild atrial enlargement.
2. Very mild mitral regurgitation.
3. Mild tricuspid regurgitation.
4. Normal left ventricular size and function.
5. No apparent thrombus in the left atrium or the left ventricle.

COLONOSCOPY

INDICATIONS: The patient is a 65-year-old white male, guaiac positive, recently having lower abdominal pain.

Prior to the procedure the patient underwent physical examination and was found to have a height of 5 feet 8 inches, weight of 183 pounds, a blood pressure of 164/86, a pulse of 93, and respirations of 12; afebrile, alert and oriented x 3. Throat clear. Lungs clear. Cardiac examination shows regular rate and rhythm. Abdomen is soft and nontender, positive bowel sounds. Extremities are symmetrical without cyanosis, clubbing, or edema.

DESCRIPTION OF PROCEDURE: The Olympus CF-100 TL colonoscope was used. With premedication of 35 mg of Demerol and 5 mg of Versed IV, the colonoscope was advanced to the cecum in a well-prepped colon. In the cecum there was a lobulated polypoid mass, which was flat and approximately 3 x 3 cm in size. Actually several polyps were removed with a snare, but a large amount were left in place.

Further removal of the scope revealed in the mid-ascending colon what appeared to be a small fold, but on return biopsy it could be seen that this was another villous-appearing lesion that was a flat sessile polyp about 2 cm in diameter. Biopsies were obtained. No attempt at removal was carried out because if the patient is referred for surgery this could be included in the operative segment and removed at that point. Further withdrawal revealed a normal transverse colon.

The descending colon and sigmoid colon showed widespread diverticulosis with no evidence of polyps in this area. The rectum appeared normal, and large external hemorrhoids were removed that were present on the examination before the procedure.

ASSESSMENT
1. Multiple colon polyps in the right colon that have the appearance of villous adenomas and will probably require surgical removal.
2. Diverticulosis.
3. External hemorrhoids.

PLAN: Continue Anusol suppositories and await biopsy results. A discussion will be carried out concerning possible surgical options.

ECHOCARDIOGRAM #1

M-MODE ECHOCARDIOGRAM: M-mode echocardiographic study demonstrates a left atrial size of 2.8 cm with an aortic root dimension of 3.3 cm. The left ventricular internal diastolic dimension is 4.4 cm, while the internal systolic dimension is 2.7 cm. The intraventricular septum measures 8 mm, and the posterior wall measures 10 mm.

2D ECHOCARDIOGRAM: The mitral valve is a normal-appearing structure without systolic anterior motion or mitral valve prolapse. The aortic valve is a normal-appearing trileaflet structure. The tricuspid valve appears normal. The pulmonic valve was not well seen.

All four cardiac chambers and the aortic root are normal in size. Left ventricular wall thickness appears normal.

Right and left ventricular wall motion appears normal. The estimated left ventricular ejection fraction is 65%.

No intracardiac masses, thrombi, or vegetations are apparent. The intraventricular septum and intraatrial septum were visually intact. No pericardial effusion is present.

IMPRESSION: Overall normal study.

ECHOCARDIOGRAM #2

PROCEDURE PERFORMED: Echocardiogram.

INDICATIONS: Echocardiography requested for evaluation of cardiac function and to evaluate for possible infective endocarditis in the face of an osteomyelitis.

FINDINGS: Study was of good technical quality.

The aortic root is of normal diameter. The aortic valve leaflets move freely. There is no stenosis or regurgitation. The left atrium is enlarged with an internal diameter of 5.5 cm. The mitral valve leaflets move freely. Diastolic flow is normal. There is no regurgitation identified. The left ventricle is normal size with a mild concentric hypertrophy and normal function. The right ventricle is normal size. The right atrium is borderline enlarged. No tricuspid regurgitation is identified. Some of the subcostal views reveal narrowing of the pleural spaces, suggesting a pleural effusion; correlation with chest x-ray is required.

IMPRESSIONS
1. Left ventricular hypertrophy with normal size and contractility.
2. No vegetation or other evidence suggesting infective endocarditis seen.
3. Bi-atrial enlargement, left greater than right.
4. Possible pleural effusion; correlation with chest x-ray required.

ECHOCARDIOGRAM #3

M-mode and 2-dimensional echocardiograms were performed which were technically adequate studies. A screening Doppler study was also performed at no charge to the patient.

ECHOCARDIOGRAPHIC FINDINGS

1. The left ventricle is within normal limits in terms of overall wall thickness and internal dimensions at both end-systole and end-diastole. No high-grade segmental wall motion abnormalities or contractions were identified. Overall left ventricular function is normal with estimated ejection fraction of 55–60%.
2. The left atrium is normal in size at 3.6 cm. The right atrium and right ventricle are normal in size. Right ventricular systolic function is normal.
3. The aortic valve is a trileaflet structure with minimal commissural edge thickening and normal systolic leaflet excursion of 1.9 cm. The aortic root size is normal at 2.6 cm. Aortic root wall motion is normal.
4. The mitral and tricuspid valves are structural and functional. Specifically, there is no evidence of prolapse or stenosis and no B notch was seen on the M-mode tracing of the anterior mitral valve leaflet. The pulmonic valve cannot be well imaged, owing to technical limitation.
5. No pericardial abnormality or significant pericardial effusion was seen. There was some systolic "lifting" posteriorly near the base.
6. No intracavitary mass, lesion, or thrombi were detected.
7. The intraatrial septum and intraventricular septum are visually intact.
8. The inferior vena cava does not appear to be dilated on a limited subcostal view.

A screening Doppler study showed no hemodynamically significant abnormality flow patterns.

IMPRESSION: Technically adequate echocardiogram demonstrating normal left ventricular size and function without high-grade segmental wall motion abnormality. The estimated ejection fraction is 55–60%. No chamber enlargement was seen. No hemodynamically significant valvular abnormalities were apparent. No obvious cardiac source of chest pain was seen on this tracing.

ELECTROCARDIOGRAM #1

Ventricular rate 79 bpm. PR interval 0.19. QRS duration 0.97. QT corrected 0.42. QRS axis −40 degrees.

OVERALL INTERPRETATION: Normal sinus rhythm. She has a left anterior fascicular block and nonspecific ST wave changes. Abnormal electrocardiogram. No previous tracings for comparison.

ELECTROCARDIOGRAM #2

Ventricular rate 53 bpm. PR interval 0.17. QRS duration 0.14. QT corrected 0.50. QRS axis −30 degrees.

OVERALL INTERPRETATION: Pattern of sinus bradycardia, left ventricular hypertrophy, and left bundle branch block. No significant change from previous tracings, however.

ELECTROCARDIOGRAM #3

Rate 53. PR 0.17. QRS 0.08. Axis normal. Nonspecific ST-T changes compatible with drug, metabolic, or ischemic effects. No change from prior tracings.

ELECTROCARDIOGRAM #4

EKG reveals a normal sinus rhythm with a ventricular rate of just over 70 beats per minute. There is a first-degree AV block with a PR interval of greater than 200 ms. There does appear to be an old septal MI, age undetermined. The QRS duration, QT interval, and QRS axis all appear within normal limits. There are some nonspecific ST and T-wave changes noted. Therefore, this should be considered an abnormal EKG.

ELECTROENCEPHALOGRAM

PROCEDURE PERFORMED: Electrodiagnostic laboratory electroencephalogram.

PURPOSE OF THE STUDY: Assess for encephalopathy.

TECHNICAL REMARKS: This is a technically satisfactory 10-channel EEG done using disc electrodes. Differential and referential runs and an estimated international 10–20 placement system was used.

DESCRIPTION: During the awake state, a background rhythm of approximately 5 to 6 cycles/second was seen intermittently during the tracing. Most prominent in the tracing was the presence of diffuse 4- to 7-Hz theta activity. There was some mixed delta activity in the 1- to 3-Hz range, but this was much less frequent, and all of the slowing was diffuse and nonlateralizing. Noted in the tracing were some triphasic waves which were of low voltage and seen intermittently. During drowsiness, there was some decrease in voltage of the recording. There continued to be mostly theta slowing but with some less frequent delta activity and occasional triphasics as described above.

ASSESSMENT: This is an abnormal electroencephalogram during the awake and drowsy states, consistent with a moderate degree of encephalopathy. It is noted that triphasic waves have been classically seen in hepatic encephalopathy; however, the findings of triphasic waves have subsequently been determined to be nonspecific. Please note that the absence of epileptiform activity on an electroencephalogram does not fully rule out the presence of a seizure disorder.

ELECTRONEUROMYOGRAPHY REPORT #1

CLINICAL INFORMATION: Rule out carpal tunnel syndrome.

NERVE CONDUCTION VELOCITIES

Left Median Motor	Elbow to Wrist	54.3 m/sec
	Distal Delay	3.9 ms
Left Median Sensory	Elbow to Wrist	62.5 m/sec
	Distal Delay	3.3 ms
Left Ulnar Motor	Across the Elbow	62.5 m/sec
	Below Elbow to Wrist	61.3 m/sec
	Distal Delay	2.6 ms
Right Median Sensory	Elbow to Wrist	51.1 m/sec
	Distal Delay	3.1 ms
Right Median Motor	Elbow to Wrist	52.3 m/sec
	Distal Delay	3.5 ms

ASSESSMENT: Normal nerve conduction velocities and distal delays, although the left median motor distal delay is 3.9 ms, which is on the slow side of normal.

ELECTRONEUROMYOGRAPHY REPORT #2

CLINICAL INFORMATION: Rule out carpal tunnel syndrome.

NERVE CONDUCTION VELOCITIES

Right Median Motor	Elbow to Wristz	56.4 m/sec
	Distal Delay	5.2 ms

Right Median Sensory	Elbow to Wrist	62.8 m/sec
	Distal Delay	4.8 ms
Right Ulnar Motor	Across the Elbow	70.5 m/sec
	Below Elbow to Wrist	62.6 m/sec
	Distal Delay	2.7 ms
Left Median Motor	Elbow to Wrist	61.1 m/sec
	Distal Delay	4.1 ms
Left Median Sensory	Elbow to Wrist	64.7 m/sec
	Distal Delay	4.4 ms

Muscles	**Insertional & Resting Activity**	**Volitional Activity**
RIGHT		
Opponens	Normal	Polyphasic potentials noted on volition.
LEFT		
Opponens	Normal	Normal

ASSESSMENT: Patient has prolongation of the distal delay of the median nerve across the wrists bilaterally, suggestive of carpal tunnel syndrome, with evidence of axonal degeneration noted on needle EMG study on the right side.

SUMMARY: Bilateral carpal tunnel syndrome, right worse than left.

ELECTRONEUROMYOGRAPHY REPORT #3

CLINICAL INFORMATION: Rule out tarsal tunnel syndrome.

NERVE CONDUCTION VELOCITIES

Right Posterior Tibial	Knee to Ankle	48.7 m/sec
	Distal Delay	
	Pick-up at abductor hallucis	5.9 ms
	Pick-up at abductor digiti quinti	5.5 ms
Left Posterior Tibial	Knee to Ankle	50.1 m/sec
	Distal Delay	
	Pick-up at abductor hallucis	6.2 ms
	Pick-up at abductor digiti quinti	6.9 ms

ASSESSMENT: Prolongation is noted of the distal delay of the posterior tibial nerve on the left side, both the medial and lateral plantar nerves. The right side is slightly prolonged on the medial plantar portion.

SUMMARY: Tarsal tunnel syndrome noted on the left. Borderline findings on the right.

ELECTRONEUROMYOGRAPHY REPORT #4

CLINICAL INFORMATION: Rule out peripheral neuropathy versus radiculopathy.

NERVE CONDUCTION VELOCITIES

Left Posterior Tibial	Knee to Ankle	26.8 m/sec
	Distal Delay	8.3 ms
	Evoked Action Potentials	400 mv
Left Peroneal	Knee to Ankle	33.3 m/sec
	Distal Delay	5.3 ms
	Evoked Action Potentials	400 mv
Right Posterior Tibial	Knee to Ankle	31.5 m/sec
	Distal Delay	6.4 ms
	Evoked Action Potentials	500 mv

Muscles	Insertional & Resting Activity	Volitional Activity
LEFT		
Anterior Tibialis	Normal	Polyphasic potentials and giant motor units noted on volition.
Extensor Hallucis Longus	Normal	Polyphasic potentials and giant motor units noted on volition.

ASSESSMENT: Patient has significant slowing of nerve conduction velocities, suggestive of peripheral neuropathy with changes indicative of an axonal degeneration on limited EMG. In the face of a peripheral neuropathy with abnormalities on EMG, there is no way that any assessment can be made regarding a more proximal lesion, such as a nerve root irritation. If that is considered, a MRI scan could be performed.

ESOPHAGOGASTRODUODENOSCOPY

PROCEDURE: Esophagogastroduodenoscopy.

INDICATIONS FOR PROCEDURE: Previous vomiting and history of hematemesis.

ANESTHESIA: Topical Cetacaine, Demerol 100 mg, and Versed 6 mg IV.

INSTRUMENT USED: Olympus adult videoendoscope.

FINDINGS: Under direct vision, the endoscope was advanced into the esophagus without difficulty. Mucosa in the esophagus was normal without esophagitis and no varices, masses, strictures, or tears. The Z line was at 36 cm from the incisor level. The scope was then advanced into the stomach with a very small hiatus hernia noted. Retroflex view of the cardia and fundus was normal. Views in the body and antrum revealed normal gastric mucosa, with the exception of just some minimal gastritis of the body of the stomach. There was no bleeding and no ulcers, masses, or vascular abnormalities. The pylorus was normal. First and second portions of the duodenum revealed normal duodenal mucosa without duodenitis or duodenal ulcers. There were no masses in the duodenum and no bleeding sites. Upon withdrawal of the scope, I looked at the vocal cords, epiglottis, and surrounding areas, and everything was normal.

ASSESSMENT
1. Small hiatus hernia.
2. Minimal gastritis of the body of the stomach with no bleeding.

HISTORY & PHYSICAL

HISTORY OF PRESENT ILLNESS: This 73-year-old female recently had biopsy of a skin lesion of her right chest wall, which revealed metastatic breast carcinoma. The patient originally had a modified radical mastectomy followed by adjuvant chemotherapy. She had a small skin lesion on her chest wall and was started on treatment with Nolvadex. Lately, however, the chest wall lesion has increased in size, and she is admitted for excision of the area after biopsy-proven metastatic disease. She has had a chest film and bone scan performed, which were normal. Her Nolvadex has been discontinued, and she has been started on Megace by her oncologist.

PAST MEDICAL HISTORY
Major illnesses: None.

Operations: Removal of ovarian cyst, hysterectomy, and mastectomy.

ALLERGIES: None.

MEDICATIONS: Megace.

REVIEW OF SYSTEMS: HEENT: Notes no frequent headaches, epistaxis, or chronic colds. Cardiac: No history of chest pain, shortness of breath, or pedal edema. Respiratory: No history of chronic cough, hemoptysis, or night sweats. Gastrointestinal: No history of nausea and vomiting, hematemesis, or melena. Genitourinary: No history of frequency, urgency, or dysuria.

PHYSICAL EXAMINATION: Vital signs: Blood pressure 140/80. Pulse of 88. Respirations of 20. Temperature of 99.2°F. Height: 5 feet 1–1/2 inches. Weight of 140 pounds. General: This is a well-developed, well-nourished white female in no acute distress. Integument: Skin warm and dry. Turgor good. HEENT: Pupils were equal, round, and reactive to light. Extraocular movements are intact. Pharynx benign. Neck: No thyromegaly or cervical adenopathy. Chest: Clear to percussion and auscultation. Cardiac: Normal sinus rhythm; no thrills or murmurs. Breasts: The right breast is missing. The left breast is normal to examination. There is a 1.5- x 2.5-cm nodular erythematous area of the right anterior chest in the area of the old mastectomy site. Abdomen: Soft; no organomegaly, no masses, and no tenderness. Extremities: Full range of motion of all joints. No pedal edema.

IMPRESSION: Recurrent breast carcinoma, right anterior chest wall.

DISPOSITION: Admit for surgery.

HOLTER MONITOR

INTERPRETATION: Monitor was worn for 24 hours; quality of the tracing was good. Patient reported palpitations and weakness on several occasions. She has very occasional PVCs and some PACs. No particular tachyarrhythmias are noted.

Of interest were multiple pauses, the longest exceeding 4 seconds. These pauses appear to be prompted by a high degree of AV block, and the 4-second pause has at least 4 nonconducted P waves. The shorter pauses of 2 to 3 seconds also have 2 to 3 nonconducted P waves. There are occasional isolated blocked P waves. There does not appear to be any lengthening of the PR interval to suggest a Wenckebach-type phenomenon. Patient did record feeling a little lightheaded on one of these occasions.

IMPRESSION: Several pauses in the range of 2 to 4 seconds with multiple nonconducted P waves, which appear to be related to a high degree of AV block. They seem to come paroxysmally throughout the day. Otherwise, occasional PVCs. No significant tachyarrhythmia is noted.

MODIFIED BARIUM SWALLOW STUDY

STUDY: Modified barium swallow with fluoroscopy and study of the thoracic esophagus and cervical spine.

The patient was placed in a lateral projection and upright position and given 7 consistencies with 13 swallows performed.

FINDINGS

1. There is some penetration seen with both thick and thin liquids with a straw. No aspiration identified.
2. Oral phase showed mild-to-moderate abnormalities of bolus formation and tongue pumping with moderate-to-severe premature spillage. Mastication, bolus transit time, palatal movement, and labial closure were within functional limits.
3. Pharyngeal phase showed moderate-to-severe abnormalities of swallowing response with mild abnormalities of peristalsis. Transit time and tongue propulsion were within functional limits.
4. Moderate-to-severe pooling is seen within the valleculae and piriform sinuses.
5. A volitional and reflexive swallow and cough are present.
6. Cervical spine showed mild-to-moderate degenerative changes from C2-C6 with anterior and posterior spurs, which are most severe at C5-C6. Generalized osteoporosis is present.
7. Thoracic esophagus exam was performed in both lateral and AP projections. Mild calcification is seen within the aortic arch which is only very slightly indenting the midesophagus. Mild decrease in peristalsis is seen with mild tertiary contractions and mild stasis with some pooling seen in the midesophagus. No hiatal hernia or reflux seen. No evidence of other motility disturbances or mucosal abnormalities. No fixed masses, constricting, or obstructing lesions. No evidence of other intrinsic or extrinsic abnormalities.

STRESS TEST #1

The patient underwent stress testing today for some atypical chest pain. His exercise tolerance was excellent. No ST changes were seen. The test appears to be negative. Results reviewed with the patient. Recheck with his family practice doctor on his cholesterol.

STRESS TEST #2

INTERPRETATION OF THE STRESS TEST: The patient was stressed according to Bruce protocol. He completed 12–1/2 minutes of testing without difficulty. No chest pain or unusual symptoms. Blood pressure response was appropriate. No ST changes seen during exercise or recovery.

IMPRESSION: Negative maximal stress test with good tolerance.

SWALLOWING STUDY

STUDY: Swallowing study.

The patient was challenged with thin liquids, nectar, and puree.

ORAL PHASE: Good oral coordination and strength with good formation of bolus and propulsion of bolus.

PHARYNX: Moderate delay in swallowing reflex with weak pharyngeal contraction and poor closure. Significant pooling of material in the valleculae and piriform sinuses with eventual spill of piriform sinus material into the glottis. Frank aspiration following particularly large residual. Moderate clearance of residual material with repeated dry swallows. No cricopharyngeal discoordination.

IMPRESSION: Weak pharyngeal contraction with residual material building in the piriform sinuses, eventually spilling into the glottis with frank aspiration, most pronounced with thin liquids.

VENOUS DOPPLER ULTRASOUND

PROCEDURE PERFORMED: Venous Doppler ultrasound, bilateral lower extremities.

BRIEF HISTORY: The patient has respiratory failure. Venous Doppler ultrasound is performed to exclude deep venous thrombosis.

DESCRIPTION OF PROCEDURE: Bilateral deep venous Doppler ultrasound of the lower extremities was performed, including common femoral, superficial femoral, greater saphenous vein, popliteal vein, and posterior tibial vein. On the right side there was no area of thrombosis noted. On the left side there was a thrombosis of the common femoral as well as the superficial femoral vein noted. This seems to be a fresh thrombosis. There was no collateralization noted. There is still some flow around the right superficial femoral vein.

CONCLUSIONS

1. No thrombosis of the left side noted.
2. There is a thrombosis of the right common femoral as well as the superficial femoral vein seen.
3. The patient will need to be anticoagulated.
4. The results were discussed with the patient's primary care physician.

Herbarium

HERB	**CONDITION**
acetyl-L-carnitine (ALC)	Alzheimer disease; depression; diabetic peripheral neuropathy.
adrenal extract	Fatigue, stress.
alder buckthorn	See buckthorn bark.
alfalfa (*Medicago sativa*)	Anemia; antifungal; antiinflammatory; balances hormones; bleeding disorders; bone and joint disorders; colon and digestive disorders; detoxifier; diuretic; hypercholesterolemia; promotes pituitary function; skin disorders; ulcers.
aloe (*Aloe barbadensis*)	Healing agent in wounds, minor burns, and other minor skin irritations; short-term treatment of occasional constipation.
alpha-lipoic acid	Antioxidant; diabetes, diabetic neuropathy; glaucoma, prevention of cataracts; prevention of neurologic disorders including stroke.
androstenedione	Increases strength and muscle mass.
angelica root (*Angelica archangelica*)	Loss of appetite; peptic discomforts such as mild spasms of the gastrointestinal tract, feeling of fullness, and flatulence.

HERB	**CONDITION**
aortic extract	Enhancement of function, structure, and integrity of arteries and veins; helps protect against various forms of vascular disease, including athero-sclerosis, cerebral and peripheral arterial insufficiency, hemorrhoids, varicose veins, and vascular retinop-athies, such as macular degeneration.
arabinoxylane	Decreases chemotherapy-induced leukopenia; immune system enhancement (antiviral and anticancer activity); reported useful in HIV infection.
arginine (amino acid)	Helps lower elevated cholesterol; improves circulation; increases lean body mass; inflammatory bowel disease; immune enhancement; male infertility; sexual vitality and enhance-ment; surgery and wound healing.
artichoke leaf (*Cynara scolymus*)	Bloating, nausea, and impairment of digestion; lipid-lowering agent.
ashwagandha (*Withania somnifera*)	Adaptogen; chemotherapy and radiation protection; general tonic; stress, fatigue, nervous exhaustion.
astragalus (*Astragalus membranaceus*)	Adaptogen (tonic-enhanced endurance, stamina); improvement in immune function and disease resistance; improvement in tissue oxygenation; support for chemotherapy and radiation.
Autumn crocus	See colchicum.
bacopa (*Bacopa monniera*)	Memory enhancement, improvement of cognitive function.

HERB	**CONDITION**
barberry (*Berberis vulgaris*)	Decreases heart rate; kills bacteria on skin; reduces bronchial constriction; slows breathing.
bayberry (*Myrica cerifera, M. gale*)	Astringent; clears congestion; eyes; helps circulation; hypothyroidism; immune system; reduces fever; ulcers.
beard-moss	See usnea.
beta-carotene (fat-soluble vitamin)	Cancer prevention, cervical dysplasia; immunostimulant; photoprotection (erythropoietic protoporphyria).
betaine hydrochloride	Digestive aid (hypochlorhydria and achlorhydria).
betony	See wood betony.
bilberry fruit (*Vaccinium myrtillus*)	Local therapy for mild inflammation of the mucous membranes of the mouth and throat; nonspecific, acute diarrhea.
biotin / vitamin B_7 (water-soluble vitamin)	Brittle nails; diabetes, diabetic neuropathy; seborrheic dermatitis; uncombable hair syndrome.
birch (*Betulae folium*)	Antiinflammatory; diuretic; pain reliever, joint pain; urinary tract infections.
black cohosh (*Cimicifuga racemosa*)	Arthritis; mild depression; premenstrual syndrome; vasomotor symptoms of menopause.
black elder	See elder.
blackberry root (*Rubus fruticosus*)	Antidiarrheal agent.
bladderwrack (*Fucus vesiculosus*)	Fibrocystic breast disease; hypothyroidism; rich source of iodine, potassium, magnesium, calcium, and iron.

HERB	**CONDITION**
blessed thistle (*Cnicus benedictus*)	Anorexia; dyspepsia; loss of appetite.
boldo leaf (*Peumus boldus*)	Mild dyspepsia; spastic gastrointestinal complaints.
boron (trace mineral)	Osteoarthritis; osteoporosis; rheumatoid arthritis.
boswellia (*Boswellia serrata*)	Antiinflammatory; arthritis; ulcerative colitis.
box holly	See butcher's broom.
buchu (*Barosmae folium*)	Bladder and kidney problems; decreases inflammation of colon, gums, mucous membranes, prostate, sinuses, vagina; diabetes; digestive disorders; fluid retention.
buckthorn bark (*Rhamnus frangula*)	Constipation; stool softener.
butcher's broom (*Ruscus aculeatus*)	To treat discomforts of chronic venous insufficiency (such as pain and heaviness, leg cramps, itching, and swelling); hemorrhoids.
calcium (bulk mineral)	Blood pressure regulation; cancer prevention; elevated cholesterol; hypertension; kidney stones; pregnancy; premenstrual syndrome; prevention of osteoporosis.
calendula (*Calendula officinalis*)	Antibacterial; antifungal; antiprotozoal; antiviral; vulnerary; wound-healing agent.
carnitine (amino acid)	Congestive heart failure; enhanced athletic performance; hyperlipidemia; male infertility; weight loss.
cascara / cascara sagrada bark (*Rhamnus purshiana*)	Constipation; stool softener.

HERB	**CONDITION**
cassia / cassia cinnamon	See Chinese cinnamon bark.
cat's claw (*Uncaria tomentosa*)	Antiinflammatory; antimicrobial (antibacterial, antifungal, antiviral); antioxidant; immunostimulant.
cayenne (*Capsicum annuum*)	Cardiovascular circulatory support; digestive stimulant; inflammation and pain (topical).
celery (*Apium graveolens*)	Antioxidant; appetite; arthritis; kidney problems; muscle spasms; reduces blood pressure; sedative.
chamomile flower (*Matricaria recutita, Chamomilla recutita*)	Used internally as symptomatic treatment of digestive ailments such as dyspepsia, epigastric bloating, impaired digestion, and flatulence. Used externally for irritation of the mouth and gums and for hemorrhoids.
chaste berry (*Vitex agnus-castus*)	Irregularities of menstrual cycle; mastodynia; premenstrual complaints.
Chinese cinnamon bark (*Cinnamomum aromaticum*)	Bloating; colic; dyspepsia; flatulence; gastrointestinal tract spasm; loss of appetite.
chittem bark	See cascara.
chondroitin sulfate	Osteoarthritis.
chromium (trace mineral)	Atherosclerosis; elevated cholesterol; elevated triglycerides; glaucoma; hypoglycemia; type 1 diabetes, type 2 diabetes; weight loss.
coenzyme Q_{10}	Angina; adjunct in chemotherapy; chronic fatigue syndrome; congestive heart failure; hypertension; muscular dystrophy; obesity; periodontal disease.

HERB	**CONDITION**
colchicum (*Colchicum autumnale*)	Gout. Not available over the counter.
coleus (*Coleus forskohlii*)	Asthma, allergies; congestive heart failure; eczema; hypertension; psoriasis.
collagen (type II)	Arthritis; diabetic ulcers resulting from arterial insufficiencies; first- and second-degree burns; pressure ulcers; surgical and traumatic wounds; topical application for wound healing; venous stasis ulcers.
comfrey (*Symphytum officinale*)	Healing of wounds and skin conditions.
common balm	See lemon balm.
conjugated linoleic acid (CLA)	Increases metabolism, decreases body fat.
copper (trace mineral)	Anemia; osteoporosis; rheumatoid arthritis.
coriander seed / coriander fruit (*Coriandrum sativum*)	Dyspeptic complaints and loss of appetite.
corn silk (*Zea mays*)	Diuretic; aids bladder, kidneys, small intestine; carpal tunnel syndrome; edema; obesity; premenstrual syndrome; prostate disorders.
cranberry (*Vaccinium macrocarpon*)	Treatment and prevention of urinary tract infections.
curled dock	See yellow dock.
dehydroepiandrosterone (DHEA) (hormone)	Antiaging; depression; diabetes; fatigue; lupus.

HERB	**CONDITION**
devil's claw root (*Harpagophytum procumbens*)	Used internally to treat allergies, arthritis, blood diseases, fever, headache, indigestion, lumbago, neuralgia, painful arthroses, rheumatism, and tendinitis; used externally to treat boils, skin lesions, sores, and ulcers.
docosahexaenoic acid (DHA)	Alzheimer disease; attention deficit disorder and attention deficit hyperactivity disorder; Crohn disease; diabetes; eczema, psoriasis; elevated triglycerides; hypertension; rheumatoid arthritis.
dong quai (*Angelica sinensis*)	Amenorrhea; anemia; dysmenorrhea; phytoestrogen; premenstrual syndrome.
Echinacea purpurea herb	Supportive therapy for colds and chronic infections of the respiratory tract and lower urinary tract. Used externally for wounds and chronic ulcerations that heal poorly.
elder (*Sambucus nigra*)	Berry used as antiviral and antioxidant and for influenza; flower used as antiinflammatory, diaphoretic, diuretic, and for colds and influenza.
English walnut leaf	See walnut leaf.
ephedra (*Ephedra sinica*)	Bronchodilator in asthma; decongestant in allergies, sinusitis, hay fever; thermogenic aid in weight loss.
evening primrose (*Oenothera biennis*)	Attention deficit disorder; diabetic neuropathy; eczema, dermatitis, psoriasis; endometriosis; hyperglycemia; irritable bowel syndrome; multiple sclerosis; omega-G6 fatty acid supplementation; premenstrual syndrome, menopause; rheumatoid arthritis.

HERB	**CONDITION**
fennel oil/seed (*Foeniculum vulgare*)	Catarrh of the upper respiratory tract; dyspepsia, fullness, and flatulence.
fenugreek seed (*Trigonella foenum-graecum*)	Anorexia, dyspepsia, gastritis; used topically for furunculosis, gout, leg ulcers, lymphadenitis, myalgia, and wounds.
feverfew (*Tanacetum parthenium*)	Antiinflammatory, rheumatoid arthritis; prevention of migraine headaches.
fish oil	Crohn disease; diabetes; dysmenorrhea; eczema, psoriasis; hypertension; hypertriglyceridemia; memory enhancement; rheumatoid arthritis.
folic acid (water-soluble vitamin)	Alcoholism; anemia; atherosclerosis; cancer prevention (colon and breast); cervical dysplasia; Crohn disease; depression; gingivitis; osteoporosis; pregnancy (prevention of birth defects), lactation.
frangula	See buckthorn bark.
garlic (*Allium sativum*)	As an adjuvant to dietetic management in treatment of hyperlipidemia; mild hypertension; prevention of age-dependent vascular changes.
ginger root (*Zingiber officinale*)	Prophylaxis of nausea and vomiting associated with motion sickness, postoperative nausea, and seasickness.
ginkgo (*Ginkgo biloba*)	Alzheimer disease, dementia; asthma; increases peripheral blood flow (cerebral vascular disease, peripheral vascular insufficiency, impotence, tinnitus, and resistant depression); intermittent claudication; macular degeneration; memory enhancement; sexual dysfunction (antidepressant-induced).

HERB	**CONDITION**
ginseng, Asian (*Panax ginseng*)	Adrenal tonic; enhancement of physical and mental performance, energy levels; adaptation to stress; supports immune function; adjunct support for chemotherapy and radiation.
ginseng, Siberian (*Eleutherococcus senticosus*)	Adaptogen; beneficial in athletic performance; adaptation to stress (decreased fatigue); support of immune function.
glucosamine (amino sugar)	Osteoarthritis; rheumatoid arthritis and other inflammatory conditions.
glutamine (amino acid)	Adjunct therapy for cancer, HIV; alcoholism; catabolic wasting processes; peptic ulcers; performance enhancement; postsurgical healing; ulcerative colitis and other forms of inflammatory bowel disease.
gotu kola (*Centella asiatica*)	Hemorrhoids (topical); memory enhancement; psoriasis; support/ modulation of connective tissue synthesis; venous insufficiency; wound healing (topical).
grape seed (*Vitis vinifera*)	Antiinflammatory; antioxidant; antiplatelet; arterial/venous insufficiency (intermittent claudication, varicose veins); improves circulation; improves capillary fragility; treatment of allergies, asthma.
gravel root (*Eupatorium purpureum*)	Diuretic and urinary tract tonic; fluid retention; prostate disorders.

HERB	**CONDITION**
green tea (*Camellia sinensis*)	Adjunct support for chemotherapy and radiation; anticarcinogenic activity; antioxidant; may lower cholesterol; platelet-aggregation inhibitor; support in cancer prevention and cardio-vascular disease.
hawthorn (*Crataegus laevigata, Crataegus monogyna*)	Angina; cardiotonic; congestive heart failure; hypotension, hypertension; peripheral vascular disease; tachycardia.
holy thistle	See blessed thistle.
hops (*Humulus lupulus*)	Mood disturbances; sleep disturbances.
horehound (*Marrubium vulgare*)	Acute bronchitis, non-productive coughs, and catarrh of the respiratory tract; loss of appetite, bloating, and flatulence.
horse chestnut (*Aesculus hippocastanum*)	Deep venous thrombosis; lower extremity edema; used topically and orally for varicose veins, hemorrhoids, and other venous insufficiencies.
horseradish (*Armoracia rusticana*)	Catarrhs of respiratory tract; supportive therapy for urinary tract infections.
huckleberry	See bilberry fruit.
hydrangea (*Hydrangea arborescens*)	Diuretic; bladder infection; kidney disease; obesity; prostate disorders; kidney stones (combined with gravel root).
hyssop (*Hyssopus officinalis*)	Circulatory problems; congestion; blood pressure; epilepsy; fever; gout; weight problems; used topically to promote wound healing.
Iceland moss (*Cetraria islandica*)	Irritation of oropharyngeal mucous membranes; cough; loss of appetite.

HERB

iodine (trace mineral)

ipriflavone

iron (trace mineral)

isoflavone (soy)

kava kava (*Piper methysticum*)

Lactobacillus acidophilus (bacteria)

lapacho

lavender (*Lavandula angustifolia*)

lemon balm (*Melissa officinalis*)

licorice root (*Glycyrrhiza glabra*)

lutein

lycopene

lysine (amino acid)

CONDITION

Fibrocystic breast disease; goiter prevention; mucolytic agent.

Prevention of and use in osteoporosis (men and women).

Anemia; menorrhagia; pregnancy; restless leg syndrome.

Cancer prevention; chemotherapy support; decreases bone loss; hypercholesterolemia; menopausal symptoms.

Anxiety; postischemic episodes; sedation; skeletal muscle relaxation.

Constipation; enhances immunity; hypercholesterolemia; lactose intolerance; recolonizes the GI tract with beneficial bacteria during and after antibiotic use; vaginal candidiasis.

See pau d'arco.

Nervous stomach irritation; restlessness or insomnia.

Gastrointestinal complaints; nervous sleeping disorders; tenseness, restlessness, irritability.

Bronchitis; catarrhs of the upper respiratory tract; gastric or duodenal ulcers; rheumatism and arthritis.

Cataracts; macular degeneration.

Atherosclerosis; cancer prevention, especially prostate; macular degeneration.

Angina pectoris; herpes simplex; osteoporosis.

HERB	**CONDITION**
magnesium (bulk mineral)	Asthma; cardiovascular disease; congestive heart failure; diabetes; epilepsy; fatigue; high blood pressure; kidney stones; migraine headaches; mitral valve prolapse; muscle cramps; nervousness; osteoporosis; premenstrual syndrome.
ma huang	See ephedra.
manganese (trace mineral)	Diabetes; epilepsy; osteoporosis.
marshmallow (*Althaea officinalis*)	Bladder infection; digestive upset; diuretic; expectorant; fluid retention; headache; intestinal disorders; kidney problems; sinusitis; soothes and heals skin and mucous membranes; sore throat.
maté (*Ilex paraguariensis*)	Mental and physical fatigue; headache from fatigue.
melatonin (hormone)	Insomnia; recovery from jet lag.
melissa	See lemon balm.
milk vetch root	See astragalus.
mint oil (*Mentha arvensis*)	Used internally for flatulence, functional gastrointestinal and gallbladder disorders, and catarrhs of the upper respiratory tract; used externally for myalgia and neuralgic ailments.
molybdenum (trace mineral)	Nervous system; process waste; energy.
mullein (*Verbascum thapsus*)	Asthma; bronchitis; earache; hay fever; laxative; painkiller; sleep aid; soothes kidney inflammation; swollen glands.
mustard (*Brassica alba, Brassica nigra*)	Digestion; metabolism of fat. Externally, helpful for joint pain, inflammation, chest congestion.

HERB	**CONDITION**
nicotinamide adenine dinucleotide (NADH)	Chronic fatigue; Parkinson disease; stamina and energy.
oak bark (*Quercus robur*)	Inflammatory skin diseases; local treatment of mild inflammation of the genital and anal area; nonspecific, acute diarrhea.
oat straw (*Avenae stramentum*)	Antidepressant; insomnia; skin disorders.
old man's beard	See usnea.
olive leaf (*Olea europaea*)	Antibiotic, antifungal, antiviral; anti-hypertensive activity; hypoglycemic activity.
onion (*Allium cepa*)	Loss of appetite; prevention of atherosclerosis.
orange peel, bitter (*Citrus aurantium*)	Loss of appetite and dyspeptic ailments; minor sleeplessness; neurotonic disorders.
Oregon grape (*Mahonia aquifolium*)	Blood purifier; cleanses liver; skin conditions.
papaya (*Carica papaya*)	Aids digestion; heartburn; inflammatory bowel disorders; loss of appetite.
passion flower (*Passiflora incarnata*)	Sedative; anxiety; hyperactivity; insomnia; neuritis; stress-related disorders.
pau d'arco (*Tabebuia heptaphylla*)	AIDS; allergies; antibacterial; cancer; candidiasis; cardiovascular; infection; inflammatory bowel disease; rheumatism; smoker's cough; tumors; ulcers; warts.
phosphorus (bulk mineral)	Essential for bone formation; heart and kidney function; muscle contraction; tissue repair.

HERB	**CONDITION**
potassium (bulk mineral)	Cardiac arrhythmias; congestive heart failure; hypertension; kidney stones.
pregnenolone	Arthritis; improved mental performance.
progesterone (hormone)	Endometriosis; menopause symptoms; osteoporosis; premenstrual symptoms; prevention of breast cancer.
pumpkin seed (*Cucurbita pepo*)	Irritable bladder and micturition problems of benign prostatic hyperplasia stages 1 and 2; functional disorders of the bladder; difficult urination; childhood enuresis nocturna; irritable bladder; also used to eradicate tapeworms.
pygeum (*Prunus africana*)	Symptoms associated with benign prostatic hyperplasia.
raspberry leaf (*Rubus idaeus*)	Diarrhea; painful and profuse menstruation.
red clover (*Trifolium pratense*)	Liquid extract used for liver detoxification, kidney detoxification; menopausal symptoms.
red yeast rice (*Monascus purpureus*)	Hypercholesterolemic agent; may lower triglycerides and low-density lipoprotein cholesterol and raise high-density lipoprotein cholesterol.
rehmannia (*Rehmannia glutinosa*)	Immunosuppressive agent in rheumatoid arthritis.
rose (*Rosa centifolia*)	Bladder problems; infections.
rose hip tea (*Rosa canina*)	Diarrhea.
rosemary (*Rosmarinus officinalis*)	Dyspepsia; supportive therapy for rheumatic diseases and circulatory problems.

HERB	**CONDITION**
sacred bark	See cascara.
sad dock	See yellow dock.
sage leaf (*Salvia officinalis*)	Dyspeptic symptoms; excessive perspiration; gingivitis; stomatitis.
selenium (trace mineral)	AIDS; atherosclerosis; bronchial asthma; cancer prevention; cardiomyopathy; cataracts; chemotherapy/radiation support; eczema.
senna leaf/fruit (*Senna alexandrina*)	Short-term treatment of occasional constipation.
shark cartilage	Cancer therapy; osteoarthritis; rheumatoid arthritis.
skullcap (*Scutellaria lateriflora*)	Aids sleep; anxiety and fatigue; cardiovascular disease; headache; hyperactivity; improves circulation; muscle cramps; nervous disorders; rheumatism; treatment of barbiturate addiction and drug withdrawal.
soy lecithin / phospholipid (*Glycine max*)	Anemia; diabetes; hypercholesterolemia; poor nutrition; rickets; tuberculosis.
sparrowgrass	See asparagus root.
St. John's wort (*Hypericum perforatum*)	Antibacterial; antiinflammatory; antiviral activity in increased doses; mild-to-moderate depression, melancholia, and anxiety; used topically for minor wounds and infections; may be used topically for bruises, muscle soreness, and sprains.
sulfur (trace mineral)	Blood clotting; metabolism, blood sugar regulation.

HERB	**CONDITION**
suma (*Pfaffia paniculata*)	AIDS; anemia, fatigue, stress; cancer; high blood pressure; immune system booster; liver disease.
sweet balm	See lemon balm.
taheebo	See pau d'arco.
tea tree (*Melaleuca alternifolia*)	Disinfectant; skin conditions.
thyme (*Thymus vulgaris*)	Antifungal; coughs and upper respiratory congestion.
usnea (*Usnea barbata*)	Mild inflammation of oropharyngeal mucosa.
uva ursi leaf (*Arctostaphylos uva-ursi*)	Inflammatory disorders or mild infections of the urinary tract.
valerian (*Valeriana officinalis*)	Sedative or hypnotic; nervous tension during premenstrual syndrome, menopause; restless motor syndromes and muscle spasms.
walnut leaf (*Juglans regia*)	Skin rashes (topical).
white horehound	See horehound.
white oak (*Quercus alba*)	Soothing agent in mild inflammation of the throat and mouth.
whortleberry	See bilberry fruit.
wild yam (*Dioscorea villosa*)	Contains steroidal precursors; used for female vitality. Conversion to progesterone in the body is poor.
willow / white willow (*Salix alba*)	Antiinflammatory; antipyretic; reduces fever and arthritic complaints.

HERB	CONDITION
witch hazel (*Hamamelis virginiana*)	Local inflammation of skin, mucous membranes and hemorrhoids; minor skin injuries; varicose veins.
wood betony (*Betonica officinalis*)	Cardiovascular disorders; hyperactivity; neuritis.
wormwood (*Absinthii herba*)	Intestinal parasites; migraine; mild sedative; vascular disorders.
yarrow (*Achillea millefolium*)	Fever, common cold; mild spastic discomforts of the gastrointestinal tract; used topically for slow-healing wounds and skin inflammations.
yellow dock (*Rumex crispus*)	Anemia; blood purifier and cleanser; colon and liver function; eczema, psoriasis, rashes.
yerba maté	See maté.
yohimbe bark / yohimbine (*Pausinystalia yohimbe*)	Erectile dysfunction; exhaustion.
yucca	Arthritis; blood purifier; inflammatory disorders; osteoporosis.

Appendix 7
Profiles of Common Medical Conditions

ALCOHOLISM

DESCRIPTION: Any pattern of alcohol use causing significant physical, mental, or social dysfunction; key features are tolerance, withdrawal, and persistent use despite problems.
System(s) affected: Nervous, gastrointestinal

SPECIAL TESTS:
Psychological questionnaires:
- CAGE (Ewing & Rooss alcohol use questionnaire): 4 items; score > 2 is 74–89% sensitive, 79–95% specific for alcohol use disorder; less sensitive (43–73%) for early problem drinking or heavy drinking
- MAST (Michigan Alcohol Screening Test): 25 items, score > 5 indicates alcohol use disorder, sensitivity 90%, specificity 74%
- AUDIT (Alcohol Use Disorders Identification Test): 10 items, score = 5 is 70–92% sensitive, 73–94% specific

DRUG(S) OF CHOICE:
For detoxification and management of alcohol withdrawal syndrome (multiple regimens):
- Chlordiazepoxide 25–100 mg t.i.d.-q.i.d.
- Diazepam 5–20 mg b.i.d.-t.i.d.
- Lorazepam 1–4 mg t.i.d.-q.i.d.; lorazepam preferred in elderly, severe liver disease, or for IV drip
- Phenobarbital: may be safer in pregnancy
- Use parenteral route only for delirium tremens or when medicines cannot be given by mouth

Adjuncts to detoxification:
- Beta blockers for tachycardia
- Clonidine 0.1 mg t.i.d. for autonomic hyperactivity
- Haloperidol for psychosis, agitation
- Phenytoin for seizures

Adjuncts to rehabilitation:
- Naltrexone 25–100 mg p.o. q.d., opiate antagonist shown to reduce craving and chance of heavy drinking with relapse
- Disulfiram 250–500 mg p.o. q.d., lack of proven efficacy, may provide psychologic deterrent to drinking

Supplements to all:
- Thiamine 100 mg p.o./IV q.d. (first dose IV)
- Folic acid 1 mg p.o./IV q.d.
- Multivitamin p.o. q.d.

- Magnesium sulfate 1 gram IM q.6h. (especially if history of delirium tremens or withdrawal seizure)

ALZHEIMER DISEASE (AD)

DESCRIPTION: A degenerative organic mental disease characterized by progressive intellectual deterioration and dementia, usually occurring after age 65. The diagnosis is made on clinical grounds after ruling out treatable disorders with similar characteristics. Long-term care cost to the nation is approximately $100 billion/year. Usual course—progressive, chronic.
System(s) affected: Nervous

PATHOLOGICAL FINDINGS:
- Gross—diffuse cerebral atrophy in association areas, hippocampus, amygdala, and some subcortical nuclei
- Micro—pyramidal cell loss
- Micro—decreased cholinergic innervation (other neurotransmitters variably decreased)
- Micro—neuritic senile plaques
- Micro—degeneration of locus ceruleus and basal forebrain nuclei of Meynert
- Neurofibrillary tangles
- Amyloid angiopathy common
- Inflammatory cells present

SPECIAL TESTS:
- Cerebrospinal fluid (depending on circumstances and clinical information).
- Extensive neuropsychological battery, only needed if clinical picture is confusing.
- Controversy exists about need for routine cerebral imaging. MRI or CT clearly needed if cognitive decline is recent, there is history of stroke, or focal neurologic signs are present.

DRUG(S) OF CHOICE:
For wandering, restlessness, fidgeting, uncooperativeness, hoarding, irritability:
- Use behavioral techniques.

For depression (occurs in 1/3 of patients):
- Selective serotonin reuptake inhibitors (SSRIs) or trazodone (Desyrel). Start with one-half the usual adult dose.

For insomnia:
- Trazodone 25–100 mg q.h.s., zolpidem (Ambien) 5 mg q.h.s., zaleplon (Sonata) 5–10 mg q.h.s., or temazepam (Restoril) 7.5–15 mg q.h.s.

For moderate anxiety/restlessness:
- Low-dose, short-acting benzodiazepines or buspirone; efficacy unproven.

For severe aggressive agitation, especially if psychotic features present (delusions, hallucinations):

- Low-dose butyrophenones or phenothiazines. Risperidone (Risperdal) 0.5–1.0 mg b.i.d. and other newer atypical antipsychotic agents useful in this setting due to better side effect profile. Attempt periodic dose reductions or discontinuation, especially in nursing home patient.
- Carbamazepine (Tegretol) 100 mg b.i.d.-t.i.d., propranolol (Inderal) 10–40 mg b.i.d.-t.i.d., trazodone 200 mg/day and valproic acid 250–1500 mg/day. Also anecdotally reported in literature to help with severe aggressive agitation. Selective serotonin reuptake inhibitors (SSRIs) also being tried.

For memory enhancement:

- Donepezil (Aricept) 5–10 mg q.d. has supplanted tacrine (Cognex) as the agent of choice. Can be tried in mild-to-moderate disease, but only 30% of patients will respond.
- A recent study supported modest efficacy of selegiline 5 mg b.i.d. and/or vitamin E 1000 IU b.i.d. in slowing progression of disease.
- NSAIDs and estrogen replacement therapy (ERT) are consistently related to lesser incidence and slower progression of Alzheimer disease. Cyclooxygenase-2 (COX-2) NSAIDs offer theoretical advantage due to COX-2 expression in AD. No standards for routine use exist.

SYNONYMS:

- Presenile dementia
- Senile dementia, Alzheimer type (SDAT)
- Primary degenerative dementia

ANGINA

DESCRIPTION: Symptom complex resulting from mismatch of myocardial oxygen demand and supply.

- *Classic angina*—a sense of choking or of pressure or heaviness deep to the precordium, usually brought on by exertion or anxiety and relieved by rest.
- *Anginal equivalent*—exertional dyspnea or exertional fatigue which results from myocardial ischemia and is relieved by rest or nitroglycerin.
- *Variant angina*—also referred to as Prinzmetal angina; describes angina occurring at rest or in atypical patterns, such as after exercise or nocturnally. Prinzmetal angina is caused by coronary artery spasm and is associated with electrocardiogram (ECG) changes (usually ST elevation) during symptoms.
- *Unstable angina*—pain which is new or which is changed in character to become more frequent, more sever, or both. Unstable angina portends myocardial infarction in a certain percentage of patients.

System(s) affected: Cardiovascular

SPECIAL TESTS:
- Electrocardiogram (ECG)—may show evidence of prior myocardial infarction. Other findings are nonspecific and tracings are frequently normal. Bundle-branch block, Wolff-Parkinson-White syndrome, or intraventricular conduction delay may make the ECG unreliable.
- Exercise stress testing

DRUG(S) OF CHOICE:
- Aspirin, 81–325 mg q.d. for all patients with coronary disease in whom this medication is not contraindicated (i.e., warfarin usage).
- Beta-blockers—atenolol 25–100 mg q.d., metoprolol 25–100 mg b.i.d., or propranolol 30–100 mg b.i.d.-t.i.d. Beta-blockers are effective in reducing the heart rate and thereby decreasing oxygen consumption and reducing angina.
- Nitroglycerin 0.3–0.6 mg sublingually is the most effective therapy for acute anginal episodes.
- Nitrates—long-acting nitrates (mononitrates or transdermal nitrates) should be used with allowance for drug-free interval of 10–14 hours to prevent tolerance. A beta-blocker or calcium channel blocker should be used in conjunction with the nitrates during the drug free interval.
- Calcium antagonist—long-acting formulations of verapamil 160–480 mg q.d., diltiazem 90–360 mg q.d., nifedipine 30–120 mg q.d., or amlodipine 5–20 mg q.d. are available. Neither verapamil nor diltiazem should be used in patients with compromised ventricular function (left ventricular ejection fraction < 40%).
- HMG-CoA reductase inhibitors (e.g., pravastatin, lovastatin, and others) should be started for hypercholesterolemia. The new statin drug atorvastatin is particularly effective in lowering total cholesterol, low-density lipoprotein (LDL), and triglycerides.
- Heparin—intravenously in therapeutic doses should be initiated in patients hospitalized with unstable angina.
- Combination therapy—especially nitrates plus calcium antagonists may be used. Triple therapy with addition of beta-blockers may be necessary. Combination therapies should be used with care to avoid impairment of LV function.

SYNONYMS:
- Stenocardia
- Heberden syndrome

ARTERIOSCLEROTIC HEART DISEASE (ASHD)

DESCRIPTION: Arteriosclerosis is a group of diseases characterized by thickening and loss of elasticity of the arterial walls which progressively blocks the coronary arteries and their branches. Arteriosclerosis is the most common form of coronary arteriosclerosis. The process is chronic, occurring over many years, and is the most common cause of cardiovascular disability and death. Other forms of arteriosclerosis include arteriolosclerosis and medial calcific stenosis, both of which are uncommon in the coronary vasculature.

System(s) affected: Cardiovascular

SPECIAL TESTS:
- Echocardiogram (ECG)—variable. May be normal or may see ST segment elevation/depression and/or T wave inversion.
- Exercise stress test—positive

DRUG(S) OF CHOICE:
- Aspirin, 160–325 mg/day, unless contraindicated
- Cholesterol-lowering agents
  - Cholestyramine or colestipol, (bile acid sequestrants) 12–32 grams orally b.i.d.-q.i.d.
  - Niacin 2–6 grams daily in divided doses (highly efficacious, but side effects restrict use)
  - Gemfibrozil 600 mg b.i.d.
  - Probucol 500 mg b.i.d.
  - HMG-CoA reductase inhibitors (dose varies with product): atorvastatin (Lipitor), cerivastatin (Baycol), fluvastatin (Lescol), lovastatin (Mevacor), pravastatin (Pravachol), simvastatin (Zocor)

SYNONYMS:
- Coronary artery disease (CAD)
- Coronary heart disease
- Coronary arteriosclerosis

ARTHRITIS, OSTEO

DESCRIPTION: Osteoarthritis (OA) is the most common form of joint disease. Involves progressive loss of articular cartilage and reactive changes at joint margins and in subchondral bone.

Primary:
- Idiopathic
- Divided into subsets depending on clinical features

Secondary:
- Childhood anatomic abnormalities (e.g., congenital hip dysplasia, slipped femoral epiphyses)
- Inheritable metabolic disorders (e.g., alkaptonuria, Wilson disease, hemochromatosis)

- Neuropathic arthropathy (Charcot joints)
- Hemophilic arthropathy
- Acromegalic arthropathy
- Paget disease
- Hyperparathyroidism
- Noninfectious inflammatory arthritis (e.g., rheumatoid arthritis, spondyloar-thropathies)
- Gout, calcium pyrophosphate deposition disease (pseudogout)
- Septic or tuberculous arthritis
- Posttraumatic

System(s) affected: Musculoskeletal

DRUG(S) OF CHOICE:

Pain relief:
- Acetaminophen; if not effective, nonacetylated salicylates (e.g., salsalate, choline-magnesium salicylate), or low-dose ibuprofen ≤ 1600 mg/day.
- Other NSAIDs can be used and have similar efficacy. Their prolonged use is associated with significant side effects, especially in the elderly. Since pain in osteoarthritis varies from day to day, brief courses of a short-acting NSAID is preferable.
- A new class of NSAIDs referred to as cyclooxygenase-2 (COX-2) specific inhibitors has recently become available. They are less likely to cause stomach ulcers and they work as well as the nonspecific NSAIDs in reducing arthritis inflammation and pain.

Treatment of acute episodes of pain:
- Opioid analgesics (e.g., codeine, oxycodone, propoxyphene)

SYNONYMS:

- Osteoarthrosis
- Degenerative joint disease

ARTHRITIS, RHEUMATOID (RA)

DESCRIPTION: A chronic systemic inflammatory disease of unknown etiology with a predilection for joint involvement. Articular inflammation may be remitting, but if continued usually results in joint damage and disability. Certain extraarticular manifestations are characteristic, including rheumatoid nodules, arteritis, neuropathy, scleritis, pericarditis, and splenomegaly.

System(s) affected: Musculoskeletal, hematologic/lymphatic/immunologic, pulmonary, cardiovascular, nervous

DRUG(S) OF CHOICE:

If patient has ongoing joint pain/morning stiffness, active synovitis, or persistent increase in ESR/CRP despite appropriate dose NSAIDs:

- Start disease modifying antirheumatic drugs (DMARDs) within 2 months.

Early disease or acute/chronic inflammation:

- Aspirin or other NSAID
- COX-2 inhibitors—celecoxib (Celebrex) and rofecoxib (Vioxx)

Severe disease or to minimize disease activity while awaiting DMARDs to act, decrease activity for a short period of time, or control active disease when NSAIDs/DMARDs have failed:

- Prednisone 5–15 mg q.d.

Persistent disease activity (chronic synovitis, a.m. stiffness, increased ESR/CRP, extraarticular disease):

- Intraarticular steroid injections—use judiciously and as rarely as possible (due to long-term effects).
- Antimalarials—hydroxychloroquine (HCQ, Plaquenil) 400 mg q.h.s. for 2–3 months, then 200 mg q.h.s.; 6-month trial usual.
- Auranofin 6–10 mg/day p.o.; reevaluate in 6 months or 1 gram total. Injectable gold—weekly for 22 weeks, then every 2–4 weeks.
- Sulfasalazine (SSZ)—500 mg/day, increase to 2 grams/day over one month; max 2–3 grams/day; 6-month trial.
- Penicillamine (d-penicillamine)—250 mg/day, increase slowly to 750–1000 mg/day; 9 month trial with 8–12 weeks at maximum dosage.
- Azathioprine
- Methotrexate—5–15 mg/week p.o.; 3–6 month trial—for steroid-dependent disease or after other measures unsuccessful.
- Celecoxib (Celebrex), rofecoxib (Vioxx)—perhaps best agents for patients with history of ulcers or GI bleeding.
- Etanercept (Enbrel)—first in the class of tumor necrosis factor (TNF) inhibitors. Given twice weekly SQ.
- Protein A immunoabsorption (Prosorba)—for moderate-to-severe RA. Removes antibodies responsible for RA activity. Primarily for patients who have failed other DMARDs, including MTX.
- Sodium hyaluronate (Hyalgan, Hyalgan G-F20)—hyaluronic acid substitutes. Increases the "quality" of joint fluid, although exact mechanism is unclear. Primarily for pain relief. Expected duration of therapy 6 months to 1 year.
- Infliximab (Remicade)—biologic response modifier which inhibits tumor necrosis factor (TNF). Administered IV once a month.
- Leflunomide (Arava)—modifies T-cell function by inhibiting a key enzyme in pyrimidine synthesis, to decrease autoimmune activity. Benefits are similar to MTX but with much lower incidence of malaise, nausea, and altered mental status; 20 mg daily reported comparable to sulfasalazine at 2 mg daily.

ALTERNATIVE DRUGS: Combinations of methotrexate and cyclosporine, gold salts and prednisone, and methotrexate and hydroxychloroquine all may be useful for resistant disease. Use of methotrexate and either gold or sulfasalazine (SSZ) is not currently supported by clinical trials.

BREAST CANCER

DESCRIPTION: Malignant neoplasm in the breast. Breast cancers are classified as noninvasive (in situ) or invasive (infiltrating) with approximately 70% of all breast cancers possessing a component of invasion.
System(s) affected: Skin/exocrine, pulmonary, gastrointestinal, musculoskeletal, nervous

SPECIAL TESTS:
- Bone scan should be performed if symptoms suggest bony metastasis, if alkaline phosphatase is elevated, or if widespread disease is suspected.
- CT or ultrasound of the abdomen may be indicated if widespread or recurrent disease is suspected.

DRUG(S) OF CHOICE:
- Metastatic disease is considered incurable but treatable, with remissions occurring in 30–40% of patients.
- Chemotherapy reduces the risk of recurrence 22–37% and death 14–27%.
- The process of deciding when to use chemotherapy or hormonal therapy is complex and is dependent on tumor type, size, node status, hormone receptor status, and other factors; practice guidelines are available.
- Combination chemotherapy is preferred over single agents.
- Tamoxifen reduces the risk of recurrence and death for women of all ages; treatment should be continued for 5 years. It should be discontinued if tumor growth continues. It probably is not of benefit to women with estrogen receptor negative tumors.

CATARACT

DESCRIPTION: Any opacity of the lens, either localized or generalized. Single largest cause of blindness in the world, blinding an estimated 17 million people. Types include:
- Age-related ("senile")—over 90%
- Congenital—1/250 newborns, 10–38% of childhood blindness
- Toxic/nutritional
- Systemic disease associated, e.g., myotonic dystrophy, atopic dermatitis

- Metabolic—diabetes (accelerated sorbitol pathway), hypocalcemia, Wilson disease
- "Complicated"—secondary to associated eye disease, e.g., uveitis (juvenile rheumatoid arthritis, sarcoid, etc.); also secondary to occult tumor (melanoma, retinoblastoma)
- Trauma—heat (infrared), electrical shock, radiation, concussion, perforating eye injuries, intraocular foreign body

System(s) affected: Nervous

SPECIAL TESTS:

- Visual quality assessment—glare testing and contrast sensitivity are sometimes indicated. (Hyperglycemic state, as in poor diabetic control, creates osmotic change within lens and may alter measurement of visual acuity and refractive state.)
- Retinal/macular function assessment—potential acuity meter testing, fluorescein retinal angiography sometimes required.

CONGESTIVE HEART FAILURE (CHF)

DESCRIPTION: Congestive heart failure (CHF) is the principal complication of heart disease. It is a pathophysiologic state produced by an abnormality in cardiac pump function (either transient or prolonged). The heart is unable to transport blood in a sufficient flow to meet metabolic needs. CHF occurs at some time in most cases of severe heart disease.

CHF produces a variety of clinical circumstances from acute left ventricular dysfunction (due to tachyarrhythmia, bradyarrhythmia, and acute myocardial infarction) to chronic left ventricular dysfunction (due to chronic volume/pressure overload as seen in valvular heart disease).

Two physiologic components explain most of the clinical findings of CHF—most patients have findings consistent with both mechanisms:
- an inotropic abnormality resulting in diminished systolic emptying (systolic failure)
- a compliance abnormality in which the ability of the ventricles to accept blood is impaired (diastolic failure)

System(s) affected: Cardiovascular, pulmonary

DRUG(S) OF CHOICE:

Diuretics, usually in combination with digitalis, are used to initiate therapy. Angiotensin-converting enzyme (ACE) inhibitors have become a mainstay of therapy. For acute pulmonary edema, IV morphine remains cornerstone of therapy.
- Digoxin
  - Improves contractility, slows ventricular rate in atrial fibrillation.
  - May be harmful in acute MI, hypertrophic cardiomyopathy.
  - Loading dose should be sufficient to have early beneficial effect, especially in

atrial fibrillation with a rapid rate, e.g., 0.5–1.0 mg IV/p.o., then another 1.0–1.5 mg in divided doses q.4–6h.
- Diuretics
  - Furosemide (Lasix)—IV or p.o., depending on severity of pulmonary congestion. May require continuous drip.
  - Metolazone (Zaroxolyn)—excellent addition when furosemide does not seem to be sufficient.
  - Spironolactone—when used carefully, to avoid hyperkalemia. May be proper addition to difficult chronic cases.
- ACE Inhibitors
  - Used to decrease afterload.
  - Improve general symptomatology and overall exercise capacity.
- Beta blockers
  - Carvedilol (Coreg) 3.125 mg p.o. b.i.d. for 2 weeks, then 6.25 mg b.i.d. for 2 weeks, increased to maximum 25 mg b.i.d. for class I to III CHF.
  - Bisoprolol (Zebeta) 5–20 mg/day: in CIBIS-II study significantly decreases all-cause mortality and sudden death.
- Vasodilators
  - IV nitroglycerin may be of short-term benefit to decrease preload, afterload, and systemic resistance.
  - Oral medications (e.g., hydralazine, prazosin, and isosorbide dinitrate) demonstrate tachyphylaxis.

SYNONYMS:
- Heart failure
- Dropsy
- Circulatory failure
- Cardiac failure

DEMENTIA

DESCRIPTION: A pathologic process defined as a persistent impairment of a prior level of intellectual functioning.
- Dementia of Alzheimer type (DAT) is the most common form and characterized by a relentless deterioration of higher cortical functioning. The rate of deterioration is variable.
- Ischemic vascular dementia (IVD), formerly multiinfarct dementia, occurs as a result of clinical or subclinical cerebral infarcts secondary to atherosclerosis. Deterioration is stepwise with periods of clinical plateaus.
- Frontotemporal dementia (FTD)—insidious change in personality with cognitive dysfunction. Onset usually prior to age 65.

- Secondary dementias—also referred to as "reversible dementias" because the cognitive impairment may reverse with treatment of the primary disorder.
- Dementia with Lewy bodies (DLB)—early-onset dementia with associated psychosis, depression.

System(s) affected: Nervous

SPECIAL TESTS:

- Mental status testing
- Neuropsychologic testing
- Electroencephalogram (EEG) for patients with altered consciousness or associated seizures

DRUG(S) OF CHOICE:

Secondary causes, such as hypothyroidism or vitamin B_{12} deficiency:

- Treat appropriately. With other causes, drugs are used to treat behavioral symptoms after nonpharmacologic therapy has failed.

Sundowning, aggressive behavior:

- Antipsychotics such as haloperidol (Haldol) or risperidone (Risperdal) 0.5–1.0 mg at bedtime are reasonable choices in a nonemergency situation.

Depression:

- Nortriptyline (Pamelor) 20–50 mg, desipramine (Norpramin) 25 mg b.i.d., or serotonin reuptake inhibitors sertraline (Zoloft), fluoxetine (Prozac), paroxetine (Paxil), or fluvoxamine (Luvox).

Sleep disturbance:

- Intermittent use of temazepam (Restoril) 15 mg, zolpidem (Ambien) 5 mg, trazodone (Desyrel) 25–50 mg, or chloral hydrate 500 mg at bedtime is occasionally warranted.

Mild-to-moderate DAT:

- Donepezil (Aricept)—5–10 mg every morning.
- Tacrine (Cognex)—10–40 mg q.i.d. (doses >100 mg/day appear to be associated with increased risk of hepatotoxicity). Increase dose in 40 mg/day increments every 6 weeks.
- Vitamin E—2000 IU per day.

SYNONYM: Senility

DIABETES MELLITUS, TYPE 2

DESCRIPTION: Nonketosis-prone hyperglycemia and glucose intolerance due to defects in insulin secretion and peripheral insulin action; accounts for 80% of diabetic cases.

System(s) affected: Endocrine/metabolic, nervous, renal/urologic, cardiovascular

SPECIAL TESTS:
- Glucose tolerance test usually not necessary, except when diagnosing gestational diabetes.
- Hemoglobin A_{1C} not recommended for diagnosis but helpful in management.

DRUG(S) OF CHOICE:
The following classes of agents may be used alone or in combination:
- Biguanide
  - Metformin (Glucophage) 500–850 mg b.i.d.-t.i.d.
- Sulfonylureas
  - Glimepiride (Amaryl) 1–8 mg/day in 1 dose
  - Glipizide (Glucotrol) 2.5–40 mg/day in 1–2 doses (1st 20 mg in a.m.)
  - Glipizide extended-release tablets 5–20 mg/day in 1 dose
  - Glyburide (DiaBeta, Micronase) 1.25–20 mg/day in 1–2 doses (1st 10 mg in a.m.)
- Thiazolidinediones
  - Pioglitazone (Actos) 15–45 mg q.d.
  - Rosiglitazone (Avandia) 2–4 mg b.i.d. Monitor serum transaminase every 2 months for 1st year.
- Alpha-glucosidase inhibitors
  - Acarbose (Precose) 25–100 mg t.i.d.
  - Miglitol (Glyset) 25–100 mg t.i.d. taken at beginning of meals to decrease post-prandial glucose peaks.

SYNONYMS:
- Adult-onset diabetes mellitus
- Nonketotic diabetes mellitus
- Non-insulin-dependent diabetes mellitus (NIDDM)

GASTROESOPHAGEAL REFLUX DISEASE (GERD)

DESCRIPTION: Reflux of gastroduodenal contents into the esophagus with or without esophageal inflammation
System(s) affected: Gastrointestinal

SPECIAL TESTS:
- Esophageal pH monitoring (antacids, H_2 blockers, proton pump inhibitors, and other antisecretory agents can give false negative pH monitoring)
- Esophageal manometry (anticholinergics, theophylline, calcium channel blockers, meperidine, and diazepam may give falsely low LES pressure on manometry)
- Acid perfusion (Bernstein) test
- Gastric analysis (exclude gastric hypersecretion)

DRUG(S) OF CHOICE:

Mild-to-moderate disease:

- H$_2$ blockers in equipotent oral doses, e.g., cimetidine (Tagamet) 800 mg b.i.d. or 400 mg q.i.d.; ranitidine (Zantac) 150 b.i.d.; famotidine (Pepcid) 20 mg b.i.d.; or nizatidine (Axid) 150 mg b.i.d.
- Proton pump inhibitors, e.g., omeprazole 20 mg/day newly indicated in initial heartburn symptom therapy.

Erosive esophagitis:

- Omeprazole (Prilosec) 20 mg q.d.; rabeprazole (Aciphex) 20 mg q.d.; lansoprazole (Prevacid) 30 mg q.d.; or higher dose H$_2$ receptor antagonist (e.g., ranitidine 150 mg q.i.d. or famotidine 40 mg b.i.d.) with or without cisapride for up to 12 weeks.

Severe disease (refractory to initial therapy):

- Proton pump inhibitor given twice daily or higher.

SYNONYMS:

- Reflux esophagitis
- Peptic esophagitis
- Barrett esophagus
- Symptomatic hiatal hernia

HYPOTHYROIDISM, ADULT

DESCRIPTION: A clinical state resulting from decreased circulating levels of free thyroid hormone or from resistance to hormone action. Myxedema connotes severe hypothyroidism.

System(s) affected: Endocrine/metabolic

SPECIAL TESTS: Radioimmunoassay

DRUG(S) OF CHOICE:

- Levothyroxine (Synthroid, Levothroid)
- 50–100 mcg/day. Increase by 25 mcg/day every 4–6 weeks until TSH is in normal range.
- Dosage requirements may vary with age, sex, residual secretory capacity of thyroid gland, other drugs being taken by patient, and intestinal function.
- Elderly patients may require lower dose because clearance is decreased.

SYNONYM: Myxedema

IRRITABLE BOWEL SYNDROME

DESCRIPTION: Altered bowel habits, abdominal pain, gaseousness, in the absence of organic pathology (divided into four types):
- Alternating diarrhea with constipation
- Diarrhea predominant
- Constipation predominant
- Upper abdominal bloating and discomfort

System(s) affected: Gastrointestinal

DRUG(S) OF CHOICE:

Use from among this list according to need or response:
- Bulk-producing agents—psyllium-containing products (Metamucil) 1 Tbsp b.i.d. or t.i.d.
- Constipating agents (if diarrhea is significant)—loperamide (Imodium) 4 mg initial dose, then 2 mg after each unformed stool or diphenoxylate/atropine (Lomotil) 2.5–5.0 mg (1–2 tablets) after each unformed stool
- Antispasmodics/anticholinergics—dicyclomine (Bentyl) 10–20 mg b.i.d. to q.i.d. or lactase (LactAid) 1–3 caplets a.c. for lactose intolerance
- Anticholinergics/sedatives—chlordiazepoxide/clidinium (Librax) 1 or 2 a.c. and q.h.s.; phenobarbital/hyoscyamine/atropine/hyoscine (Donnatal) 1 or 2 tablets a.c. and q.h.s.; amitriptyline HCl (Elavil) 25–50 mg q.h.s.
- Antiflatulents—simethicone (Mylicon) 2 or 4 tablets p.c. and q.h.s.
- For milk intolerance—lactase capsules or tablets; 1–2 tablets prior to ingesting milk products

SYNONYMS:
- Mucous colitis
- Spastic colon
- Irritable colon

MENOPAUSE

DESCRIPTION: The cessation of spontaneous menstrual cycles.
- *Perimenopause*—period of time where there is a decline in ovarian function. Although a woman may continue to have periodic uterine bleeding, such cycles may be anovulatory. During this time estrogen production diminishes and a woman may experience early signs of estrogen deficiency.
- *Postmenopause*—the period after menopause usually accounting for more than one-third of a woman's total life.
- *Premature menopause*—occurring before age 30; may be associated with sex chromosome abnormalities.

System(s) affected: Reproductive, endocrine/metabolic, musculoskeletal, cardiovascular

SPECIAL TESTS:
- Endometrial biopsy and/or D&C in patients who have intermenstrual or postmenopausal bleeding—may be accompanied by hysteroscopy. Investigation for endometrial cancer is necessary even in the presence of an atrophic vagina (usually the cause of the bleeding).
- Bleeding may also be evaluated by vaginal sonography; if double wall thickness of endometrial stripe is less than 5 mm, endometrial carcinoma is highly unlikely.

DRUG(S) OF CHOICE:
- Estrogens—commonly oral estrogen, conjugated (Premarin), or estradiol
  - For retarding osteoporosis 0.625 mg q.d.; lesser doses not effective.
  - If vasomotor symptoms persist at 0.625 mg, increase to 0.9 mg or 1.25 mg; however, optimal cardioprotective effect is 0.625 mg.
  - Other forms of oral estrogen or the transdermal patch may be used and appear to be equally effective.
- Progestogen—commonly medroxyprogesterone (Provera, Depo-Provera)
  - Because estrogens are carcinogenic to the endometrium, a progestogen should be added for its protective effect against endometrial cancer. (If the uterus has been removed, a progestogen is not needed.)
- Administration:
  - Estrogens and progestogens may be administered continuously (no withdrawal bleeding expected) or cyclically.
  - Common regimens—Premarin 0.625 mg plus Provera 2.5 mg q.d. *or* Premarin 0.625 mg for 25 days per month plus Provera 5 mg during the last 14 days of estrogen therapy *or* Premarin 0.625 mg daily plus Provera 5 mg during 14 days of month. Fixed combinations (Prempro, Premphase) may be convenient. Another option is Premarin and micronized progesterone.

SYNONYMS:
- Climacteric
- Ovarian failure

MYOCARDIAL INFARCTION (MI)

DESCRIPTION: Acute myocardial infarction (AMI) is the rapid development of myocardial necrosis resulting from a sustained and complete reduction of blood flow to a portion of the myocardium, produced by a superimposed thrombosis, generated by a ruptured atherosclerotic plaque.
- Clinical consequences—dependent on the size and location of the infarction and

the rapidity with which blood flow can be reestablished by pharmacologic or mechanical modalities.

- After total occlusion, myocardial necrosis is complete in 4–6 hours. Flow to ischemic area must remain above 40% of preocclusion levels for that area to survive.
- Infarctions can be divided into Q wave and non Q wave, with the former being transmural and associated with totally obstructed infarct-related artery and the latter being nontransmural and associated with patent, but highly narrowed, infarct-related artery.
- Total occlusion of the left main coronary artery, which usually supplies 70% of the LV mass, is catastrophic and results in death in minutes.

System(s) affected: Cardiovascular

SPECIAL TESTS:

- Electrocardiography
  - ST-segment elevation in a regional pattern—typical of acute transmural ischemia.
  - ST-segment depression with T wave inversions—typical of subendocardial ischemia.
  - ST-segment elevation and depression are early findings of myocardial ischemia. A significant percent of patients will have nonspecific findings on presentation, such as peaked T waves and ST-segment elevation less than 0.1 mv. A small percentage of patients, with transmural infarction, present with normal ECG.
  - Q waves representing transmural myocardial necrosis appear with 24–48 hours.
- Echocardiography
  - 2D and M-mode echocardiography useful in evaluating wall motion abnormalities in MI and overall left ventricular function.
  - Useful in delineating and assessing mechanical complications.

DRUG(S) OF CHOICE:

Coronary reperfusion:

- Alteplase (Activase); tissue plasminogen activator (t-PA). 15 mg IV bolus, 50 mg over 30 minutes, then 35 mg over 60 minutes
- Heparin by standard or weight-adjusted protocol
- Aspirin 325 mg p.o. acutely

Acute MI, general

- Nitrates 5 mcg/min IV, increase slowly. Do not lower arterial blood pressure beyond 90 mm Hg. Change to oral or topical when patient stable.
- Lidocaine 1–2 mg/kg once, then 1–4 mg/min. Use for ventricular arrhythmias only. Do not expect arrhythmia prophylaxis.
- Oxygen (2–4 L/minute)
- Oxazepam 10 mg p.o. or lorazepam 0.5 mg IV if needed for sedation, every 4–6 hours.
- Morphine 2–6 mg IV q.2–4h. p.r.n. pain/sedation.

- Metoprolol (Lopressor) 5 mg IV x 3, 2 minutes apart followed by 50 mg p.o. q.6h. starting 15 minutes after past IV dose.
- Stool softeners—milk of magnesia, docusate sodium (dioctyl sodium sulfosuccinate) 100 mg b.i.d., etc., to avoid straining and constipation secondary to immobility and narcotic use.

Post-MI

- Beta blockers reduce mortality.
- Nitrates may be needed for angina.
- ACE inhibitors prevent adverse remodeling, may improve longevity.

SYNONYMS:
- Coronary thrombosis
- Coronary occlusion
- Heart attack

OBESITY

DESCRIPTION: A condition of increased body weight (consisting of both lean and fat tissue) that leads to increased morbidity and mortality. Also defined as weight 20% greater than an individual's desirable weight as defined by the Metropolitan Life Insurance Company or BMI > 28.

Android obesity (male pattern or abdominal obesity) is higher risk and *gynecoid obesity* (female pattern or gluteal obesity) is lower risk for long-term health problems.

Obesity threshold (BMI=28)	
Height	**Weight (lb)**
5′ 0 ″	143
5′ 2 ″	153
5′ 4 ″	163
5′ 6 ″	173
5′ 8 ″	184
5′ 10 ″	195
6′ 0 ″	206
6′ 2 ″	218
6′ 4 ″	230

System(s) affected: Gastrointestinal, endocrine/metabolic

SPECIAL TESTS:
- Body mass index (BMI) = body weight (kg) divided by the square of body height (m). Obesity is BMI > 28 kg/m^2.
- Determine fat distribution pattern by measuring waist and hips circumferences and calculating the waist to hips ratio (WHR).
- Android (male pattern or abdominal obesity) has WHR greater than 0.85 for females; 0.95 for males.
- Gynecoid (female pattern or gluteal obesity) has WHR less than 0.85 for females; 0.95 for males.

DRUG(S) OF CHOICE:
Drug treatment is not usually recommended, although appetite suppressants may be indicated for short-term use (few weeks) in conjunction with a weight loss regimen.
- Schedule III drugs:
  - Phendimetrazine
  - Benzphetamine
- Schedule IV drugs:
  - Diethylpropion
  - Phentermine
  - Mazindol
  - Sibutramine 5–15 mg q.d. (starting dose 10 mg) is approved without restriction on length of use

SYNONYMS:
- Overweight
- Adiposis
- Adiposity

PEPTIC ULCER DISEASE

DESCRIPTION: A chronic ulcer in the lining of the gastrointestinal tract.
- *Duodenal ulcer* (DU)—most located in the duodenal bulb. Multiple ulcers, and if distal to the bulb, raise the possibility of Zollinger-Ellison syndrome.
- *Gastric ulcer* (GU)—much less common than DU (in the absence NSAIDs). Most commonly located along the lesser curvature of the antrum near the incisura and in the prepyloric area.
- *Esophageal ulcer*—a peptic ulcer in the distal esophagus may be part of Barrett epithelial change due to chronic reflux of gastroduodenal contents.
- *Ectopic gastric mucosal ulceration*—may develop in patients with Meckel diverticula or other sites of ectopic gastric mucosa.
System(s) affected: Gastrointestinal

SPECIAL TESTS: Serology or urea breath test for *Helicobacter pylori*

DRUG(S) OF CHOICE:
Acute healing of DU and GU:
- Acid suppression
  - H_2 blocker—ranitidine or nizatidine 150 b.i.d. or 300 mg q.h.s.; cimetidine 400 mg b.i.d. or 800 mg q.h.s.; famotidine 150 mg b.i.d. or 300 mg q.h.s. for 8–12 weeks
  - Proton pump inhibitor, e.g., omeprazole 20 mg, lansoprazole 15 mg q.d. or rabeprazole 20 mg daily for 4 weeks
- Eradication of *H. pylori* (HP), single antibiotic regimens discouraged. Currently optimal HP eradication regimens:
  - Omeprazole 20 mg or lansoprazole 30 mg b.i.d. plus 2 antibiotics (e.g., clarithromycin 500 mg b.i.d. and amoxicillin 1 gram b.i.d. for 2 weeks)
  - Ranitidine-bismuth-citrate 400 mg b.i.d. plus clarithromycin 500 mg b.i.d. and amoxicillin 1 gram b.i.d. for 2 weeks
  - Alternative antibiotics—tetracycline
Treatment of *H. pylori*-negative ulcers:
  - Most are due to NSAIDs; treat acutely with H_2-receptor antagonists or proton pump inhibitor for 4–12 weeks. Optimally, the NSAID should be discontinued.
Unhealed refractory ulcers:
  - Higher doses of H_2 blockers or proton pump inhibitors or surgery

SYNONYMS:
- Duodenal ulcer
- Gastric ulcer
- *H. pylori* gastritis

PLEURAL EFFUSION

DESCRIPTION: A pleural effusion occurs when there is excessive fluid released into the pleural space or if there is lymphatic obstruction precluding normal drainage. Under normal conditions there is a small volume of pleural fluid in the pleural space which functions as a lubricant. Under pathological conditions, effusions develop and are classified as either transudates or exudates. Transudates are due to an imbalance between hydrostatic and oncotic pressures (as in hepatic cirrhosis, congestive heart failure, nephrotic syndrome, and obstruction of the superior vena cava). Exudates are secondary to a disturbance of the systems regulating pleural fluid formation and absorption/drainage (as in bacterial, viral, or fungal infection, rheumatologic disease, or malignancy). Distinguishing between these types of effusions, when etiology is uncertain or if there is inadequate response to therapy, can be helpful.
System(s) affected: Pulmonary, cardiovascular

SPECIAL TESTS:

- Evaluation of pleural fluid withdrawn by thoracentesis. Transudates and exudates must be distinguished. A transudate has none of the following characteristics; however, an exudate must meet one:
  - Pleural fluid protein/serum protein
  - Pleural fluid LDH/serum LDH > 0.6
  - Pleural fluid LDH > 2/3 upper limit of that in serum
- All exudates must be evaluated for:
  - Differential cell count
  - Amylase level
  - Glucose level
  - Comprehensive microbiologic culturing and Gram staining
  - Cytology for tumor cells
- Additional studies: pH, RBC count (hemorrhagic effusion if >100,000/cc, consider trauma as etiology for effusion)
- In the absence of a known primary tumor and/or there is a high index of suspicion for malignancy, the cells harvested from an effusion can be evaluated for a variety of tumor markers (VIM, CD15, CA19–9, CA125, CEA, HBME-l, etc.)

DRUG(S) OF CHOICE:

- Antimicrobial therapy according to pathogens and associated sensitivities
- Chemical pleurodesis with doxycycline 500 mg, bleomycin 60 units, or talc in a slurry, as indicated
- Chemotherapy according to current oncologic protocols
- Steroids and nonsteroidal antiinflammatory drugs for rheumatologic and inflammatory etiologies
- Diuresis as appropriate for effusions secondary to congestive heart failure and ascites

POSTTRAUMATIC STRESS DISORDER (PTSD)

DESCRIPTION: A condition seen in people who experienced an event that would be extremely distressing to most human beings, e.g., serious threat to one's life or physical or psychological integrity; serious threat or harm to one's children, spouse, siblings, parents, or other close relatives or friends; sudden destruction of one's home or community; seeing another person who has recently been (or is being) injured or killed as a result of a man-made violent act or natural disaster.

- The person's response involved intense fear, helplessness, or horror. Note: In children, this may be expressed instead by disorganized or agitated behavior.
- Symptoms of this condition did not exist prior to the trauma, and symptoms persist for at least one month following the trauma.

- There is a subtype of posttraumatic stress disorder (PTSD) with a delayed onset of the symptoms which starts at least 6 months after the trauma.
- The acute form of PTSD has a duration of less than 3 months.
- Chronic form has a duration of more than 3 months.

System(s) affected: Nervous

SPECIAL TESTS:

- Neuropsychological testing is helpful in cases of dementia and more subtle cognitive dysfunction.
- EEG to rule out any brain damage (results may be altered by any drug affecting EEG patterns such as sleeping pills, antidepressants, neuroleptics, and other psychotropic medications).
- Psychological testing and a thorough mental status examination are valuable in a complete, thorough assessment of the patient.
- Sleep lab studies (8-hour EEG) help in diagnosis of sleep disorders.
- Through an examination and interview, assisted by amobarbital (Amytal) (given intravenously) or similar substances, one may uncover traumatic material in patients with amnesia. Similarly, an examination assisted by hypnosis may help in the diagnosis.
- Tests may be affected by withdrawal or intoxication from drugs and alcohol, or any organic brain syndromes, such as multiple infarct dementia, other forms of dementia, and forms of epilepsy.

DRUG(S) OF CHOICE:

- Selective serotonin reuptake inhibitors (SSRI) (this group has recently been proven to be safe and effective for the control of many symptoms of PTSD):
  - Fluoxetine 20–80 mg/day
  - Sertraline 50–200 mg/day
  - Paroxetine 20–60 mg/day
  - Citalopram 20–60 mg/day
  - Venlafaxine 75–325 mg/day
- Tricyclic antidepressants:
  - Doxepin 50–150 mg/day
  - Nortriptyline 30–100 mg/day
  - Imipramine 50–300 mg/day
  - Desipramine 50–300 mg/day
  - Amitriptyline 50–300 mg/day
  - Trimipramine 50–300 mg/day
  - Protriptyline 15–60 mg/day
  - Amoxapine 50–300 mg/day
  - Maprotiline 50–225 mg/day (increased risk of seizures with higher doses)

- Monoamine oxidase inhibitors:
  - Phenelzine 45–75 mg/day is useful especially in PTSD patients with panic attacks
- Others:
  - Trazodone 100–400 mg/day, given mostly at bedtime is helpful in patients with insomnia
  - Nefazodone 200–600 mg/day in patients with insomnia improves REM sleep
  - Small doses of neuroleptics are helpful in selective patients
  - Bupropion 100–450 mg/day
  - Neuroleptics—small doses are helpful in selective patients
  - Benzodiazepines should be used selectively and with caution

SYNONYMS:
- Trauma syndrome
- Battle fatigue
- Shell shock
- Postdisaster syndrome
- Trauma survivor's syndrome
- Traumatic neurosis

PROSTATIC CANCER

DESCRIPTION: The prostate is composed of acinar glands and their ducts arranged in a radial fashion with the stroma containing blood vessels, lymphatics and nerves. Ninety-five percent of prostate cancers are acinar adenocarcinomas.
Tumor grading:
- A1, A2, B1, B2—confined within capsule
- C1—extension beyond the capsule
- C2—involving the seminal vesicles
- D1—metastatic disease in regional lymph nodes
- D2—metastatic disease in bone or other organs

System(s) affected: Reproductive

SPECIAL TESTS:
- Prostate-specific antigen (PSA)
- Free PSA

DRUG(S) OF CHOICE:
In androgen-dependent tumors a reduction in serum testosterone is helpful in reducing tumor size, and bone pain, and for improving survival. Orchiectomy is the simplest androgen ablation method; however, medical castration can alternatively be utilized.
- CAB or MAB (combined or maximum androgen blockade)—often recommended

although some studies have shown no survival advantage over orchiectomy alone. Reduction in pain (54% versus 37% in patients with orchiectomy alone) is significant, although the side effects of the antiandrogens (hot flashes, night blindness, diarrhea, etc.) may be troublesome.

- For androgen ablation (medical castration), in patients without orchiectomy:
  - Leuprolide (Lupron) 1 mg subcutaneously daily or 7.5 mg IM depot monthly or 30 mg IM depot 4 months sustained every 4 months
  - Goserelin (Zoladex) 3.6 mg every month
- Nonsteroidal antiandrogens (to block testosterone produced outside the testes, i.e., used with androgen ablation or orchiectomy)
  - Bicalutamide (Casodex) 50 mg q.d.

SYNONYM: Carcinoma of the prostate

PULMONARY EDEMA

DESCRIPTION: Pulmonary interstitial and/or alveolar fluid accumulation that results when the forces moving fluid out of the pulmonary capillary exceed the forces restraining that fluid.
System(s) affected: Cardiovascular, pulmonary

SPECIAL TESTS:
- Arterial blood gas
- Electrocardiogram
- Pulmonary function tests
- Mixed venous oxygen saturation

DRUG(S) OF CHOICE:
Acute cardiogenic pulmonary edema:
- Morphine sulfate 2–5 mg IV
- Furosemide 20–80 mg IV
- Nitroglycerin paste 1–2 inches
- In selected cases: Nitroglycerin drip beginning at 5 mcg/min and increasing by 5–10 mcg/min every few minutes, titrating to blood pressure, etc. Nitroprusside IV drip beginning at 10 mcg/min and increasing by 5–10 mcg/min every few minutes, titrating to blood pressure, etc. Dobutamine 2 mcg/kg/min IV titrating to blood pressure, cardiac output, pulmonary capillary wedge pressure, etc.

Chronic management of cardiogenic pulmonary edema:
- Furosemide 20–400 mg daily
- Angiotensin-converting enzyme inhibitors (e.g., captopril 6.25–25 mg p.o. t.i.d., lisinopril 2.5–20 mg p.o. q.d., enalapril 2.5–15 mg p.o. q.d.-b.i.d.)
- Digoxin 0.125–0.25 mg p.o. q.d.

- Carvedilol 3.125–25 mg p.o. b.i.d.
- Isosorbide dinitrate 10–60 mg p.o. t.i.d.-q.i.d.
- Thiazide diuretics (e.g., hydrochlorothiazide [HCTZ] 25–50 mg p.o. q.d.)
- Spironolactone 25–200 mg daily

Noncardiogenic pulmonary edema:
- Oxygen
- Selected cardiovascular drugs to optimize tissue oxygen delivery

RENAL FAILURE, ACUTE (ARF)

DESCRIPTION: A syndrome of rapidly deteriorating kidney function with the accumulation of nitrogenous wastes
System(s) affected: Renal/urologic, cardiovascular

SPECIAL TESTS:
- Angiogram (renal vascular disease)
- Cystoscopy—retrograde
- Bleeding time

DRUG(S) OF CHOICE:
Prior to fixed renal failure—IV volume expansion with normal saline followed by mannitol, furosemide (Lasix), and calcium channel blockers. Low-dose dopamine has not been shown to have a beneficial effect on survival. Volume expansion alone is beneficial in contrast injury. Dopamine-1 selective agonists may have promise for future treatment.

SEIZURE DISORDERS

DESCRIPTION: A sudden alteration of behavior, characterized by a sensory perception or motor activity with or without change in awareness or consciousness, due to aberrant cortical electrical activity.
- Classification of seizures
  I. Partial seizures (seizures begin locally)—(A) without impairment of consciousness, (B) with complex symptoms (with impairment of consciousness)
  II. Generalized seizures (bilaterally symmetrical and without local onset)
  III. Unclassified epileptic seizures

System(s) affected: Nervous

SPECIAL TESTS:
- Electroencephalogram (EEG)—a negative EEG does not rule out a seizure disorder. Sensitivity, specificity, and predictive value of the test depend on the underlying cause and anatomic location of the seizure focus.

A131

- 24-hour ambulatory EEG—allows for continuous monitoring of cortical activity during regular activities
- Video monitoring—useful in conjunction with simultaneous EEG monitoring in separating true events from pseudoseizures

DRUG(S) OF CHOICE:

To avoid a particular side effect, one drug may be preferred within one of the seizure groups listed below.

Generalized seizures—tonic clonic:
- Phenytoin (Dilantin)—200–400 mg/day in 1–3 doses; therapeutic range: 10–20 mcg/mL
- Phenobarbital—100–200 mg/day in 1–2 doses; therapeutic range: 10–30 mcg/mL
- Carbamazepine (Tegretol)—600–1200 mg/day in 2–4 doses; therapeutic range: 4–12 mcg/mL
- Valproic acid (Depakene)—750–3000 mg/day in 1–3 doses (begin at 15 mg/kg/day; increase in one week by 5–10 mg/kg/day; split at 250 mg; maximum 60 mg/kg/day); therapeutic range 50–150 mcg/mL

Generalized seizures—absence:
- Ethosuximide (Zarontin)—250–1500 mg/day in 1–2 doses; therapeutic range: 40–100 mcg/mL
- Valproic acid—dose noted above; therapeutic range: 50–100 mcg/mL
- Clonazepam (Klonopin)—0.01–0.3 mg/kg/day in 2–3 doses (maximum 20 mg/day); therapeutic range: 20–80 ng/mL (63–254 nmol/L)

Partial seizures:
- Phenytoin (Dilantin)
- Carbamazepine (Tegretol)
- Phenobarbital

SYNONYMS:

- Convulsions
- Epilepsy
- Fits
- Spells

STROKE (BRAIN ATTACK)

DESCRIPTION: The sudden onset of a focal neurological deficit resulting from either infarction or hemorrhage within the brain
System(s) affected: Nervous, cardiovascular

SPECIAL TESTS:
- Duplex carotid ultrasonography
- Cerebral angiography
- Echocardiogram (ECG)
- Transthoracic echocardiogram (TTE); if normal and a cardiac source is suspected, followup with transesophageal echocardiogram
- Holter monitoring
- Electroencephalogram (EEG) for suspected seizure
- International normalized ratio (INR) and partial thromboplastin time (PTT). Coumadin prolongs PTT.
- Antiphospholipid antibodies

DRUG(S) OF CHOICE:
- Enteric-coated aspirin (EC ASA) 50–325 mg/day.
  or
- Dipyridamole-aspirin (Aggrenox)—extended release, 200 mg/25 mg capsule p.o. b.i.d.; more efficacious than aspirin alone.
- Clopidogrel (Plavix) 75 mg/day is a descendent of ticlopidine and has fewer side effects, but shows only a slight advantage over ASA.

SYNONYMS:
- Cerebrovascular accident (CVA)
- Reversible ischemic neurological accident (RIND)

THROMBOSIS, DEEP VEIN (DVT)

DESCRIPTION: Development of single or multiple blood clots within the deep veins of the extremities or pelvis, usually accompanied by inflammation of the vessel wall. The major clinical consequence is embolization, usually to the lung, that is frequently life threatening.
System(s) affected: Cardiovascular

DRUG(S) OF CHOICE:
Immediate therapy:
- Heparin 80 units/kg intravenous bolus followed by continuous IV infusion starting at 18 units/kg/hr. Adjust dosage based on activated partial thromboplastin time (APTT) to achieve APTT of approximately 3 times control value.

Maintenance therapy:
- Warfarin (Coumadin) beginning 1–3 days after starting heparin, in a single daily dose starting at 5–10 mg daily and adjusting based on prothrombin time (PT) with a target value of PT of 1.5–2 times control value. Patient should remain on

heparin until target PT level is achieved. Physicians should use international nor-malized ratio (INR), if available, to guide therapy. Aim for INR 2.0–3.0.

SYNONYM: Deep venous thrombophlebitis

TRANSIENT ISCHEMIC ATTACK (TIA)

DESCRIPTION: The sudden onset of a focal and transient (< 24 hours) neurological deficit due to brain ischemia.
System(s) affected: Nervous

SPECIAL TESTS:
- Duplex carotid ultrasonography
- Cerebral angiography
- Echocardiogram (ECG)
- Transthoracic echocardiogram (TTE); if normal and a cardiac source is suspected, follow with transesophageal echocardiogram
- Holter monitoring
- Electroencephalogram (EEG) for suspected seizure
- International normalized ratio (INR) and partial thromboplastin time (PTT); Coumadin prolongs INR
- Antiphospholipid antibodies

DRUG(S) OF CHOICE:
- Enteric-coated aspirin (EC ASA) 50–325 mg/day,
  or
- Clopidogrel (Plavix) 75 mg daily; descendent of ticlopidine and has fewer side effects; shows a slight advantage over ASA
- Dipyridamole/aspirin (Aggrenox)—extended release, 200 mg/25 mg capsule p.o. b.i.d.; more efficacious than aspirin alone, but more costly

SYNONYM: Mini-stroke

URINARY TRACT INFECTION (UTI)—FEMALES

DESCRIPTION: Inflammation of bladder mucosa. This topic refers primarily to infectious cystitis.
System(s) affected: Renal/urologic

DRUG(S) OF CHOICE:
First, rare, or infrequent UTIs in adolescents and adults who are not pregnant, non-

diabetic, afebrile, nonimmunocompromised and have no abnormality of the urinary tract (i.e., uncomplicated):

- 3-day treatment with trimethoprim/sulfamethoxazole (TMP/SMX) or fluoroquinolone. Increasing resistance being reported to TMP/SMX. Use local sensitivity patterns to dictate first-choice antibiotic.

Postcoital:

- Single-dose TMP/SMX or cephalexin may reduce frequency of UTI in sexually active women.

Pregnant patients:

- 10–14 days or longer of treatment with pregnancy-safe antibiotic chosen based on culture/sensitivity results. May begin with cephalosporin, amoxicillin, or other antibiotic while awaiting culture/sensitivity results.

All other patients:

- 10–14 days of treatment with antibiotic chosen based on culture/sensitivity results. May begin with fluoroquinolone, TMP/SMX, cephalosporin, or other antibiotic while awaiting culture/sensitivity results.

SYNONYM: Cystitis

URINARY TRACT INFECTION (UTI) — MALES

DESCRIPTION: Cystitis is an infection of the lower urinary tract, usually resulting from a single gram-negative enteric bacteria.
System(s) affected: Renal/urologic

SPECIAL TESTS: Urologic investigations necessary to rule out other disorders

DRUG(S) OF CHOICE:

Acute UTI, first infection, no risk factors for treatment:

- 7–10 days of oral antibiotics either empirically or based on cultures and sensitivity results. For empiric therapy, trimethoprim-sulfamethoxazole (TMP/SMX) b.i.d. will usually treat the most likely pathogens.

Complicated or recurrent UTI:

- 14–21 days of antibiotics based on antimicrobial sensitivities with repeat urine check after treatment

SYNONYM: Cystitis

Adapted from Dambro MR. *Griffith's 5-Minute Clinical Consult 2001.* Philadelphia: Lippincott Williams & Wilkins, 2001.